Pharmacotherapeutics for Veterinary Dispensing

Pharmacotherapeutics for Veterinary Dispensing

Edited by

Katrina L. Mealey, BS (Pharm), DVM, PhD
Diplomate ACVIM, Diplomate ACVCP
Fellow, National Academy of Inventors
Professor and Ott Endowed Chair
College of Veterinary Medicine
Washington State University
Pullman, WA, USA

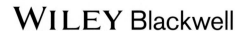

Registered Office
John Wiley & Sons, Inc., 111 River Street, Hoboken, NJ 07030, USA

Editorial Office
111 River Street, Hoboken, NJ 07030, USA

For details of our global editorial offices, customer services, and more information about Wiley products visit us at www.wiley.com.

Wiley also publishes its books in a variety of electronic formats and by print-on-demand. Some content that appears in standard print versions of this book may not be available in other formats.

Library of Congress Cataloging-in-Publication Data

Names: Mealey, Katrina L., editor.
Title: Pharmacotherapeutics for veterinary dispensing / edited by Katrina L. Mealey.
Description: Hoboken, N.J. : Wiley Blackwell, 2019. | Includes bibliographical references and index. |
Identifiers: LCCN 2018033848 (print) | LCCN 2018034804 (ebook) | ISBN 9781119404552
    (Adobe PDF) | ISBN 9781119532576 (ePub) | ISBN 9781119404545 (pbk.)
Subjects: LCSH: Veterinary drugs. | MESH: Veterinary Drugs | Pharmaceutical Services |
    Veterinary Medicine | Animal Diseases–drug therapy
Classification: LCC SF917 (ebook) | LCC SF917 .P43 2019 (print) | NLM SF 917 | DDC 636.089/51–dc23
LC record available at https://lccn.loc.gov/2018033848

Cover Design: Wiley
Cover Images: © Rachael Householder; © Henry Moore

Set in 10/12pt Warnock by SPi Global, Pondicherry, India
Printed and bound in Singapore by Markono Print Media Pte Ltd

10 9 8 7 6 5 4 3 2 1

Contents

List of Contributors

Terri L. Alessio, DVM, DACVO
Veterinary Medical Teaching Hospital
College of Veterinary Medicine
Washington State University, Pullman,
WA, USA

Joe Bartges, DVM, PhD, DACVIM, DACVN
Department of Small Animal Medicine
and Surgery, College of Veterinary
Medicine, University of Georgia, Athens,
GA, USA

Eden Bermingham, DVM, MS, DACVCP
Clinical Pharmacology Team, Division
of Scientific Support, Office of New
Animal Drug Evaluation, FDA Center
for Veterinary Medicine, Rockville,
MD, USA

**Annie Chen-Allen, DVM MS, DACVIM
(Neurology)**
Neurology and Neurosurgery, College of
Veterinary Medicine, Washington State
University, Pullman, WA, USA

Gigi Davidson, BSPharm, DICVP
Clinical Pharmacy Services, College of
Veterinary Medicine, North Carolina State
University, Raleigh, NC, USA

**Jennifer L. Davis, DVM, PhD, DACVIM (LA),
DACVCP**
Department of Biomedical Sciences and
Pathobiology, Virginia-Maryland (VA-MD)
College of Veterinary Medicine, Virginia
Tech, Blacksburg, VA, USA

Virginia R. Fajt, DVM, PhD, DACVCP
Veterinary Physiology and Pharmacology
College of Veterinary Medicine &
Biomedical Sciences, Texas A&M University
College Station, TX, USA

Lauren Eichstadt Forsythe, PharmD, FSVHP
Veterinary Medical Teaching Hospital
School of Veterinary Medicine, University of
California, Davis, CA, USA

Alice M. Jeromin, RPh, DVM, DACVD
Private practice, Richfield, OH, USA

Margo J. Karriker, PharmD, FSVHP, DICVP
University of California Veterinary Medical
Center–San Diego, UC Davis School of
Veterinary Medicine, San Diego, CA, USA

Butch Kukanich, DVM, PhD, Diplomate ACVCP
Department of Anatomy and Physiology
College of Veterinary Medicine, Kansas
State University, Manhattan, KS, USA

**Sunshine M. Lahmers, DVM, PhD, DACVIM
(Cardiology)**
Department of Small Animal Clinical
Sciences, Virginia-Maryland (VA-MD)
College of Veterinary Medicine, Virginia
Tech, Blacksburg, VA, USA

Cory Langston, DVM, PhD, DACVCP
ORCID ID 0000-0002-4644-1616
College of Veterinary Medicine, Mississippi
State University, Mississippi State, MS, USA

Stephen W. Mealey
Washington State University, Pullman,
WA, USA

**Katrina L. Mealey, BS (Pharm), DVM, PhD,
Diplomate ACVIM, Diplomate ACVCP**
College of Veterinary Medicine, Washington
State University, Pullman, WA, USA

**Karen L. Overall, MA, VMD, PhD,
Diplomate ACVB**
Department of Biology, University of
Pennsylvania, Philadelphia, PA, USA
Department of Health Management
Atlantic Veterinary College, UPEI
Charlottetown, PE, Canada

Mark G. Papich, DVM, MS, Diplomate ACVCP
Clinical Pharmacology, College of
Veterinary Medicine, North Carolina State
University, Raleigh, NC, USA

**Patricia A. Talcott, MS, DVM, PhD,
Diplomate ABVT**
Integrative Physiology and Neuroscience
and Washington Animal Disease Diagnostic
Laboratory, College of Veterinary Medicine
Washington State University, Pullman,
WA, USA

Andrea S. Varela-Stokes, DVM, PhD
ORCID ID 0000-0002-3991-9730
College of Veterinary Medicine, Mississippi
State University, Mississippi State, MS, USA

**Katrina R. Viviano, DVM, PhD, DACVIM,
DACVCP**
Department of Medical Sciences, School
of Veterinary Medicine, University of
Wisconsin, Madison, WI, USA

Valerie J. Wiebe, PharmD, FSVHP, DICVP
Department of Medicine and Epidemiology,
School of Veterinary Medicine, and
Veterinary Medical Teaching Hospital
University of California, Davis, CA, USA

Michael D. Willard, DVM, MS, DACVIM
Department of Small Animal Clinical
Sciences, College of Veterinary Medicine
& Biomedical Sciences, Texas A&M
University, College Station, TX, USA

Preface

The greatness of a nation and its moral progress can be judged by the way its animals are treated.

Mahatma Gandhi

A number of in-depth veterinary pharmacology resources have been written that are aimed at the veterinary profession (veterinarians, veterinary students, and veterinary researchers). Similarly, there are a multitude of clinical pharmacology and pharmacotherapeutics resources available on the human side aimed at physicians and pharmacists. To our knowledge, this book represents the first effort to "marry" the disciplines of veterinary medicine and pharmacy.

Veterinary medicine, and veterinary pharmacotherapeutics in particular, are undergoing immense changes. No longer is veterinary pharmacology an inexact extension of human pharmacology. Veterinary pharmaceutical products are no longer discarded human drug candidates that are subsequently developed for animals. Targeted enzyme pathway inhibitors (tyrosine kinase and JAK kinase) and even species-specific monoclonal antibody therapies have been developed by the veterinary pharmaceutical industry and are currently marketed for veterinary patients. The companion animal pharmaceutical market is a multibillion dollar per year industry. In an effort to gain part of this market share, corporate (traditionally "human") pharmacies have actively lobbied to introduce legislation at both state and federal levels that requires veterinarians to provide prescriptions to pet owners rather than dispense drugs directly to pet owners. Veterinarians have independently started writing more outpatient prescriptions rather than dispensing drugs from their own formulary because (i) carrying a large drug inventory is expensive, and (ii) a number of human-approved formulations are used off-label for companion animal disorders.

Consequently, pharmacists are increasingly encountering pet owners in their pharmacies, dispensing drugs for veterinary patients, and being asked to provide counseling on veterinary pharmacotherapeutics. Unfortunately, most pharmacists are not adequately trained to provide these services for veterinary patients. The wealth of information pharmacists acquire in pharmacy school regarding "human" medicine, pharmacology, therapeutics, and so on is often not applicable to other species. Because the pharmacy oath is not limited to one species (i.e. human patients), all pharmacists have an obligation to gain the knowledge and skills necessary to assure optimal outcomes for *all* patients (human and animal).

The primary goal of this book, therefore, is to improve safety and efficacy of pharmacotherapeutics in veterinary patients – to minimize mistakes based on the presumption that human pharmacology applies to all species, and to maximize therapeutic efficacy by enabling pharmacists to be an integral member of the veterinary healthcare team. The book is not intended (nor is it possible) to include every drug and indication for each veterinary species. The book is not intended to rehash information that pharmacists and pharmacy students have already mastered (i.e. mechanisms of action of drugs used in humans). To emphasize important points, text boxes are used throughout the book. Yellow boxes indicate "Practiced but Not Proven" use of medications by veterinarians (common use of a particular drug without strong evidence supporting that use). Gray boxes indicate when there is a "Dramatic Difference" between species with respect to drug disposition, particularly between humans and animals. Pink boxes indicate "Mandatory Monitoring" for a particular drug, providing the reader with information that can be used to counsel pet owners.

Each contributor, whether a veterinarian, pharmacist, or both, is a recognized expert in his or her field, having received advanced training, achieving certification in their discipline, and most importantly having acquired extensive clinical experience. Collectively, we hope this text will enable more Schools of Pharmacy to provide courses in veterinary (or comparative) pharmacology and/or veterinary pharmacotherapeutics because it isn't enough to know that a dog is not a small person and a cat is not a small dog.

1

Introduction to Veterinary Pharmacy

Gigi Davidson

Clinical Pharmacy Services, College of Veterinary Medicine, North Carolina State University, Raleigh, NC, USA

Key Points

- Several organizations exist that support veterinary pharmacy practice, including a training and credentialing process that culminates in the designation of Diplomate, International College of Veterinary Pharmacy (ICVP).
- Veterinary pharmacists are uniquely trained specialists that provide competent care and drug products to nonhuman species and can be resources for community pharmacists dispensing drugs to animals.
- Veterinary pharmacotherapy is rapidly entering the mainstream of pharmacy practice, despite the fact that most pharmacists are not adequately trained in the field.

- Veterinary drug law is significantly different from human drug law. For example, there is not currently a legal avenue for pharmacists to recommend human over-the-counter (OTC) drug products for veterinary patients.
- Veterinary pharmacy residency training programs have grown substantially since 1989.
- Core competencies for veterinary pharmacy education must be standardized and uniformly implemented across pharmacy school curricula.

1.1 Introduction

Although the practice of providing medicinal therapy to animals dates back to the Mesopotamian healer Urlugaledinna in 3000 BCE (Royal College of Veterinary Surgeons 2017), it took society nearly 5000 years to realize that pharmacists were well-placed medical professionals that could provide safe and effective pharmacotherapy and monitoring to animal patients as well as to humans. In 1761, the first college of veterinary medicine was established in Lyon, France (Larkin 2010); and from that time until the mid-twentieth century, the preparation, dispensing, and monitoring of medicinal agents for animals were almost exclusively performed by veterinarians. In the late twentieth century, the practice of clinical pharmacy for human medicine was established, and veterinary professionals began to recognize the unique therapeutic contributions made by clinically trained Doctors of Pharmacy. Veterinary pharmacy, which is practiced by pharmacists, is unique from the field of veterinary pharmacology, which is practiced by veterinarians, because it encompasses a three-pronged approach that utilizes medicinal chemistry, pharmacology, and species-specific pharmacotherapeutics to evaluate the best action plan for a specific patient.

Pharmacotherapeutics for Veterinary Dispensing, First Edition. Edited by Katrina L. Mealey.

"I promise to devote myself to a lifetime of service to others through the profession of pharmacy. In fulfilling this vow:

- I will consider the welfare of humanity and relief of suffering my primary concerns.
- I will apply my knowledge, experience, and skills to the best of my ability to assure optimal outcomes for my patients.
- I will respect and protect all personal and health information entrusted to me.
- I will accept the lifelong obligation to improve my professional knowledge and competence.
- I will hold myself and my colleagues to the highest principles of our profession's moral, ethical, and legal conduct.
- I will embrace and advocate changes that improve patient care.
- I will utilize my knowledge, skills, experiences, and values to prepare the next generation of pharmacists.

I take these vows voluntarily with the full realization of the responsibility with which I am entrusted by the public."

Figure 1.1 The pharmacist's oath.

Beginning with a handful of pharmacists interested in veterinary medicine, veterinary pharmacy has now evolved into a globally impactful specialty area of pharmacy practice and residency training programs and encompasses a broad spectrum of practice settings, including veterinary teaching hospitals, veterinary medical practices, community pharmacies, governmental agencies, and the pharmaceutical industry.

While most pharmacists are not trained as veterinary pharmacy specialists, most community pharmacists will encounter prescriptions for nonhuman patients in their practice. A survey of more than 13 000 licensed pharmacists in North Carolina revealed that 77% of respondents filled prescriptions for animal patients in their practice (Sorah et al. 2015). A similar survey of pharmacists in Oregon also revealed that 77% of respondents filled prescriptions for veterinary patients (Mingura 2017). Pharmacists are the only healthcare professionals expected by society – and legally permitted by regulatory authorities – to provide pharmaceutical care and drug products for all species. Yet despite this unique position, only 4% of pharmacy students who graduated in 2015 reported receiving any training in veterinary pharmacotherapy (Arnish et al. 2015). In fact, the pharmacy oath (Figure 1.1) does not distinguish between human patients and veterinary patients. Despite the lack of standardized education in veterinary

pharmacy, a US Food and Drug Administration (FDA) guidance document released in 2015 estimated that 75 000 pharmacies fill 6 350 000 compounded prescriptions for animal patients annually (FDA 2015). It is important to note that this estimate was only for *compounded* veterinary prescriptions and did not account for the number of all prescriptions dispensed from pharmacies to animals. Because most pharmacists have not received adequate training in comparative pharmacology and veterinary pharmacotherapeutics, one would have to question whether pharmacists are fulfilling the oath's obligations when it comes to dispensing drugs to veterinary patients.

Drugs that achieve desired therapeutic effects in humans do not always produce the same effects in nonhuman patients, and vice versa. Using the wrong drug or the wrong dose of medications in animals can result in therapeutic failure or serious adverse events. In addition, statutes, regulations, rules, and guidance for drug use in animals are significantly different from those for humans, particularly with respect to animal species whose tissues or milk may be consumed by humans. Consequently, there is a critical need for community pharmacists to understand basic comparative pharmacology principles, laws surrounding drug use in food animal species, and pharmacotherapy of common veterinary diseases in order to serve the needs of the pet-owning public. There is an additional need for a designated veterinary pharmacy specialty to meet the unique needs of providing legally compliant pharmaceutical products, compounds, counseling, and monitoring of veterinary patients on an in-patient basis, as well as serving as a resource for community pharmacists outside of the veterinary practice setting.

1.1.1 History

Historically, the role of pharmacists in veterinary medicine was limited to incidental compounding of medications and dispensing human-approved prescription drugs for pets within the community pharmacy practice. Veterinary pharmacy, as an exclusive practice, originated in colleges of veterinary medicine in North America. In 1965, Laurence Reed Enos, PharmD, became the first veterinary pharmacist when he was hired by the University of California (UC) Davis School of Veterinary Medicine (Laurence Reed Enos, personal communication, May 9, 2011; Jeanne Enos, personal communication, June 13, 2016). Clinical pharmacy was just beginning in human medicine at that time, and Dr. Enos was hired to serve a clinical role providing pharmaceutical care for veterinary patients and to provide education in pharmacotherapeutic principles to veterinary students. He held administrative, teaching, and service roles within both the School of Veterinary Medicine and the College of Pharmacy during his 37 years of practice there. His philosophy was to develop a strong clinical program in veterinary pharmacy that emphasized teaching, research, and therapeutics. In 1968, Faye Kernan, BSP, MTS, became Canada's first veterinary pharmacist, hired by the Western College of Veterinary Medicine at the University of Saskatchewan (Faye Kernan, personal communication, May 9, 2011). Like her US counterpart at UC Davis, Ms. Kernan established a model for veterinary pharmacy practice and earned tremendous respect from her veterinarian and pharmacist peers. Fifty years later,

Kernan remains an active and vital contributor to veterinary pharmacy practice. Several other veterinary schools followed suit in hiring pharmacists in the late 1970s and early 1980s, and today all but one of the veterinary schools in the USA and Canada employ at least one pharmacist in a faculty, administrative, or professional staff position. In 1982, a group of veterinary pharmacists, including Kernan, met in Lincoln, Nebraska, to establish the Society of Veterinary Hospital Pharmacists (SVHP), the first professional organization representing veterinary pharmacists. The organization has steadily grown and now hosts more than 165 veterinary pharmacist members practicing throughout the world. In 1989, the Auburn University College of Veterinary Medicine and College of Pharmacy collaborated to create the first veterinary pharmacy residency program, and selected Dr. Bobbi Anglin as the first veterinary pharmacy resident (Dr. Sue Duran, personal communication, Auburn University College of Veterinary Medicine, March 19, 2017). Since then, UC Davis, North Carolina State University, Purdue University, and the University of Wisconsin have all established veterinary pharmacy residency training programs, producing many residency-trained veterinary pharmacists. Compared to their humble beginnings in 1965, today's veterinary pharmacists provide a significant and positive impact on animal healthcare.

1.2 Veterinary Pharmacy Professional Organizations

1.2.1 Society of Veterinary Hospital Pharmacists

The SVHP is an organization of pharmacists who work exclusively in the veterinary field, primarily at veterinary teaching hospitals in colleges of veterinary medicine (see www.svhp.org). Membership is international; the USA, Canada, the Netherlands, Denmark, South Africa, Australia, Spain, Austria, and New Zealand are currently represented.

The SVHP membership meets annually to participate in the Accreditation Council for Pharmacy Education (ACPE) and accredited continuing education activities, and to exchange ideas and information about veterinary pharmacy practice. While membership as an SVHP Fellow is restricted to licensed pharmacists who practice in nonprofit veterinary institutional settings providing professional service, teaching, or research (or some combination thereof), associate membership is open to pharmacists, veterinarians, and other animal health professionals who have an interest in veterinary pharmacy. The number of practicing veterinary hospital pharmacists continues to grow steadily.

1.2.2 International College of Veterinary Pharmacy

In 2000, the International College of Veterinary Pharmacy (ICVP) was established by the SVHP to develop a recognized specialty college and certification for veterinary hospital pharmacy. Appropriately trained SVHP Fellows would qualify for specialty certification through an arduous credentialing process and would then be eligible to sit for a rigorous certification examination. In 2001, the first 13 diplomates of the ICVP were awarded the credentials of Diplomate, ICVP. Today, there are 31 diplomates of ICVP, with approximately 10 additional candidates undergoing the certification process.

1.2.3 American College of Veterinary Pharmacists

The American College of Veterinary Pharmacists (ACVP) is affiliated with the American College of Apothecaries and was established to support the efforts of independent pharmacists in developing and strengthening the services they provide for animals and strengthening the support services they provide for veterinarians. Pharmacist membership is open to any licensed pharmacist meeting ACVP Practice Standards.

ACVP develops and disseminates ACPE-accredited educational materials, sponsors programs (including compounding and disease state management courses), serves as an information resource, and works closely with allied organizations to enhance the veterinary pharmacy care offered by pharmacy practitioners.

1.3 Veterinary Organizations with Pharmacological Expertise

1.3.1 The American Academy of Veterinary Pharmacology and Therapeutics (AAVPT)

The AAVPT was founded in 1977 and consists of approximately 300 veterinary pharmacology trained professionals from over 20 countries. Members of AAVPT share a common interest in research and teaching in veterinary pharmacology. The Academy's stated objectives are to support and promote education and research in comparative pharmacology, clinical veterinary pharmacology, and other aspects of pharmacology of interest to the veterinary profession; to sponsor a journal publishing related pharmacology manuscripts; to provide educational meetings and symposia in veterinary pharmacology and therapeutics; to enhance the exchange of educational materials and ideas among veterinary pharmacologists; and to organize advisory committees of experts to address problems in veterinary therapeutics. The AAVPT has been very supportive to veterinary pharmacists since its inception and has welcomed many of them into its membership.

1.3.2 The American College of Veterinary Clinical Pharmacology (ACVCP)

Similar to the relationship between the SVHP and ICVP, the ACVCP originated from the AAVPT in 1990 as an AVMA-recognized board specialty in veterinary clinical pharmacology. Veterinarians must complete a residency, board examinations, and graduate training in veterinary clinical pharmacology to achieve diplomate status. The logo of ACVCP demonstrates the college's commitment to advancing the practice of clinical pharmacology in veterinary medicine: "To cure with compassion, knowledge, and diligence." More than 60 veterinary pharmacologists have achieved diplomate status in ACVCP, with many more pursuing certification. ACVCP-boarded veterinary pharmacologists often work collaboratively with veterinary pharmacists in veterinary teaching hospitals, and many routinely provide clinical pharmacology support to community veterinarians and pharmacists seeking their expert knowledge of clinical veterinary therapeutic strategies.

1.4 Impact of Veterinary Pharmacy Practice

Veterinary drug sales approximated $76.4 billion in 2010 (Animal Health Institute 2017). In 2010, approximately 31% of all dog owners and 18% of cat owners received prescriptions for medication from their pet's veterinarian (American Veterinary Medical Association 2010). It is unknown how many of these prescriptions were dispensed by pharmacists adequately trained in veterinary pharmacotherapy. Several recent reports describe serious errors made by pharmacists when dispensing drugs to veterinary patients, some of which resulted in patient fatalities. The author is aware of legal action directed at pharmacists because of dispensing errors. Adequate training of pharmacists in veterinary pharmacotherapy as part of a core pharmacy curriculum would prevent many dispensing errors. The pet-owning public demands and deserves high-quality medical care for their animals that does not stop abruptly at the pharmacy when they encounter a pharmacist not adequately trained in veterinary pharmacotherapy.

Although the impact of the human–animal bond cannot be measured quantitatively, the benefit animals provide to human life is great. A *Mintel Market Report* on America's pet owners (America's Pet Owners US 2016)

determined that 87% of US pet owners surveyed consider their pets as family members. Animals provide service, entertainment, protection, food, and companionship, and even answer medical research questions for humans in ways that greatly improve the quality and length of human life. Pharmacists can play a major role in maintaining animal health, and by doing so also contributing to the health and well-being of humans, whether by strengthening the human–animal bond, preventing the spread of zoonotic disease, or preventing drug residues in human food. Veterinary pharmacists (those whose practice is limited to veterinary patients) may play a larger role in these efforts, but the role of community pharmacists in maintaining animal health continues to grow.

The benefits that veterinary pharmacists provide to veterinary teaching hospitals have been measured (Jinks and Paulsen 1982), demonstrating that in addition to positive effects on patient care, veterinary pharmacists add value in areas of drug distribution, academic development, and clinical research. The impact of pharmacists adequately trained in veterinary pharmacy that are practicing in the community, industrial, and governmental sectors has not been measured, but predictably would reveal equally valuable contributions. The scope of veterinary pharmacy practice by veterinary pharmacists (those individuals who have deliberately chosen to limit their practice to veterinary patients) also continues to expand as pet owners and veterinarians recognize the valuable contributions that veterinary pharmacists make as part of the veterinary healthcare team.

The role of community and even hospital pharmacists in veterinary medicine continues to expand regardless of whether or not an individual pharmacist intended to dispense medications to veterinary patients. This is the result of both state and federal legislation (proposed and passed) that encourages or mandates veterinarians to provide prescriptions to pet owners instead of dispensing medication directly from the veterinary hospital.

1.5 Scope of Pharmacist Involvement in Veterinary Medicine

The current scope of veterinary pharmacy practice includes, but is not limited to, veterinary academia, veterinary specialty referral centers, community and online (Internet) pharmacies that serve veterinary patients only, the pharmaceutical and agricultural industry, and governmental public health and regulatory sectors. The scope of pharmacy practice that incorporates both human and veterinary patients includes community pharmacies (chain and independent) and sometimes hospital pharmacies. This section of the chapter describes the various levels of involvement pharmacists may have in veterinary medicine, from roles that require postgraduate training and documentation that a certain level of expertise has been acquired (Diplomates, ICVP) to those that only occasionally fill prescriptions for veterinary patients. It is important to note that even the latter role requires a basic level of understanding of comparative pharmacology and veterinary drug law in order to fulfill the profession's responsibility to patient care.

The desire, by veterinarians, to proactively involve pharmacists in veterinary medicine was well documented over four decades ago. In 1977, a survey of veterinarians in Wyoming demonstrated the need for pharmacist involvement in veterinary medicine and recommended the establishment of a veterinary pharmacy specialty that should require specialized education and examination for licensure (Nelson 1977). Unfortunately, the Board of Pharmaceutical Specialties (BPS) still does not include veterinary pharmacy as a pharmacy specialty practice. However, veterinary pharmacy certainly qualifies for consideration in light of BPS's overriding mission "to ensure that the public receives the level of pharmacy services that will improve a patient's quality of life (Board of Pharmaceutical Specialties 2017). BPS's stated mission does not characterize patients as being limited to the human species, nor does the pharmacist's oath. The public expects competency from pharmacists when providing pharmaceutical care for all family members, human or otherwise. As human reliance on animals increases (e.g. companionship, service, research, food, agribusiness, and entertainment), most pharmacists will eventually find themselves providing some degree of pharmaceutical care and drugs to a nonhuman patient. Many pharmacists have devoted a large portion, if not all, of their professional practice to providing pharmaceutical expertise and specialized skills to care for animals. Pharmacists desiring to effectively participate in animal care have many career options, some of which are described throughout the remainder of this section, starting with venues that require greater veterinary pharmacy expertise and then discussing those that may require less veterinary pharmacy expertise.

1.5.1 Veterinary Teaching Hospitals

The most well-established practice of veterinary pharmacy resides in veterinary academic teaching hospitals (Figure 1.2) associated with Colleges of Veterinary Medicine (Appendix A). Pharmacists in these roles provide expertise in areas of service (drug selection, distribution, and control), teaching (didactic, incidental exchanges, client counseling, in-service education, and continuing education programs for pharmacists and veterinarians), and research (clinical trial development and administration, compounded preparation quality assurance, adverse drug reaction and medication error reporting, publication of articles in scientific and professional journals, and responding to drug information queries).

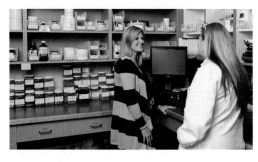

Figure 1.2

A typical day for a veterinary teaching hospital pharmacist involves attending service rounds with clinical veterinary faculty, house officers, and students; preparing and delivering lectures for veterinary, pharmacy, and veterinary technology students; providing drug utilization reviews and therapeutic interventions; maintaining hospital pharmacy operations (inpatient and outpatient drug distribution, preparing sterile and nonsterile compounds, and admixture of intravenous and chemotherapeutic therapies); and engaging in a variety of incidental teaching and consultative activities with students, veterinary practitioners, and animal owners. *Veterinary pharmacists at teaching hospitals, and their staff, are valuable resources for community pharmacists.*

1.5.2 Veterinary Specialty Referral Centers

Many pharmacists are not aware that veterinary specialization exists. Specialty training programs (generally three years) and certification examinations exist in veterinary ophthalmology, oncology, anesthesiology, cardiology, neurology, surgery, dentistry, and so on. While veterinary teaching hospitals often employ many of these specialists, there are an increasing number of large, private veterinary hospitals that limit their practice to specialized veterinary medicine. These are called referral hospitals or referral centers because the primary care veterinarian "refers" patients to these hospitals. Small-animal (canine and feline) oncology, internal medicine, cardiology, neurology, and ophthalmology are among the most common specialties at these private veterinary hospitals. Recently, veterinary specialty referral centers are employing veterinary pharmacists. Interventions by these pharmacists have a direct and positive impact on patient care, patient well-being, and practice revenue (Dorsey n.d.). Some veterinary pharmacists in these settings are species specialists and are noted for their expertise and skills in providing pharmaceutical care for a single species, such as pharmacists caring for horses

in exclusively equine veterinary practices. A typical day for a veterinary pharmacist practicing in a specialty referral center involves many of the distributive and consultative duties that are performed by pharmacists at veterinary teaching hospitals but with less emphasis on teaching and research.

1.5.3 "Community" Veterinary Pharmacies

One of the most rapidly growing areas of veterinary pharmacy practice is in the community pharmacy setting. When the Animal Medicinal Drug Use Clarification Act (AMDUCA) of 1996 codified the extra-label use of human drugs in animals, veterinarians began prescribing more and more human drugs for use in animal patients. As a result, pharmacists in chain and independent pharmacies were presented with an unprecedented number of prescriptions for animals. The professional rewards of helping animals combined with the financial rewards of cash-paying customers (third-party payment for veterinary patients is rare in the USA) caused retail pharmacy market analysts to set their sights on the veterinary prescription market. Independent pharmacies also began actively collaborating with veterinarians to provide compounded preparations for animal patients, and large retail chains began allowing pets into the discounted generics plans traditionally offered for human prescriptions. The result has been the emergence of several veterinary-only pharmacies catering solely to animal patients, and most recently, veterinary-only online pharmacies are becoming more prevalent. In 2011, the Fairness to Pet Owners Act was debated by the US Congress, proposing legislation that would force veterinarians to provide written prescriptions to all pet owners, giving them the option to purchase prescription drugs outside of the veterinary clinic. Failing to get out of committee in 2011, the bill was reintroduced in 2014 as HR4203. While the fate of the bill is not yet determined, discussion did prompt the Federal Trade Commission to examine the portability of pet medications. This is anticipated to further increase the flow of veterinary prescriptions into retail pharmacies. A critical point that has not been part of the debate around the Fairness to Pet Owners Act is the lack of competence of most pharmacists in veterinary pharmacology. Instead, the debate has been centered on potential cost savings for pet owners if drugs are purchased at chain pharmacies rather than veterinary hospitals. For community pharmacists to provide the same level of expertise for veterinary patients as they do for human patients, additional education is necessary. Optimally, veterinary pharmacotherapeutics would become a core curricular requirement in accredited US colleges of pharmacy.

1.5.4 Industry (Pharmaceutical and Agricultural)

Pharmacists with veterinary expertise are valuable to the animal health industry.

Because of their unique training that combines pharmacological expertise, clinical decision making, and marketing skills, pharmacists with specialized veterinary training make excellent professional representatives for the veterinary pharmaceutical industry. They can easily explain the pharmacodynamics and clinical advantages of new drugs to veterinarians and can serve as consultants for adverse event monitoring and reporting. Veterinary pharmacists also serve in research and development roles in the veterinary pharmaceutical industry by designing and overseeing pre- and postmarketing clinical trials for veterinary drugs. Veterinary pharmacists with expertise in the livestock or poultry industry are contracted by producers to consult in areas of medication management, specialized compounding, and avoidance of drug residues in the tissues of food-producing animals. As pharmacists are well trained in pharmacokinetic principles, they are able to collaborate with producers to predict drug depletion profiles for therapeutic agents used in food-producing animals.

1.5.5 Government Sectors (FDA, CDC, NIH, and Disaster Relief)

Veterinary pharmacists provide valuable services to governmental and regulatory sectors. The Center for Veterinary Medicine of the US Food and Drug Administration (FDA CVM) employs many veterinary pharmacists in areas of compliance, surveillance, adverse event reporting, and medication error prevention. The Centers for Disease Control and Prevention (CDC) also employ veterinary pharmacists who are charged with overseeing the distribution and use of biological agents and drugs used to prevent or treat rare diseases that are zoonotic. The National Institutes of Health (NIH) employ a veterinary pharmacist responsible for providing conventionally manufactured drugs, compounds, and consultation for research animals in NIH-funded protocols. Among other responsibilities, pharmacists in this role may focus their efforts on minimizing the stress that drug administration can cause to research animals, which involves developing combination drug dosage forms (to avoid multiple administrations) and transmucosally absorbed drugs for nasal and buccal administration.

Veterinary pharmacists may also serve on disaster relief teams. These specially trained pharmacists are parts of multidisciplinary teams that also may include veterinarians and veterinary technicians that are ready to be deployed regionally. When called upon, these teams of veterinary professionals are deployed to stricken areas to provide triage, medical care, and treatment for displaced and injured animals. One of the largest deployments of a Veterinary Medical Assistance Team (VMAT) was during the Hurricane Katrina recovery in 2005. Many veterinary pharmacists were involved in these efforts.

1.5.6 Animal Poison Prevention and Consultation

Veterinary pharmacists may also serve as poison control specialists at animal poison control centers such as the Pet Poison

Helpline (www.petpoisonhelpline.com). Pharmacists often are the last line of defense in recognizing and preventing potential animal poisoning. Unfortunately, pharmacists traditionally are trained only in human toxicology, which can be vastly different from veterinary toxicology. In fact, canine toxicology can be vastly different from feline toxicology, which can be vastly different from equine toxicology. Factors that affect the risk of toxicity vary greatly among species; they include (but are not limited to) differences in absorption, distribution, metabolism, and elimination; anatomical characteristics, such as the inability to vomit; the age and size of the animal; and seasonal and environmental influences. Veterinary pharmacists possess a working knowledge of species-specific susceptibilities to toxins and can work with boarded veterinary toxicologists (DVMs with specialty training in veterinary toxicology) for more unusual toxic exposures. The American Society for the Prevention of Cruelty to Animals reported that 16% of pet poisonings in 2015 were attributable to human drugs (American Society for the Prevention of Cruelty to Animals 2017). Lack of knowledge on the part of pet owners can result in inadvertent poisonings when pets are accidentally or intentionally exposed to drugs. In some instances, pet owners attempt to treat animals with human OTC products or their own prescription drugs; pharmacists who are adequate trained in veterinary pharmacology are ideally positioned to intervene and provide valuable post-ingestion consultation.

Dramatic difference

It is important for community pharmacists to understand that emetics that are effective for inducing vomiting in one species may not be effective for another species (Chapter 6).

1.6 Veterinary Pharmacy Practice Considerations

1.6.1 Basic Considerations

The two most profound differences between human and animal patients are that animal patients do not communicate using spoken words, and animals and their byproducts are consumed as food by humans. These two differences drive many of the rules and regulations regarding drug use in animals. A complete discussion on drug therapy in food-producing animals is provided in Chapter 22.

To fully appreciate the differences in veterinary pharmacy practice as compared to human pharmacy practice, it is also important to consider the unintended impact of human healthcare systems and human behaviors on veterinary medicine. The complex systems of private, and state or federally mandated, third-party payor programs are mostly unique to human medicine, and although private third-party insurance is available to animal owners, it is rarely encountered by pharmacists. Because most payment for veterinary healthcare is out of pocket, animal owners must carefully consider the expense of purchasing medications for their animals. This consideration often drives them out of the veterinary practice to large discount outlets or the Internet to find the least expensive options for therapy. The lack of veterinary pharmacology knowledge and risk of poor-quality drugs in some of these outlets can result in disastrous consequences for pet owners who are trying to save money. For example, purchasing a cheap or compounded version of the immunomodulating therapy cyclosporine instead of the FDA-approved version for a dog with life-threatening immune-mediated disease can result in subtherapeutic blood concentrations or often therapeutic failure. As a result, the pet owner is forced to spend considerably more money back at the veterinary clinic trying to re-stabilize the animal or is forced to opt for humane euthanasia. Unlike human medicine, veterinary practitioners and animal owners have the option of humane euthanasia to end suffering when circumstances (financial or medical) necessitate.

State and federal third-party payor systems for Medicare and Medicaid (Center for Medicare and Medicaid Services [CMS]) also strongly influence the human medical system through approved reimbursement formularies and a mandate for pharmacists to substitute generic drugs when filling prescriptions for CMS patients. As a result, human pharmacy software programs require a national prescriber identification number (NPI) that verifies that prescriber in the CMS database before new prescriptions can be processed. Community pharmacists often request NPI numbers from veterinarians and find it difficult to proceed in the software without this verification number. The alternative verification is through the prescriber's DEA [Drug Enforcement Administration] number, but DEA has stated that it "strongly opposes the use of a DEA registration number for any purpose other than the one for which it was intended, to provide certification of DEA registration in transactions involving controlled substances. The use of DEA registration numbers as an NPI is not an appropriate use and could lead to a weakening of the registration system" (DEA n.d.). Veterinarians express significant frustration when asked for NPI or DEA numbers or when pharmacists automatically substitute generic medications even when the veterinarian has indicated that therapeutic substitution is not permitted. Community pharmacists should be prepared for a different approach when filling prescriptions for animals: (i) Instead of NPI or DEA numbers, identify an alternate prescriber verification number (e.g. the state veterinary license number), (ii) do not substitute generically without the veterinarian's authorization, and (iii) only require DEA numbers for prescriptions for controlled substances.

As mentioned in this chapter, opioid shortages may occur due to manufacturing shortages or interruption of the supply chain during and after natural disasters. However, human behavior also strongly influences the availability of opioids. Because of the rampant rise of human addiction to opioids, all 51 states and territories in the USA have Prescription Drug Monitoring Programs (PDMPs) that closely monitor and often severely restrict the quantity of opioids that a prescriber can give to a human for use outside of a hospital admission. To decrease supplies of opioids, federal mandates have also been issued to reduce manufacturing of opioids. The unintended consequence for veterinarians and animal patients is an increasing difficulty in obtaining opioids to meet patient needs. In 16 of the states with PDMPs, veterinarians have been specifically excluded from these restrictions, but community pharmacists often do not realize that opioid prescriptions for animals may be exempt from their state PDMP rules. It is critical that community pharmacists remain current and informed of all state and federal rules and regulations that may affect animal patients.

Key Points for Processing Veterinary Prescriptions

1) Instead of NPI or DEA numbers, identify an alternate prescriber verification number (e.g. the state veterinary license number).
2) Do not substitute generically without the veterinarian's authorization.
3) Only require DEA numbers for prescriptions for controlled substances.

The third-party payor system also heavily influences the drug approval and marketing process. The human pharmaceutical industry (Pharmaceutical Researchers and Manufacturers of America [PhRMA]) consistently ranks as the most profitable industry in the USA, and was relatively resistant to the economic crisis that affected the USA in 2009. The insurance industry also remains relatively lucrative (Kaiser Health News 2009). Because third-party payors almost always cover the costs of human drug therapy for their constituents, there is little incentive to reduce the astronomical prices that are charged for new human drug therapies. Profits by the pharmaceutical industry are used to subsidize drug approval fees for new submissions, and the approval system is largely subsidized by these profits. In 2017, there were more than 35 000 drugs approved for humans, while only 1564 were approved for use in animals. The FDA approved 45 new human drugs in 2015 and consistently averages about 28 new drug approvals annually. In comparison, FDA CVM approved five new animal drugs in 2015 and was praised in the 2017 budget for "exceeding all performance goals" in 2015 (FDA 2017). Comparing the 2015 FDA budgets for human and animal new drug approval, the human drug approval budget was almost eight times larger than that for animal drugs. Considering the vast number of species and diseases requiring new drug therapy in veterinary medicine, the ratio of expenditure and drug availability for humans versus animals seems upside down. The priority of human need over animal need is also evident during shortages of human drug supplies. Manufacturing problems, mergers, and natural disasters all contribute to significant drug shortages, which grow steadily every year. When drug supplies are short, many drug manufacturers and wholesalers operate in a distribution mode known as "allocation," whereby human providers get top priority for receiving drugs, and amounts are based on the provider's purchasing history of the shorted item. During shortages of intravenous fluids, electrolytes, chemotherapy drugs, and opioids, many veterinary providers are denied access to drugs because their patients are not human. Because community pharmacists are well positioned to serve all species of patients, they serve a valuable role in helping veterinarians and pet owners identify affordable and available drug therapy for their patients.

Postmarketing adverse drug events are also more likely in animal patients, since cohorts of only 50–300 animals are required for animal drug approval. Human drug approval is based on cohorts of several thousand humans. Occasionally, a drug intended to be marketed for humans is successful in Phase I (animal) testing but is determined to be toxic to humans in Phase II or III (human) premarketing studies. To attempt to recoup some of the research and development investment for these drugs, they are sometimes taken up by the animal pharmaceutical industry (Animal Health Institute [AHI]) for development for animal use. Some examples of these drugs include flunixin meglumine, enrofloxacin, and tilmicosin for which the FDA CVM approved labeling bears a strong warning that these products are not for use in humans. It is important to note that these warnings or potential drug interactions with other drugs will not be included in any drug interaction/pharmacy alert software. The vast number of species, breeds, and genetic polymorphisms encountered in veterinary pharmacotherapy have thus far prevented the development of any intelligent drug interaction software for animal patients. As mentioned further in this chapter, community pharmacists must become familiar with the pharmacology and toxicity of veterinary-only drugs and employ methods that will prevent them from being erroneously dispensed to humans.

Finally, there are many sound-alike drugs that can be problematic for community pharmacists accepting verbal prescriptions from veterinarians. For example, Soloxine® (oral levothyroxine tablets) sounds identical to Ciloxan® (ciprofloxacin ophthalmic ointment or solution). Usually, the instructions would prompt a pharmacist to request clarification, but if the veterinarian states "use as directed" without distinction to route of administration, then dispensing errors may occur. Another common and more consequential mistake is when veterinarians are phoning in prescriptions for Hycodan® for cough suppression in dogs, to be followed by a written or faxed prescription. Instead of Hycodan, the pharmacist thinks he hears the more commonly prescribed drug for humans, Vicodin®. Vicodin contains a fatal dose of acetaminophen for cats and a potentially fatal dose of acetaminophen for small dogs. Although the paper prescription would eventually alert the pharmacist to this error, severe morbidity or death could have likely ensured in the few days between verbal and written orders. Community pharmacists are well advised to have veterinarians spell out drug names if there is any doubt at all as to what the veterinarian is prescribing.

1.6.2 Veterinary Drug Law

It is important for pharmacists to understand that regulations for veterinary drug use are different from those that apply to human drug use, but it is even more complicated than that. There are a specific set of regulations that apply to only some animals (food animal species) but not others. Detailed information about drug use in food animals is presented in Chapter 22, but a summary is in this chapter. All other veterinary drug regulations apply to both food animals and companion animals.

Veterinary pharmacists must work within the boundaries for drug use established by a number of agencies at both the federal and state levels. These agencies include the FDA, DEA, US Department of Agriculture (USDA), and Environmental Protection Agency (EPA) (see Table 1.1, "Classes of Veterinary Products Approved by Agency"), in addition to the state boards of pharmacy and veterinary medicine. In the USA, regulations governing veterinary drugs have much in common with the regulations that govern human drugs. For example, both human and animal drugs are

regulated by the FDA under the Federal Food, Drug, and Cosmetic (FDC) Act. New animal drugs must have an approved New Animal Drug Application (NADA), similar to the New Drug Application (NDA) for human drugs. Animal drugs, like human drugs, must be shown to be safe and effective for their intended uses. Generic copies of new animal drug products can be approved pursuant to submission of an Abbreviated New Animal Drug Application (ANADA).

1.6.3 Regulations for Drugs Intended for Food-Producing Animals

Regulations for human and "food-producing" animal drugs differ in important ways because humans may consume animal tissues and byproducts. The administration of drugs to food-producing animals (see Chapter 22 for additional information), including drugs in animal feed or water, has the potential to generate residues of the parent drug or its metabolites that could be consumed by (and pose health hazards to) humans. It is necessary to determine when it is safe for the public to consume tissues from an animal that has been treated with a drug. This information is part of the FDA-mandated approval process for drugs labeled for use in food animals. That is why there are major differences in regulations related to extra-label use of drugs (i.e. use for an indication that has not received FDA approval) in food animals compared to humans. After a drug is approved for human use, the FDA does not limit or control how physicians prescribe medications. In contrast, extra-label use of drugs in food animals is permitted only under limited conditions to ensure public safety. For some drugs, extra-label use is expressly prohibited (see Chapter 22).

1.6.4 Regulations for Drug Use in Companion Animals

In 1996, a milestone veterinary drug law, AMDUCA, was enacted, permitting extra-label

Table 1.1 Classes of veterinary products approved by agency.

Agency	Product class
FDA	Drugs
EPA	Topically administered pesticides
USDA	Biologics and vaccines
DEA	Controlled substances

use of many approved animal and human drugs by or on the lawful order of a veterinarian within the context of an established set of conditions known as a "veterinarian–client–patient relationship" (VCPR; see Figure 1.3, "Elements of the Veterinarian–Client–Patient Relationship"). Prior to AMDUCA, the law required veterinarians to use drugs exactly as labeled for the approved indication, at the approved dose, by the approved route, for the approved duration, and only in the approved species. This effectively rendered any other drug use, including use of any human-labeled drug, illegal. Because AMDUCA grants veterinarians the ability to prescribe human-labeled drugs for use in animals, the need for pharmacists trained in veterinary pharmacotherapy has emerged as a needed discipline. The quality of medical care for companion animals is substantially enhanced with access to human-approved drugs because there are so few approved veterinary drugs in comparison.

Prescription and OTC drugs approved by the FDA for use in animals are listed in the *Green Book*, also known as *Animal Drugs@ FDA* (http://www.fda.gov/animalveterinary). All drugs in the *Green Book* have an assigned NADA number for new animal drugs or an ANADA number for generic animal drugs. If a "drug" cannot be located in the *Green Book*, it is not FDA approved for use in animals. National Drug Code (NDC) numbers for drugs only identify the manufacturer, specific product (e.g. strength, dosage form, and formulation), and package size and type: They do not denote legal approval by the FDA. Although categories of veterinary drugs are similar to those for human drugs, there are some notable differences in their use. For example, megesterol acetate, a hormonal agent, is used almost exclusively as an antineoplastic therapy in humans but is used for behavior modification in animals. A pharmacist receiving a prescription for megesterol for a cat cannot assume that the cat has cancer.

1.6.4.1 Prescription Drugs

Prescription animal drugs (also known as legend drugs) are restricted by federal law to use by or on the order of a licensed veterinarian, according to Section 503(f) of the FDC Act. The law requires that such drugs be labeled with the statement "Caution: Federal law restricts this drug to use by or on the order of a licensed veterinarian" (see Figure 1.4) within the confines of a VCPR (see Figure 1.3). The VCPR primarily evolved because animal patients cannot communicate verbally with their healthcare providers. While a human patient can phone a prescriber and describe symptoms that can lead to a reasonable diagnosis, animal patients cannot. For this reason, veterinarians must have either physically examined the animal or visited the site where the animal is housed.

Elements of the Veterinarian–Client–Patient Relationship

A Veterinarian–Client–Patient relationship. A VCPR means that **all of** the following are required:

a. The veterinarian has assumed the responsibility for making medical judgments regarding the health of the patient, and the client has agreed to follow the veterinarian's instructions.

b. The veterinarian has sufficient knowledge of the patient to initiate at least a general or preliminary diagnosis of the medical condition of the patient. This means that the veterinarian is personally acquainted with the keeping and care of the patient **by virtue of**:

   i. a timely examination of the patient by the veterinarian, or

   ii. medically appropriate and timely visits by the veterinarian to the operation where the patient is managed.

c. The veterinarian is readily available for follow-up evaluation or has arranged for the following:

   i. veterinary emergency coverage, and

   ii. continuing care and treatment.

d. The veterinarian provides oversight of treatment, compliance, and outcome.

e. Patient records are maintained.

Figure 1.3

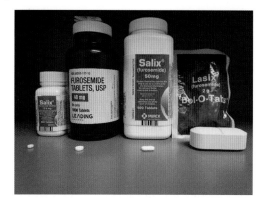

Figure 1.4

All states except Alaska, Connecticut, Delaware, Maine, Washington, and the District of Columbia currently have laws in place that require a VCPR before a veterinarian can prescribe a drug for use in an animal (American Veterinary Medical Association 2017). Even if a VCPR is not mandated at the state level, it is required by federal law when drugs are prescribed for extra-label use in animal patients (21 CFR 530.10), when veterinary feed directive drugs are used in animal patients [21 CFR 558.6 (a)(2)], and when autologous biologics are used in animal patients (9 CFR 113.113).

1.6.4.2 Over-the-Counter Drugs

Unlike human OTC drugs, veterinary OTC drugs undergo full approval by the FDA. The FDA is responsible for determining whether an animal drug product will be available by prescription only or sold directly to laypersons. OTC status hinges on whether it is possible to prepare "adequate directions for use" under which a layperson can use the drug safely and effectively. Safe use includes safety to the animal, safety of food products derived from the animal, safety to persons administering the drug or otherwise associated with the animal, and safety in terms of the drug's impact on the environment.

Dramatic difference

It is important for the pharmacist to understand that human OTC drugs are not labeled for use in any species other than humans. Consequently, federal law prohibits the use

---

of a human OTC drug in an animal unless such use is specifically pursuant to a prescription order by a licensed veterinarian within the context of a valid VCPR. This means that there is not currently a legal avenue for pharmacists to recommend human OTC drug products for veterinary patients. Hopefully, this can change as the pharmacy profession adopts veterinary pharmacotherapeutics as a core competency.

1.6.5 Veterinary Drug Compounding

Drug compounding is the process by which a veterinarian or pharmacist prepares a medication in a manner not stipulated in the product labeling to create a compound specifically tailored to the needs of an individual patient. Compared with the number of drugs approved by the FDA for use in humans, the number of drugs approved for use in veterinary species is low, so the need for compounded therapies to treat animals is consequently high. Even though current federal law permits veterinarians to use and prescribe drugs that are FDA approved for human use in an extra-label fashion, many human medications are only available in formulations impractical or unsafe for use in pets (e.g. the use of xylitol as an artificial sweetener). Compounding also allows access to medications that are not currently commercially available, such as drugs discontinued by pharmaceutical companies for economic reasons or as a result of voluntarily or federally mandated withdrawals (e.g. cisapride, potassium bromide, and diethylstilbestrol), and drugs unavailable for use due to temporary shortages (e.g. electrolytes and fluids, and opioid injections). A comprehensive discussion on compounding is provided in Chapter 3.

1.6.6 Veterinary Adverse Drug Event Reporting

Recognizing and reporting adverse drug events (ADEs) in animal patients comprise an integral role for the veterinary pharmacist.

While not mandated by regulation in the USA, the American Animal Hospital Association (AAHA) considers adverse drug experience reporting a standard for accreditation. Responsibility for this important task could easily be assigned to the veterinary pharmacist, who can develop, implement, and monitor systems for adverse drug experience surveillance. Community pharmacists are often the first healthcare professional that pet owners reach out to regarding a suspected ADE. Pharmacists lacking training in veterinary pharmacotherapy are not likely familiar with recognizing adverse events in animals but can play a key role in referring the owner to seek immediate evaluation from their veterinarian when adverse events are known or suspected.

An ADE is defined by the FDA CVM as "any observation in animals, whether or not considered to be product-related, that is unfavorable and unintended and that occurs after any use of veterinary medical products (off-label and on-label uses). Included are events related to a suspected lack of expected efficacy according to approved labeling or noxious reactions in humans after being exposed to veterinary medical product(s)" (FDA 2006). Monitoring for and reporting ADEs comprise a multidisciplinary responsibility and are accomplished through a combined effort of veterinarians, pharmacists, veterinary technicians, and all other members of the veterinary healthcare team. Although not mandated by the FDC Act, monitoring and reporting of ADEs are required by the Joint Commission for Accreditation of Healthcare Organizations, the American Society of Health-Systems Pharmacists, and the American Animal Hospital Association.

ADEs in animals can be reported to the manufacturer or through the FDA Adverse Drug Event Reporting Form 1932a (FDA 2017). ADE monitoring is required by the FDA for all approved veterinary drugs. Additionally, the manufacturer (sponsor) is required to report ADEs to the FDA.

Pharmacists, particularly veterinary pharmacists at teaching hospitals or specialty referral hospitals, can enhance pharmacotherapy by instituting an adverse event monitoring system. The primary purpose of instituting a monitoring system is to improve detection of ADEs (including lack of efficacy) associated with the use of approved drugs in animals. Compared to human drugs, there is a greater need for an adverse event monitoring system because of the limited number of patients included in pre-approval clinical trials (a few dozen to a few hundred). Because only a limited number of animals are exposed to the drug prior to its commercial release, ADEs that are uncommon may not be discovered until after the drug has been administered to a large number of animals. Additionally, veterinary clinical trials do not include all breeds of a species, nor do they include animals receiving many concurrent drugs. Therefore, unexpected breed-specific ADEs (Chapter 5) and drug–drug interactions are likely to occur, even though they are not indicated on the label. Pharmacist-driven adverse event monitoring systems can improve patient care, educate the veterinary staff concerning ADEs, and provide drug regulatory agencies with statistical information regarding the incidence, types, and impact of adverse drug experiences on patient outcomes.

For veterinary pharmacists interested in instituting an adverse event monitoring system, the type of information collected is critical. It is important that veterinarians and staff can easily access the reporting forms, whether they are electronic or paper. While forms may vary between hospitals, the data indicated in Table 1.2 are recommended.

Once the ADE is submitted to the veterinary pharmacist, formal acknowledgment of receipt should be returned to the reporter. Once the internal report is evaluated for completeness, a notation should be made in the patient's permanent medical record and appropriate reports on appropriate forms to (i) the attending veterinarian, (ii) the FDA, (iii) the drug manufacturer or compounding pharmacy, and (iv) the institutional Pharmacy and Therapeutics Committee or equivalent. Note that reporting to FDA simultaneously accomplishes notifying the

Table 1.2 Elements of a veterinary adverse event report.

Patient signalment
Time and date
Identity of reporter
Attending veterinarian
Diagnosis
Organ system involvement/clinical signs
Suspected drugs
Concurrently administered drugs and therapies
Relevant tests and laboratory data
Date and time of onset
Treatment and follow-up
Previous reactions to similar agents
Instructions for where to send the completed form

drug manufacturer. ADEs associated with biologicals and vaccines should be reported to the US Department of Agriculture, Center for Veterinary Biologics (USDA, CVB). ADEs caused by pesticides should be reported to the EPA. Adverse events from products that are not approved by the FDA (e.g. grooming aids) should be reported to the US Consumer Product Safety Commission (CPSC). Links to these agencies are listed in Table 1.3.

1.6.7 Veterinary Terminology

Veterinary medical terminology is largely grounded in the same Latin system that applies to human medicine; however, significant differences have developed between veterinary and human medical terminology. Chapter 25 and Appendix B provide information about differences in anatomic terminology that are necessary to describe species that walk on four legs compared to species that walk on two legs. There are other phrases, terminology, and just plain "jargon" that are standard in a veterinary hospital but that most pharmacists are not aware of. Until recently, veterinarians almost exclusively dispensed medications to pet owners themselves, so they had no need to learn to write prescriptions properly. Consequently, many veterinary colleges did not teach veterinary students how to write prescriptions using standard Latin abbreviations, so non-veterinary-trained pharmacists frequently misinterpret unknown veterinary abbreviations. This has resulted in disastrous consequences. For example, "once daily" is almost exclusively abbreviated as SID (*semel in die*) by veterinary prescribers, and pharmacists have misinterpreted this abbreviation to read TID, QID, and even 5/D, usually resulting in serious toxicity (even death). Table 1.4 lists abbreviations that might be encountered by community pharmacists filling prescriptions for veterinary patients.

1.6.8 Drug Administration

As described in Chapter 25, there are major differences in drug administration techniques between human and veterinary patients as well as between veterinary species. These

Table 1.3 Adverse event reporting by product category.

Product type	Agency	Link
Drugs	FDA	http://www.fda.gov/AnimalVeterinary/SafetyHealth/ReportaProblem/ucm055305.htm
Vaccines	USDA	www.aphis.usda.gov/aphis/ourfocus/animalhealth/veterinary-biologics/adverse-event-reporting/ct_vb_adverse_event
Pesticides	EPA	http://www.epa.gov/enforcement/report-environmental-violations
Grooming aids	CPSC	http://www.cpsc.gov

Table 1.4 Common veterinary abbreviations in prescription writing.

Common veterinary abbreviations in prescription writing	
Term or abbreviation	**Translation**
Bolus	Large, solid, oral dosage form, usually for horses or livestock
Divided BID	The total daily dose is calculated and then administered over 2 equally divided doses 12 hours apart
DLH	Domestic Longhaired (cat)
Drench	Large volume of oral liquid administered as a single dose (usually livestock)
DSH	Domestic Shorthaired (cat)
EOD	Every other day
Fe	Feline or cat
FS or F/S	Female spayed
Intact	A non-neutered animal
K9	Canine or dog
MC or M/C	Male castrated
MN or M/N	Male neutered
OD	Once daily *or* right eye, depending on context
Paste	Viscous oral liquid dosage form (frequently for horses)
Pinnae	The inner, hairless part of an animal's ears
QOD	Every other day
SID	*Semel in die* (once daily)
TD	Transdermal

differences are based on the size of the animal, its temperament, anatomical differences, and others. A pharmacist's knowledge of compounding (Chapter 3) can be lifesaving for some veterinary patients by enabling an owner or veterinarian to treat a fractious, aggressive, or fearful animal. Examples of creative manipulations that veterinary pharmacists use to allow drug delivery include enhancing palatability, formulating transmucosally or transdermally absorbed drugs, and creating combination therapy capsules.

Dosage forms and descriptive terminology also vary for drugs administered to animals. In veterinary medicine, "pastes," "boluses," and "drenches" are exclusively intended for oral use when referring to horses, cattle, sheep, goats, and/or pigs. Sometimes, the term "bolus" is also intended for intravenous drug boluses (as the term is typically used in human medicine) in dogs or cats. The pharmacist should confirm with the veterinarian what the intended route of administration is prior to dispensing.

1.6.9 Veterinary-Only Drugs

Many drugs may be used legally in both human and animal patients, including furosemide, many beta lactam antimicrobials, corticosteroids, and many others. Other drugs have unique human toxicities and are approved for use only in animals or in some cases only in one species. Some drugs were approved initially for use in humans but withdrawn after serious adverse effects emerged (Table 1.5). In other cases, these drugs were identified as toxic to humans

Table 1.5 Veterinary indications for drugs withdrawn for humans for safety reasons.

Drug	Human toxicity	Indications for animal use
Potassium bromide	Bromism – CNS toxicity	Canine epilepsy
Cisapride	Fatal arrhythmias	Prokinetic
Diethylstilbestrol	Carcinogenic in offspring of user	Urinary incontinence
Dipyrone	Hepatotoxicity	Antipyretic
Phenylbutazone	Nephrotoxicity	Anti-inflammatory
Phenylpropanolamine	Hypertensive crisis/stroke	Urinary incontinence

Table 1.6 Therapeutic plasma concentrations of selected drugs by species.

Drug	Species	Therapeutic concentration
Bromides (potassium and sodium)	Canine	1–3 mg/mL
Cyclosporine	Canine, feline	400–600 nanogram/mL (trough)
Phenobarbital	Canine, feline	15–45 microgram/mL
Digoxin	Canine, feline	0.8–1.2 nanogram/mL
Theophylline	Canine, feline	8–10 microgram/mL (trough)

early in development and never approved for human use.

More than 1400 drugs are approved by the FDA CVM for use in animals. Veterinary pharmacists must possess a working knowledge of the names, mechanisms of action, indications, dosing, adverse effects, safety profiles, and counseling points for veterinary-only drugs that may belong to similar therapeutic classes as those used in humans but may cause serious adverse effects if accidentally dispensed to a human. For example, enrofloxacin is a commonly prescribed veterinary-only fluoroquinolone antibiotic known to cause severe central nervous system (CNS) disturbances (e.g. auditory and visual hallucinations) in humans. To avoid erroneous dispensing of veterinary-only drugs to humans, most retail pharmacies that stock veterinary-only drugs segregate them from human drug inventory. Because medication administration to animals by necessity involves a human, veterinary pharmacists

must be able to advise human caregivers about possible risks from exposure to veterinary drugs.

1.6.10 Monitoring Veterinary Patients for Response to Drug Therapy

Pharmacists who are well trained in pharmacokinetic/pharmacodynamic principles and therapeutic drug monitoring can use those skills as veterinary pharmacists. Therapeutic drug monitoring in animals is performed for many reasons, including but not limited to determining if the current drug dose is achieving target therapeutic plasma concentrations. Therapeutic plasma concentrations of several drugs are well defined in dogs and cats (Table 1.6). For performance animals (Chapter 24), plasma and urine samples are collected to screen for the presence of banned substances. Other samples that may be collected include hair and saliva. Veterinary pharmacists should be familiar with sample collection and handling methods and protocols.

Veterinary pharmacists can help educate pet owners to monitor for drug efficacy and toxicity. Veterinary pharmacists should be familiar with how to monitor vital signs in each veterinary species. For example, pulse rate may be a good indicator of drug efficacy or toxicity for many drugs (sympathomimetics, tricyclic antidepressants, selective serotonin reuptake inhibitors, beta adrenergic receptor antagonists, etc.) and is best determined in cats by palpating the femoral artery in the inner thigh. That would definitely not be recommended for horses! The mandibular artery beneath the lower jawbone in horses is a much safer location. Neither of those are appropriate access points for monitoring human pulse rate. The body temperature that constitutes a "fever" in humans may be quite normal or even hypothermic in animals, and a respiratory rate that is normal in humans may indicate tachypnea in horses. Veterinary pharmacists should be familiar with normal ranges for vital signs in most domestic species (Appendix C) and the implications for values that fall out of range.

1.7 Species Specifics

Competent veterinary pharmacists must be well versed in practice considerations that are vastly different from those for human pharmacotherapy. As detailed in Chapter 4, comprehensive knowledge of species anatomy and physiology, species metabolic and toxicologic susceptibilities, and veterinary medical terminology, as well as legal and regulatory boundaries (Chapter 2), drug depletion profiles for food-producing animals (Chapter 22), intended use of animals (Chapter 24), behavioral characteristics (Chapter 16), dietary preferences, drug administration techniques (Chapter 25), and drug-monitoring techniques, will enable the veterinary pharmacist to more accurately predict drug disposition and effect in individual animals. In addition to a mastery of

these subjects, the veterinary pharmacist must be familiar with veterinary drug information resources and connected to references that ensure instant access to the most current evidence or conventional wisdom on any given subject. Because every veterinary species is unique and is accompanied with an intended use that may invoke specific regulatory restrictions, veterinary pharmacists must also develop a personal algorithm to approach each prescription order individually in a way that considers therapeutic management of disease as well as intended use of the patient. At the very least, the competent veterinary pharmacist knows that extrapolation directly from human pharmacology is rarely appropriate and is frequently dangerous.

1.7.1 Anatomy

Dosing of drugs in humans is, for the most part, empirical and based on stage of life. Pharmacists caring for humans are familiar with typical "adult" doses and typical "pediatric" doses and process prescription orders that are generally dosed in "units per human" instead of metrology based on body weight or surface area. The heterogeneity across veterinary species prohibits empiric dosing in most cases. Veterinary pharmacists must learn acceptable dosage ranges as applied to body weight and body surface area, and when dosing by body surface area, the veterinary pharmacist must choose the appropriate body surface area calculation formula for a given species. Veterinary patients are also horizontally oriented, as opposed to humans who are vertically oriented. Solid dosage forms administered orally to animals do not have the benefit of gravity to move them to the stomach, so veterinary pharmacists must ensure that adequate measures are taken to ensure that drugs do not become trapped on esophageal mucosa, where they may be erosive. Humans also have a relatively homogeneous skin covering, whereas fur, feathers, scales, and exoskeletons may prove to be tremendous barriers to drug administration in animal species. Digestive organs of many animal species are also vastly different from those of humans. Although humans have a simple, monogastric stomach, herbivorous species require complex, microbe-filled digestive organs such as rumens and cecums to adequately convert cellulose fibers into utilizable carbohydrate energy. Oral antibiotics must be carefully selected to introduce into these complex microbe-filled organs, or else malabsorption and endotoxemia from bacterial overgrowth may occur.

1.7.2 Physiology

Veterinary pharmacy also involves a working knowledge of species' physiological variations. Not only do digestive organs impact drug disposition across the species, but dietary habit also has significant impact. Animals that are primarily carnivores may have a relatively more acidic gastrointestinal and urinary pH than humans. Herbivores may have a relatively more basic gastrointestinal and urinary pH than humans. Both extremes will cause variation on the intestinal absorption and urinary reabsorption of weak acids and weak bases as compared to what occurs in humans. Many herbivorous species are physiologically unable to vomit (e.g. horses and rabbits). For this reason, great care must be taken to prevent unintentional oral administration of a potential toxin because induction of emesis is not likely to be effective. Animals that are unable to vomit have also evolved powerfully discerning olfactory senses that make forced oral drug administration very difficult. The thermoregulatory capability of an animal species must also be considered. Many animals cannot sweat efficiently (e.g. dogs and cats) and must therefore depend on respiration and vasodilation for dissipation of body heat. Drugs acting on these systems can have dramatic and sometimes lethal effects on body temperature. Other animals (e.g. reptiles and fish) cannot voluntarily maintain a preferred body temperature (poikilotherms) and are vulnerable to environmental conditions. Drug metabolism in these species is likely to vary with the temperature of the animal's habitat. Veterinary pharmacists must also consider other physiological variants such as normal body temperature or preferred body temperature range, respiratory and pulse range, glomerular filtration rate, intravascular blood volume, and cellular idiosyncrasies such as hemoglobin structure when considering appropriate therapeutic regimens for animals.

1.7.3 Metabolic Capacity

In addition to the vast amount of drug metabolism knowledge that pharmacists must commit to memory for human therapeutics, veterinary pharmacists must also master the metabolic capabilities, microsomal enzyme systems, and p-glycoprotein substrate interactions for all veterinary species. As animal species have evolved differently from humans, so has their capacity to metabolize xenobiotics. A drug substance such as acetaminophen may be safe and therapeutically effective in humans but is metabolized to lethal hemotoxins and hepatotoxins in cats.

1.7.4 Pharmacogenomics

Pharmacogenomics are beginning to play a large role in human pharmacotherapy, but genetic and cultural factors have always been considered significantly in veterinary pharmacotherapy. Veterinary pharmacists must carefully consider breed-specific disease predispositions and drug tolerances in animal species. For example, many herding breeds (e.g. Border Collies, Australian Shepherds, and Shetland Sheepdogs) lack the MDR1 gene that prevents drugs from crossing the blood–brain barrier and are very susceptible to the adverse CNS effects of heartworm preventatives and other anthelmintic drugs (Washington State University College of Veterinary Medicine Veterinary Clinical Pharmacology Lab 2017). Veterinary pharmacists must also consider an animal's behavior and habitat when providing drug therapy. Cats are notorious groomers of themselves and of other household cats. For this reason, a topically administered drug will become systemically available not only in the cat to which it is applied, but also to any other household cat that helped groom the medication off the treated cat's skin. Finally, animals housed exclusively outside are particularly vulnerable to weather extremes, and drug therapy must be planned accordingly.

1.8 Critical Evaluation of Published Veterinary Literature

Given the relative shortage of approved drugs for all needs in veterinary medicine compared to human medicine, veterinary pharmacists frequently aid in evaluating and providing novel drug therapies for animal patients. Veterinary pharmacists should be capable of reviewing and evaluating published literature to support the use of novel therapies in animals, rather than merely reading and accepting investigator conclusions. Accordingly, veterinary pharmacists possess a basic knowledge of study design and should be able to determine if the methods employed in a particular study were appropriate. They should be familiar with the intent and validity of statistical presentations, as well as possible sources of error and limitations of the investigation.

It is important to note that many of the assumptions regarding the validity of human trials – for example, rational selection of cohort size – do not necessarily apply to animal studies. Because animal subjects do not "volunteer" for investigational studies as humans do, Institutional Animal Care and Use Committees (IACUCs) must ensure that a sufficient number of animals is included to accomplish investigator aims without using animals unnecessarily. This requires careful balancing of multiple considerations: rational selection of group size (e.g. for a pilot study or power analysis), careful experimental design, maximizing use of each animal, minimizing loss of animals, and efficient statistical analysis (maximum information from the minimum number of animals). Pharmacists must appreciate these limitations when they evaluate and/or participate in veterinary research.

1.9 Veterinary Pharmacy Information Resources

Drug dosing in nonhuman patients is not as straightforward as it is in human patients. Dosing in animals often is species specific or indication specific. For example, the labeled dose of firocoxib, a veterinary-only non-steroidal anti-inflammatory agent, for horses is 0.1 mg/kg, while the labeled dose for dogs is 5 mg/kg, a 50-fold difference. The labeled dose of maropitant, an antiemetic veterinary-only drug, is 2 mg/kg orally to prevent vomiting in dogs, and 8 mg/kg orally to prevent motion sickness in dogs. Consequently, it is imperative that pharmacists are aware of and have access to current and credible veterinary drug information resources. When consulting veterinary references, veterinary pharmacists determine the most recent publication date and consider the frequency with which the material is revised. Many new veterinary information reference books and databases are published each year. This section describes drug information resources that veterinary pharmacists most commonly use.

1.9.1 Veterinary Drug Information Reference Handbooks

The resource known familiarly as "Plumb's" comprises two reference products: the print-version *Plumb's Veterinary Drug Handbook* and the electronic *Plumb's Veterinary Drugs*. The author (Donald C. Plumb, PharmD) and contributors all are well-known authorities in the veterinary medical field, and this publication is widely utilized as a formulary by practicing veterinary pharmacists.

The *Saunders Handbook of Veterinary Drugs: Small and Large Animal* is written by board-certified veterinary pharmacology expert Mark G. Papich, DVM, PhD, Diplomate,

American College of Veterinary Clinical Pharmacology. It currently is in its fourth edition. This book is available in both traditional print and e-book formats.

The Exotic Animal Formulary, currently in its fourth edition, is the only drug formulary that exclusively addresses drug treatment of exotic animals. It is written by clinical and research veterinarian James W. Carpenter, with contributions from more than 20 expert veterinary authors.

The Compendium of Veterinary Products (CVP) is a comprehensive collection of veterinary product information, including FDA-approved labeling for veterinary drugs. CVP is particularly helpful for pharmacists seeking to associate brand names with generic contents for veterinary drugs.

The Food Animal Residue Avoidance Databank (FARAD; www.farad.org) is of critical importance to veterinary pharmacists who provide drug products and care for food-producing animals. FARAD is a congressionally mandated drug residue avoidance risk management program supported by the USDA. Its primary mission is to provide scientifically based expert advice to help mitigate unsafe chemical residues (e.g. drugs, pesticides, and biotoxins) in products derived from food animals. FARAD is maintained by a consortium of universities, including the University of California Davis, University of Florida, Kansas State University, and North Carolina State University. The program employs veterinary pharmacologists and veterinary pharmacists to evaluate drug depletion profiles in edible animal products.

1.9.2 Veterinary Journals

As with human medicine, new and emerging information in veterinary medicine is published in primary literature (i.e. journals). Pharmacists likely are accustomed to seeing impact factors reported for healthcare journals. The impact factor reflects the average number of citations received per paper published in that journal during the two preceding years (e.g. a journal's 2015 impact factor is the average number of citations from that journal in 2013 and 2014). Impact factors were designed to indicate the quality of journals. For example, the *New England Journal of Medicine* had an impact factor of 59.558 in 2015, considered to be the highest among general medicine journals (*New England Journal of Medicine* 2017).

Impact factors for human journals cannot be applied comparably to veterinary journals. In 2015, the *Journal of Veterinary Internal Medicine* (JVIM) – one of the most widely read and respected veterinary journals – had an impact factor of 1.821. While this pales in comparison to the *New England Journal of Medicine*, one must consider that JVIM publishes a narrower scope of articles (no articles on public health, policy, surgery, radiology, etc.). Another reason for the relatively low impact factor of veterinary journals is the fact that human journals are focused on intensive research for specific diseases in a single species. Veterinary journals publish research for hundreds of diseases in dozens of species, so multiple citations of any one article are less likely. To the point, an impact factor of 1.5–2 is excellent for a veterinary journal.

1.10 Veterinary Pharmacy Educational Core

Although veterinary pharmacy is rapidly moving into the mainstream of pharmacy practice, and related test questions are now included in the national pharmacy licensure examination (NABPLEX), veterinary pharmacy education is lagging. At the time of writing, only a handful of veterinary pharmacy educational opportunities (didactic and experiential) are offered during the Doctor of Pharmacy program and only in a few schools of pharmacy. Pharmacists wishing to provide competent medical care for nonhuman patients have largely had to acquire this knowledge through postgraduate continuing education programs. Unfortunately, the quality of veterinary pharmacy continuing education programs is heavily dependent on the credentials of the author/presenter, and while many of those individuals are interested in veterinary pharmacy topics, they possess no specialty credentials and have no authentic veterinary pharmacy experience. Pharmacists wishing to learn the principles of veterinary pharmacy practice through continuing education programs are well advised to inquire about and confirm the qualifications of these authors/presenters. For authors who are pharmacists, diplomate status in ICVP is a good indicator, as well as employment in a veterinary teaching hospital or veterinary-focused institution. Veterinarians who provide continuing education to pharmacists should ideally be diplomates of the American College of Veterinary Clinical Pharmacology or diplomates in another specialty college (e.g. American College of Veterinary Internal Medicine or American College of Veterinary Ophthalmology). Content can also betray lack of expertise. For example, veterinary pharmacy continuing educational programs that include information on how pharmacists can counsel pet owners in using human OTC products are clearly lacking an understanding of the legal restrictions placed on use of OTC drugs in animals. Similarly, content that provides only "recipes" for compounding veterinary products but does not provide evidence for efficacy of the compounded products in veterinary species lacks an understanding of the importance of pharmacotherapeutics.

While some schools and colleges of pharmacy have been quick to offer veterinary pharmacy electives, this material is not offered in all pharmacy school curricula. For pharmacy schools to produce the most competent practitioners, structured learning programs containing core principles of veterinary pharmacy practice should be standardized with the goal of achieving uniform competency across pharmacy school graduates. The following outline for basic core competencies in veterinary pharmacy is offered here for those institutions wishing to offer complete veterinary pharmacy education in their programs:

1) Veterinary Drug Information Resources
2) Principles of Drug Disposition in Nonhuman Species
3) Principles of Toxicology in Nonhuman Species
4) Veterinary Drug Law and Ethical Considerations
5) Species Specific Anatomical and Physiological Considerations for Dogs, Cats, Horses, Food Animals, and Exotic Species
6) Species-Specific Disease State Management Principles
7) Top 50 Veterinary-Only Drugs Review
8) Compounding Considerations for Nonhuman Species.

The primary purpose of this book is to provide colleges of pharmacy with a text that can be used to create a core course in veterinary pharmacy.

1.11 Summary

Pharmacists are the only healthcare professionals who are legally allowed to and expected by society to provide competent pharmaceutical care and products to all species. However, most pharmacists have not received formal training in comparative pharmacology, veterinary pharmacotherapy, or veterinary drug laws and regulations. Pharmacists specially trained in veterinary pharmacotherapy can support community pharmacists as well as veterinarians and their patients in many important therapeutic aspects, including drug therapy selection, compounding, therapeutic monitoring, counseling of pet owners, drug information research, and adverse drug event reporting.

References

American Society for the Prevention of Cruelty to Animals. (2014). Ten most common pet toxins of 2014. http://www.aspca.org/news/ten-most-common-pet-toxins-2014.

American Veterinary Medical Association (2010). *US Pet Ownership and Demographics Sourcebook*. Schaumburg, IL: American Veterinary Medical Association.

American Veterinary Medical Association. (2017). Does every state require a valid VCPR to exist before a veterinarian can write a prescription? https://www.avma.org/Advocacy/StateAndLocal/Documents/VCPR_state_chart.pdf.

America's Pet Owners US. (2016). Mintel market reports. http://www.store.mintel.com/americas-pet-owners-us-august-2016.

Animal Health Institute (2017). *Industry statistics*. Washington, DC: Animal Health Institute http://www.ahi.org/about-animal-medicines/industry-statistics.

Arnish CE, Davidson GS, Royal K. (2015). Veterinary pharmacy education: prevalence and perceptions. Poster presented at the Society of Veterinary Hospital Pharmacists 34th Annual Meeting, June 14–17, Portland, ME.

Board of Pharmaceutical Specialties. (2017). History [of the Board of Pharmaceutical Specialties]. https://www.bpsweb.org/about-bps/history.

Dorsey M. (2001). Impact of a clinical pharmacist on pain management in a veterinary specialty referral practice. Paper presented at the American Society of Health-System Pharmacists (ASHP) 36th Midyear Clinical Meeting, New Orleans, LA, December, abstr. no. p-45d.

Drug Enforcement Agency (DEA). (N.d.). General requirements. In Practitioner's Manual, sect. II. https://www.deadiversion.usdoj.gov/pubs/manuals/pract/section2.htm.

Food and Drug Administration (FDA). (2006). Pharmacovigilance of veterinary medicinal products: management of adverse event reports (AERs) – VICH GL24. https://www.fda.gov/downloads/AnimalVeterinary/GuidanceComplianceEnforcement/GuidanceforIndustry/UCM052657.pdf.

Food and Drug Administration (FDA). (2015). Compounding animal drugs from bulk drug substances; draft guidance for industry; availability; withdrawal of Compliance Policy Guide; Section 608.400 Compounding of drugs for use in animals. Federal Register. https://www.federalregister.gov/articles/2015/05/19/2015-11982/compounding-animal-drugs-from-bulk-drug-substances-draft-guidance-for-industry-availability.

Food and Drug Administration (FDA). (2017). FDA budget. https://www.fda.gov/AboutFDA/ReportsManualsForms/Reports/BudgetReports/ucm559364.htm.

Jinks, M.J. and Paulsen, L.M. (1982). Pharmaceutical services in a veterinary hospital and clinic. *Am. J. Hosp. Pharm.* 39 (4): 619–621.

Kaiser Health News. (2009). Pharmaceutical industry ranks as "Most Profitable" in "Fortune 500." https://khn.org/morning-breakout/dr00004161.

Larkin M. (2010). Pioneering a profession. JAVMA News. https://www.avma.org/News/JAVMANews/Pages/110101a.aspx.

Mingura M. (2017). Community pharmacists and veterinary prescriptions: an analysis of prevalence, type, training, and knowledge retention. Poster presentation at the Society of Veterinary Hospital Pharmacists 36th Annual Meeting, Portland, OR, June 12–14.

Nelson, R.B. (1977). The role of the pharmacist in drug information for the agricultural sector. *Fed. Proc.* 36 (1): 127–129.

New England Journal of Medicine. (2017). Media Center fact sheet. http://www.nejm.org/page/media-center/fact-sheet.

Royal College of Veterinary Surgeons. (2017). History of the veterinary profession. https://knowledge.rcvs.org.uk/heritage-and-history/history-of-the-veterinary-profession.

Sorah E, Davidson G. Royal K. (2015). Dispensing errors for non-human patients in the community pharmacy setting: a survey of pharmacists and veterinarians. Poster presentation at the Society of Veterinary Hospital Pharmacists 34th Annual Meeting, Portland, ME, June 14–17.

Washington State University College of Veterinary Medicine Veterinary Clinical Pharmacology Lab. (N.d.). Problem drugs. https://vcpl.vetmed.wsu.edu/problem-drugs.

2

Regulation of Veterinary Pharmaceuticals

Eden Bermingham

Clinical Pharmacology Team, Division of Scientific Support, Office of New Animal Drug Evaluation, FDA Center for Veterinary Medicine, Rockville, MD, USA

Key Points

- Veterinary pharmaceuticals in the USA are regulated by the US Food and Drug Administration (FDA). There are many similarities in the drug approval process for human and veterinary drugs.
- Animal health companies are required to conduct safety and effectiveness studies under the same quality standards as used for human drugs.

- Veterinary drugs are manufactured according to the same standard as used for human drugs.
- Important differences between veterinary and human drugs include the number of animal species regulated, the number of animals used in field studies, and the need to demonstrate human food safety for drugs used in food animals.

Disclaimer: This chapter was written by Eden Bermingham in her private capacity. No official support or endorsement by the FDA is intended or should be inferred.

2.1 Introduction

Pharmaceuticals and biologics intended for use in human patients are regulated by the US Food and Drug Administration (FDA). In contrast, there are three government agencies that have regulatory oversight of veterinary medical products: pharmaceuticals are regulated by the Center for Veterinary Medicine (CVM) within the FDA, biologics (including vaccines) are regulated by the Center for Veterinary Biologics (CVB) within the US Department of Agriculture (USDA), and pesticides are regulated by the Environmental

Protection Agency (EPA). The Virus-Serum-Toxin Act (VSTA) was passed in 1913 to ensure the safe supply of animal vaccines and is enforced by the Animal and Plant Health Inspection Service (APHIS) of the USDA. The FDA CVM is located in Rockville, Maryland, and the USDA CVB is located in Ames, Iowa.

Some products to control external parasites come under the jurisdiction of the EPA. The FDA and EPA work together to ensure adherence to all applicable laws and regulations. In general, flea and tick products that are given orally or by injection are regulated by the FDA.

Immunomodulators may be regulated by CVM or CVB. The jurisdiction of this category of products is determined by a committee composed of members of both centers, and the decision is based primarily on the

Pharmacotherapeutics for Veterinary Dispensing, First Edition. Edited by Katrina L. Mealey.
© 2019 John Wiley & Sons, Inc. Published 2019 by John Wiley & Sons, Inc.

product's mechanism of action (MOA) and proposed indication. In general, products will be regulated as biologics if they are intended for use in the diagnosis, cure, mitigation, treatment, or prevention of animal disease and the mechanism of action is primarily through an immune process. Products will generally be regulated as drugs if they are intended for use in the diagnosis, cure, mitigation, treatment, or prevention of animal disease and the primary mechanism of action is not immunological or is unknown, or if they are intended to affect the structure or function of the body of animals.

The jurisdiction for an ectoparasiticide generally depends on whether or not the product has internal or external effects. Although a few topical flea and tick products have been approved by the EPA, any topical product intended to act systemically or with an indication for treating endoparasites would be regulated by CVM.

2.1.1 FDA Center for Veterinary Medicine Organizational Structure

The FDA is composed of the Office of the Commissioner and four directorates. Oversight for human medical products is the function of the Office of Medical Products and Tobacco, while oversight of veterinary medicinal products is a function of the Office of Foods and Veterinary Medicine. The Office of Foods was created in 2009 by the FDA to unify the FDA foods program, and then was reorganized as the Office of Foods and Veterinary Medicine. The two centers under this office are the Center for Food Safety and Applied Nutrition (CFSAN) and CVM. General information about CVM can be found at www.fda.gov under "About the Center for Veterinary Medicine." CVM is the veterinary equivalent of the Center for Drug Evaluation and Research (CDER), which is the FDA center primarily responsible for the approval of human drugs.

Within CVM, there are several offices that are responsible for veterinary drug approval and research: the Office of New Animal Drug

Evaluation (ONADE), Office of Surveillance and Compliance (OS&C), Office of Research (OR), and Office of Minor Use and Minor Species Animal Drug Development (OMUMS). ONADE is responsible for the pre-approval of veterinary drugs and will be the focus of this chapter.

OS&C monitors approved drugs, food additives, and veterinary devices, and assists the FDA Field Offices, who conduct inspections of medicated feed manufacturers and perform audits of animal studies. Within OS&C, the Division of Animal Feeds monitors and establishes standards for feed contaminants, approves safe food additives, reviews Generally Recognized as Safe (GRAS) ingredients, and manages the FDA's medicated feed and pet food programs.

OMUMS was established in response to the Minor Use and Minor Species Animal Health Act of 2004 to facilitate the approval of drugs for species other than the seven major species (dogs, cats, horses, cattle, pigs, chickens, and turkeys) and for minor use, which are drugs used in a major species for a disease that occurs infrequently or in only a small number of animals each year.

OR has research programs that perform analysis of compounds in animal tissue or feed that could pose a potential health risk, conduct applied and basic research in animal health, and identify and characterize pathogens, including programs to monitor the development of bacterial resistance to antimicrobials.

Within ONADE, there are divisions dedicated to companion animals (e.g. dogs, cats, and horses), food animals (e.g. cattle, swine, chickens, and turkeys), production drugs (drugs that increase feed or reproductive efficiency), chemistry and manufacturing, human food safety (drug residues in food animals), and generic veterinary drugs. The role of these divisions in the drug approval process will be described in more detail in this chapter.

In 2003, the Federal Food, Drug, and Cosmetic Act (FFDCA) was amended to include the Animal Drug User Fee Act of 2003 (ADUFA I), which authorized FDA to collect fees from animal health companies for specific animal drug applications, establishments, products, and sponsors. The fees serve as a revenue source to enhance the performance and predictability in review times for the animal drug industry and provide FDA with resources to improve its review of applications for new animal drugs, with the result that safe and effective new products will be more readily available. This strategy of supplementing FDA's resources through drug user fees was based on the Prescription Drug User Fee Act (PDUFA) and Generic Drug User Fee Amendment (GDUFA), which were passed in 1992 and 2012, respectively, for human drug approvals. The fees paid by drug companies are intended to supplement, not replace, direct appropriations, and allow CVM to hire additional reviewers and decrease application review times. In return, CVM is required to adhere to certain performance goals, and has to review and act on 90% of the New Animal Drug Applications (NADA) within 60, 120, or 180 days after submission date, depending on the type of submission. ADUFA is renegotiated every five years: ADUFA II was passed in 2008, ADUFA III in 2013, and negotiations for ADUFA IV are ongoing.

A similar drug user fee amendment, the Animal Generic Drug User Fee Act (AGDUFA), was first passed in 2008 for generic animal drugs. This amendment is also renegotiated every five years, but performance goals are slightly different, in that CVM is required to review and act on 90% of Abbreviated New Animal Drug Applications (ANADA) within 270 days after submission date. The proposed AGDUFA III deadline is 180 days after the submission date.

2.2 Veterinary Drug Approval Process

2.2.1 Regulatory Framework

The regulatory framework that governs the veterinary drug approval process consists of four tiers. As with human drugs, the overarching law is the Federal Food, Drug, and Cosmetic Act (FFDCA), which is a set of laws passed by Congress in 1938 giving authority to the FDA to regulate the safety of food, drugs, and cosmetics. The act has been amended many times, and some of the most important amendments for veterinary drugs were the Generic Animal Drug and Patent Term Restoration Act (GADPTRA) of 1988, the Animal Medicinal Drug Use Clarification Act (AMDUCA) of 1994, the Animal Drug Availability Act (ADAA) of 1996, the Animal Drug User Feed Act (ADUFA) of 2003, and the Minor Use and Minor Species Animal Health Act (MUMS) of 2004.

The second tier is the Code of Federal Regulations (CFR), which is the codification or application of the FFDCA published in the *Federal Register*. The CFR "translates" the FFDCA by providing specific regulations for animal drugs in Title 21, chapter 1, subchapter "E-Animal Drugs, Feeds, and Related Products". The information contained in this subchapter is considered to be law and therefore comprises the requirements in the approval process.

The third tier is the Guidance for Industry (GFI). These are documents that represent CVM's current thinking on a topic, and are not legally binding. In some cases, CVM will consider an alternative approach to the one described in a GFI, as long as the approach satisfies the requirements of the applicable regulations. The list of GFIs is too extensive for the scope of this chapter, but it can be found at: https://www.fda.gov/AnimalVeterinary/GuidanceComplianceEnforcement/GuidanceforIndustry/default.htm.

Many of the GFIs have been revised under the principles of the International Cooperation on Harmonization of Technical Requirements for Registration of Veterinary Medicinal Products (VICH) to provide a unified standard for the European Union (EU), Japan, and the USA to facilitate the mutual acceptance of clinical data by the relevant regulatory authorities. VICH is based on similar principles as the International Council for Harmonization of Technical Requirements for Pharmaceuticals for Human Use. The global harmonization of the veterinary drug approval has become even more important over the past decade, as more animal health companies have consolidated.

The fourth tier is the Policy and Procedures, which provide information more specific to internal processes and assist in maintaining consistency within the center while providing transparency to CVM's stakeholders. These are also publicly available at https://www.fda.gov/AnimalVeterinary/GuidanceCompliance Enforcement/PoliciesProceduresManual/default.htm.

CVM adheres to the same international scientific quality standards as for human drugs: Good Clinical Practice (GCP) as described in GFI #85 GL 9, "Good Clinical Practice," and Good Laboratory Practice (GLP) as codified in 21 CFR Part 58. Compliance with GCP provides public assurance about the integrity of the clinical study data, and helps to protect both the animals and personnel involved in the study. Although GCP procedures for designing, conducting, monitoring, recording, auditing, analyzing, and reporting clinical studies are essentially the same as for human trials, there are some obvious differences, such as requesting informed consent from the owner to enroll their animals in the study and disposal of study animals. One of the most important differences between GCP and GLP standards is that GLP is enforceable as a regulation, but GCP is not enforceable. GLP is the standard for laboratory studies in purpose-bought animals in contrast to GCP, which is the standard for the conduct of clinical studies in client-owned animals.

2.2.2 Original Application or Pioneer Drugs

A brief overview of the veterinary drug approval process can be found at https://www.fda.gov/animalveterinary/resourcesforyou/ucm268128.htm. New animal drugs are referred to as Investigational New Animal Drugs (INADs), while new human drugs are referred to as Investigational New Drugs (INDs). Once a veterinary drug is approved, it is assigned a New Animal Drug Approval (NADA) number.

For original or pioneer drug approvals, there are seven technical sections that need to be completed before a drug can be approved:

1) Effectiveness
2) Target animal safety
3) Human food safety for food animals, such as cattle, swine, chicken, and turkeys
4) Chemistry, manufacturing, and controls
5) Environmental impact
6) Labeling
7) All other information.

The animal health company or "sponsor" can choose to submit all of the technical sections at once, or independently of each other as "phased" submissions. This flexibility decreases the sponsors' risk by allowing them to submit technical sections as they are completed, or to submit a more problematic technical section earlier to allow for a multiple-cycle review if needed. Unlike human studies, CVM does not refer to the studies as Phase I, II, III, or IV. Instead, the studies are described with respect to the objective, such as dose determination or dose confirmation studies, target animal safety studies, or field studies. The term "field study" is synonymous with clinical trial.

2.2.2.1 Effectiveness Technical Section

This section consists of the studies conducted to demonstrate the effectiveness of the drug for a specific indication in a particular species and, if applicable, class of animal (e.g. lactating or beef cow). Depending on the indication, effectiveness studies can be conducted in laboratory or purpose-bought animals (e.g. cattle), or in client-owned animals (e.g. dogs and cats) that are enrolled in clinical trials.

As in the human drug approval process, the first step in the drug development program is usually to identify a dose. The effectiveness technical section also includes the studies or supporting evidence used for dosage characterization. There are three areas in which veterinary dosage characterization differs substantially from human drug approval: the sponsor's responsibility in choosing a dose, the requirement for pharmacokinetic (PK) data, and dosage based on the weight of the animal (mg/kg). Unlike in CDER, an animal health company (sponsor) is not required to have ONADE's approval of a dose prior to study conduct. As stated in the Animal Drug Availability Act of 1996, there are no requirements for how a sponsor chooses the dose, and a dose can be based on clinical data and/or scientific literature. However, for the majority of animal drugs, sponsors conduct exploratory effectiveness and/or PK studies to determine a dose. Dosage characterization studies, such as PK studies, are usually conducted in a small number of healthy animals, ranging from 5 to 24 animals.

Because of the large diversity between and within (e.g. dog breeds) species, most veterinary drugs are dosed by body weight, unlike many human drugs, which are dosed based on a 70 kg person. After the dose has been chosen, many sponsors then conduct a small exploratory clinical study in affected animals. These exploratory effectiveness studies can be performed in laboratory or purpose-bought animals using a disease model or in client-owned animals that are already affected.

Under 21 CFR Part 514.117, one or more adequate and well-controlled studies are required to establish, by substantial evidence, that a new animal drug is effective. Characteristics of an adequate and well-controlled study include, among others, a study protocol, an appropriate standard of conduct (e.g. GCP), a study design that permits a valid comparison of drug effects, and the use of a new animal drug that is produced in accordance with appropriate manufacturing practices. CVM does not require concurrence for a study protocol, but most sponsors choose to submit the protocol for review prior to the start of the study, because it decreases their risk that the study design would be found unacceptable

by CVM. The clinical studies that demonstrate effectiveness in compliance with GCP are described as "pivotal," whereas exploratory studies are considered "nonpivotal."

The pivotal field studies are designed to demonstrate the effectiveness of a drug for a specific indication under conditions of use. The conditions of use not only include the species and/or type of animal and disease, but also could include a specific management practice. For example, many cattle drugs have indications for pastured versus feedlot cattle because of the substantial differences in husbandry. Safety data, such as adverse reactions, are also collected in field studies.

In general, veterinary clinical trials are much smaller than human trials. Companion animal field studies typically range from 100 to 200 animals in number. Food animal field studies are larger; cattle and swine studies are usually conducted in several hundred animals. While quantitative aspects of animal field studies differ from those of human clinical trials, the qualitative aspects are similar. As in human trials, animals are enrolled according to inclusion and exclusion criteria, are randomized to treatment groups (which may include placebo groups), receive the designated treatment provided by the sponsor, and are evaluated for treatment response based on prespecified clinical endpoints.

2.2.2.2 Target Animal Safety Technical Section

There are two major categories of safety data in the target animal safety (TAS) technical section: a TAS study or studies conducted in healthy laboratory or purpose-bought animals, and the field safety data collected from the affected target population during an effectiveness study. The major difference between the TAS and field safety data is that the field study data reflect safety in a larger population of diseased animals treated at the proposed dose and dosing interval and in use with concomitant medications.

The design of the pivotal TAS study, as described in GFI #185/VICH GL43, "Target Animal Safety for Veterinary Pharmaceutical

Products," provides data to allow CVM to establish a margin of safety around the proposed dose. The TAS studies are generally conducted in young, healthy animals that are age-matched to the youngest age for the proposed indication. The number of animals in each of the four treatment groups is relatively small, usually with eight animals (four males and four females, unless the drug is indicated for a single sex) in each treatment group. Typically, TAS studies are conducted using four treatment groups: a negative control (0×), the proposed dose (1×), and two multiples of this dose (e.g. 3× and 5×). Although 3× and 5× are commonly used for the exaggerated doses, CVM will consider alternative doses, such as 2× and 3×, for drugs with more narrow therapeutic margins, such as non-steroidal anti-inflammatory drugs (NSAIDs). The duration of the study is 3× the proposed duration, up to a maximum of 90 days. However, if the drug is expected to be administered for a period longer than three months, then the safety study duration may be up to six months or longer.

Safety studies are conducted according to GLP, as described in 21 CFR Part 58, to assure data integrity. In most safety studies, animals are randomized to treatment groups prior to drug administration, they undergo physical examinations by the study veterinarian, and samples for hematology, blood chemistry, and urinalysis are collected. Physical examinations and clinical pathology sample collections are repeated at appropriate intervals throughout the study. In most (but not all) safety studies, the animals are humanely euthanized at the end of the study, and necropsies are performed. Tissues are examined for gross pathology, and samples are collected for histopathology (the organs to be sampled are listed in GFI #185/VICH GL43, "Target Animal Safety for Veterinary Pharmaceutical Products"). CVM's recommendations for the statistical analysis of the safety data are described in GFI#226, "Target Animal Safety Data Presentation and Statistical Analysis."

More specific safety studies, such as an injection site reaction or reproductive safety studies, may also be performed depending on the drug indication. An injection site safety study is most commonly used to support the local safety of injectable drugs in food animals, such as cattle. Most animal drugs are not evaluated in pregnant, breeding, or lactating animals, and therefore have a warning on the label not to use the drug under these conditions. However, drugs used for reproduction, such as hormones used to facilitate cattle breeding, may need additional safety data to determine that there aren't any adverse reactions in the animal itself or its offspring. Generally, the reproductive safety studies are conducted using a negative control (0×) and 3× the proposed dose throughout the reproductive phase (follicular phase until conception) and gestation. The number and viability of the offspring (e.g. the number of pigs in a litter) are also documented.

The TAS technical section also includes human user safety, which is the safety for anyone who is administering the drug. The type of information or data needed for this section depends on several factors, including the formulation, drug toxicity (e.g. chemotherapeutics), route of administration (e.g. oral or transdermal), and indication (e.g. single or multiple animal administrations, as in a feedlot situation where many animals are processed in a short span of time). Chemotherapeutics are considered to be among the most toxic drugs, and the user safety information for these drugs includes recommendations for the owners to avoid contact with the animal's saliva, vomit, urine, or feces for a period of time after dosing. For transdermal formulations, sponsors generally conduct residual drug studies, where the amount of drug that can be wiped off the animal's skin is measured over time to determine a post-administration avoidance period.

2.2.2.3 Human Food Safety Technical Section

There are several safety aspects to evaluate in this technical section: systemic toxicology, effects on human intestinal flora, tissue residues, and antimicrobial resistance for antimicrobial new animal drugs. The newly revised GFI #3, "General Principles for Evaluating the Human Food Safety of New Animal Drugs Used in Food-Producing Animals," provides an overview of the studies used to support human food safety. This GFI also describes the following:

- Determination of the human acceptable daily intake (ADI) of a drug
- Calculation of the safe concentration in the tissue that will not exceed the ADI
- Assignment of the maximum acceptable amount of tissue drug residues (tolerance)
- Calculation of the withdrawal period and milk discard time
- Evaluation of carcinogenic compounds used in food animals.

For the toxicology component of this technical section, CVM is generally concerned with both intermittent and chronic exposure of humans to relatively low concentrations of drug residues in edible tissues. The toxicity studies described in GFI #3 are a standard set of studies designed to evaluate the oral toxicity of new animal drug residues to humans

who may be exposed to these residues through the consumption of food derived from animals treated with the new animal drug. Traditional toxicology studies are designed to determine if the new animal drug produces an adverse effect in an *in vitro* or *in vivo* biological test system and to identify the highest dose of the new animal drug that produces a no-observed-effect level (NOEL), which CVM considers to be the same as the no-observed-adverse-effect level (NOAEL).

Table 2.1 summarizes the GFIs that describe in greater detail the types of studies that may be needed to address the toxicity of a drug, depending on its physicochemical properties.

The toxicological ADI is derived by dividing the NOEL or NOAEL by an appropriate safety factor. The safety factor used in this calculation is dependent on the type of toxicity studies conducted and reflects uncertainties associated with the extrapolation of data from toxicology studies (usually conducted in rodents or dogs) to humans. Generally, the safety factor consists of multiples of 10, with each factor representing a specific uncertainty inherent in the available data.

Table 2.1 GFIs detailing the types of studies that may be needed to address toxicity of a drug.

Title	GFI #	VICH GL #
Studies to Evaluate the Safety of Residues of Veterinary Drugs in Human Food: Repeat-Dose (90-Day) Toxicity Testing in Human Food: Repeat-Dose (90-Day) Toxicity Testing	147	31
Studies to Evaluate the Safety of Residues of Veterinary Drugs in Human Food: Repeat-Dose (Chronic) Toxicity Testing in Human Food: Repeat-Dose (Chronic) Toxicity Testing	160	37
Studies to Evaluate the Safety of Residues of Veterinary Drugs in Human Food: Developmental Toxicity Testing	148	32
Safety Studies for Veterinary Drug Residues in Human Food: Reproduction Toxicity Testing	115	22
Studies to Evaluate the Safety of Residues of Veterinary Drugs in Human Food: Genotoxicity Testing (Revised)	116	23R
Studies to Evaluate the Safety of Residues of Veterinary Drugs in Human Food: Carcinogenicity Testing	141	28
Studies to Evaluate the Safety of Residues of Veterinary Drugs in Human Food: General Approach to Establish a Microbiological ADI (Revised)	159	36 R

For example, CVM has historically applied a safety factor of 100 for an ADI based on the NOEL/NOAEL from a chronic toxicity study (10-fold for extrapolating animal data to humans and 10-fold for variability in sensitivity to the toxicity of the new animal drug among humans).

The toxicological ADI is then partitioned among the edible tissues and the food consumption values for each tissue. Partitioning refers to allocating portions of the ADI across edible tissues when consumption of those tissues may contribute to the total human exposure of a new animal drug and/or its residues. Edible tissues include muscle, liver, kidney, fat or skin with fat in natural proportions (as appropriate), whole eggs, whole milk, and honey. For some products (e.g. products not used in lactating dairy cows or laying hens), the ADI can be allocated to edible muscle, liver, kidney, or fat without partitioning. When estimating the daily consumption for edible tissues, CVM assumes that, when an individual consumes a full portion of any edible tissue (e.g. muscle, liver, kidney, or fat) from one species, that individual would not consume a full portion of any other edible tissue from another species on the same day. Based on this assumption, Table 2.2 summarizes the food consumption values for each edible tissue.

Table 2.2 Food consumption values for edible tissues.

Edible tissue	Quantity consumed per day
Muscle	300 g
Liver	100 g
Kidney	50 g
Fat or skin/fat	50 g
Milk	1500 ml
Eggs	100 g
Honey	20 g

Note: "Skin/fat" refers to skin that includes fat in natural proportions. Skin with fat in natural proportions is the edible tissue for swine and poultry.

The safe concentration is the amount of total residue of a new animal drug that can be consumed from each edible tissue every day for up to the lifetime of a human without exposing the human to residues in excess of the ADI. The safe concentration of total residues of the new animal drug in each edible tissue is calculated as the ADI × human body weight (60 kg) divided by the food consumption value.

For antimicrobials, a microbiological ADI (mADI) may be necessary according to the approach described in GFI #159/VICH 36(R), "Studies to Evaluate the Safety of Residues of Veterinary Drugs in Human Food: General Approach to Establish a Microbiological ADI." This guidance describes a harmonized stepwise approach to be used to determine if residues of an antimicrobial new animal drug reach the human colon and remain active, and affect intestinal bacteria by disrupting the colonization barrier or the development/selection of antimicrobial-resistant populations. If there is a possibility that the intestinal bacteria are affected, a determination of a mADI may be necessary. Antimicrobial new animal drugs may be assigned both a microbiological ADI and toxicological ADI. The final ADI is the more appropriate of these two ADIs, which is usually the lower of the toxicological and microbiological ADIs. For some new animal drugs, CVM may not establish an ADI if it does not present a hazard to human health.

In addition to determining the ADI and the safe concentration, the sponsor has to conduct residue chemistry studies to assess the quantity and nature of residues in tissues derived from animals treated with the new animal drug. Table 2.3 summarizes the GFIs for the residue chemistry studies.

The purpose of the comparative metabolism study is to determine whether the drug metabolites in the target animal (which may be consumed in edible tissues by humans) are also produced by metabolism in the laboratory animals (e.g. rodents and dogs) used for the toxicological testing. The metabolism of a drug in both target and laboratory

Table 2.3 GFIs for residue chemistry studies.

Title	GFI #	VICH GL #
Studies to Evaluate the Metabolism and Residue Kinetics of Veterinary Drugs in Food-Producing Animals: Metabolism Study to Determine the Quantity and Identify the Nature of Residues	205	46
Studies to Evaluate the Metabolism and Residue Kinetics of Veterinary Drugs in Food-Producing Animals: Comparative Metabolism Studies in Laboratory Animals to Determine the Quantity and Identify the Nature of Residues	206	47
Studies to Evaluate the Metabolism and Residue Kinetics of Veterinary Drugs in Food-Producing Animals: Marker Residue Depletion Studies to Establish Product Withdrawal Periods (Revised)	207	48R
Studies to Evaluate the Metabolism and Residue Kinetics of Veterinary Drugs in Food-Producing Animals: Validation of Analytical Methods Used in Residue Depletion Studies (Revised)	208	49R
Studies to Evaluate the Metabolism and Residue Kinetics of Veterinary Drugs in Food-Producing Species: Study Design Recommendations for Residue Studies in Honey for Establishing MRLs and Withdrawal Periods (Draft)	243	56

animals may be determined by a radiolabeled drug study in which the amount of radioactivity in each tissue type is measured. The marker residue refers to the residue whose concentration is in a known relationship to the concentration of total residue in an edible tissue of the target animal. The target tissue refers to the edible tissue selected to monitor for residues in the target animal. The total residue and metabolism data are analyzed to determine the marker residue, the target tissue, and the marker residue–to–total residue ratio (M/T ratio). The target tissue is usually, but not necessarily, the last tissue in which residues deplete to the permitted concentration. The target tissue and marker residue are selected so that the absence of marker residue above the tolerance would confirm that each edible tissue has a concentration of total residue at or below its safe concentration. Typically, for terrestrial animals, the target tissue is liver or kidney, but could also be fat.

Once a final ADI, safe concentration, target tissue, and marker residue are selected, a tolerance for the new animal drug can be determined. Tolerance is the maximum concentration of a marker residue, or other residue indicated for monitoring, that can legally remain in a specific edible tissue of a treated animal. The tolerance is determined by examining depletion data consisting of total residue concentrations (typically from radiolabel studies, as described in GFI #205/ VICH GL 46) and marker residue concentrations measured by the proposed analytical method (e.g. liquid chromatography/mass spectrometry).

The withdrawal period or the milk discard time is the interval between the time of the last administration of a new animal drug and the time when the animal can be safely slaughtered for food or the milk can be safely consumed. To determine the withdrawal period for meat or the milk discard time needed for the target residue to deplete to below the tolerance, the sponsor must conduct tissue residue depletion studies in the target animal. The data provided by these studies are used to calculate a meat withdrawal period or milk discard time. The recommended study design for a tissue residue depletion study is described in GFI #207/ VICH GL 48(R). Ideally, tissues from treated animals should be collected to provide residue data above the tolerance at a minimum of two sampling timepoints and below the tolerance (but above the limit of quantification of the analytical method) at a minimum of one sampling timepoint. When determining the withdrawal period, CVM uses a conservative approach by calculating the 99th percentile tolerance limit with a 95% confidence. This means that 99% or more of tissue or milk residue samples at and beyond the withdrawal period (or discard time) are expected to fall below the tolerance.

Sponsors must also provide a practicable method for analyzing tissue residues, as described in 21 CFR 514.1(b)(7). Typically, the analytical method is developed to measure the concentration of the marker residue in the target tissue. After validating the method, the sponsor must then prove that this method can be used with acceptable accuracy and precision by multiple laboratories in an interlaboratory method transfer trial. The method is tested in one FDA laboratory, the sponsor's reference laboratory that developed and validated the procedure, and two independent testing laboratories selected by the sponsor. One USDA laboratory may optionally participate in the method transfer trial.

CVM recommends that sponsors address the risk of the development of antimicrobial-resistant zoonotic pathogens of human health concern by utilizing the risk assessment model described in GFI #152. Evaluating the safety of antimicrobial new animal drugs with regard to their microbiological effects on bacteria of human health concern. The sponsor evaluates the potential effects of antimicrobial new animal drugs on nontarget bacteria in the human intestinal microflora, as described in GFI #159. As stated in GFI #152, CVM's opinion is that human exposure through ingestion of antimicrobial-resistant bacteria from animal-derived foods represents the most significant pathway for human exposure to antimicrobial-resistant bacteria that have emerged or been selected as a consequence of antimicrobial use in food animals. The objective of the microbial food safety assessment is to mitigate the risk of the development of antimicrobial resistance in pathogens of human health concern, which in turn mitigates the risk of human clinical therapy failures for human illnesses. There

are two potential approaches to address the risk associated with antimicrobial new animal drugs: (i) a hazard characterization; and (ii) a complete, qualitative antimicrobial resistance risk assessment.

The hazard has been defined in GFI #152 as human illness, caused by antimicrobial-resistant bacteria attributable to an animal-derived food commodity, and treated with the human antimicrobial drug of interest. The sponsor provides a hazard characterization by submitting information regarding the chemical, biochemical, microbiological, pharmacokinetic/pharmacodynamic, and physical properties of the drug that characterize the downstream effects of the drug. The sponsor also provides bacterial resistance information to support the hazard characterization, such as bacterial species and strains for which resistance has potential human health consequences, and known resistance determinants or mechanisms for that drug.

The qualitative antimicrobial resistance risk assessment evaluates the following components:

- *Release assessment:* Ranks factors related to an antimicrobial drug and its use in animals that contribute to the emergence of resistant bacteria or resistant determinants in the animal as High, Medium, or Low
- *Exposure assessment:* Probability for humans to ingest bacteria in question from the edible tissues, and ranked as High, Medium, or Low.
- *Consequence assessment:* Probability that human exposure to resistant bacteria results in an adverse health consequence, and ranked as Important, Highly Important, or Critically Important.

The risk estimation integrates the results from the release, exposure, and consequence assessments into an overall risk estimation from the proposed use of the drug. CVM recommends that the risk estimation rank drugs as high, medium, or low risk to represent the potential for human health to be adversely impacted by the selection or emergence of antimicrobial foodborne bacteria from the use of the drug in food animals. The risk estimation is used to determine any recommendations for restriction of use conditions. For example, antimicrobials that are considered to be high risk could have restricted use conditions in food animals, such as a prohibition against extra-label use or being limited to use by, or under the supervision of, a veterinarian. Additional risk management steps, such as post-approval resistance monitoring, may be implemented to mitigate the human exposure to high-risk antimicrobials.

2.2.2.4 Chemistry, Manufacturing, and Controls Technical Section

The chemistry, manufacturing, and controls (CMC) technical section is the technical section in which the sponsor has to prove that the drug can be manufactured under controls to ensure consistent quality, such as potency and stability. This technical section has the least difference between human and veterinary drugs, since many of the regulations and GFIs are similar to both INADs and INDs. As with human drugs, veterinary drugs are manufactured according to Good Manufacturing Practice (GMP), which is described in 21 CFR Parts 210 and 211. Applying GMP helps to ensure the drug's identity, strength, purity, quality, and performance. In addition, there are several GFIs that focus on specific manufacturing aspects, such as stability testing and specifications for modified-release parenteral dosage forms. CVM also uses the same United States Pharmacopeia (USP) standards as for human drugs if the drug has a USP monograph.

CVM recommends that the final formulation be used in the pivotal safety and effectiveness studies, and if not, then *in vitro* and/or *in vivo* data are needed to bridge nonfinal and final formulations. Depending on the formulation, the sponsor must provide data to support the following:

- Characterization of the active pharmaceutical ingredient (API) and excipients
- Release specifications to ensure interbatch consistency
- Characterization of impurities, such as degradation products and residual solvents from the manufacturing process

- Stability testing in the final packaging
- Validated methods to measure API, excipients, and impurities
- *In vitro* dissolution methods for solid dosage forms
- Sterility procedures for injectable formulations.

2.2.2.5 Environmental Impact Technical Section

The environmental impact technical section differs from the other technical sections in that it is evaluated in accordance with the requirements of the National Environmental Policy Act (NEPA). The procedures under 21 CFR Part 25 require that all applications (including NADA or ANADA) filed with CVM must evaluate the potential for environmental impacts due to the use of the proposed animal drug. In general, this is done by submitting either an environmental assessment (EA) or a claim of categorical exclusion from the requirement to prepare an EA.

A categorical exclusion from the need to prepare an EA is possible for certain animal drugs, provided that an appropriate exclusion is claimed under 21 CFR 25.33, and no extraordinary circumstances exist indicating that the animal drug may significantly affect the quality of the environment (21 CFR 25.21). Most companion animal drugs are eligible for a categorical exclusion because they are used in limited circumstances under the control of a veterinarian's order and these animals have dispersed excretion patterns over large regions where the waste is typically disposed of via landfill.

If an animal drug is not eligible for a categorical exclusion, then an adequate EA is required so that CVM can evaluate the potential for the animal drug to cause environmental impacts. The sponsor should include the following:

- Estimate the fate of the animal drug by evaluating its metabolism and excretion by the target animal, mobility (in air, soil, and water), degradation, transformation, or subsequent accumulation (or persistence).

- Determine the ecotoxicological effects resulting from exposure to the animal drug.
- Predict any potential effects upon natural resources or endangered species.
- Identify methods to mitigate or reduce any potential effects.

If the information in the EA is sufficient and demonstrates that no significant environmental impacts are expected, then CVM prepares a finding of no significant impact (FONSI). If the information in the EA demonstrates that significant environmental impacts are expected, then CVM prepares an environmental impact statement (EIS) and record of decision (ROD). Examples of drugs that may require an EA are drugs for food animals, because of the high risk of environmental exposure due to excretion of the drug from a large number of animals in a small area.

2.2.2.6 Labeling Technical Section

The labeling and "all other information" (AOI) technical sections are referred to as the minor technical sections. The labeling section includes the package insert and labels for the bottles and cartons of each strength. With the completion of each major technical section, such as safety and effectiveness, draft label language for that section is added and discussed with the sponsor. Both CVM and the sponsor have to agree on the label language, whereas CVM is the only author of the Freedom of Information summary. Several sections of Title 21 of the CFR address specific parts of both veterinary and human labels, such as the expiration date and warnings to keep from children. For human labels, there are multiple GFIs addressing the content and format of sections of the label to provide consistency and facilitate the use of the label by the physician or pharmacist. In contrast, there is no GFI for veterinary labels, so the type of information may be more variable and may have fewer details than human drug labels. However, most veterinary drug labels contain the following sections, which can be valuable sources of information for pharmacists:

- *Description:* Strength of tablets; concentration of injectable drugs
- *Indication:* Disease, species, and class of animal
- *Dosage and administration:* Drug concentration, dosage, dosing tables, route(s) of administration, dosing interval, and information on whether the animal should be fed or fasted when administering the drug
- *Precautions:* Information that does not warrant a warning or contraindication statement, but still needs to be communicated for the safe and effective use of the drug. For example, recommended screening or diagnostic tests, information about drug interactions, carcinogenesis, adverse reactions in other species, reproductive safety, or use in specified subgroups (e.g. pediatric, geriatric, or specific disease states) may be included as a precaution. A precaution statement stating that the drug has not been tested in specified subgroups such as pregnant or lactating animals may be included on the label.
- *Caution statement:* Prescription drugs contain the following statement: "Federal law restricts this drug to use by or on the order of a licensed veterinarian" For some food animal drugs, there is also a caution statement against extra-label use.
- *Warning:* A warning may address user safety, human food safety (residue warnings for meat and milk withdrawal times), environmental safety, or serious adverse reactions and potential safety hazards to the animal receiving the drug. This section may also describe steps that should be taken following human exposure.
- *Contraindications:* A contraindication is a statement making it clear that a drug should not be used in certain circumstances because of the substantial risk of its use in the animal.
- *Clinical pharmacology:* Mechanism of action, PK, metabolism, and fed/fasted bioavailability. This section may not appear on all labels because it is not required.

- *Effectiveness:* A brief description of the study and summary of the results, such as the number of animals, the dosing regimen, the primary clinical endpoints, and treatment success and failure rates
- *Safety:* A brief description of the study and a summary of the results, with focus on any adverse reactions or abnormal pathology
- *NADA number and statement "Approved by FDA"*
- *Storage conditions.*

2.2.2.7 All Other Information
Technical Section
The all other information technical section contains the final study report of any study (no data) that wasn't previously submitted under a specific technical section, and the results of a literature search for any studies using the new animal drug in the target animal. In addition, any new pharmacovigilance reports, both domestic and global, are submitted in this technical section.

Freedom of Information Summary (FOI): This is not a technical section, but is an important public document. The FOI is a summary of the safety and effectiveness information that the FDA relied upon to support approval. Exploratory or supportive studies considered to be nonpivotal are not summarized in the FOI. FOIs are available to the public under the drug's NADA or ANADA number at https://www.fda.gov/AnimalVeterinary/ Products/ApprovedAnimalDrugProducts/ FOIADrugSummaries/default.htm.

2.2.3 Generic Animal Drugs

The approval process of generic veterinary drugs is very similar to that of generic human drugs; instead of conducting safety and effectiveness studies, the generic company conducts a bioequivalence study, which compares the PK of the pioneer or reference listed new animal drug (RLNAD) to the generic drug. If the two PK parameters, C_{max} (maximum plasma drug concentration) and AUC (area under the plasma concentration vs. time curve), meet the statistical criteria described in GFI #224/VICH GL 52 ("Bioequivalence: Blood Level Bioequivalence"), then the two drugs are considered to be bioequivalent. The PK parameters and statistical analysis used to determine bioequivalence are the same for both veterinary and human drugs. If the two drugs are bioequivalent, then the generic sponsor can reference the target animal safety and effectiveness data of the pioneer. For generic food animal drugs, CVM has concluded that the tissue residue depletion of a generic food animal drug is not adequately addressed through bioequivalence studies, so both a bioequivalence and tissue residue depletion study are required.

The bioanalytical method to measure the plasma concentrations must be validated for that species according to the GFI for Bioanalytical Method Validation, and the same GFI is used for both veterinary and human drugs. The label for the generic drug will be exactly the same as that of the RLNAD, with some permissible differences such as expiration date or sponsor information, and, if approved, a generic animal drug will be given an ANADA number.

Similar to human bioequivalence studies, most veterinary bioequivalence studies are conducted in a small number (e.g. 16–24) of healthy animals using a single-dose, randomized, two-treatment, two-sequence, two-period crossover study design. Blood drug level bioequivalence is considered to be the most sensitive approach to detect a difference between the generic and RLNAD formulations. However, there are veterinary drugs with negligible systemic absorption, such as some locally acting antiparasitics, for which a blood level study would not be appropriate. In these cases, CVM will consider a pharmacological or clinical endpoint bioequivalence study, with the stipulation that these alternative endpoints have to be sensitive enough to detect a difference between the generic and RLNAD formulations.

For some drugs, a waiver from the requirement to perform a bioequivalence study may be requested. As described in GFI #35 "Bioequivalence Guidance," the requirement for an *in vivo* bioequivalence study may be waived for certain generic products. Categories of products that may be eligible for waivers include, but are not limited to, the following:

1) Parenteral solutions intended for injection by the intravenous, subcutaneous, or intramuscular routes of administration
2) Oral solutions or other solubilized forms
3) Topically applied solutions intended for local therapeutic effects or other topically applied dosage forms intended for local therapeutic effects in non-food animals only
4) Inhalant volatile anesthetic solutions.

In general, the generic drug being considered for a waiver contains the same active and inactive ingredients in the same dosage form and concentration as the RLNAD. However, CVM will consider bioequivalence waivers for nonfood animal topical products with certain differences in the inactive ingredients between the pioneer and generic products.

Unlike human drugs, the concentrations of API and excipients are typically listed only on injectable formulations, so that a generic sponsor must "reverse engineer" oral or topical dosage forms to match the RLNAD. In general, the requirements for the CMC technical section of the generic drug are the same as those for the RLNAD, although the generic sponsor may be required to conduct additional tests to demonstrate that the generic drug performs the same as the RLNAD.

2.3 Prescription versus Over-the-Counter Status of Animal Drugs

CVM is responsible for determining the marketing status (prescription, over-the-counter [OTC], or Veterinary Feed Directive [VFD]) of animal drug products based on whether or not it is possible to prepare "adequate directions for use" under which a layperson can use the drug safely and effectively. The classification of prescription and OTC designation is described in the public *Policy and Procedures Manual Guide 1240.2220*. Prescription products can be dispensed only by or upon the lawful written order of a licensed veterinarian. Prescription products must bear the following legend:

> Caution: Federal law restricts this drug to use by or on the order of a licensed veterinarian.

CVM considers "safe use" to include the safety of the animal, food products derived from the animal, people associated with the animal, and the drug's impact on the environment. For the effective use of a drug, CVM assumes that an accurate diagnosis can be made with a reasonable degree of certainty, that the drug can be properly administered, and that the course of the disease can be followed so that the success or lack of success of the product can be observed. Therefore, the same drug can be marketed in a number of different dosage forms, intended for use by different routes of administration and in different species of animals. Consequently, some drugs may be appropriately labeled prescriptions for some species and indications and OTC for others. Examples of drugs with both prescription and OTC labels include many of the horse and cattle antiparasitics, which can be administered safely and effectively by laypeople.

2.3.1 Animal Feeds

The FFDCA defines "food" as "articles used for food or drink for man or other animals," and "drug" as "articles intended for use in the diagnosis, cure, mitigation, treatment, or prevention of disease in man or animals." Medicated animal feeds with indications to treat a disease or that have a production claim (weight gain and feed efficiency) are regulated as drugs under Section 201(g) of the FFDCA, and are reviewed by ONADE. Products marketed as dietary supplements or "feed supplements" for animals still fall under the FFDCA (i.e. they are considered "foods" or "new animal drugs," depending on the intended use). The regulatory status of a product is determined by CVM on a case-by-case basis, using criteria provided in the public *Policy and Procedures Guide 1240.3605*.

CVM carries out its responsibility for the regulation of nonmedicated animal feed in cooperation with state and local partners through cooperative agreements, contracts, grants, memoranda of understanding, and partnerships. For instance, CVM cooperates with the Association of American Feed Control Officials (AAFCO) and the individual states for the implementation of uniform policies for regulating the use of nonmedicated animal feed products. This includes the establishment of uniform feed ingredient definitions and proper labeling to assure the safe use of feeds. The ingredient definitions are important because medicated and non-medicated animal feeds and feed ingredients must be correctly labeled when they are marketed. Although CVM has the responsibility for regulating the use of nonmedicated animal feed products within the Division of Animal Feeds, the ultimate responsibility for the production of safe animal feed products lies with the manufacturers and distributors of the products.

Like nonmedicated animal feeds, pet foods are not required to have pre-market approval by CVM. However, CVM does ensure that the ingredients used in pet food are safe. The meat, poultry, and grains are generally considered to be safe. Additional ingredients, such as minerals, vitamins, flavorings, and preservatives, may be generally recognized as safe or must be approved as food additives. Food additives must have an approved food additive petition to be legally marketed. The petition describes the chemical identity of the additive and the manufacturing process. The petition also includes safety data and the proposed labeling. If CVM agrees with the sponsor's information in the petition, then the food additive is approved for its intended use.

For animal feeds containing antimicrobials that are of importance to human health, the Animal Drug Availability Act (ADAA) of 1996 was amended to implement the VFD to help ensure the judicious use of these antimicrobials. A VFD is a written statement issued by a licensed veterinarian for the use of a specific drug (e.g. an antimicrobial), in or on an animal feed, and requires that the veterinarian have a valid veterinarian–client–patient relationship. The VFD specifies the amount of drug to be mixed in or on the feed, the name and address of the client, the identity and number of animals to be fed, and the last day that the feed can be used. The veterinarian or client then sends the VFD drug directly to the feed distributor, who mixes the drug into the feed as directed.

2.3.2 Extra-Label Drug Use in Veterinary Patients

In 1994, the FFDCA was amended to include the AMDUCA to allow extra-label drug use in animals. Extra-label use is essential for the practice of veterinary medicine, because so few FDA-approved animal drugs exist in comparison to approved human drugs. Under AMDUCA, veterinarians can legally prescribe approved human and animal drugs for extra-label use under the following specific conditions as described in Title 21 CFR Part 530:

- There must be a veterinary–client–patient relationship.
- The veterinarian has sufficient knowledge of the animals for at least a general or preliminary diagnosis.
- The veterinarian is available for follow-up in case of adverse reactions or failure of therapy.
- The veterinarian must maintain records of the extra-label use for two years. The records should include the drug, condition treated, species and number of animals treated, dosage, treatment duration, and meat and/or milk withdrawal times if appropriate.

However, there are several limitations under AMDUCA, such as:

- Extra-label use is restricted to veterinarians or under the supervision of a veterinarian.
- Extra-label drugs cannot be used in animal feeds.
- Extra-label use cannot result in a residue that presents a risk to human health or is present at a concentration above the tolerance.

There are also restrictions on the extra-label use of compounded drugs (see the "Compounded Drugs" section of this chapter).

The following drugs, as listed in 21 CFR Part 530.41, are prohibited from extra-label use in food animals due to concerns about the residue safety for humans who might consume tissues from the treated animal. The associated risks in humans for each drug are not included in the CFR, but they are listed here as explanation for the extra-label prohibition:

- *Chloramphenicol:* Aplastic anemia in humans
- *Clenbuterol:* Cardiac arrhythmias
- *Diethylstilbestrol (DES):* Carcinogen
- *Dimetridazole:* Carcinogen
- *Ipronidazole and other nitroimidazoles:* Carcinogen
- *Furazolidone and nitrofurazone:* Carcinogen
- *Sulfonamide drugs in lactating dairy cattle, except for the approved use of sulfadimethoxine, sulfabromomethazine, and sulfaethoxypyridazine:* Thyroid hyperplasia and cancer
- *Fluoroquinolones:* Antimicrobial resistance
- *Glycopeptides:* Antimicrobial resistance
- *Phenylbutazone in female dairy cattle 20 months of age or older:* Aplastic anemia *Cephalosporins (not including cephapirin) in cattle, swine, chickens, or turkeys:*

  - For disease prevention purposes: Antimicrobial resistance;
  - At unapproved doses, frequencies, durations, or routes of administration; *or*

  - If the drug is not approved for that species and production class.

- The following drugs, or classes of drugs, that are approved for treating or preventing influenza A are prohibited from extra-label uses in chickens, turkeys, and ducks to prevent the emergence of resistant strains of influenza A viruses:

  - Adamantane
  - Neuraminidase inhibitors.

There are no approved drugs that are prohibited from extra-label use in companion animals.

2.4 Nutritional Supplements for Veterinary Patients

In 1994, the Dietary Supplement Health and Education Act (DSHEA) amended the FFDCA to create the new category of dietary supplements, under the general umbrella of "foods" instead of under food additives or drugs – both of which require the FDA's pre-market review. Therefore, DSHEA allows companies to market dietary supplements or nutraceuticals without a pre-market review. In 1996, the FDA determined that DSHEA wasn't meant to apply to products for use in animals. Therefore, products marketed as dietary supplements for animals don't fall under DSHEA, and the FDA doesn't recognize them as a special category. Rather, the agency classifies these products as either food for animals or animal drugs, depending on their intended use.

2.5 Compounded Drugs for Veterinary Patients

The FFDCA does not generally differentiate between compounding and other methods of animal drug manufacturing. Animals drugs that are not approved or not included on the Index of Legally Marketed Unapproved New Animal Drugs for Minor Species are considered to be "unsafe" under Section 512 (a)(1) and "adulterated" under Section 501(a)(5) of the FFDCA. Animal drugs compounded from bulk drug substances are considered to be new animal drugs.

The FDA acknowledges the necessity of veterinary compounding, but it is concerned about the use of animal drugs compounded from bulk drugs when an approved alternative exists that can be used as labeled or in an extra-label manner consistent with the FDA's extra-label provisions. Compounded drugs have not undergone premarket CVM review for safety, effectiveness, and manufacturing quality; therefore, the FDA is concerned that unrestricted compounding of animal drugs from bulk drug substances has the potential to compromise food safety, increase the risk of unsafe or ineffective treatment, or undermine incentive to develop new animal drugs.

The FDA allows the extra-label use from compounding of approved new animal or human drugs as described in Title 21 CFR Part 530.13. It is important to note that nothing in this part should be construed as permitting compounding from bulk drugs. Extra-label use from compounding of approved new animal or human drugs is permitted if:

- There is no approved new animal or human drug in the available dosage form and/or concentration that will appropriately treat the condition diagnosed. Compounding from a human drug for use in food animals will not be permitted if an approved animal drug can be used for the compounding.
- The compounding is performed by a licensed pharmacist or veterinarian within the scope of a professional practice.
- Adequate procedures and processes are followed that ensure the safety and effectiveness of the compounded product.
- The scale of the compounding operation is commensurate with the established need for compounded products (e.g. similar to that of comparable practices).
- All relevant state laws relating to the compounding of drugs for use in animals are followed.

On May 19, 2015, the FDA revoked the *Compliance Policy Guide*'s Section 608.400, "Compounding of Drugs for Use in Animals," and published a draft guidance that provided information to compounders of animal drugs and other interested stakeholders on the FDA's enforcement approach with respect to the compounding of animal drugs from bulk drug substances. *Compliance Policy Guide* §608.400 was withdrawn because it was no longer consistent with the FDA's current thinking. After reviewing the comments submitted to the docket, the FDA decided not to finalize the current draft guidance, and will instead develop and issue a new draft guidance. In developing the new draft, the FDA will carefully consider the issues that are specific to compounding of animal drugs, including the significance of using compounded drugs as a treatment option in various veterinary settings and animal species. Until the FDA publishes final guidance on this issue, they intend to look at the totality of the circumstances when determining whether to take enforcement action for unlawful animal drug-compounding activities.

2.6 Conclusion

As outlined in this chapter, the drug approval process for human and animal drugs has many similarities. There are several offices within the FDA CVM that are responsible for reviewing the safety, effectiveness, and manufacturing data to determine if an animal drug is safe and effective, and can be manufactured under adequate quality controls to ensure potency and stability. Animal health companies are required to conduct safety and effectiveness studies under the same quality standards (GCP and GLP) as those used for human drugs. Similarly, the manufacturing standards used for the review of veterinary drugs are the same as for human drugs, which ensures batch-to-batch consistency of approved animal drugs. The approval process for generic animal drugs is also similar to that for human generics, where the generic sponsor has to demonstrate bioequivalence of the generic product to the reference-listed new animal drug product using the same statistical criteria as used for human generics. Like physicians, veterinarians are allowed to use extra-label drugs under specific conditions. This is absolutely necessary considering that there are fewer FDA-approved animal drugs compared to human drugs.

There are also several important differences between the human and animal drug approval processes, such as the number of animal species regulated, the number of animals used in the field studies, and the need to demonstrate human food safety for drugs intended for food animals. The FDA CVM recognizes seven major species of animals, and many more minor species, and sponsors provide safety and effectiveness data for each species and indication proposed in the labeling. In addition, there can be different classes of the same species, such as dairy and beef cows, that may require separate safety and effectiveness studies. Field studies for animal drugs generally have fewer numbers of subjects than human clinical trials. For safety studies with purpose-bought (non-client-owned) animals, necropsies are usually performed to provide tissues for histopathology evaluation. For food animal drugs, sponsors must demonstrate the safety of edible tissues when consumed by humans, and the lack of impact on human gastrointestinal microflora for antimicrobials.

Abbreviations

ADAA	Animal Drug Availability Act of 1996
ADI	Acceptable daily intake
ADUFA	Animal Drug User Fee Act
AGDUFA	Animal Generic Drug User Fee Act
AMDUCA	Animal Medicinal Drug Use Clarification Act of 1994
CFR	Code of Federal Regulations
CVM	Center for Veterinary Medicine
FFDCA	Federal Food, Drug, and Cosmetic Act
GADPTRA	Generic Animal Drug and Patent Term Restoration Act of 1988
GCP	Good Clinical Practice
GLP	Good Laboratory Practice
ONADE	Office of New Animal Drug Evaluation
TAS	Target animal safety
VICH	International Cooperation on Harmonization of Technical Requirements for Registration of Veterinary Medicinal Products

3

Compounding for Animals

Gigi Davidson

Clinical Pharmacy Services, College of Veterinary Medicine, North Carolina State University, Raleigh, NC, USA

Key Points

- The prevalence of pharmacists compounding medications for use in animals is widespread.
- Veterinary pharmacotherapy and compounding principles and skills are conspicuously absent from the pharmacy educational curriculum.
- The current regulatory environment for veterinary compounding is significantly incongruous with the human compounding regulatory environment.
- Compounding standards and best practices observed for preparing human compounds must be utilized when preparing compounds for animals.

- Prior to dispensing compounded drugs to pet owners, pharmacists must ensure that pet owners are aware of the risks (i.e. lack of safety and efficacy data, lack of stability data, etc.) compared to US Food and Drug Administration (FDA)-approved drug products.
- Component selection for nonhuman patients is dependent on many species-specific and patient-specific factors.
- Specialized training programs in veterinary compounding vary widely in credentialing and content.

3.1 Introduction

The spectrum of therapeutic need in veterinary medicine is great, while the availability of approved drug products for all veterinary species and indications is small. A recent search of the AnimalDrugs@FDA database revealed a total of 1564 approved new animal drugs for all nonhuman species (see https://animaldrugsatfda.fda.gov/adafda/views/#/search). A similar search of the Orange Book Data Files at the US Food and Drug Administration (FDA) revealed more than 35000 approved new drugs for humans (see https://www.fda.gov/downloads/Drugs/InformationOnDrugs/UCM163762.zip). Because of the paucity of approved drugs for use in animal patients, compounding is of great importance to fill therapeutic gaps for nonhuman species. In May 2015, the FDA estimated that 75 000 pharmacies fill 6 350 000 compounded prescriptions for animals in the USA each year (FDA 2015). Estimates for other countries are not available;

Pharmacotherapeutics for Veterinary Dispensing, First Edition. Edited by Katrina L. Mealey.

however, a survey of veterinarians in Czechoslovakia revealed that surveyed veterinarians prescribe about one compounded preparation per day (Agelova and Maceskova 2005). Although no other specific data are available, considering the many roles that animals play for humans, the prevalence of compounded drug products prepared for animals worldwide is likely to be large. Competence in providing pharmaceutical expertise and compounded drugs for animal patients is critical for pharmacists, because pharmacists are the only healthcare providers that are expected by society to provide care for all species, both humans and nonhumans, and are the only healthcare providers that are legally allowed to do so. Pharmacists are also well positioned to consult with veterinarians and pet owners to collaborate to provide a high-quality compounded formulation that is safe for the intended patient and has optimal composition to potentially provide the desired therapeutic effect.

Use of a compounded drug may be an option when an FDA-approved veterinary or human drug product is not available for the therapeutic need. Compounding can include activities such as mixing two or more approved drug products together into a single dosage form (e.g. mixing two anesthetic drugs in the same syringe), changing the dosage form (e.g. crushing oral tablets to make an oral liquid suspension), or adding patient-preferred flavoring to an approved drug product. If no approved drug exists for the desired therapy, compounding can also include starting with bulk chemical active ingredients and other excipients such as suspending agents, fillers, binders, and flavors.

The information presented in this chapter is intended to provide an overview of the current landscape of compounding for animals; a discussion on associated benefits, risks, and challenges; and resources to aid in sourcing components and formulas for preparing animal compounds of the highest possible quality.

3.2 Definitions of Compounding

Terminology to describe the extemporaneous preparation of medicines varies widely across the global community. The practice may be referred to as "extemporaneous manufacturing," "extemporaneous preparation," "extemporaneous compounding," or simply "compounding" depending on the national directives of the individual countries (Council of the EEC 1965; World Health Organization 2016; Food and Drug Administration 2018c). For the purposes of this chapter, the term "compounding" will be used. Legal definitions for compounding are often nonspecific and broad. The FDA's Center for Veterinary Medicine (FDA CVM) currently lacks a definition for compounding and simply states that "to be legally marketed, new animal drugs must be approved under Section 512 of the US Food, Drug, and Cosmetic Act (FDC) Act, conditionally approved under Section 571 of the FDC Act or included on the Index of Legally Marketed Unapproved New Animal Drugs for Minor Species under Section 572 of the FDC Act" (FDA 2018a). Compounded preparations are considered unapproved by the FDA, and to be legally marketed, they require approval by the statutorily established process. The FDA recognizes the need for compounded medicines and has issued various guidances and policy guides for compounding for animals since 1996, but none of those documents are currently in effect, nor was compounding defined in any of the documents. The FDA announced an intention to complete a new draft guidance for compounding, Guidance for Industry #256 (Guidance for Industry 2017), and ideally this will contain a definition of compounding. The definition of compounding for humans is statutorily defined with both a positive definition, "Compounding is defined as combining, admixing, mixing, diluting, pooling, reconstituting, or otherwise altering of a drug or bulk drug substance to create a drug," and a negative definition, "Compounding does not include mixing, reconstituting, or other such acts that are performed in accordance with directions contained in approved labeling provided by the product's manufacturer and other manufacturer directions consistent with that labeling" (Drug Quality and Security Act 2013). The United States Pharmacopeia (USP) defines compounding as "the preparation, mixing, assembling, altering, packaging, and labeling of a drug, drug-delivery device, or device in accordance with a licensed practitioner's prescription, medication order, or initiative based on the practitioner/patient/pharmacist/ compounder relationship in the course of professional practice" (USP Legal Recognition 2017). The USP definition does not distinguish compounding for humans from that for animals. The only government that appears to specifically address compounding for animals is New Zealand. The New Zealand government defines compounding for animals as "a means to make up, prepare, produce, or process a veterinary medicine into a preparation for treatment of animals under the care of the compounding veterinarian" (New Zealand Ministry for Primary Industries 2017). The American Veterinary Medical Association (AVMA) aligns its definition of compounding with the FDA CVM's Extra Label Drug Use Guidance and states that compounding is the "customized manipulation of an approved drug(s) by a veterinarian, or by a pharmacist upon the prescription of a veterinarian, to meet the needs of a particular patient" (AVMA 2017). Note that AVMA's definition, like FDA CVM regulations, is silent on the use of bulk drug substances for compounding, a regulatory void that will be addressed later in this chapter. Pharmacists preparing compounds for use in nonhuman patients are well advised to check with their respective state board of pharmacy to determine the jurisdictional definitions and boundaries before extrapolating any agency or organizational definition of compounding to veterinary medicine.

3.3 Scope of Veterinary Compounding

Although in its withdrawn Guidance for Industry #230, the FDA estimated that 75 000 pharmacies fill 6 350 000 compounded prescriptions for animals in the USA each year, the exact extent to which drugs are compounded for veterinary patients is unknown. The Brakke Company conducted a survey of veterinary compounding in 2013 and claims to answer the question "How big is the veterinary drug compounding market?" However, results of this survey are only available by purchase for US$8995.00 (Veterinary Drug Compounding 2017). An Internet search for "veterinary compounding pharmacy in the United States" reveals 208 000 hits (search performed on Google in 2017). A 2017 publication revealed that there were almost 68 000 community pharmacies in the USA in 2015 (Qato et al. 2017), so it is not likely that there are 208 000 veterinary compounding pharmacies in the USA; however, the large number of Internet links to "veterinary compounding pharmacy" indicate a strong presence of pharmacies preparing compounded drugs for veterinary patients. Statistical numbers based on reporting to the FDA are not available, because unlike veterinary drug manufacturers, veterinary compounding pharmacies do not have to register with the FDA. While pharmacies must register with state boards of pharmacy in the USA, the data collected by state boards of pharmacy are not aggregated or comprehensive, and many boards of pharmacy do not distinguish prescription activity for humans from that activity for nonhumans. While several countries require that pharmacists follow regulations or guidelines for compounding medicines and some may impose reporting requirements for the number and type of compounds prepared (FDA 2018b), these requirements appear to be limited to only sterile compounds prepared for humans.

Considering that 77% of community pharmacists report filling prescriptions for animals (Sorah et al. 2015; Mingura 2017), it is likely that many of these prescriptions are for compounded medications.

3.4 Potential Benefits of Compounded Drugs for Veterinary Patients

Compounded medications provide treatment options for animal patients when no suitable government-approved (e.g. FDA) drugs are available. Drug products approved for use in certain species may be commercially available in dosage forms (e.g. large chewable tablets) that are not suitable for use in other species (e.g. cats or exotic animal patients). Likewise, approved products may be available in flavors that are not accepted by certain animal species (e.g. citrus and sweetly flavored human pediatric medicines are not accepted by cats). In these instances, compounding can be used to modify an approved product into an acceptable dosage form or flavor to increase adherence in an individual patient, particularly in species that are difficult to medicate (e.g. cats, and exotic and wild animal species).

In addition to optimizing drug formulations to better suit the needs of an individual animal patient, compounded preparations can also provide therapeutic options when there are no approved drugs available (for either humans or animals) for an indication. For example, cisapride, a prokinetic, was withdrawn from the US human market for safety reasons in 2000, but it is considered the best available treatment option for non-obstructive chronic constipation or megacolon in cats (Figure 3.1) (Washabau and Holt 1999). Even though the human safety issues with cisapride have not been observed in cats, to date no veterinary drug companies have elected to submit applications for cisapride approval for animals, so compounding remains the only option for veterinarians to obtain cisapride for animals in need of effective prokinetic drug therapy. Drugs containing bromides were also removed from the

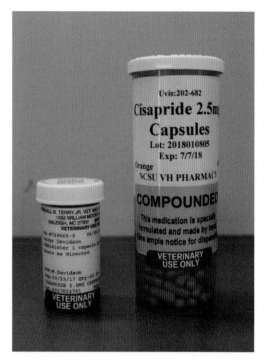

Figure 3.1 Compounded cisapride capsules (right) used to fill a prescription to be dispensed for a feline patient (left).

human market in the 1970s, and potassium bromide remains unavailable in a legally marketed and approved animal dosage form. Pharmacokinetic and pharmacodynamic parameters are well described to support the therapeutic use of bromides for treating idiopathic epilepsy in dogs (Trepanier et al. 1998), and veterinarians commonly prescribe compounded potassium bromide for canine epileptic patients. It is unlikely that any veterinary pharmaceutical company will elect to pursue approval for drugs like cisapride and potassium bromide because the cost of approval far outweighs any potential profits from sales to the small patient populations requiring these therapies.

Although economic reasons are also often cited by veterinarians as a benefit of using compounded drugs, *regulatory agencies and professional veterinary organizations state that using a compounded preparation over an approved product strictly for economic reasons is inappropriate.* Very few animal patients are covered by medical insurance policies, so cost of medical care for animals is completely out of pocket for most animal owners. Veterinarians often find themselves having to choose between treatment options based on an owner's financial constraints, and pharmacists will face this dilemma as well. Practicing within strict legal compliance (i.e. dispensing an expensive approved product) or practicing outside the confines of the law (i.e. dispensing a compounded drug instead of the approved product) is a decision that pharmacists will need to make on a case-by-case basis. The information provided in this chapter is intended to help pharmacists weigh their options.

One example of a compounded drug that has recently been prescribed by veterinarians for economic reasons is the chemotherapeutic drug chlorambucil, which is used to treat lymphoma, a common neoplastic disease in dogs and cats. Chlorambucil is not available as a veterinary approved drug but has been used in an extra-label manner in veterinary patients for decades. Recently, the price of chlorambucil has risen dramatically – from approximately one US dollar per tablet to 23 US dollars per tablet. The consequence of this price increase for the pet owner means that a six-month course of treatment that had previously cost the owner well under $100 will now cost the pet owner a few thousand dollars. Because of third-party payment systems for human patients, the actual cost of chlorambucil is usually not realized by human patients, but it certainly is for most pet owners. Most veterinarians, pharmacists, and pet owners would agree that a quality compounded product (with assured strength and stability, free from contaminants, and equally bioavailable) would be a reasonable and justifiable option to provide the pet owner. If there are no FDA-approved veterinary drugs for treating these diseases, a quality compounded drug could be a reasonable option. It is more difficult to justify dispensing a compounded drug when an FDA-approved veterinary product with proven safety and efficacy data is available and the

cost differences are not in the several-thousand-dollar range. For example, veterinary pharmaceutical companies, after years of research and development, have recently gained FDA approval for drugs to treat canine atopic dermatitis (oclacitinib; Apoquel®) and hyperadrenocorticism (trilostane; Vetoryl®). There are no equivalent human products. The recent market availability of these products provides improved therapeutic options for veterinarians and improved outcomes for patients. Unlike the previous examples, these FDA-approved veterinary products do not cost several thousand dollars for a single course of therapy. Thus, it is difficult to justify dispensing a compounded drug (with no safety, efficacy, bioavailability, or stability data) to save some money. What is *not* justifiable is dispensing a compounded drug when numerous, reasonably priced FDA-approved products are available. Examples of the latter include heartworm preventives and antiparasitic drugs, among many others. I am aware of a fatal adverse event resulting from a compounded ivermectin heartworm preventive product (Katrina L. Mealey, DVM, PhD, personal communication, December 16, 2017). The dog received a 1000-fold overdose of ivermectin because the compounding pharmacy mistakenly dispensed a milligram, rather than a microgram, dose of ivermectin, and the dog died of severe neurological toxicity as a direct result of the ivermectin overdose. The difference in price between safe and effective FDA-approved heartworm preventives and antiparasitic agents versus compounded products is negligible (roughly $10 per month, depending on the size of the animal).

Regardless of potential cost savings, the risk of poor quality (contaminants, impurities, and incorrect strength), unknown bioavailability, unknown stability, and subsequent therapeutic failure from these compounded mimics is significant and predictably may increase overall costs to the pet owner due to lack of clinical response or overt toxicity. Pharmacists preparing compounds for veterinary patients must engage in dialogue with veterinarians prescribing compounded drugs for economic reasons to determine potential therapeutic risks of using compounded drugs instead of commercially available, approved drugs. Prior to dispensing compounded drugs to pet owners, pharmacists must ensure that pet owners are aware of not only the potential cost savings but also the risks (e.g. lack of safety and efficacy data, lack of stability data, etc.).

3.5 Risks Associated with the Use of Compounded Drugs in Animals

While the benefits of specific compounded drugs for animals are well established (Papich 2005; Frank 2006), risk of serious harm including therapeutic failure from compounded preparations is significant and well established. The deaths of 64 humans from contaminated sterile compounds in the USA in 2012 (Centers for Disease Control and Prevention [CDC] 2012) caused sweeping regulatory oversight for compounds prepared for humans (Drug Quality and Security Act 2013); however, little regulatory action has been undertaken to minimize risks posed by compounded drugs to animal patients. Headlines of animal deaths resulting from compounded drugs have become more common in the world media. The deaths of 21 Polo Ponies in Florida from a 10-fold overdose of selenium in a compounded drug product (Belainesh et al. 2011), the deaths of four horses and permanent injury to six others in Florida and Kentucky from superpotent concentrations of compounded pyrimethamine (Veterinary Practice News Editors 2014), and the deaths of three horses from a 70-fold superpotent compounded clenbuterol product (Thompson et al. 2011) gained wide attention and prescriber concern, but little has been accomplished on the US regulatory front to reduce the risk of harm from compounded preparations for animals. Furthermore, there are no specific data regarding lack of efficacy that has resulted from compounded drug products dispensed to veterinary patients due to lack of bioavailability, lack of potency, or poor stability.

Animal suffering and death from compounded drugs may be attributed to many factors, including preparation errors, contamination, chemical and physical instability, lack of bioavailability in the target patient, and low stability. Poor quality due to compounding error has been widely investigated and reported for compounded drugs prepared for animals (Stanley et al. 2003; Cook et al. 2012; Scott-Moncrief et al. 2012; Umstead et al. 2012). Although no distinction was made between compounds prepared for humans and animals, the Missouri Board of Pharmacy recently found that as many as one-fifth of randomly selected compounds from Missouri licensed pharmacies did not contain the amount of active ingredient (range, 0–450%) indicated on the prescription label (Missouri Board of Pharmacy 2017). At the time of writing, no legal requirements exist in any country that require testing to demonstrate that compounded preparations meet the strength as indicated on the prescription labeling.

While extensive studies have been conducted to establish safety, efficacy, bioavailability, stability, and consistent quality for drugs receiving FDA approval for animal use, there are no equivalent assurances for these attributes in compounded preparations. Ample evidence does exist, however, proving that many compounded preparations are not bioequivalent to approved products in animal patients, and that even when administered by the same route, they are not bioavailable compared to FDA-approved products. One example worth discussion is compounded transdermal preparations. Although some may ultimately achieve effective blood concentrations, compounded transdermal drug products are consistently less bioavailable than the commercially available orally administered counterparts

(Ciribassi et al. 2003; Krotscheck et al. 2004; Mealey et al. 2004; Bennett et al. 2005; MacGregor et al. 2008). Compounded preparations prepared from active pharmaceutical ingredients (e.g. itraconazole) have also been proven to be less (or not at all) bioavailable compared to the approved products when given at the same dose by the same route of administration (Smith et al. 2010; Mawby et al. 2014). Other studies have demonstrated a significant increase in oral bioavailability of approved drugs when compounded into different dosage forms. The bioavailability of intact mitotane tablets in Beagles was shown to increase 38-fold when crushed and suspended in an oil vehicle (Watson et al. 1987), posing a significant risk for life-threatening adrenal damage in dogs switched from the FDA-approved tablets to compounded oral suspensions.

Humans may also face risk from compounded drugs prepared for use in animals. Drug depletion profiles from tissues of treated food-producing animals have not been determined for compounded preparations, and humans may be exposed to drug residues when consuming tissues or byproducts (e.g. milk, eggs, or honey) from treated animals. Veterinarians and pharmacists sometimes fail to consider the risk of human exposure to compounded medications. Animals do not self-medicate. Even those dosage forms that animals self-administer, such as medicated feeds and water, are prepared by humans, so the risk of drug exposure to human caregivers is always great. Compounded formulations of drugs that were removed from the human market for safety reasons (e.g. cisapride, bromides, diethylstilbestrol, and trilostane) can cause serious adverse events in humans who may be exposed. Community pharmacists providing compounded drugs to pet owners should include counseling points (described further in this chapter) to minimize human exposure when administering potentially toxic compounds to their pets. This may be particularly important for some compounded transdermal formulations intended for household pets. Pet owners, including children, may be exposed "secondhand" to the drug by intentional or unintentional physical contact with the drug application site when playing with the animal or if the animal rubs up against exposed skin of someone in the household.

Finally, compounded mimics of FDA-approved drugs negatively affect veterinary medical therapy in the long term, because such mimics destroy incentive for veterinary pharmaceutical companies to perform research and development to seek FDA approval for new animal drugs.

3.6 Current Regulatory Environment for Compounding

Regulatory oversight for compounded veterinary drugs varies widely from country to country. The Parsemus Foundation, a small private foundation interested in compounded contraceptive drugs, recently surveyed the veterinary drug regulatory landscape of various countries. In their report surveying legal use for a compounded injectable chemical neutering agent for male dogs, *Regulatory Status of Compounded Treatments, by Country* (Parsemus Foundation 2016), Parsemus characterizes countries as those "with a strong veterinary regulatory culture" (European Union countries, Canada, China, South Africa, Australia, and Japan), those "without a strong veterinary regulatory culture" (Nigeria, Trinidad and Tobago, Bangladesh, Fiji, Ghana, Iraq, Kenya, Nepal, Tanzania, and Sierra Leone), and those "with a special situation" regarding veterinary regulatory culture (Mexico, Bolivia, Panama, Colombia, and the USA). The report states that the USA generally falls into the category of "with a strong veterinary regulatory culture" but that "great ambiguity exists around compounding in the USA, with nearly all small-animal veterinarians ordering drugs compounded from bulk substances in situations that are technically contrary to FDA regulations" (Parsemus Foundation 2016). Although the Parsemus survey was not validated or analyzed for statistical significance, its conclusions are consistent with opinions widely held by all relevant stakeholders for veterinary compounding in the USA. Since veterinary pharmacotherapy and law are not included in US pharmacy school core curricula, community pharmacists are largely oblivious to the trafficking of "office use" compounded drugs in veterinary practice.

Specific regulations for veterinary compounding outside of the USA are described for only a few countries. The Pharmacy Board of Australia has provided comprehensive guidelines for compounding of medicine (Pharmacy Board of Australia 2016), which includes a section on compounding veterinary medicines. The Australian guidelines instruct pharmacists to be educated in the principles of compounding for animals, and to maintain suitable information resources regarding veterinary medicine, including consultations with veterinary surgeons. Australian pharmacists are also encouraged to seek legal advice to ensure that they are compounding within the parameters of the Australian AgVet Code. The Irish Pharmacy Practice Guidance Manual includes veterinary pharmacy in its guidance and requires that compounded veterinary preparations be prepared only in response to a veterinarian's order; no anticipatory compounding is allowed (Pharmacy Practice Guidance Manual 2016). Denmark allows compounding for animals only pursuant to a veterinarian's prescription and only if there is no suitable registered veterinary medical product available (Danish Veterinary and Food Administration 2017). The Ontario College of Pharmacists publishes compounding guidelines that include some of the most specific guidance on veterinary compounding and require the same standards used when preparing compounds for humans; specific auxiliary labeling for veterinary compounded drugs, including the veterinarian's stated

withdrawal time for food-producing animals; and a prohibition of selling compounded drugs to third parties outside of the veterinarian–client–patient relationship (Ontario College of Pharmacists 2017). Considering the global efforts to standardize and improve the quality of drugs compounded for animals, community pharmacists in the USA are well advised to follow the models provided by these initiatives, while US regulatory agencies struggle to initiate change.

Although veterinarians may compound drugs for animal patients, compounding practice is primarily performed by pharmacists. In most countries, pharmacy practice is regulated by provincial or national boards of pharmacy, and compounding activities are very well regulated. However, in the USA, pharmacies are solely regulated by state boards of pharmacy, and unless pharmacies are engaging in behavior that more closely resembles manufacturing, the FDA has little jurisdiction of compounding pharmacies. Consequently, surveillance and compliance for veterinary compounding vary widely from state to state, and because pharmacies may register with multiple state boards of pharmacy and engage in interstate commerce of compounded veterinary drugs, regulatory action has historically been extremely difficult to accomplish. This lack of control is exacerbated by the fact that state Boards of Pharmacy often assume, incorrectly, that regulations for drug use in animals are the same as those for humans. The magnitude of veterinary compounding in the USA and the lack of regulatory consistency confirm the Parsemus assessment that much ambiguity exists and that veterinarians can prescribe and dispense compounded drugs that are technically at odds with FDA regulations. Compounding pharmacies may prepare quantities of compounded drugs for sale to veterinary practices, which are outside the jurisdiction of boards of pharmacy. Veterinarians subsequently dispense these compounds as if they were FDA-approved products, and the extent of this activity occurs, for the most part, beneath the regulatory radar. To further complicate matters, sweeping reform and enforcement of compounding through the US Drug Quality and Security Act of 2013 (DQSA) dramatically increased the regulatory oversight of compounding for humans, but was written to specifically exclude regulation of compounding for animals. The resultant regulatory void for veterinary compounding has further contributed to great ambiguity in surveillance and determination of compliance in the USA. While it is currently still legally acceptable in most states for pharmacists to provide compounded drugs for use in a veterinarian's office, pharmacists must assume responsibility for recognizing what drug quantities and dispensing behaviors constitute acceptable office use.

The US Animal Medicinal Drug Use Clarification Act of 1996 (AMDUCA) codified the extra-label use of drugs, including compounded drugs, in animal patients, but was silent on the use of bulk drug substances for compounding. Consequently, in 1996, the FDA promulgated rules for compounding affirming that compounded drugs prepared for animal patients must use FDA-approved products as the starting ingredients, and that nothing in the regulation "shall be construed as permitting compounding from bulk drugs." No other countries appear to have mandated a prohibition on the use of bulk drug substances for compounding and, as stated in this chapter, have only required that veterinary compounded drugs be prepared in the absence of a suitable approved product. From 1996 to 2015, the FDA practiced regulatory discretion toward compounding with bulk drug substances through an internal compliance policy guide, CPG 608.400 (FDA Manual of Compliance Policy Guides 2017). However, to harmonize enforcement with the DQSA, the FDA rescinded CPG 608.400 in May 2015 and proposed a new draft guidance for industry (GFI) (FDA Draft Guidance for Industry #230 2017) for public comment regarding use of bulk drug substances for animal compounding. However, in 2017, after receiving extensive and diverse

public comments on the proposed guidance, the FDA CVM withdrew the guidance, stating that they would develop a new guidance and "will carefully consider the issues that are specific to compounding of animal drugs, including the significance of using compounded drugs as a treatment option in various veterinary settings and animal species" (FDA Withdraws Guidance for Industry 2017). Availability of this new guidance is anticipated by the end of 2018, and until then, veterinary compounding enforcement in the USA regarding use of bulk drug substances continues to remain in regulatory limbo. Pharmacists compounding drugs for animals should consider that comparison of the CPG and the GFI documents indicates that the FDA's primary concerns regarding compounding with bulk drug substances are the following: (i) copies of FDA-approved drugs, (ii) resale of office stock compounds, and (iii) use of bulk drug substances to compound for food-producing animals. Hopefully, future guidance or a legislative initiative will provide clarity with respect to these three concerns for a country where more than six million compounded drugs are prepared for animals annually by pharmacy professionals who have little to no training in veterinary drug law.

The FDA has inspected some compounding pharmacies on a "for cause" basis and has consequently issued warning letters to pharmacies found to be out of compliance. Unfortunately, a September 2015 audit by the US General Accounting Office (GAO) (Government Accounting Office 2017) found that the FDA had not consistently documented the basis for citing these veterinary compounding infractions, and the warning letters have had little effect on improving the quality of compounded drugs provided for veterinary patients. Another unfortunate regulatory void in the USA is the FDA's lack of statutory authority to mandate drug recalls, including recalls for compounded drugs found to be of unacceptable quality during inspections. Consequently, when the FDA discovers compounded drugs that may potentially cause harm, suffering, or death to animal patients, they must rely upon the willingness of the compounding pharmacy to issue a voluntary recall. *This is in direct contrast to the FDA's clear statutory authority to mandate drug recalls for FDA-approved drug products, even if the violation is more minor than what is identified in a compounded drug product.* The FDA does provide a list of voluntarily recalled veterinary compounds (see http://www.fda.gov/AnimalVeterinary/SafetyHealth/RecallsWithdrawals/default.htm). Pharmacists should be familiar with the recalls listed at this link to facilitate recall efforts with local veterinarians and pet owners if necessary.

3.7 Compounding for Food-Producing Animals

Meat, milk, eggs, honey, and many other food products come from livestock species such as cattle, swine, sheep, goats, chickens, turkeys, fish, and honeybees. Animal by-products (e.g. fur, skin, bone meal, manure, hooves, horns, blood, internal organs, and beeswax) are used extensively in hundreds of other products used by humans. Because the use of animal tissues in human foods and products is so widespread, great care must be taken to avoid residues caused by drug administration to animals. The FDA CVM is responsible for ensuring that drugs do not contaminate the human food supply and has clear rules for extra-label drug use and drug compounding for food-producing animal species. Contrary to the situation in companion animals, compounding of drugs for use in food animals is highly actionable by the FDA.

The FDA considers the major food-producing animal species to be cows, pigs, chickens, and turkeys; however, since any animal (except endangered species) may be consumed by humans as food, US Congress has never statutorily defined a food-producing animal by species, but instead by its intended use. For example, rabbits may be food-producing, pelt-producing, pets, or laboratory animals. Pigs may be either consumed as meat or kept as pets (e.g. potbellied and miniature pigs). Consequently, the intended use of any rabbit or pig must be carefully considered before drugs are administered. Drug distribution into tissues is an extensive area of scientific investigation in veterinary medicine, and depletion profiles of drugs from muscle, organs, blood, milk, and eggs are carefully characterized for drugs that are FDA approved for use in food-producing species. The time that must lapse after administration of the last dose until the food is safe to consume by humans is called a "withdrawal time" and is described thoroughly in Chapter 22. If a veterinarian deems it necessary to utilize a compounded drug product for a food animal, the veterinarian must ensure that there is no suitable FDA-approved product available for the treatment, that the desired drug class is not banned for use in a food-producing species, that no illegal drug residues occur, and that the owner of the animal is aware of the withdrawal time. Veterinarians may confirm that use of a compound is permissible by contacting the FDA for compassionate use (e.g. antidotes for poisoned livestock) and should indicate this to the pharmacist who will be preparing the compounded prescription.

Pharmacists filling prescriptions for animal patients must be aware of the intended use of the animal patient (pet, performance, or food-producing) and follow all regulations and guidance when providing drugs for animals intended for use as food. For example, if a pharmacist receives a prescription for a pet chicken, the pharmacist should look for an egg withdrawal time to be indicated on that prescription because even if the chicken is a pet, the owners are still likely to consume the eggs.

Certain drugs are prohibited from ELDU in any food animal species and must never be used to prepare compounds for food-producing animals. Chapter 22 describes these drugs in detail. Additionally, Chapter 22 provides resources available for pharmacists and veterinarians for determining withdrawal times following drug use in food-producing animals.

3.8 Compounding Controlled Substances

While compounding of controlled substances is permitted under federal compounding law, there are additional federal requirements that must be followed. In addition to FDA regulations, prescribing and dispensing must comply with Drug Enforcement Administration (DEA) rules and regulations and comply with all pertinent state controlled substances laws. It is strongly recommended that pharmacists familiarize themselves with these regulations to avoid violating DEA controlled substance laws. Pharmacies compounding controlled substances for office use must register with the DEA as a controlled substance manufacturer. Pharmacies compounding controlled substances for individual patients do not have to register with the DEA as a controlled substance manufacturer but *must dispense the product directly to the client and may not send the controlled substances to the veterinary practice for dispensing.* For example, a prescription for compounded tramadol oral suspension must be written for an individual patient and dispensed to that patient's owner. It may not be distributed to the prescribing veterinary practice for dispensing. If the compounded medication enters a practice (brought in by a client or prepared for office use) or is prepared in a practice (by practice personnel), it must be logged into appropriate controlled substance inventory and dispositioned from receipt to administration just as with DEA requirements for non-compounded controlled substances. Because of the combined influences of drug shortages and decreased production of opioids due to the opioid crisis, pharmacists are being requested to compound controlled

substances more and more frequently (e.g. morphine, methadone, fentanyl, hydromorphone, etc.). Community pharmacists who compound controlled substances for veterinarians and veterinary patients serve a valuable role in averting drug shortages and even more so by accurately communicating DEA requirements to veterinarians to help them avoid penalties and fines for noncompliance.

3.9 Quality Standards for Compounded Drugs

3.9.1 USP Compounding Standards

The USP is a private, science-driven, non-governmental standards-setting organization established in 1820 that develops and publishes enforceable quality standards for drugs, chemicals, foods, dietary supplements, and healthcare. USP standards are developed by committees of experts and undergo a period of public comment before they become officially adoptable and enforceable by state, federal, and organizational authorities (e.g. state boards of pharmacy, the FDA, and the Joint Commission). The USP develops enforceable standards but does not engage in any regulatory or enforcement activities itself. USP standards are called out in the Food, Drug, and Cosmetic Act (the FDC Act), and pharmaceutical manufacturers and compounders are required to abide by the USP's published standards in their respective jurisdictions.

USP standards take two overarching forms: monographs and general chapters. Monographs provide standards for identity, quality, purity, strength, packaging, and labeling for bulk substances, drug products, compounded preparations, and other ingredients that are used by the pharmaceutical industry and compounding practitioners. USP compounded preparation monographs are verified formulas and processes that allow compounders to prepare compounded drug preparations of known purity, strength, quality, and stability. They are named by the USP's nomenclature convention, which consists of *Generic Drug Name, Compounded, Dosage Form*, and *Veterinary* if for veterinary use only (e.g. "*Enrofloxacin, Compounded, Oral Suspension, Veterinary*"). Over 200 compounding monographs are currently available from the USP, and approximately 10% are earmarked for veterinary use. Pharmacists intending to compound drugs for veterinary use should have the applicable monographs readily available.

General chapter nomenclature is designated by a number in <brackets> next to the italicized *Name of the Chapter* (e.g. <797> *Pharmaceutical Compounding – Sterile Preparations*). General chapters numbered below <1000> are mandatory and enforceable by regulatory authorities (e.g. the FDA and Boards of Pharmacy). General chapters numbered greater than <1000> are interpretive and are intended to provide information on, give definition to, or describe best practices for a subject. If a below <1000> general chapter cites an above <1000> general chapter, the informational chapter may then become enforceable in that context. Mandatory general chapters typically describe general processes, methods, tests, assays, and other requirements that are applicable to the articles described in USP monographs, while informational chapters do not contain mandatory methods, tests, assays, or requirements. Table 3.1 describes the USP general chapters related to compounding. Table 3.2 lists examples of veterinary-use compounded preparation monographs.

USP standards are published in print and electronic compendia and are available by subscription. USP compendia include the *USP/NF*, which contains all currently official USP general chapters and monographs for drugs, excipients, and dietary supplements; the *USP Compounding Compendium*, which contains all general chapters and monographs relevant to compounding; the *Dietary Supplements Compendium*, which contains monographs, regulatory guidances, and reference tools relevant to the dietary

supplement supply chain; and the *Food Chemicals Codex*, which contains standards for identifying the quality, purity, and identity of food ingredients. USP also publishes other useful databases including the *Food Fraud Database*, which provides records of incidents, surveillance, and analytical methods that can be used to mitigate food fraud. See Table 3.3 for a summary of how each of the USP's compendia may be used by pharmacists preparing compounds for animals.

3.10 Component Considerations for Veterinary Patients

When using verified compounding formulas, pharmacists must use the ingredients listed in the monograph or peer-reviewed study. Although the FDA currently requires that only approved products be used as the starting ingredients for compounds for animals, many medically necessary therapies are not available as approved products (e.g. cisapride, bromide salts, diethylstilbestrol, and metronidazole benzoate). Even if available, the approved product is sometimes not appropriate for compounding (e.g. marbofloxacin powder must be used to compound aqueous marbofloxacin oral suspensions because the excipients in the approved tablets destabilize to a foul-smelling degradant within 24 hours of compounding) (Marbofloxacin, Compounded, Oral Suspension, Veterinary Monograph n.d.).

Species and breed differences in drug absorption, distribution, metabolism, and excretion (and, consequently, toxicological differences) are also important considerations for nonhuman compounding (Baggot 2001). Glomerular filtration rate, hepatic drug-metabolizing enzymes, protein transporters, and efflux pumps in nonhuman species and breeds vary widely. Understanding nonhuman drug disposition differences is critical to preparing compounds for animal species. Chapters 4 and 5, respectively,

Table 3.1 USP compounding general chapters.

General chapter	Subject matter	Legal status
<795> *Pharmaceutical Compounding – Nonsterile Preparations*	Standards and requirements for the compounding process, facilities, equipment, components, documentation, quality controls and training; standards for assigning BUDs	Enforceable
<797> *Pharmaceutical Compounding – Sterile Preparations*	Standards and requirements for responsibilities of compounding personnel, training, facilities, environmental monitoring, and storage and testing of finished preparations; standards for assigning BUDs	Enforceable
<800> *Hazardous Drugs – Handling in Healthcare Settings*	Standards and requirements for responsibilities of personnel handling hazardous drugs; facility and engineering controls; procedures for deactivating, decontaminating and cleaning; spill control; and documentation; applies to all healthcare personnel who receive, prepare, administer, transport, or otherwise come in contact with hazardous drugs and all the environments in which they are handled	Enforceable
<1160> *Pharmaceutical Calculations in Prescription Compounding*	Provides information for a variety of determinations, including quantities of ingredients, dosages, infusion rates, endotoxin load, stability, and expiration dates, and provides illustrative sample calculations	Informational
<1163> *Quality Assurance in Pharmaceutical Compounding*	Defines integrated components that should comprise a robust quality assurance program, including training; standard operating procedures; documentation; verification; testing; cleaning, disinfecting and safety; containers, packaging, repackaging, labeling and storage; outsourcing (if used); and responsible personnel	Informational
<1176> *Prescription Balances and Volumetric Apparatus Used in Compounding*	Describes tests for balances and guidance on selection of volumetric apparatuses (i.e. medicine droppers, dispensing bottles, syringes, pipets, and volumetric flasks)	Informational
<1168> *Compounding for Phase 1 Investigational Studies*	Describes considerations such as training, facilities, equipment and components, release testing, quality assurance, quality control, and documentation for compounding investigational preparations	Informational

discuss species and breed differences in drug disposition that pharmacists should be aware of.

For example, cats perform some, but not all, glucuronyl transferase conjugations inefficiently. Therefore, drugs, excipients, flavors, and dyes cleared by this mechanism can be toxic and are often deadly at very low doses in cats. Pharmacists should evaluate any drug, excipient, preservative, flavor, or dye carefully before using it to compound a preparation for a feline patient. Alcohols, benzoic acid derivatives, and azo dyes are particularly problematic. If a colored tracer (a colored powder added to inspect homogeneity visually) is required when triturating powders to compound capsules for cats, a naturally colored powder such as cyanocobalamin should be used instead of an artificially colored dye. It is also very important to note that cats groom themselves and other cats, so these same principles should also be applied to all topical therapies to prevent unintended systemic adverse effects from topically administered compounds.

Dogs are relatively deficient in the enzymes that acetylate drugs, and pharmacists should beware of this deficiency before compounding for dogs. Dogs also have significant genetic anomalies that predispose them to

Table 3.2 USP monographs for veterinary compounded preparations.

Currently official USP veterinary compounded preparation monographs
Atenolol Compounded Oral Suspension, Veterinary
Benazepril Hydrochloride Compounded Oral Suspension, Veterinary
Buprenorphine Compounded Buccal Solution, Veterinary
Cisapride Compounded Injection, Veterinary
Cisapride Compounded Oral Suspension, Veterinary
Cyclosporine Compounded Ophthalmic Solution, Veterinary
Doxycycline Compounded Oral Suspension, Veterinary
Enalapril Maleate Compounded Oral Suspension, Veterinary
Enrofloxacin Compounded Oral Suspension, Veterinary
Marbofloxacin Compounded Oral Suspension, Veterinary
Pergolide Compounded Oral Suspension, Veterinary
Potassium Bromide Compounded Oral Solution, Veterinary
Prednisolone Compounded Oral Suspension, Veterinary
Sodium Bromide Compounded Injection, Veterinary
Sodium Bromide Compounded Oral Solution, Veterinary
Spironolactone Compounded Oral Suspension, Veterinary
Tramadol Hydrochloride Compounded Oral Suspension, Veterinary
Voriconazole Compounded Ophthalmic Solution, Veterinary

Table 3.3 Examples of useful compounding information in USP's compendia.

Compendium	Contents	Example uses
USP/NF	Monographs for drug substances, products, dietary supplements, general chapters	Comparing the USP substance monograph for Cisapride to an accompanying certificate of analysis for bulk chemical cisapride powder to see if it complies
Compounding Compendium	Compounded preparation monographs, general chapters related to compounding	Using the Cisapride Compounded Oral Suspension, Veterinary monograph to prepare a prescription of cisapride for oral use in a cat
Dietary Supplements Compendium	Monographs for dietary supplements	Dietary supplements do not undergo the FDA approval process; monographs could be examined to determine standards for OTC dietary supplement products of milk thistle for a patient who requires hepatoprotection after mushroom ingestion.
Food Chemicals Codex	Monographs for food ingredients and general information tables useful in the food ingredient supply chain	Search the database to determine if any of the food dyes listed on a box of gelatin are azo dyes to use the gelatin to compound a medicated treat for a cat; determine the chemical nature of artificial strawberry flavoring (aldehyde).

Table 3.4 Toxicity of select substances and foods by species.

Substance or food	Species affected	Toxicity
Alcohols	Dogs, cats, birds	Central nervous system toxicity/depression
Avocado	Birds	Pulmonary congestion, nonsuppurative inflammation of the liver, kidney, pancreas, skin, and proventriculus
Azo dyes	Cats	Hemolytic anemia, Heinz body formation
Benzocaine, benzoic acid derivatives	Cats	Red blood cell oxidative injury, hemolytic anemia
Chocolate	Dogs, birds	Cardiovascular and central nervous system stimulation
Cremophor	Dogs	Histamine release, anaphylaxis
Fat, high-fat foods	Dogs	Increased risk of pancreatitis
Garlic, onions	Dogs, cats	Hemolytic anemia, Heinz body formation
Grapes, raisins	Dogs	Renal toxicity
Macadamia nuts	Dogs	Lethargy, hyperthermia, ataxia, vomiting
Pennyroyal oil	Cats	Hepatotoxicity
Polysorbate 80	Dogs	Histamine release, anaphylaxis
Propylene glycol	Cats	Hemolytic anemia and Heinz body formation from concentrations >5–10%
Yeast, raw yeast dough	Dogs	Alcohol poisoning, gastrointestinal dilatation and volvulus
Xylitol	Dogs, birds	Profound hypoglycemia and hepatocellular necrosis

unique toxicities. While the artificial sweetener xylitol is generally recognized as safe in most species, it is rapidly and completely absorbed across the gastrointestinal–blood barrier in dogs. In dogs, the pancreas reacts to xylitol as it does to glucose, by releasing insulin resulting in profound, often fatal, hypoglycemia. Chronic xylitol exposure can also cause severe hepatic necrosis in dogs (Piscitelli et al. 2010). Many drugs approved for use in humans contain xylitol as an inactive ingredient, and pharmacists may receive prescriptions for xylitol-free compounded preparations of commercially available drugs, such as gabapentin (Neurontin˚) oral solution, which contains xylitol (Pfizer 2009). Canine mast cells are reactive to surfactants and preservatives commonly used in human drugs (e.g. polysorbate 80 and Cremophor EL), and their use in dogs can result in serious, life-threatening anaphylactic reactions (Lorenz et al. 1977; Varma et al. 1985). While

a comprehensive discussion of species-specific metabolic differences is beyond the scope of this activity (see Chapter 4), Table 3.4 illustrates excipients, flavors, preservatives, and dyes that should be avoided in select species.

Dietary and behavioral considerations are also important when providing safe, palatable, compounded drugs for veterinary patients. Animal flavor preferences correlate strongly with their natural diets. For example, cats are obligate carnivores (i.e. they depend on the nutrients found only in animal flesh for their survival), typically preying on small rodent species, birds, and fish. They are relatively uninterested in flavors associated with carbohydrates (e.g. sweet or aromatic). Cats' tongues lack sweet taste receptors (Li et al. 2006) and primarily prefer meat-based or organ flavors, such as tuna, salmon, chicken, or liver. Dogs evolved with a more omnivorous dietary habit after preying on species with large quantities of herbivorous matter in their gastrointestinal tracts. As a result, dogs have a wider spectrum of flavor preferences, including sweet, salty, and meat-based flavors.

Birds' wide variety of flavor and texture preferences are related to their species and natural diets. Herbivorous and omnivorous birds, such as caged birds and poultry, often prefer color and movement over flavor and texture (GamberaleStille and Tullberg 2001). For example, chickens usually prefer a colorful, wiggly medicated gummy worm offered by hand over a flavored, colorless, oral suspension delivered from an oral syringe.

Horses' carbohydrate-rich diets lead them to prefer sweet and aromatic flavors. Horses select food based on visual cues, odor, taste, texture, availability, and variety. A flavor-preference study performed at the University of Southampton identified some surprising favorite flavors for horses, with the top-ranked favorite being fenugreek (a spice with a maple fragrance and bitter-to-sweet taste) (Goodwin et al. 2005).

Comprehensive reviews of animal taste preferences have been published for companion animals (Thombre 2004; Koppel 2014). Table 3.5 describes flavor preferences by species; however, the pharmacist should always consult the animal's caregiver to confirm which flavors are most likely to be accepted.

Table 3.5 Species differences in flavor preferences.

Species	Preference
Cat	Meat, organ meat, fish
Dog	Meat, salty, sweet
Horse	Sweet, fruit, aromatic herbs/grasses
Bird	Dietary dependent
Cow	Sweet, aromatic herbs/grasses
Rabbit	Herb, vegetable, sweet
Pig	Sweet, fruit, vegetable
Ferret	Meat, fish, sweet
Reptile	Dietary dependent

Finally, pharmacists must consider impact on drug stability and bioavailability when adding flavors to compounds. Before including flavoring agents in compounded preparations, pharmacists should ensure that it does not alter drug bioavailability or activity by changing pH, altering solubility or suspendibility, or binding to or chelating active ingredients.

3.11 Sourcing Verified Formulas for Compounds

While many verified and peer-reviewed formulas are available for compounded dosage forms intended for humans, these formulas may be inappropriate for use in veterinary species. As mentioned, the USP has developed many verified compounded preparation formulas specifically for veterinary use. Many of the almost 200 USP-developed compounded preparations not specified for veterinary use may also be appropriate for animal patients if species- and patient-specific criteria are used to evaluate them appropriately.

When a USP formula monograph is unavailable, drug manufacturers may sometimes provide extemporaneous compounding information for their products; however, this information is rarely available, and manufacturers – concerned about liability – are often unwilling to share this information. Pharmacists can locate other compounding formulas by searching secondary-source collections of published peer-reviewed compounded preparation stability studies (Trissel and American Pharmacists Association 2012), again with the caveat that they must review species-specific considerations for each component used. If peer-reviewed evidence cannot be located in secondary resources, a search of primary peer-reviewed literature may reveal a stability-tested formula suitable for use in animal patients. The *International Journal of Pharmaceutical Compounding* is a bimonthly scientific and

Table 3.6 USP <795> Default beyond-use dates for nonsterile compounds.

Type of Preparation	BUDs (days)	Storage Temperature
Non-preserved aqueous dosage forms[a]	14	Refrigerator
Preserved aqueous dosage forms[a]	30	Controlled room temperature or refrigerator
Nonaqueous dosage forms[b]	90	Controlled room temperature or refrigerator
Solid dosage forms[c]	180	Controlled room temperature or refrigerator

[a] An aqueous preparation is one that has a water activity (Aw) of > 0.6 (e.g., emulsions, gels, creams, solutions, sprays, or suspensions). See USP – *Application of Water Activity Determination to Nonsterile Pharmaceutical Products <1112>*.
[b] Any preparation other than solid dosage forms that have a reduced Aw of ≤ 0.6 (e.g., suppositories, ointments, fixed oils, or waxes).
[c] Capsules, tablets, granules, powders.

professional journal that frequently features stability-tested formulas for veterinary compounds (International Journal of Pharmaceutical Compounding [IJPC] n.d.).

When no evidence is available to support stability and ingredient compatibility for a compounded preparation, pharmacists should apply USP compounding defaults. They must consider the active drug's inherent stability, the suitability of components for the target patient/species, the and potential adverse effects if the compound is not stable throughout the labeled beyond-use date (BUD) and intended therapy period. USP default BUDs for nonsterile compounds are listed in Table 3.6. An illustrative example for applying USP defaults to a non-evidence-based compounded preparation for animals follows in Table 3.6.

In all situations, pharmacists should counsel veterinarians and pet owners about the limitations of the compounded preparation with respect to stability, bioavailability, and potential risks to the patient.

3.12 Compounded Veterinary Dosage Forms and Compounding Techniques

Regarding compounding drugs for veterinary patients, most prescriptions presented to community pharmacists by the animal's caregiver will be for simple, nonsterile drug preparations. The compounded drug requested will often have evidence-based formulas and usually involve making oral liquids, capsules, medicated treats, or transdermal gels. Less often, community pharmacists will be asked to perform complex nonsterile compounding (e.g. preparing core-coated targeted-release tablets). A discussion of considerations for the most commonly prescribed compounded dosage forms for use in animals is presented in the remainder of this section.

3.12.1 Oral Suspensions

The most commonly compounded drug preparations for animal patients are oral liquids. This dosage form allows concentration or dilution of strength, as compared to the FDA-approved products, and allows flexible dose adjustment necessitated by growth or desired therapeutic effect. Many cat, horse, and exotic animal pet owners also prefer oral liquids as they are easier to administer than other forms. Oral suspensions are more commonly prepared than oral solutions. When compounding oral suspensions, pharmacists must consider two critical factors about drugs' particle size in suspension (from active pharmaceutical ingredients [APIs] or FDA-approved product tablets or capsules): (i) Particle size should be small enough to keep the drug sufficiently suspended to allow caregivers to withdraw uniform doses; and

Table 3.7 Compounding oral suspensions.

Directions for compounding oral suspensions for veterinary patients
1) Comminute (grind) dry ingredients to a fine, uniform powder in a mortar and pestle.
2) Wet the powder with the smallest volume of vehicle to accomplish a thick paste (too much liquid at this point defeats the high shear necessary to reduce particle size further and completely wet the powder).
3) Geometrically add vehicle and triturate to a pourable liquid.
4) Add any flavoring at this point.
5) Transfer the pourable liquid to a calibrated dispensing container.
6) Rinse the mortar with vehicle, and bring forward to the dispensing container to bring to final volume.
7) Shake well before dispensing.
8) Affix appropriate labels and auxiliary labels (Appendix D).

(ii) particle size should not be so small that it settles on the bottom of the container and forms a hard, nondispersible cake (United States Pharmacopeial Convention 2015). Appropriate vehicle viscosity is critical. Aqueous vehicles such as methylcellulose or simple syrup are usually employed and are frequently listed in USP compounded preparation monographs as *Vehicle, NF* or *Syrup, NF*, respectively. Commercially available suspending vehicles containing methylcellulose and preservative systems are available (e.g. OraBlend˚ and SyrSpend®) in both sweetened and sugar-free presentations. Anhydrous vehicles include *Corn oil, NF* and *Cod liver oil, NF*. Silica gel can be used as a suspending agent. Note that silica gel should be avoided in animals with a propensity to develop silicate uroliths, a condition that can be confirmed with the prescriber prior to compounding. When selecting a suspending vehicle, pharmacists should ensure appropriateness of all ingredients in the suspending vehicle for use in the target species. For example, Simple Syrup, NF is often preserved with benzoic acid derivatives, which may not be appropriate for chronic administration to cats as they inefficiently metabolize these substances. Pharmacists should also assess pH of the vehicle, vehicle compatibility with drug (e.g. does not contain divalent cations when compounding fluoroquinolones), excipient compatibility with drug, and container

compatibility with drug if a verified evidence-based formula is not available. The preparation of oral suspensions is generally accomplished by the steps listed in Table 3.7.

3.12.2 Oral Pastes

As mentioned in Chapter 1, veterinarians almost always classify pastes as oral dosage forms and rarely administer them topically. Oral pastes are moderately complex nonsterile dosage forms. Veterinarians frequently prescribe them for horses or other animals where a high viscosity is desired (to keep the drug from running back out of a patient's mouth), but dosing flexibility is still required. Pharmacists compound pastes using a process almost identical to that for oral suspensions. However, the suspending vehicle's viscosity must be high enough to prevent drug settling, and the pharmacist must ensure that the drug remains completely suspended in the vehicle before dispensing because pastes are too viscous to allow shaking to resuspend. Anhydrous paste bases include various concentrations of polyethylene bases, and aqueous bases are generally made from high concentrations (4–5%) of methylcellulose. Pastes are generally dispensed in single-dose oral syringes, or in multiple-dose, calibrated syringes that may or may not have a dial to control the amount of paste delivered (Figure 3.2).

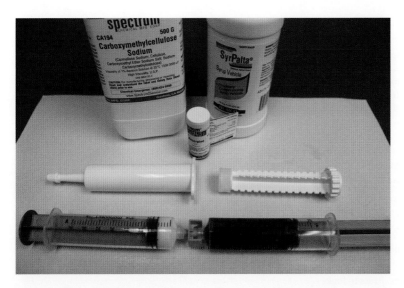

Figure 3.2 Compounding an oral paste to dispense in a "Dial-A-Dose" syringe that is typically used for administering drugs orally to horses.

3.12.3 Oral Capsules

Compounding oral capsules is generally considered to be of moderate complexity. However, once the pharmacist creates a Master Formulation Record that can be followed exactly with no calculations and no calibrations, then compounded capsules can be prepared by qualified nonpharmacist personnel. Compounded capsules offer significant advantages over liquid dosage forms as they contain an exact dose, and pet owners have fewer measuring tasks than with liquids or pastes. Capsules also may contain powders or liquids, and since they can be sealed and locked, they may mask the taste of drugs that animals find unpalatable. Caregivers may also open capsules and sprinkle the contents on moist food or mix them with a small amount of palatable compatible liquid in an oral-dosing syringe immediately before administration. The USP default stability BUD for capsules is 180 days or the manufacturer's API expiration date, whichever is shorter, so capsules are ideal for chronic conditions that require only occasional follow-up appointments with the prescribing veterinarian. Capsules are available in many

inert and dissolvable materials (e.g. gelatin and vegetable cellulose) and colors, making them pharmaceutically elegant and appealing to pet owners. Pharmacists can prepare capsules from approved solid dosage forms (tablets or capsules) or API powders if approved products are not available or are inappropriate for compounding. Instead of a liquid vehicle, the diluent vehicle is usually an inert powder such as *Lactose, USP* or *Hypromellose, USP*. For capsules that will be opened by pet owners and sprinkled on the pet's food, pharmacists can comminute finely ground dried kibble (pet food) to a fine powder and use it as the capsule diluent (provided the drug is compatible with ingredients in the kibble). The typical procedure for compounding capsules is explained in Table 3.8 (see also Figure 3.3).

3.12.4 Medicated Treats

Many FDA-approved veterinary medications are available in chewable tablet forms. Because pets tend to like them, pet owners and veterinarians often ask pharmacists to prepare a similar dosage form when

Table 3.8 Compounding capsules.

Directions for compounding oral capsules for veterinary patients

1) Calculate the total amount of active ingredient required using commercially available tablets, capsules, or API powder. Remember to account for any inert ingredients in starting tablets or capsules, and waters of hydration, salt forms, and percentage strength from the certificate of analysis for API powders.

2) Calculate total amount of diluent powder required to mix with active drug ingredients to ensure that the finished weight completely occupies the calibrated volume of the empty capsule. *Note:* If a colored tracer is used to estimate uniform mixing, cyanocobalamin powder (magenta color and nontoxic) should be used and the amount used accounted for.

3) Working in a powder hood with appropriate protective clothing, weigh all calculated components, and place in mortar using geometric dilution of API powders with excipients.

4) Comminute (grind) dry ingredients into a uniformly fine particle size.

5) Using a capsule machine or packing individually by hand, fill the long end of each capsule to the calibrated capacity.

6) Replace the capsule tops. Press to lock.

7) Weigh at least 20 capsules or 10% of the final number of capsules (whichever is less) to ensure that they are within ±10% of the target filled-capsule weight range, remembering to account for the weight of the empty capsule before it was filled.

8) Capsules should be dispensed in light- and moisture-resistant childproof containers, and pet owners instructed to store capsules at controlled room temperature (or under refrigeration if required for the active drug) out of the reach of pets and children.

9) Affix appropriate labels and auxiliary labels (Appendix D).

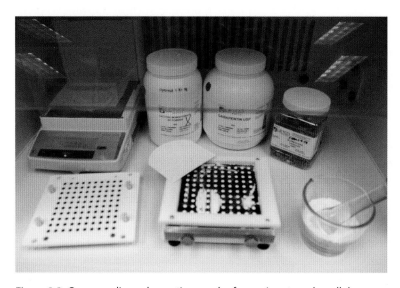

Figure 3.3 Compounding gabapentin capsules for use in cats and small dogs.

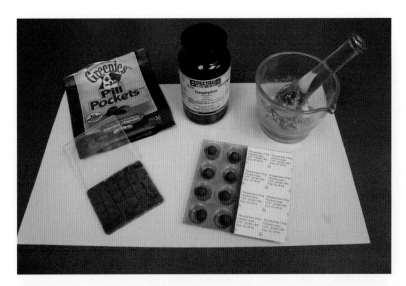

Figure 3.4 Compounded medicated "treats" (flavored chewables), troche mold, and blister packaging.

compounded medications are needed (Figure 3.4). Medicated chewable treats are commonly requested for dogs, cats, and horses, and frequently exotic animal patients as well. Medicated treat bases may be prepared using semimoist pet treats as the base, or by mixing glycerin, gelatin, and polyethylene base with flavors that the pet prefers. Pharmacists prepare medicated treats similarly to capsules. They use a mold of known calibrated final weight (similar to the known calibrated final weight of an empty capsule) and an appropriate ratio of drug-to-treat base to achieve the desired final dose. Used less often, another method is to calibrate the weight of a punched shape (e.g. like a cookie cutter) cut from a sheet of treat base rolled to a uniform thickness and performed with calculations similar to the molded treat process. It is important to note that many semimoist treats marketed for dogs contain propylene glycol. Propylene glycol has been banned for

Table 3.9 Compounding medicated treats.

Directions for compounding medicated treats for veterinary patients

---

1) Calculate the total amount of active ingredient required using commercially available tablets, capsules, or API powder. Remember to account for any inert ingredients in starting tablets or capsules, and waters of hydration, salt forms, and percentage strength from the certificate of analysis for API powders. *Note:* If a colored tracer is used to estimate uniform mixing, cyanocobalamin powder (magenta color and nontoxic) should be used and the amount used accounted for.

2) Calculate the total amount of treat base required to mix with active drug ingredients to achieve the total weight of the calibrated mold or cutout.

3) Working in a powder hood with appropriate protective clothing, weigh all calculated components, and place in mortar.

4) Comminute (grind) ingredients into a uniformly mixed dough.

5) Using a treat mold, fill each mold evenly to capacity, or roll out dough uniformly and cut to appropriate size.

6) Weigh at least 10% of the final number of treats to ensure that they are within ±10% of the target weight range.

7) Affix appropriate labels and auxiliary labels (Appendix D).

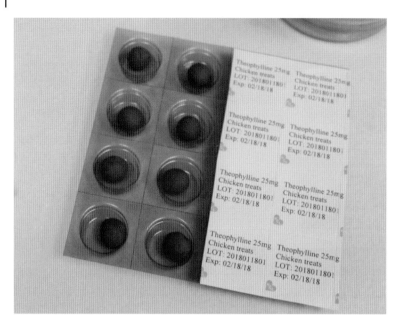

Figure 3.5 Unit dose blister packaging of individual doses of compounded theophylline "treats" or flavored chewables. Moisture loss changes the texture of the treat, and many pets will reject treats if this occurs; therefore, appropriate packaging is necessary.

addition to cat food or treats since 1996, as concentrations of 5–10% propylene glycol have caused Heinz body anemia in cats (Christopher et al. 1989). Medicated chewable treats are ideally packaged in closed troche molds or in individual blister packs to prevent exposure to mold and moisture loss. Moisture loss changes the texture of the treat, and many pets will reject treats if this occurs. The procedure for compounding medicated treats is illustrated in Table 3.9.

Medicated treat compounds are ideally individually packaged into blister-type unit doses to preserve taste, texture, and stability, and to deter unintended mass ingestion of medicated treats by pets. Blister packaging and labeling systems are widely available from various healthcare suppliers. See Figure 3.5.

3.12.5 Transdermal Gels

Transdermal gels are included in the complex category of nonsterile compounding. They are formulated in penetration-enhancing percutaneous vehicles (e.g. pluronic-lecithin-organogel [PLO] or Lipoderm®) intended to achieve systemic bioavailability after topical application to intact skin. The drug's molecular weight (ideally 300 Da or less), therapeutic index, lipid solubility, target plasma concentration, human caregiver sensitivity, and likelihood of causing local irritation are all important factors in considering a drug for transdermal administration. Veterinary transdermal gels are used most often in cats, because they are notoriously difficult to medicate orally. The most common application site is the hairless pinna inside the cat's ear (Davidson 2001). To accomplish transdermal penetration, drugs are usually compounded in concentrations that deliver doses in volumes of 0.1–0.2 mL. For example, methimazole transdermal gel is compounded in a concentration of 50 milligrams (mg) per mL to allow delivery of 5 mg in 0.1 mL.

Veterinarians will frequently consult compounding pharmacists for advice as to whether a drug is a good candidate for transdermal administration. While a comprehensive discussion of the use of transdermal gels in veterinary medicine is beyond the scope of this chapter, note that drugs with narrow therapeutic indices, drugs with known safety issues for humans, and drugs that are listed as contact irritants in the Material Safety Data Sheet are generally considered inappropriate candidates for transdermal administration. Figure 3.6 illustrates chemical burns caused by transdermal application of fluoxetine to a feline patient.

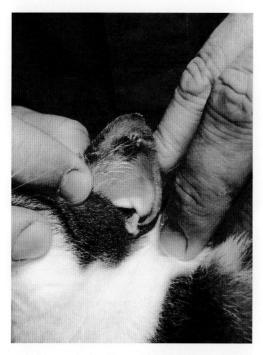

Figure 3.6 Chemical burns of the inner pinna caused by transdermal administration of fluoxetine to a cat.

> **Mandatory monitoring**
>
> Pharmacists should advise pet owners that transdermal drugs may cause inflammation or contact irritation. Pet owners should monitor for this potential adverse reaction and cease applying the transdermal product should this occur. Ample evidence exists demonstrating incomplete or erratic absorption of transdermally administered drugs, and drug administration by the transdermal route is considered a therapy of last resort. Transdermal gels are generally prepared as shown in Table 3.10.

Unless data on the specific drug and vehicle are available, pharmacists should counsel veterinarians and pet owners that bioavailability may be inadequate to attain sufficient drug concentrations in the patient with this compounded formulation. For example, antimicrobials should never be applied transdermally because even if they are completely absorbed, the time to achieve an effective inhibitory concentration in the blood or infected tissue may take days, during which time the risk for antimicrobial resistance is increased. Likewise, drugs that exert their effects by achieving serum concentrations in mg/mL are not as likely to achieve those concentrations as drugs that exert their effects in serum concentrations of nanograms (ng)/mL.

Transdermal gels are typically dispensed in 1 mL amber dosing syringes with 0.1 mL calibration marks, so each syringe contains

Table 3.10 Compounding transdermal gels.

Directions for compounding transdermal gels for veterinary patients

---

1) Weigh or measure the appropriate amount of API powder required to prepare the prescribed volume of the transdermal gel.

2) In a suitable container (syringe or mortar), wet the API with a suitable solvent, such as diethylene glycol, to a smooth paste.

3) Add the appropriate percutaneous penetration-enhancing vehicle (e.g. lecithin–isopropyl palmitate solution and Pluronic F127 [PLO] or Lipoderm® Base) to volume.

4) Mix using a shearing action by using an ointment mill or with a sufficient number of syringe-to-syringe transfers to accomplish uniform mixing.

5) Affix appropriate labels and auxiliary labels (Appendix D).

---

approximately 10 doses. Twist-and-click delivery systems are available for delivery of transdermal gels, but these administration devices must be calibrated carefully to ensure uniform dose delivery. Since transdermal drugs do not discriminate between patient skin and caregiver skin, pharmacists should counsel caregivers to use protective gloves or finger cots when applying transdermal medications and to wash hands thoroughly after.

3.13 Quality Assurance for Compounded Drugs

USP compounded preparation monographs provide exact instructions for mixing exact quantities of known substances to produce a compound of known purity, identity, quality, and strength over the designated BUD. To ensure that the preparation maintains these characteristics, USP compounded preparation monographs require specific tests for pharmacists to perform for each finished compound. Tests to determine pH, content uniformity of dosage units, endotoxin and sterility testing, and so on all provide quality assurance for finished compounds and allow the compounder to assign the BUD in the monograph. For those compounds that do not have a USP compounded preparation monograph, the same tests can be performed to determine compound quality. Extending the BUD for a nonmonographed compound beyond USP defaults requires consideration of five types of stability: chemical, physical, microbiological, therapeutic, and toxicological. Chemical, physical, and toxicological stability can only truly be determined by stability-indicating methods. Stability-indicating methods impose forced degradation of a compound (chemical, thermal, UV light, and acid/base/peroxide exposure) to identify degradant products and impurities. Stability-indicating assays are not the same as strength-over-time (potency) studies. Strength-over-time does not detect or distinguish quantities of degradants or impurities. Figures 3.7 and 3.8 illustrate the difference between a stability-indicating chromatogram and a strength-over-time chromatogram, respectively (Kupiec et al. 2008). Pharmacists may also consult peer-reviewed stability-indicating studies when extending BUDs past USP defaults if the ingredients, process, and container are the same as those used in the study. It is important for pharmacists to understand method suitability when extending BUDs beyond USP defaults.

3.14 Animal-Friendly Dispensing and Administration Devices for Compounded Drugs

Oral liquids for humans are often labeled and dosed in concentrations that reflect imperial system spoon measurements (e.g. teaspoonfuls and tablespoonfuls). While imperial units may be useful for dosing human patients when pouring liquid doses into a spoon, they are impractical for dosing animal patients who do not ingest medications or foods in this manner. Animal patients also vary greatly in size, making spoon measurements even less relevant when delivering accurate doses for very small or very large animals. For this reason, compounded veterinary liquid drug formulations should be dispensed with oral-dosing syringes and special adapter caps or inserts to allow liquids to be removed accurately and cleanly. Oral-dosing syringes resemble injectable syringes in all aspects with the exception that the hub is too large to accept standard hypodermic needles. This will prevent accidental injection of oral medications by owners who may be administering multiple medications by multiple routes. The hub of an oral-dosing syringe is inserted into the adapter cap aperture, the bottle inverted, and liquid withdrawn to the desired dosing mark. Figure 3.9 demonstrates this procedure. Pharmacists can wrap "dose mark" auxiliary labels around the oral-dosing syringe, clearly indicating the intended dose

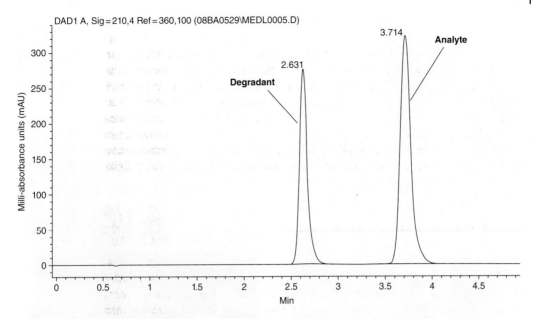

Figure 3.7 An example chromatogram of a stability-indicating high-performance liquid chromatography (HPLC) method that evaluates the analyte and degradant peaks that are fully resolved from one another.

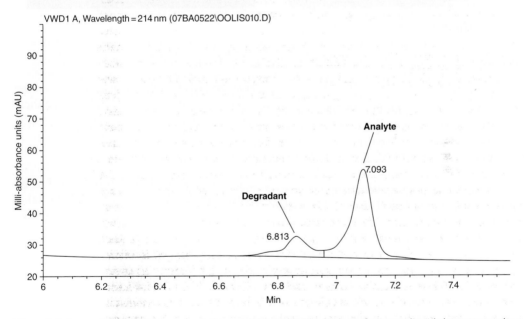

Figure 3.8 An example chromatogram of a non-stability-indicating high-performance liquid chromatography (HPLC) method that evaluates the analyte and degradant peaks that are not fully resolved from one another.

with a black line. Adapter caps, button inserts, dose mark auxiliary labels, and oral syringes are widely available from human healthcare suppliers.

The viscosity of a liquid formulation must also be taken into consideration when dispensing medications to pet owners. For oil-based formulations, screw-on adapter caps

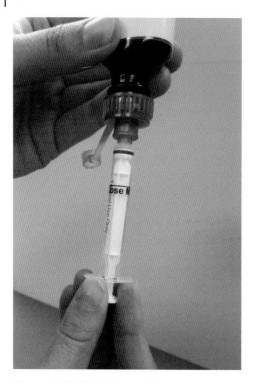

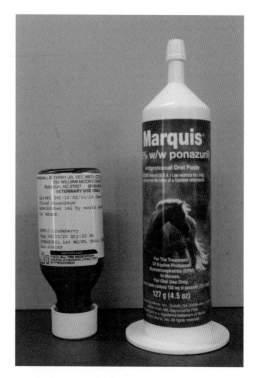

Figure 3.9 The hub of an oral-dosing syringe is inserted into the adapter cap aperture, the bottle inverted, and the liquid medication withdrawn to the indicated dosing mark.

Figure 3.10 Ponazuril paste in dispensing bottle labeled "upside down" to allow for easier removal of drug from the container.

are more secure, as the button-type inserts can easily be pushed down into the bottle once lubricated by the oil vehicle. Button-type inserts are more appropriate for aqueous vehicles. Extremely viscous liquids that adhere to the sides of the dispensing bottle (e.g. atovaquone or ponazuril paste) are best labeled to encourage the owner to store the medication with the top down. This will allow for only a quick inversion to remove the lid without disturbing the medication, which has settled near the dispensing adapter. Affixing the label upside down on the container will allow the owner to read instructions without having to invert the bottle (see Figure 3.10).

Prescription labels are often too small to accommodate all information necessary for safe and accurate drug administration by pet owners. For this reason, auxiliary labels are affixed directly to either the prescription container or external packaging. Hundreds of

auxiliary labels are available for dispensing medication for human use, and many of these are appropriate for use with veterinary prescriptions (e.g. Shake Well, Keep in Refrigerator, Keep out of Reach of Children, and For External Use Only). Some veterinary-specific auxiliary labels are also available (e.g. Do Not Use on Cats, and Veterinary Use Only). In other instances, a word-processing program and blank labels can be used to create customized and drug-specific auxiliary labels. A comprehensive list of auxiliary labels cross-referenced by drug can be found in Appendix D.

3.15 Owner Counseling Points for Compounded Veterinary Drugs

Pet owners are often distracted when picking up medications from a pharmacy and are anxious to get back to their pets who are

Table 3.11 Counseling points for compounded drugs in veterinary patients.

10 Essential counseling points for pet owners when dispensing compounded drug formulations[a]
1) Emphasize that the medication is a compounded preparation, and provide its limitations compared to an FDA-approved product.
2) Review drug name, indication, and route of administration.
3) Review frequency of administration, and duration of therapy.
4) Demonstrate administration devices and accurate dose markings for each drug.
5) Discuss storage and handling of medication, including any caregiver precautions.
6) Describe proper disposal of unused compounded drug.
7) Emphasize observation of compounded drug for any change in physical characteristics (color, consistency, or odor) or pet refusal to take compounded drug after initial acceptance.
8) Inform the caregiver of any drugs or foods to avoid, and remind them to check for any performance drug rules for animal athletes (Chapter 24).
9) Emphasize the importance of returning to the veterinarian for recheck appointment.
10) Describe monitoring signs for efficacy (or lack thereof) and toxicity (including allergic reactions), and advise to contact the veterinarian immediately if noticed.

[a] More detailed information about counseling the pet owner is provided in Chapter 25.

either waiting in the car or at home. Distraction can be even greater for pet owners who have brought their pets into the pharmacy to pick up medications. Since they are not evaluated for safety and efficacy by the FDA, compounded drugs require additional counseling to educate pet owners to observe for any adverse effects that may be caused by changes in the compounded drug's quality – and this includes lack of efficacy. For this reason, it is very important for pharmacists to learn to deliver quick and effective verbal counseling and to provide written client education handouts for pet owners to review when they are less distracted at home. Table 3.11 summarizes 10 counseling points essential to patient well-being and therapeutic success. Chapter 25 includes more detailed information about counseling.

Client educational veterinary medical guides are available from numerous sources and describe topics such as drug information, drug administration techniques, poisonous substances, as well as management of several common disease states.

3.16 Adverse Event Reporting for Compounded Drugs

Community pharmacists are often the first healthcare providers to recognize or suspect adverse drug events related to compounded drugs. As a result, community pharmacists can play a valuable role in collecting, investigating, and reporting this valuable information to the prescribing veterinarian and/or the FDA Adverse Event Reporting System.

Adverse events resulting from compounded drugs are often caused by poor compound quality and may manifest as lack of expected therapeutic response (e.g. from subpotent, unstable, or non-bioavailable compounds), a new unexpected symptom or behavior (e.g. rash, swelling, hypersalivation, sneezing, vomiting, or diarrhea), or symptoms of toxicity (e.g. from superpotent compounds or species-specific toxic excipients). Veterinarians may not associate new or worsening clinical signs with defects in compounded drug quality, so community pharmacists should carefully investigate the compounding records and formulation to determine whether the adverse events may be due to poor quality. Poor compounded-drug quality has sometimes perpetuated myths of inefficacy for drugs that were not stable or were not prepared correctly. For example, when the human drug pergolide was withdrawn from the market for safety reasons, veterinarians treating equine pituitary pars dysfunction were forced to use compounded forms of pergolide. Pharmacists commonly provided this drug as an oral suspension and assigned inappropriately long beyond-use dates. Many horses relapsed after one to two months of treatment with compounded pergolide despite receiving steadily increasing doses. As a result, veterinarians assumed that these horses were refractory to pergolide and switched to other therapeutic agents. such as cyproheptadine. A stability study for compounded pergolide suspension was published demonstrating that pergolide suspensions are stable for only 30–35 days and must be stored in the refrigerator protected from light (Davis et al. 2009). Only after this study was published did veterinarians realize that their patients were not refractory to pergolide but rather were being treated with a compounded preparation that contained little to no active pergolide due to an inappropriately labeled preparation.

Unlike pharmaceutical manufacturers who must report adverse events, adverse event reporting by veterinarians is voluntary. The FDA's voluntary adverse event reporting form, the *Veterinary Adverse Drug Reaction, Lack of Effectiveness, or Product Defect Report* (Form 1932a), is a complex five-page report designed for adverse event reporting for FDA-approved products. Form 1932a does not include a prompt to determine if the adverse drug event was due to a compounded preparation, and the form is too sophisticated for most pet owners to be able to complete; however, community pharmacists should easily be able to complete the form with the prescribing veterinarian's assistance. The FDA's adverse drug event reporting system for animals is not aggregated or comprehensive, and it is currently being revised. Since 2001, only 62 adverse events related to compounded drug products in animals have been reported to the FDA. The wealth of information regarding reported adverse events from veterinary compounded drugs is likely with state boards of pharmacy. However, various privacy and confidentiality laws in the states prevent boards of pharmacy from sharing this information, even if they collect adverse events from compounded drugs in animal patients. The community pharmacist is often the first healthcare provider to learn of or suspect adverse events associated with use of a compounded drug, and as such they have a responsibility to collect and report this valuable information to the FDA's database. FDA Form 1932a can be found in Appendix E.

3.17 Veterinary Compounding Training Opportunities

Pharmacists desiring to acquire training in compounding for veterinary patients should consider several factors when selecting a program. One of the most important factors to consider are the credentials of the instructors. Do they possess expertise in compounding techniques as well as in veterinary pharmacotherapy? Credentials for expertise in veterinary pharmacotherapy were discussed in Chapter 1. Regarding compounding expertise, there is currently no Board of Pharmaceutical Specialties–recognized specialty for pharmacy compounding, nor any other credentialing programs that lead to diplomate status in a compounding specialty college. Factors to consider regarding compounding expertise include: academic training in pharmaceutical compounding (e.g. faculty members teaching compounding in pharmacy schools) or accreditation status in a compounding accreditation organization (e.g. the Pharmacy Compounding Accreditation Board). While many instructors have been preparing veterinary compounds for years, this does not necessarily provide assurance of expertise. Another factor to consider is whether the training is evidence based, and if not, does the program teach the candidate to search for and evaluate evidence to support the quality and stability of a compound? Other factors to consider are the advertised focus of the training program. Does the program put primary emphasis on using veterinary compounding to promote financial gain? Or does the program state an objective to improve patient outcomes through evidence-based quality compounding? Does the program include material on state and federal veterinary compounding regulations? Finally, any veterinary compounding training program should offer training in critical evaluation of novel compounded veterinary dosage forms, such as medicated treats, transdermal gels, antibiotic-impregnated implants, and long-acting or targeted delivery systems, and whether use of each dosage form is appropriate in a given patient.

3.18 Summary

Pharmacists are expected by society to provide the same level of expertise in preparing compounds for animal patients as they do when compounding for human patients. Pharmacists who prepare compounds for nonhumans should be thoroughly familiar with regulatory boundaries for use of drugs in animals as well as knowledgeable of all the unique tolerances and toxicities for individual species and breeds. Best practices and national standards should always be followed when compounding for animal patients, and great care should be taken in finding verified compounding formulas and selecting high-quality, species-appropriate compounding components. Finally, to maintain confidence and competence in preparing compounds for veterinary patients, pharmacists must keep abreast of changes in veterinary drug laws and stay informed regarding new therapeutic trends in veterinary medicine.

References

Agelova, J. and Maceskova, B. (2005). Analysis of drugs used in out-patient practice of veterinary medicine. *Ceska Slova. Farm.* 54: 34–38.

AVMA. (2017). Veterinary compounding. https://www.avma.org/KB/Policies/Pages/Compounding.aspx.

Baggot, J.D. (2001). *The Physiological Basis of Veterinary Clinical Pharmacology*. Malden, MA: Blackwell.

Belainesh, D., Maldonado, G., and Reid, H. (2011). Acute selenium toxicosis in polo ponies. *J. Vet. Diagn. Investig.* 23: 623–628.

Bennett, N., Papich, M.G., Hoenig, M. et al. (2005). Evaluation of transdermal application of glipizide in a pluronic lecithin gel to healthy cats. *Am. J. Vet. Res.* 66: 581–588.

Centers for Disease Control and Prevention (CDC) (2012). Multistate outbreak of fungal infection associated with injection of methylprednisolone acetate solution from a single compounding pharmacy: United States, 2012. *MMWR Morb. Mortal. Wkly Rep.* 61: 839–842.

Christopher, M.M., Perman, V., and Eaton, J.W. (1989). Contribution of propylene glycolinduced Heinz body formation to anemia in cats. *J. Am. Vet. Med. Assoc.* 194 (8): 1045–1056.

Ciribassi, J., Luescher, A., Pasloske, K.S. et al. (2003). *Am. J. Vet. Res.* 64: 994–998.

Cook, A.K., Nieuwoudt, C.D., and Longhofer, S.L. (2012). Pharmaceutical evaluation of compounded trilostane products. *J. Am. Anim. Hosp. Assoc.* 4: 228–233.

Council of the EEC. (1965). Council Directive 65/65/EEC of 26 January 1965 on the approximation of provisions laid down by Law, Regulation or Administrative Action relating to proprietary medicinal products (European Directive 65/65/CE; 31965L0065). http://eur-lex.europa.eu/LexUriServ/

LexUriServ.do?uri= CELEX:31965L0065: EN:HTML.

Danish Veterinary and Food Administration. (2017). Distribution and use of veterinary drugs in Denmark. https://www. foedevarestyrelsen.dk/english/Animal/ AnimalHealth/Veterinary_medicine/Pages/ default.aspx.

Davidson, G. (2001). Evaluating transdermal medication forms for veterinary patients, part 1. *Int. J. Pharm. Compd.* 5 (2): 95–96.

Davis, J.L., Kirk, L.M., Davidson, G.S. et al. (2009). Effects of compounding and storage conditions on stability of pergolide mesylate. *J. Am. Vet. Med. Assoc.* 234 (3): 385–389.

Drug Quality and Security Act (2013). *US Public Law 113-54*. Washington, DC: Government Printing Office.

FDA Draft Guidance for Industry #230. (2017). https://www.fda.gov/AnimalVeterinary/ NewsEvents/CVMUpdates/ucm580525. htm.

FDA Manual of Compliance Policy Guides. (2017). http://www.fda.gov/ICECI/ ComplianceManuals/CompliancePolicyGui danceManual.

FDA Withdraws Guidance for Industry. (2017). https://www.fda.gov/AnimalVeterinary/ NewsEvents/CVMUpdates/ucm580525. htm.

Food and Drug Administration (FDA). (2015). Compounding animal drugs from bulk drug substances; draft guidance for industry; availability; withdrawal of Compliance Policy Guide; Section 608.400 Compounding of Drugs for Use in Animals. https://www.federalregister.gov/ articles/2015/05/19/2015-11982/ compounding-animaldrugs-from-bulk-drug-substances-draft-guidance-for-industry-availability.

Food and Drug Administration (FDA). (2018a). Index of Legally Marketed Unapproved New Animal Drugs for Minor Species. https:// www.fda.gov/animalveterinary/ resourcesforyou/ucm268128.htm.

Food and Drug Administration (FDA). (2018b). Information for outsourcing facilities. http://www.fda.gov/Drugs/Guidan ceComplianceRegulatoryInformation/ PharmacyCompounding/ucm393571.htm.

Food and Drug Administration (FDA). (2018c). What is compounding? http://www.fda.gov/ Drugs/GuidanceComplianceRegulatoryInfo rmation/PharmacyCompounding/ ucm339764.htm#what.

Frank, H. (2006). Compounding in the exotic practice. *J. Exot. Pet Med.* 15: 116–121.

GamberaleStille, G. and Tullberg, B. (2001). Fruit or aposematic insect? Context dependent colormetric preferences in domestic chicks. *Proc. Biol. Sci.* 268 (1485): 2525–2529.

Goodwin, D., Davidson, H.P.B., and Harris, P. (2005). Selection and acceptance of flavors in concentrate diets for stabled horses. *Appl. Anim. Behav. Sci.* 95 (3–4): 223–232.

Government Accounting Office. (2017). Drug compounding for animals. http://www.gao. gov/assets/680/672748.pdf.

Guidance for Industry. (2017). https://www. fda.gov/AnimalVeterinary/ GuidanceComplianceEnforcement/ GuidanceforIndustry/ucm042451.htm?utm_ campaign=2-13-2018-Guidances&utm_ medium=email&utm_source=Eloqua&elqTr ackId=42C9247A3637FF3F51098D1611F8A 60D&elq=f74cb636d68445859fd7e95ee85ec 3d6&elqaid=2417&elqat=1&elqCampaig nId=1721.

International Journal of Pharmaceutical Compounding (IJPC). (N.d.). https://www. ijpc.com.

Koppel, K. (2014). Sensory analysis of pet foods. *J. Sci. Food Agric.* 94 (11): 2148–2153.

Krotscheck, U., Boothe, D.M., and Boothe, H. (2004). Evaluation of transdermal morphine and fentanyl pluronic lecithin organogel administration in dogs. *Vet. Ther.* 5: 202–211.

Kupiec, T, Skinner, R., and Lanier, L. (2008). Stability versus potency testing: The madness is in the method. Intl J Pharm Compounding 12(1), p.50.

Li, X., Li, W., Wang, H. et al. (2006). Cats lack a sweet taste receptor. *J. Nutr.* 136 (7 Suppl.): 1932S1934S.

Lorenz, W., Reimann, H.J., Schmal, A. et al. (1977). Histamine release in dogs by

Cremophor E1 and its derivatives: oxethylated oleic acid is the most effective constituent. *Agents Actions* 7 (1): 6367.

MacGregor, J.M., Rush, J.E., Rozanski, E.A. et al. (2008). Comparison of pharmacodynamic variables following oral versus transdermal administration of atenolol to healthy cats. *Am. J. Vet. Res.* 69: 39–44.

Marbofloxacin, Compounded, Oral Suspension, Veterinary Monograph. (N.d.). USP40–NF35, p. 4965.

Mawby, D.I., Whittemore, J.C., Genger, S. et al. (2014). Bioequivalence of orally administered generic, compounded, and innovator-formulated itraconazole in healthy dogs. *J. Vet. Intern. Med.* 28: 72–77.

Mealey, K.L., Peck, K.E., Bennett, B.S. et al. (2004). Systemic absorption of amitriptyline and buspirone after oral and transdermal administration to healthy cats. *J. Vet. Intern. Med.* 18: 43–46.

Mingura M. (2017). Community pharmacists and veterinary prescriptions: an analysis of prevalence, type, training, and knowledge retention. Poster presentation, Society of Veterinary Hospital Pharmacists 36th Annual Meeting, Portland, OR, June 12–14.

Missouri Board of Pharmacy. (2017). Annual reports from 2006–2014. http://pr.mo.gov/pharmacists-annual-reports.asp.

New Zealand Ministry for Primary Industries. (2017). Developing a documented system for compounded veterinary preparations. http://www.foodsafety.govt.nz/elibrary/industry/Compounding-Veterinary-Preparation.pdf.

Ontario College of Pharmacists. (2017). Guidelines for compounding preparations. http://www.ocpinfo.com/regulations-standards/policies-guidelines/compounding.

Papich, M.G. (2005). Drug compounding for veterinary patients. *AAPS J.* 7: E281–E287.

Parsemus Foundation. (2016). Regulatory status of compounded treatments, by country. https://www.parsemusfoundation.org/wp-content/uploads/2015/03/CaCl2_Regulatory_Status_Opinion_10-14-2016.pdf.

Pfizer (2009). *Neurontin (Gabapentin) oral solution package insert*. New York: Pfizer.

Pharmacy Board of Australia. (2016). Guidelines on compounding of medicines. https://www.google.com/search?q=australian+guidelines+on+compounding+medicines&oq=australianguidelines+on+compounding+medicines&aqs=chrome.69i57.13710j0j8&sourceid=chrome&ie=UTF-8.

Pharmacy Practice Guidance Manual. (2016). Veterinary pharmacy. http://www.thepsi.ie/libraries/publications/pharmacy_practice_guidance_manual.sflb.ashx.

Piscitelli, C.M., Dunayer, E.K., and Aumann, M. (2010). Xylitol toxicity in dogs. *Compend. Contin. Educ. Vet.* 32 (2): E1E4.

Qato, D.M., Zenk, S., Wilder, J. et al. (2017). The availability of pharmacies in the United States: 2007–2015. *PLoS One* 12 (8): e0183172.

Scott-Moncrief, J.C., Moore, G.E., Coe, J. et al. (2012). Characteristics of commercially manufactured and compounded protamine zinc insulin. *J. Am. Vet. Med. Assoc.* 240: 600–605.

Smith, J.A., Papich, M.G., Russell, G. et al. (2010). Effects of compounding on pharmacokinetics of itraconazole in blackfooted penguins (*Spheniscus demersus*). *J. Zoo Wildl. Med.* 41: 487–495.

Sorah E, Davidson G. Royal K. (2015). Dispensing errors for non-human patients in the community pharmacy setting: a survey of pharmacists and veterinarians. Poster presentation, Society of Veterinary Hospital Pharmacists 34th annual meeting, Portland, ME, June 14–17.

Stanley SD, Thomas SM, Skinner W. (2003). Comparison for pharmaceutical equivalence of FDA-approved products and compounded preparations of ketoprofen, amikacin, and boldenone. In Proceedings of the 49th Annual Convention of the American Association of Equine Practitioners, New Orleans, LA, USA, November 21–25.

Thombre, A.G. (2004). Oral delivery of medications to companion animals; palatability considerations. *Adv. Drug Deliv. Rev.* 56 (10): 1399–1413.

Thompson, J.A., Mirza, M.H., Barker, S.A. et al. (2011). Clenbuterol toxicosis in three quarter horse racehorses after administration of a compounded product. *J. Am. Vet. Med. Assoc.* 239: 842–849.

Trepanier, L.A., Van Schoick, A., and Schwark, W.S. (1998). Therapeutic serum drug concentrations in epileptic dogs treated with potassium bromide alone or in combination with other anticonvulsants: 122 cases (1992–1996). *J. Am. Vet. Med. Assoc.* 213: 1449–1453.

Trissel, L.A. and American Pharmacists Association (2012). *Trissel's Stability of Compounded Formulations*, 4e. Washington, DC: American Pharmacists Association.

Umstead, M.E., Boothe, D.M., Cruz-Espindola, C. et al. (2012). Accuracy and precision of compounded ciclosporin capsules and solution. *Vet. Dermatol.* 23 (5): 431–482.

United States Pharmacopeial Convention. (2015). USP General Chapter <795> Pharmaceutical Compounding – Nonsterile Preparations. In United States Pharmacopeia 38/National Formulary 33. United States Pharmacopeial Convention, Rockville, MD.

USP Legal Recognition. (2017). http://www.usp.org/about/legal-recognition/standard-categories#compounded-prep.

Varma, R.K., Kaushal, R., Junnarkar, A.Y. et al. (1985). Polysorbate 80: a pharmacological study. *Arzneim. Forsch.* 35 (5): 804–808.

Veterinary Drug Compounding. (2017). http://www.brakkeconsulting.com/news_article/771.aspx.

Washabau, R. and Holt, D. (1999). Pathogenesis, diagnosis, and therapy of feline idiopathic megacolon. *Vet. Clin. North Am. Small Anim. Pract.* 29: 589–603.

Watson, A.D.J., Rijnberk, A., and Moolenaar, A.J. (1987). Systemic availability of o′-DDD in normal dogs, fasted and fed, and in dogs with hyperadrenocorticism. *Res. Vet. Sci.* 43: 160–165.

World Health Organization. (2016). WHO Expert Committees 18th Expert Committee on the Selection and Use Medicines: extemporaneous review. http://www.who.int/selection_medicines/committees/expert/18/policy/policy5/en.

4

Comparative Pharmacokinetics and Pharmacodynamics

Katrina L. Mealey[1] and Margo J. Karriker[2]

[1] *College of Veterinary Medicine, Washington State University, Pullman, WA, USA*
[2] *UC Davis School of Veterinary Medicine, University of California Veterinary Medical Center–San Diego, San Diego, CA, USA*

Key Points

- Remarkable physiological species differences contribute to variations in drug absorption, distribution, metabolism, and excretion, such that pharmacokinetic data from one species should not be applied to another.
- Many factors that affect oral drug absorption (gastric pH, gut microbiome, transit time, gastrointestinal anatomy, and the presence or absence of certain drug-metabolizing enzymes) are a reflection of the animal's diet (true carnivore, omnivore, herbivore, or scavenger).
- Tremendous species differences exist in phase II drug metabolism, resulting in extreme differences among species with regard to susceptibility to severe adverse drug reactions.
- Biliary and renal excretion of many drugs depends on active efflux by drug transporters, many of which vary between species.

4.1 Introduction

Among veterinarians, it is appreciated that tremendous species differences exist in drug absorption, distribution, metabolism, and excretion. Drugs with a wide therapeutic margin in some species can be fatal if administered to another species at a fraction of the dose. This is the case with two of the most commonly used drugs in people, acetaminophen and aspirin. Both drugs have a fairly wide therapeutic window in both dogs and humans, but are highly toxic to cats even after a single low dose. It is often said by veterinarians that "cats are not small dogs" with regard to their physiology and pharmacology. It can also be said that dogs are not small people. While there are an amazing number of similarities between canine, feline, and human patients, pharmacists must be especially cognizant of the differences to ensure drug efficacy and avoid toxicity. This chapter will provide specific examples of some drug disposition differences between cats, dogs, and humans, as well as the physiologic and/or molecular genetic mechanisms that explain these differences. It is important to note, however, that some interesting species differences in drug response are still unexplained.

Unfortunately, there is not a simple rule that pharmacists can apply to predict drug disposition differences between dogs, cats, and humans. At first glance (Table 4.1), it appears haphazard – some drugs are eliminated more slowly in cats, intermediate in dogs, and fastest in humans, while other drugs are eliminated fastest in cats, intermediate in humans, and slowest in dogs. As it turns out, the elimination half-life of a drug in humans is poorly predictive of the elimination half-life in dogs or cats. However, if information about each drug's elimination mechanism (e.g. conjugation, oxidative metabolism, and excretion of the parent drug) is taken into consideration, then a pattern starts to emerge – at least for some of the drugs in Table 4.1. With some exceptions, drugs that undergo conjugation tend to be eliminated much more slowly in cats than in dogs or humans, whereas the elimination half-lives of drugs that undergo oxidative metabolism or excretion tend to be similar between cats, dogs, and humans or may even be eliminated more rapidly in cats. For some drugs, the elimination half-life can differ 10-fold between species. The mechanisms responsible for some of these differences in drug clearance will be discussed in Section 4.2.3, "Species Differences in Drug Metabolism."

It is important for pharmacists to appreciate that physiologic differences between species can greatly affect drug absorption, distribution, metabolism, and excretion, and that recognizing these differences allows one to better predict drug disposition in various species and use this information to predict clinical impact. Physiologic differences that result in variability in drug absorption, distribution, metabolism, and excretion are referred to as pharmacokinetic species differences. Alternatively, pharmacodynamic species differences result from differences in drug receptor quality or quantity. Pharmacodynamic species differences can also create variation in drug efficacy and toxicity. This chapter will focus on major known pharmacokinetic and pharmacodynamic species differences in dogs and cats compared to humans. Chapter 21 will cover pharmacokinetic and pharmacodynamic considerations for horses, Chapter 22 for livestock, and Chapter 23 for some of the

Table 4.1 Mechanism of elimination and elimination half-life values reported for a variety of drugs in dogs and cats relative to elimination half-life values of those same drugs in humans.

Drug	Mechanism of elimination	Dog	Cat
Diazepam	Oxidized		
Gentamicin	Excreted		
Ketamine	Oxidized		
Lorazepam	Conjugated		
Doxycycline	Excreted		
Piroxicam	Oxidized		
Clomipramine	Oxidized		
Fluconazole	Excreted		
Meperidine	Oxidized		
Acetaminophen	Conjugated		
Buprenorphine	Oxidized		
Chloramphenicol	Conjugated		
Digoxin	Excreted		
Ketoprofen	Conjugated		
Midazolam	Oxidized		
Cephalexin	Excreted		
Ciprofloxacin	Excreted		
Ivermectin	Excreted		
Meloxicam	Oxidized		
Acetylsalicylic acid	Conjugated		
Propofol	Conjugated		

Note: Drugs that are eliminated much more slowly in cats (red cells) compared to dogs and humans are conjugated. Green, Elimination half-life more than 5× faster than that of humans; white, elimination half-life similar to that of humans (±2×); yellow, elimination half-life 2–5× slower than humans; red, elimination half-life >5× slower than humans.

less traditional pet species, including small mammals, reptiles, and birds. It is beyond the scope of this book to provide detail on every drug in every species (much of that information is not even available). Instead, the goal is to illustrate the concept that dogs and cats are not small humans and that treating them as such is likely to result in adverse drug events.

4.2 Pharmacokinetic Species Differences

4.2.1 Species Differences in Drug Absorption

Absorption is defined as the movement of drug from the site of administration into the systemic circulation (blood or plasma). As in people, there are multiple possible routes of drug administration that generally result in consistent, predictable systemic drug concentrations, including oral, subcutaneous, intramuscular, and intravenous (which, by definition, does not require absorption). Other routes of administration and specialized topical delivery will be presented in Chapter 25. The basic biology of drug absorption is similar across species – a drug molecule crosses a series of cellular membranes composed of lipid bilayers. There are no data to suggest that the chemical composition of cell membranes differs substantially enough between humans, dogs, and cats to alter the basic process of diffusion. However, species differences in drug absorption can occur because of major differences in anatomy (overall length of gastrointestinal [GI] tract segments), in physiology (e.g. differences in pH along the GI tract and gastric emptying times), and even at the molecular level (quantitative and qualitative differences in drug transporters such as P-glycoprotein and ABCG2).

4.2.1.1 Oral (Gastrointestinal) Drug Absorption

Oral dosage forms are by far the most common drug formulations that are dispensed by community pharmacies for humans, dogs, and cats. One reason for this is their relative ease of administration, although there are exceptions. Some cats are notoriously difficult to "pill" (Chapter 25 has some suggestions for handling this situation). Another reason that oral dosage forms are popular is that, unlike most other tissue spaces within the body, the oral cavity and GI tract are not sterile environments, so drugs administered

orally do not have to be sterile. However, relative to the nominal barriers encountered by a drug molecule administered by injection (subcutaneous, intramuscular, or intravenous), there are a number of potential barriers impeding oral drug bioavailability that must be overcome, including degradation in the stomach, permeability through the intestinal wall, variability in release of drug from the formulation, and metabolism by bacterial enzymes or the patient's own enzyme systems within enterocytes and hepatocytes. Drug formulations that eventually become marketed commercial drug products are usually optimized for one particular species (usually humans). Unfortunately, oral drug bioavailability in humans does not correlate well with that in animals (Musther et al. 2014). For example, the mean oral bioavailability of ganciclovir in dogs and humans is 100 and 9%, respectively (dog 10-fold greater than human), while the mean oral bioavailability of clonazepam is essentially reversed in those species (90% in humans; 33% in dogs – dog threefold less than human). Some of the reasons for the extreme variation in oral bioavailability between species are described further here.

The anatomy and physiology of the GI tract can vary dramatically between species. The size, and therefore length, of the GI tract differs substantially between species, and sometimes even within the same species (consider a Great Dane and a Chihuahua). The relative lengths of the segments of the GI tract (stomach, duodenum, jejunum, ileum, cecum, colon, and rectum) can differ between species. These species differences may impact oral drug absorption in several ways. For example, the small intestine is the primary site for absorption of most orally administered drugs. Sustained-release formulations designed for humans are rarely appropriate for use in other species because of gastric pH differences combined with a much shorter small intestine in dogs and cats relative to people. Even the function of the various segments of the GI tract can differ between species. This is not surprising if one considers the variety in diets among different animal species from herbivores (all-plant diet: e.g. horses, cattle, and sheep) to omnivores (diet consisting of plant and animal sources: e.g. humans, dogs, and pigs) to true or obligate carnivores (cats). Herbivores require a complex GI tract to effectively digest and extract nutrients from plant materials such as cellulose. The digestive tract of herbivores sometimes includes a rumen, which is a large chamber in the proximal part of the alimentary canal, as is the case for cattle, or a larger more extensive colon than humans and other monogastric species, which is the case for horses. Animals with rumens are called ruminants and include cattle, sheep, and goats (see Chapter 22). Horses (see Chapter 21) and rabbits (see Chapter 23), while herbivores, are not ruminants because they do not have a rumen. The complex GI organs of true herbivores contain a delicate balance of microbes that are essential for these animals to digest and efficiently extract nutrients from cellulose, which is indigestible by humans. Antimicrobial drugs routinely used in dogs, cats, humans, and other monogastric animals can alter the balance of normal microbial flora in herbivores, and have devastating, often fatal, consequences.

Other species-dependent factors that can alter the rate and extent of oral drug absorption include GI transit time, the gut microbiome, and bile acid composition. The GI transit time in humans (roughly 24 hours) is much slower than in smaller monogastric animals, such as dogs and cats (roughly 12 hours). Absorption and/or stability of some drugs is affected by gastric pH, which varies tremendously among different species (Beasley et al. 2015). For example, carnivores and omnivores tend to have low gastric pH (cat, 3.6; ferret, 1.5), while herbivores tend to have the highest gastric pH (horse, 4.4; Shetland Pony, 5.9). Recalling that each pH unit represents a 10-fold difference in hydrogen ion concentration, it is not surprising that oral absorption of drugs with pK values within the range of 2–7 might differ dramatically between species. Another factor that is likely to contribute to species differences in oral drug bioavailability is the gut microbiome, which has been shown to have major reductive metabolic capacity as well as other drug-metabolizing activity. Species differences in gut microbiome–mediated drug metabolism may result in greater activation of pro-drugs to their pharmacologically active form (enhanced toxicity) or greater conversion of active drugs to inactive metabolites (decreased efficacy). The presence of bile in the GI tract tends to enhance oral drug bioavailability, particularly for lipid-soluble compounds (Yeap et al. 2013). However, differences in bile salt composition present yet another variable that must be considered when comparing oral drug bioavailability between species. The key point here is that just because a drug is orally bioavailable in people, that does not mean it will have equivalent oral bioavailability in other species. Thus, oral dosing rates for humans should not be assumed to be similar across all species because of the factors just discussed as well as other species-dependent influences.

4.2.1.2 Other Routes of Administration

Commonly used parenteral routes of administration in veterinary patients include intramuscular or subcutaneous injection. Barriers to drug absorption are minimal at these sites; therefore, species differences are few. The most important difference is that the optimal sites of administration for intramuscular and subcutaneous injection differ between species based on muscle size, tissue perfusion, volume of subcutaneous space, and anatomic location of larger nerves (inadvertent injection into a nerve must be avoided). For example, the neck is a common site for intramuscular injections in horses but not for dogs, cats, or people. Subcutaneous injection in dogs and cats often occurs in the scruff of the neck, because the skin is loose and easy to manipulate (Figure 4.1). Because the same is not true for people, subcutaneous injections are not administered at that location. Drugs can be administered via inhalation for anesthesia (not discussed further because these agents will not be dispensed by

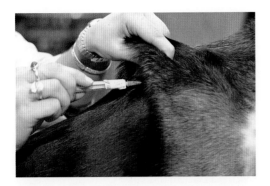

Figure 4.1 The loose skin of the scruff of the neck in dogs (and cats) can be easily "tented" to form a space for subcutaneous injection of medications. *Source:* Photo courtesy of Henry Moore Jr., Washington State University College of Veterinary Medicine, Biomedical Communications Unit.

community pharmacists) or for delivery to the respiratory tract for patients with inflammatory lung diseases such as asthma (discussed in Chapter 11). Aerosol delivery devices have been carefully designed for use in human patients taking into account particle size, sedimentation, velocity of air flow, and numerous other factors. Dogs, cats, and horses with inflammatory airway disease are often treated with metered-dose inhalers designed for human patients, but not with dry-powder inhalers, as the logistics of administering the dose is not possible. Whether or not the droplets or particles are distributed appropriately in much smaller (cats and dogs) or larger (horses) patients has not been investigated. What has been documented, however, is that systemic absorption of aerosolized particles does occur in dogs, cats, and horses, despite the fact that the intent of aerosolized drug delivery is for "topical" treatment of the respiratory tract. This is discussed in more detail in Chapters 11 and 25.

Systemic absorption of drug formulations applied to the skin may also occur. Sometimes this is intended (transdermal drug formulations), and sometimes it is not (topical treatment of dermatologic disease). Because skin structure varies tremendously not only between species but even at different body sites within the same individual,

drug products formulated for transdermal delivery in one species should not be expected to have the same absorption characteristics in another species. Local perfusion, skin structure abnormalities (like a wound), and systemic illness can also impact the distribution of a drug product across the skin. The thickness of the outermost layer of skin, the stratum corneum, is among the most important factors that contribute to variation in transdermal drug absorption. There are a number of veterinary formulations that have been designed for transdermal delivery of drugs intended to have systemic effects (pesticide "pour-ons" or "spot-ons"). Their efficacy has been demonstrated in US Food and Drug Administration (FDA)-approved preclinical and clinical trials in the target species. Examples include a pour-on formulation of ivermectin for cattle administered at a dose of 500 micrograms per kilogram of body weight. This product is indicated for the treatment of external (lice, mange, and flies) as well as internal (stomach worms and lung worms) parasites. Another example is selamectin, which is administered topically to dogs and cats for prevention and control of external (fleas and mites) and internal (gastrointestinal worms and heartworms) parasites. Both of these formulations are designed such that topical drug application results in systemic bioavailability. These formulations make it easy to deliver systemic therapy to a potentially uncooperative patient.

Because of the relative ease of administering topically applied drugs to cats, in particular, many compounding pharmacies attempt this transdermal approach using virtually any drug. While the intent is good (ease of drug administration for the owner and patient), the outcomes tend to be poor (lack of systemic absorption resulting in therapeutic failure in the patient); and the primary literature to support both the pharmacokinetics/pharmacodynamics of drugs in these formulations as well as the chemical stability of the compounded products is lacking. The reader can enter "veterinary transdermal drug" into most search engines and identify a large number of pharmacies promoting compounded transdermal formulations of dozens of drugs for veterinary patients, particularly cats. Drugs designed for transdermal drug administration tend to be highly lipophilic, which allows for penetration through the stratum corneum, but that is not the only factor that determines whether or not a transdermally administered drug can achieve therapeutic plasma concentrations. Probably one of the most important factors is drug potency. Specifically, drugs that need only achieve microgram per mL concentrations in plasma to exert their pharmacological effect are the drugs that have demonstrated efficacy after transdermal drug administration (Lee et al. 2000; Sartor et al. 2004). Conversely, drugs that require therapeutic concentrations in the milligram per mL range have generally not been effective when administered transdermally (Mealey et al. 2004; Miller et al. 2014).

Practiced but not proven

Research has shown that only a fraction of compounded transdermal products has sufficient bioavailability for the drug to reach therapeutic plasma concentrations. With very few exceptions (noted in the chapters where these drugs are discussed), compounded transdermal drug formulations should not be dispensed to dogs and cats because they lack efficacy.

One last point to be made about transdermal drug formulations for veterinary patients is safety concerns for owners and other people who may come in contact with the treated animal. This information is discussed in Chapter 25 and reviewed in greater detail elsewhere (Mills and Cross 2006; Eichstadt and Davidson 2014).

4.2.2 Species Differences in Drug Distribution

Drug distribution, or movement of drug from the systemic circulation to tissues (pharmacological sites of action), can differ

Table 4.2 Mean volumes of fluid compartments per unit weight for humans, dogs, and cats.

	Blood (mL/kg)	Plasma (mL/kg)	Extracellular fluid (mL/kg)
Human	80	40	300
Dog	78	50	200
Cat	66	50	200

Source: Data obtained from Wellman et al. (2012) and Roden and Dan (2014).

dramatically between species. Even relative blood, plasma, and extracellular fluid volumes can vary between species, resulting in different volumes of distribution (Table 4.2). Equally important is the fact that consequences of drug distribution to different tissues may be different in some veterinary species compared to human patients. For all species, the tissues that a drug is distributed to will hopefully include the desired target tissue so that the drug can elicit the desired pharmacological response. The drug will also be distributed to other tissues, where it may elicit undesirable pharmacological responses (toxicity). Some tissues have strong affinity for certain drug molecules, serving as a "sink" or depot. For example, aminoglycoside antimicrobial drugs, once distributed to the kidneys, are tightly bound by renal proximal tubule cells. In animals such as cattle or pigs that may become part of the food supply, the presence of aminoglycoside tissue residues can pose a food-safety risk for human consumers (Gehring et al. 2005). Tissue residues are an issue that is not typically considered in community pharmacy practice, but for veterinary species that are classified as "food animals," the presence of tissue residues constitutes a serious violation of FDA regulations. Chapters 2 and 21 provide more details on the legal aspects of drug residues in animal tissues and how the pharmacist can avoid violating these regulations.

Drug distribution depends on a number of factors, including relative blood flow to tissues, relative tissue mass, plasma protein binding, and tissue barriers to distribution. Tissue distribution is the factor that likely contributes most to species and individual differences in drug distribution. Many tissues express proteins that transport substrate drugs against a concentration gradient either into or out of cells comprising tissue barriers (e.g. the blood–brain barrier, intestinal epithelial barrier, renal tubules, and blood–placenta barrier). Two of the most well-characterized of these drug transporters are P-glycoprotein encoded by the ABCB1 (formerly MDR1) gene and the breast cancer resistance protein (BCRP) encoded by the ABCG2 gene. Both P-glycoprotein and ABCG2 are members of the ATP (adenosine triphosphate) binding cassette (ABC) superfamily of transport proteins.

4.2.2.1 P-Glycoprotein and Drug Distribution

P-glycoprotein exists in all mammalian organisms and performs essentially equivalent functions in each of them. P-glycoprotein protects the organism from potentially toxic xenobiotics encountered in the environment. P-glycoprotein efficiently exports substrate drugs at all of the tissue barriers mentioned here as well as others. P-glycoprotein limits oral drug absorption, enhances biliary and renal excretion of substrate drugs, and restricts distribution of substrate drugs to the central nervous system (CNS), testes, and fetus. Many drugs used in veterinary medicine have been identified as P-glycoprotein substrates (see Chapter 5), and the distribution and excretion of these drugs are dramatically influenced by P-glycoprotein. This is dramatically illustrated in animals that have deficient P-glycoprotein function. A well-known genetic polymorphism involving canine P-glycoprotein (MDR1 mutation or ABCB1-1Δ) and a different polymorphism affecting feline P-glycoprotein (*ABCB1*1930_1931del TC) result in complete loss of P-glycoprotein function in animals with two copies of the mutant allele or decreased P-glycoprotein function in heterozygotes. Dogs or cats

harboring these ABCB1 polymorphisms are highly susceptible to severe, potentially fatal, adverse drug reactions compared to dogs or cats with wildtype ABCB1. For example, the antiparasitic drug ivermectin, a substrate of P-glycoprotein, can be used safely in ABCB1 wildtype dogs at doses of 600 micrograms per kg per day for weeks. A single dose of 2500 micrograms in ABCB1 wildtype dogs causes pupillary dilation. Conversely, dogs that are homozygous for the ABCB1-1Δ mutation will experience CNS depression, respiratory depression, coma, and possibly death after receiving a 10-fold lower dose (200 micrograms per kilogram) even once. Differences in drug distribution are the reason. P-glycoprotein efficiently effluxes ivermectin from the brain as part of the blood–brain barrier, such that minute concentrations of ivermectin are achieved in sensitive brain tissue. In contrast, ivermectin achieves much higher concentrations in brain tissue of dogs and cats with defective P-glycoprotein function, as shown with a radiolabeled P-glycoprotein substrate in Figure 4.2. Polymorphisms in human ABCB1 have been documented, but none result in complete P-glycoprotein deficiency, as occurs in affected dogs and cats. Because these genetic defects are not present in all dogs or cats, they represent breed differences rather than pan-species differences, so their effect on drug toxicity will be discussed in detail in Chapter 5.

4.2.2.2 ABCG2 and Drug Distribution

ABCG2 is another important drug transporter that modulates drug distribution. Like P-glycoprotein, ABCG2 functions as a drug efflux pump in a variety of tissues, including the liver, intestine, blood–retina barrier, blood–brain barrier, and mammary gland, where it pumps substrates into the bile, intestinal lumen, systemic circulation, and milk, respectively. The role of ABCG2 in drug distribution has been studied in several veterinary species, including cats (Ramirez et al. 2011), sheep (Pulido et al. 2006), and cattle (Mahnke et al. 2016). ABCG2 facilitates

(a) (b)

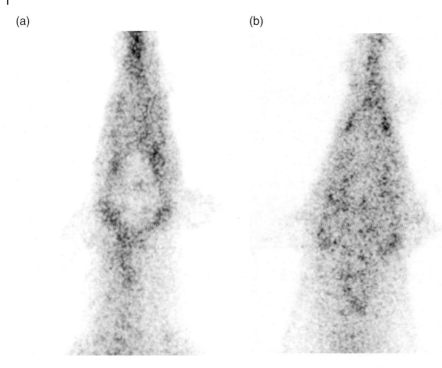

Figure 4.2 Images using nuclear scintigraphy to demonstrate the contribution of P-glycoprotein to the blood–brain barrier. A short half-life radiolabeled P-glycoprotein substrate was administered intravenously to a Collie homozygous for the wildtype MDR1 allele (Dog A) and a Collie homozygous for the mutant MDR1 allele (Dog B). The image of the head and neck of Dog A demonstrates normal P-glycoprotein function with a void of radioactivity in the brain area compared to the surrounding tissues. The image of the head and neck of Dog B demonstrates lack of P-glycoprotein function with similar density of radioactivity in the brain compared to the surrounding tissues. For orientation, the dogs' noses are at the top of the image. *Source:* Image reproduced with permission of Mealey et al. (2008).

secretion of substrate drugs into milk, affecting a number of important veterinary drugs, including some antiparasitic agents (e.g. oxfendazole and moxidectin) and antimicrobials (e.g. nitrofurantoin and fluoroquinolones). Thus, a calf nursing from a lactating cow that has been treated with an ABCG2 substrate will be inadvertently exposed to that drug. Similarly, ABCG2 also has implications for drug residues in milk intended for human consumption. In these instances, avoiding drugs that are substrates for ABCG2 is critical. This concept (avoidance of drug residues in milk) is discussed in greater detail in Chapters 2 and 22. On the other hand, patients with mastitis might benefit from the ABCG2-mediated transport of certain antimicrobial drugs into milk.

A species-wide defect in ABCG2 function has been documented in domestic cats, as well as a number of wild felids. Feline ABCG2 has several amino acid changes that occur within conserved regions of the protein compared to 10 other mammalian species (Ramirez et al. 2011). One of the amino acid changes is similar to a human variant (ABCG2 421C>A) that adversely impacts ABCG2 function in affected people. In cell culture studies, feline ABCG2 has decreased ability to transport ABCG2 substrates compared to human and canine ABCG2. Thus, one would expect that cats would be at greater risk for adverse drug reactions when treated with drugs that are ABCG2 substrates compared to other species. This is indeed the case with certain fluoroquinolones. Domestic cats

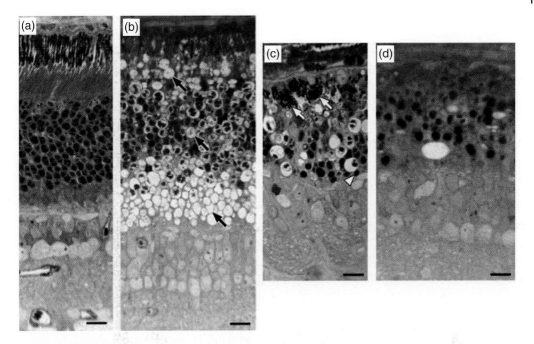

Figure 4.3 Progressive fluoroquinolone-induced retinal toxicity in cats treated with enrofloxacin. Photomicrographs of retinal tissue pretreatment (a), and at day 3 (b), day 5 (c), and day 7 (d). *Source:* Image reproduced with permission from Ford et al. (2007).

experience a peculiar but devastating adverse drug reaction associated with fluoroquinolones – acute retinal degeneration and blindness (Figure 4.3). Fluoroquinolone-induced retinal degeneration was first documented with enrofloxacin, an FDA-approved fluoroquinolone for dogs and cats, which is structurally similar to the human product ciprofloxacin. In a prospective study, all cats treated with enrofloxacin (10× label dose for seven days) developed severe retinal degeneration, while none of the control cats developed retinal lesions (Ford et al. 2007). Many other fluoroquinolones also cause retinal damage in cats (see Freedom of Information Summary NADA 141–081, www.fda.gov). The mechanism behind this unusual feline-specific adverse drug reaction is deficient ABCG2 function. Fluoroquinolones, as ABCG2 substrates, are normally restricted from retinal tissue by the blood–retina barrier. Fluoroquinolones are photoreactive compounds that, when exposed to light, generate reactive oxygen species that damage proximate tissues (recall that sensitivity to sunlight is an adverse effect of fluoroquinolones in people). Defective ABCG2 function in cats disrupts the blood–retina barrier, resulting in accumulation of photoreactive fluoroquinolone molecules in retinal tissue. When the retina is exposed to light, reactive oxygen species that are subsequently generated attack cellular lipid membranes, causing tissue damage, retinal degeneration, and blindness. It is important to note that fluoroquinolone-induced retinal toxicity occurs primarily when the label dose is exceeded or in cats with renal or liver impairment that results in impaired fluoroquinolone elimination. Extra-label use of human-approved fluoroquinolone products such as ciprofloxacin is strongly discouraged in cats because many are photoreactive. Safe dose regimens have not been determined with respect to potential retinal toxicity. Multiple fluoroquinolone products are FDA approved for cats, inclusive of oral tablets and oral suspensions, such that extra-label use of human products is generally not indicated.

4.2.2.3 Plasma Protein Binding and Drug Distribution

Drug distribution encompasses movement of drug from the systemic circulation to other tissues. As the reader would expect based on knowledge about drug distribution in human patients, the distribution of drugs bound to plasma proteins is limited to the intravascular compartment because the molecular weights of plasma proteins such as albumin and α_1 acid glycoprotein constrain their passage through capillary walls. The extent of a drug's plasma protein binding influences drug distribution, the likelihood that sufficient concentrations of drug will access the site of action, as well as the rate of metabolism and excretion of that drug. Drugs that are highly bound to plasma proteins (>95%) are the ones most likely to be involved in adverse drug events related to displacement from a carrier protein. Although a number of plasma proteins can bind xenobiotics, albumin and α_1 acid glycoprotein (also called orosomucoid) are generally considered the most important carrier proteins for drugs used in veterinary patients. Since only the unbound fraction of drug is pharmacologically active, small changes in protein binding can greatly affect efficacy and toxicity of highly protein-bound drugs such as NSAIDs, tricyclic antidepressants, selective serotonin reuptake inhibitors, propofol, and others. Consider the case with NSAIDs, which are typically ≥99% protein bound in most species. Certain clinical scenarios can decrease protein binding of the NSAID such that only 98% of the NSAID is protein bound. This seemingly innocuous change actually results in a doubling of the unbound, pharmacologically active, drug in plasma (i.e. from 1% to 2% unbound). Situations that can alter protein binding of a drug for an individual patient include drug interactions (co-administration of two highly protein-bound drugs) or changes in plasma albumin or α_1 acid glycoprotein concentrations. For example, many disease states such as liver failure or diseases of the kidney affecting the glomerulus (protein-losing nephropathy) can cause hypoalbuminemia. Conversely, rapid increases in plasma albumin concentrations can result from administration of albumin solutions or plasma transfusions. For α_1 acid glycoprotein, plasma concentrations can triple in a short time period in the face of inflammatory disease, since α_1 acid glycoprotein is an acute-phase protein.

It is important for pharmacists to know that the degree of plasma protein binding of a drug in one species may differ dramatically in other species. In one study, binding affinity of warfarin to bovine, rabbit, and rat albumin was similar to that with human albumin, whereas its binding affinity to canine albumin was much lower (Kosa et al. 1997). Conversely, for diazepam, binding parameters for bovine, rabbit, rat, and canine albumin were different than for human albumin. The mean unbound fraction of grapiprant (a drug indicated for osteoarthritis in dogs) is more than four times higher in dogs than in people (Nagahisa and Okumura 2017). The reason for these differences can be attributed to amino acid sequence differences in both the albumin and α_1 acid glycoprotein molecules among different species, particularly at drug-binding sites. What this means is that a drug that is 99% bound to human albumin is not necessarily highly bound to albumin in any other species. The reverse is also true. Drugs that are not highly protein bound in people may be highly protein bound in other species. This impacts advice pharmacists may provide about drug–drug interactions to owners of veterinary patients that are receiving multiple drugs. Drugs that are FDA approved for veterinary species often have information about protein binding included within the drug label (for the designated species that the drug is intended to treat). This is another good reason to use veterinary-approved drugs according to the label rather than substituting a human drug in an off-label manner. When predicting and discussing drug–drug interactions in animal patients, pharmacists should refer to an appropriate drug reference specific to the species of patient being treated.

4.2.3 Species Differences in Drug Metabolism

Animal studies are a routine component of pharmacokinetic, pharmacodynamic, and toxicological research in human drug development. The limitations of animal studies to accurately predict metabolism and toxicity risks for new human drugs are well known by the FDA and pharmaceutical companies alike. A drug determined to be safe in a rodent model, for example, may carry a high risk of toxicity in people. Conversely, drugs that have a high therapeutic index in human patients may have a low therapeutic index in dogs and/or cats. Species differences in drug metabolism can be profound. In fact, based on current knowledge, species differences in drug metabolism contribute more to species differences in drug response than any other factor. This shouldn't be surprising when one considers that the enzymes we call "drug-metabolizing enzymes" did not, in fact, evolve to metabolize drugs. Rather, these enzymes evolved to process xenobiotics encountered in the animal's environment and diet. In herbivores, drug-metabolizing enzymes likely evolved to detoxify chemical compounds present within plants. Organisms with the ability to detoxify more chemical compounds would enjoy a survival advantage. True carnivores, on the other hand, had less need for these detoxification enzymes and seem to have actually lost functional forms of some drug-metabolizing enzymes through an evolutionary (or de-evolutionary) mechanism (Shrestha et al. 2011). Domestic cats and wild felids, true carnivores, lack functional drug-metabolizing enzymes that are present in dogs and people (omnivores), making them exquisitely sensitive to the adverse effects of some commonly used drugs (acetaminophen and aspirin). Dogs, too, lack drug-metabolizing enzymes that are present in humans, making them susceptible to adverse effects of some drugs commonly used in people. Furthermore, even when dogs, cats, and humans each possess a particular drug-metabolizing enzyme, there are often differences in substrate specificity and/or differences in the inducibility of a particular enzyme. Thus, it is important for the pharmacist to understand that drugs that are routinely used in people (even pediatric patients) are not necessarily safe or effective for dogs or cats.

Traditionally, the liver is the organ considered to be the primary site of drug biotransformation, but it is important to at least mention that drug metabolism occurs in other tissues, including enterocytes, kidney, lung, and blood, and even within the gut microbiota. However, since research conducted to evaluate species differences in drug metabolism generally makes use of liver microsomes, the discussions in the remainder of this section will primarily reflect hepatic drug metabolism. It is reasonable to assume that future research will uncover key species differences in drug metabolism that involve drug-metabolizing enzymes in tissues other than liver.

4.2.3.1 Phase I Drug Metabolism

Oxidation, reduction, hydrolysis, and hydration are the most common phase I reactions, with oxidation mediated by cytochrome P450 (CYP) enzymes considered the most important. This is illustrated by the fact that the FDA requires pharmaceutical companies to delineate on the label of human drug products which CYPs are involved in the drug's metabolism.

Dramatic difference

In contrast to FDA requirements for human drug products, veterinary pharmaceutical companies are not currently required to provide information regarding the CYPs involved in a drug's metabolism, making it more difficult to predict CYP-mediated drug–drug interactions in veterinary patients than in human patients.

Unfortunately, the relationship of drug metabolism by human CYPs to that of canine and feline CYPs is complex, confusing, and not fully defined. Factors that contribute to complexity and confusion include the fact that a particular human CYP enzyme may

Table 4.3 Relative amounts, by rank, of cytochrome P450 subfamilies expressed in the liver of humans, dogs, and cats.

	CYP1A	CYP2A	CYP2B	CYP2C	CYP2D	CYP2E	CYP3A	Other
Human	4	5		2		3	1	
Canine			5	1	2		4	3
Feline	4	2			5	1	3	

Source: Martinez et al. (2013) and Okamatsu et al. (2017).

have the same name or a different name in other species, it may or may not share substrate specificity, and drugs that are known to induce or inhibit the human CYP enzymes may or may not have the same effect in other species (Okamatsu et al. 2017; Martinez et al. 2013). Fortunately, it is not necessary for the pharmacist to memorize specific differences among the CYP enzymes of different species. Rather, it is important for he or she to appreciate that significant differences exist and that drug-dosing regimens appropriate for a particular drug in one species are likely to be quite different for another species. Similarly, drug–drug interactions involving human CYP inducers and inhibitors may or may not apply to veterinary patients. Thus, human drug–drug interaction information software programs and websites are insufficient to prevent drug–drug interactions in veterinary patients. The discussion here provides some examples of just how diverse and unpredictable drug metabolism can be between dogs, cats, and humans.

The CYPs are grouped and named based on gene sequence similarity. Since there are enough differences in gene sequence between species, each species largely ended up with uniquely named CYPs for what are thought to be the same functional enzyme. For example, the most important CYP in human drug metabolism is CYP3A4. The canine ortholog is CYP3A12 (Court 2013a), while CYP3A131 and CYP3A132 have been proposed as feline orthologs (Honda et al. 2011). To further complicate matters, a drug, midazolam for example, metabolized by specific CYPs in one species (human CYP3A4 and CYP3A5) may

be metabolized by entirely different CYPs in another species (canine CYP 2B11). To add to the complexity, another source of variation of CYP drug metabolism between species is the relative CYP abundance in tissues, specifically liver and small intestine. Table 4.3 shows that the relative abundance of CYP enzymes in human, canine, and feline liver is disparate and would therefore contribute to differences in drug disposition, particularly for orally administered drugs. For example, the CYP2B family appears to be of greater importance to dogs (represents 10% of expressed CYPs in canine liver) than to people or cats (represents less than 2% of expressed CYPs). To achieve the same pharmacological response, drugs metabolized by CYP2B may require higher doses or more frequent administration in dogs than in people or cats.

A number of research groups are currently investigating canine and feline CYPs to better understand which CYP families are responsible for metabolizing commonly used veterinary drugs. The benefits of this information in decreasing adverse drug reactions, minimizing drug–drug interactions, and improving drug efficacy in veterinary patients cannot be overestimated. Specific to drug–drug interactions, there is yet another CYP species difference that deserves mention. Drugs that are known to induce (i.e. phenobarbital and rifampin) or inhibit (i.e. ketoconazole, cimetidine, omeprazole, and chloramphenicol) human CYPs may or may not affect canine or feline CYPs. This is an active area of intense research with respect to canine (Martinez et al. 2013) and feline (Okamatsu et al. 2017) CYPs. We anticipate that future editions of this book will contain more detailed information about interspecies CYP relationships that will allow veterinary pharmacists and pharmacologists to begin to apply human drug metabolism data to dogs and cats.

4.2.3.2 Phase II Drug Metabolism

Among the most common phase II conjugation reactions in people and animals are glucuronidation, sulfation, acetylation, and methylation. Because conjugation reactions predominantly inactivate a drug's pharmacologic actions, defects in these metabolic enzymes can cause severe toxicity. There are numerous examples of phase II metabolic differences in cats and dogs as compared to people.

Glucuronidation deficiency in domestic cats is probably the most well-known example of a species-wide difference in drug metabolism, with the first reference to this defect occurring more than 60 years ago (Robinson and Williams 1958). Veterinarians were generally aware that cats were unable to metabolize phenolic compounds (drugs and other xenobiotics) over 30 years ago, but it wasn't until 2000 that the mechanism was elucidated (Court and Greenblatt 2000). The enzyme family UDP-glucuronosyltransferase (UGT) catalyzes the conjugation of glucuronic acid to a drug (or xenotiotic), resulting in a molecule with greater water solubility and less toxicity than the parent molecule. Two commonly used drugs in human medicine, aspirin and acetaminophen, undergo glucuronidation by one of nine active human UGT enzymes to form nontoxic metabolites. Domestic cats and other felids lack all but two of those nine UGT enzymes. The absence of these enzymes can cause slower elimination of drugs that depend on glucuronidation or, in other cases, a shift to an alternate metabolic pathway (i.e. oxidative pathways). Unlike glucuronidation that almost exclusively generates a nontoxic metabolite, oxidative metabolism can sometimes generate metabolites with greater toxicity than the parent drug. This is exactly what happens with acetaminophen in cats, even with extremely low doses. Interestingly, very high doses of acetaminophen in humans can saturate glucuronidation pathways, resulting in shunting to oxidative pathways that generate the highly toxic metabolite NAPQI. More detailed information about acetaminophen toxicity in veterinary species can be found in Chapter 6. Other compounds that undergo glucuronidation and are eliminated more slowly in cats compared to dogs and/or humans include chloramphenicol, morphine, some preservatives (benzoic acid and benzyl alcohol), and the fluoroquinolone orbifloxacin. It is important to note that glucuronidation of bilirubin, which is catalyzed by UGT1A1, is not deficient in cats.

Glycination, and potentially sulfation, are other conjugation pathways that are deficient in cats. This appears to be the most convincing mechanism proposed thus far to explain the protracted elimination of aspirin in cats relative to dogs and humans (Court 2013b). The elimination half-life of aspirin in cats (22 hours) is five times slower than that in dogs (4.5 hours) and 10 times slower than that in humans (2.3 hours). In both dogs and humans, the major salicylate conjugate formed is with glycine, whereas cats form virtually no glycine conjugate. Unlike acetaminophen, aspirin can be used safely in cats if administered at very low dose rates and quite long dosing intervals (48–72 hours).

N-acetyl transferase (NAT) catalyzes the acetylation of drugs such as hydralazine, procainamide, isoniazid, and sulfonamide antimicrobials (Trepanier et al. 1997). Two major forms of NAT are present in humans (NAT1 and NAT2), and three are present in rodents (NAT1, -2, and -3). Dogs and other members of the canid family are completely deficient in NAT activity due to the absence of NAT genes (Trepanier et al. 1997). Domestic cats and wild felids (at least the seven species that were studied) are deficient in N-acetylation activity compared to humans because they lack NAT2. A specific drug toxicity has not been definitively attributed to NAT deficiency in dogs or cats, but there is evidence to suggest that NAT deficiency contributes to acetaminophen-induced methemoglobinemia

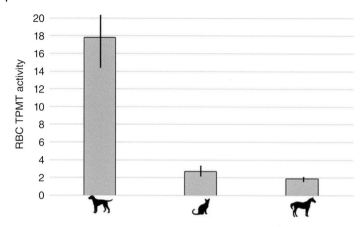

Figure 4.4 Mean red blood cell (RBC) thiopurine methyltransferase (TMPT) activity in dogs, cats, and horses. *Source:* White et al. (2000) and Salavaggione et al. (2002).

in dogs and cats (McConkey et al. 2009) and severe sulfonamide hypersensitivity reactions in dogs (Cribb and Spielberg 1990).

Thiopurine methyltransferase (TPMT) is a key enzyme in detoxifying thiopurines such as azathioprine and 6-mercaptopurine. One of the first clinically applied pharmacogenomic discoveries in people involved TMPT in patients receiving thiopurines (Lennard et al. 1989). Polymorphisms in the gene encoding TMPT in people correlate strongly with low TMPT enzymatic activity and susceptibility to thiopurine-induced myelosuppression. As is the case with people, TMPT activity in dogs can be variable, with some breeds having lower TMPT than others. In terms of species-dependent TMPT, both cats and horses appear to have low TMPT activity compared to dogs and people (Figure 4.4).

Mandatory monitoring
Generally, thiopurines are avoided in cats and horses, but if they are used, frequent assessment of neutrophil and platelet counts must be performed to avoid severe myelosuppression. Not surprisingly, cats are known to be exquisitely sensitive to azathioprine-induced myelosuppression.

4.2.4 Species Differences in Excretion

4.2.4.1 Renal Elimination

Renal function is qualitatively very similar among domestic mammals, but quantitative differences exist. For example, healthy cats concentrate urine (urine-to-plasma concentration ratio of 10:1) to a much higher extent than do healthy dogs or humans (~4–6:1). There are also urinary pH differences among species, with herbivores trending toward alkaline urine pH and carnivores typically having more acidic urinary pH. These physiologic differences contribute to some variation in renal drug excretion between species but are not likely to contribute to major differences in renal drug excretion.

Drugs can be excreted by the kidney using passive or active mechanisms, but their retention by the kidney is primarily an active process described as tubular reabsorption. Processes that favor renal drug elimination are glomerular filtration (passive) and renal tubular secretion (active). The net renal excretion of a drug is the sum of these processes. Because the kidneys receive 25% of the total cardiac output, drugs that are cleared primarily by glomerular filtration, for example aminoglycosides, can have a short plasma elimination half-life (approximately one hour in dog, cats, horses, and humans). Note that despite the physiologic differences mentioned here (urine-concentrating ability and urinary pH), the half-life of aminoglycosides is essentially the same in these four species. However, drugs that are highly bound to plasma proteins, such as albumin and α_1 acid glycoprotein, are not cleared by glomerular filtration because the proteins they are bound to are too large to be filtered by the glomerulus. Thus, species differences in the extent of a drug's plasma protein binding may influence its rate of glomerular filtration. Essentially, the filtration rate of drugs is directly proportional to the fraction of free drug in plasma, which may be 1% or less for highly protein-bound drugs. Alternatively, protein binding does not affect the rate of renal tubular secretion because this is an active, energy-dependent process. Essentially, the kinetics of drugs binding to and undergoing secretion by renal tubular transporters overcomes its binding by albumin or α_1 acid glycoprotein, so that active secretion can occur efficiently.

Several hundred transport proteins have been identified based on the human genome, with most belonging to either the ATP binding cassette (ABC) superfamily or the solute carrier (SLC) superfamily. Only a handful of these are considered clinically important with regard to drug disposition. There are seven transporters (ABCB1, ABCG2, SLCO1B1, SLCO1B3, SLC22A6, SLC22A8, and SLC22A2) that have been deemed by the FDA to be of prime importance in drug disposition (Dalgaard 2015). The European counterpart of the FDA includes those same seven and one additional transporter (SLC22A1). All but one of these are expressed by human renal tubular cells and likely contribute to active drug secretion or reabsorption. Species differences in the level of expression and substrate specificity of these transporters contribute to significant differences in renal drug excretion. For example, because dogs do not express SLCO1B1 (Dalgaard 2015), renal clearance of SLCO1B1 substrates is predicted to be prolonged in dogs compared to humans. Another factor that contributes to species differences in renal

clearance is lack of congruence in substrate specificity. Differences in substrate specificity of a given transporter in one species compared to another can be explained by amino acid differences of the same transporter in one species compared to another. For example, homology of human SLCO1B3 and SLC22A1 to the respective canine orthologs is less than 75%. Thus, it is reasonable to presume that drugs that are substrates for the human transporters may not be the same as those that are substrates for the canine, or for that matter feline, orthologs.

4.2.4.2 Biliary Elimination

The biliary system is important for clearance of both parent drug and numerous metabolites, including glucuronide and sulfate conjugates. Because conjugated drug metabolites are almost always pharmacologically inactive, we will limit our discussion to species differences in biliary excretion of parent (active) drug. Remarkable species differences in biliary clearance have been identified. Comparing published data of biliary clearance values of 19 drugs in rats and humans, clearance values ranged from 9 to more than 2500-fold greater than weight-normalized values in humans (Grime and Paine 2013). Variation between canine and human biliary drug clearance was less, with some drugs having biliary clearance values up to threefold greater in humans (methotrexate) and others having biliary clearance values up to 12-fold greater in dogs (cefazolin). Biliary drug excretion is a complex process. There are numerous physiological species differences that may translate to differences in biliary drug elimination. For example, the mean bile flow in dogs and cats (~5 mL/minute/kg) is twice that of humans. The molecular weight cutoff for biliary excretion can also vary between species (Riviere 2009). These physiologic differences have not been directly linked to species differences in the disposition of a particular drug, but one can envisage that they could certainly contribute to interspecies variation in biliary drug excretion.

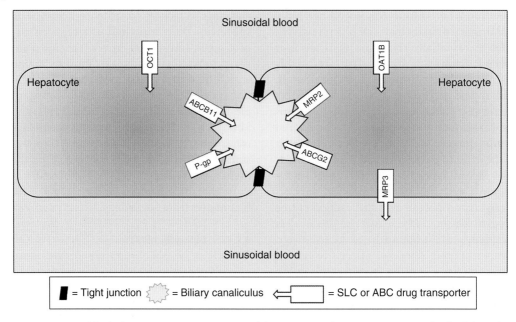

Figure 4.5 Simplified schematic representing some of the important drug transporters involved in biliary drug excretion. Many of these drug transporters belong to the solute carrier (SLC) or ATP binding cassette (ABC) carrier family of drug transporters.

Some of the more extreme species differences are likely explained by differences in active drug uptake into hepatocytes and excretion into biliary canaliculi by drug transport proteins. As shown in Figure 4.5, drug molecules present in the blood enter hepatocytes from the hepatic sinusoids either by diffusion or as substrates for transporters within the ABC or SLC transporter families. Hepatic sinusoidal blood is a mixture of blood from the portal vein and hepatic artery. In humans, genetic polymorphisms in these uptake transporters have resulted in delayed clearance of substrate drugs in patients with variant forms of ABC or SLC transporters. Deficiencies in the function of the genetic variant forms of hepatic uptake transporters result in plasma drug accumulation, ultimately causing toxicity in affected patients. Likewise, species differences in the expression or function of hepatic uptake transporters likely contribute to species differences in drug disposition. At this point, very little is known about which transporters are important for hepatic uptake of drugs from the portal vein and hepatic artery in dogs or cats.

Until we fill that knowledge gap (e.g. which drugs are substrates for particular transporters in the dog or cat, and what are the relative transport activities of the canine and feline ABC and SLC transporters compared to the corresponding human transporters), the mechanism behind many species differences in biliary drug excretion will remain unexplained.

After a drug has been taken up into the hepatocyte (by either diffusion or active transport), the next step in the process of biliary drug excretion involves yet another transporter-mediated mechanism. Several membrane-spanning ABC and SLC transporters actively efflux drugs from within hepatocytes, across the hepatocyte membrane into biliary canaliculi. Among the most important of these transporters are ABCG2, P-glycoprotein (ABCB1), and SLC47A1 (Figure 4.5), Feline ABCG2 has defective transport capacity compared to both human and canine ABCG2 (described in greater detail in Section 4.2.2.2, "ABCG2 and Drug Distribution"). Substrates for ABCG2 include fluoroquinolones, mitoxantrone, tyrosine kinase inhibitors, and other drugs. The elimination half-life of the fluoro-quinolone ciprofloxacin in cats is 1.5-fold greater than that in dogs, likely as a result of defective ABCG2-mediated efflux from hepatocyte to bile. Because ciprofloxacin relies on both renal and biliary excretion, the overall impact of defective ABCG2 function on elimination half-life is blunted. Unfortunately, since there are no data on biliary clearance of these ABCG2 substrate drugs in dogs or cats, the impact of defective ABCG2 function on biliary drug clearance in cats cannot be fully resolved. Striking individual and breed differences in P-glycoprotein function exist for both dogs and cats. These differences in P-glycoprotein function, and its impact on biliary drug excretion, lead to life-threatening adverse drug reactions that will be discussed in Chapter 5 ("Breed Differences and Pharmacogenetics").

In summary, when the biliary clearance of a drug is independent of drug transporters, species differences tend to be minimal. Biliary clearance data available for 22 drugs in both humans and rats and for 9 drugs in humans, rats, and dogs were analyzed and adjusted for differences in plasma protein binding and renal blood flow (Grime and Paine 2013). Based on their analysis, the authors discovered that only minor species differences existed in biliary drug clearance. Conversely, when drugs rely on transporters for biliary clearance, species differences in biliary clearance can be major. The impact that SLC transporters have on biliary drug elimination in humans has been well described. Until we have a basic understanding of SLC transporter expression, substrate specificity, and relative transport activity in dogs and cats, we risk causing adverse drug reactions in these patients if we simply assume that biliary drug clearance will be comparable.

4.3 Pharmacodynamic Species Differences

Pharmacodynamics is the subsection of pharmacology that explains the biochemical and physiological effects of drugs through their actions on receptors. Thus, pharmacodynamic species differences are the result of differences in the quantity or quality of drug receptors. Quantitative receptor differences between species could result from the presence of factors that upregulate or downregulate transcription of a particular receptor. The species expressing the greatest number of functional receptors would be the species predicted to experience the greatest response to a given drug concentration. Qualitative receptor differences between species would most likely result from amino acid sequence differences in a particular receptor, especially within the ligand-binding region. Pseudogenization is an extreme example of a qualitative receptor difference. Pseudogenes are essentially "faulty" DNA gene sequences in a particular species that correspond to a gene that is present and functional in most other species. Protein products of pseudogenes are defective in function, often because of accumulated mutations that have not impacted survival of the organism. Pharmacodynamic species differences likely contribute substantially to overall differences in drug response, not only between species but also between individuals within the same species. Unfortunately, there has been limited research in this area. Some of what is known is summarized in the remainder of this chapter.

In an attempt to help define the utility of dogs as a preclinical species in human drug development, a group of investigators compared the sequence of 317 human drug target genes obtained from the Pharmaprojects database (www.pharmaprojects.com) to that of a Beagle genome (Vamathevan et al. 2013). Six major drug target families were among the protein-coding sequences analyzed: kinases, proteases, nuclear hormone receptors, phosphodiesterases, ligand-gated channels, and non-olfactory G protein–coupled receptors. Results showed that 41 of the 317 genes analyzed had become pseudogenized in the Beagle, including important anti-inflammatory drug targets such as phosphodiesterase 10A. Thus, the efficacy of human drugs that rely on these 41 pathways is unlikely to translate to dogs. Conversely, the number of cyclophilin genes is more than twice as high in the Beagle compared to humans, suggesting that there are likely to be differences in response to the immunosuppressant cyclosporine, a cyclophilin inhibitor. This may explain the relative lack of cyclosporine-induced toxicity in dogs as compared to humans.

Other studies have shown substantial differences in human and canine ligand–receptor interactions, including the cannabinoid CB2 receptor (Ndong et al. 2011); estrogen receptor ERα, in a study that also assessed the feline ERα receptor (Toniti et al. 2011); and histamine H2 receptors (Preuss et al. 2007). These ligand–receptor interactions are postulated to explain such species differences as susceptibility to cannabinoid-induced adverse effects, response of mammary gland tumors to selective estrogen receptor modulators, and rate of gastric acid secretion in response to H2 receptor antagonists, respectively. Collectively, these studies indicate that species differences in ligand–receptor interactions pose limits on our ability to translate drug efficacy and safety data from one species to another. The cause of species differences in ligand–receptor interactions may be due to increased or decreased expression of receptors, structural differences in the receptor due to species-specific amino acid variations, or even species-dependent biased agonism, even though the latter has not been confirmed.

References

Beasley, D.E., Koltz, A.M., Lambert, J.E. et al. (2015). The evolution of stomach acidity and its relevance to the human microbiome. *PLoS One* 10 (7): e0134116. doi: 10.1371/journal.pone.0134116.

Court, M.H. (2013a). Canine cytochrome P450 pharmacogenetics. *Vet. Clin. North Am. Small Anim. Pract.* 43 (5): 1027–1038.

Court, M.H. (2013b). Feline drug metabolism and disposition. *Vet. Clin. North Am. Small Anim. Pract.* 43 (5): 1039–1054.

Court, M.H. and Greenblatt, D.J. (2000). Molecular genetic basis for deficient acetaminophen glucuronidation by cats: UGT1A6 is a pseudogene and evidence for reduced diversity of expressed hepatic UGT1A6 isoforms. *Pharmacogenetics* 10 (4): 355–369.

Cribb, A.E. and Spielberg, S.P. (1990). An in vitro investigation of predisposition to sulphonamide idiosyncratic toxicity in dogs. *Vet. Res. Commun.* 14 (3): 241–252.

Dalgaard, L. (2015). Comparison of minipig, dog, monkey and human drug metabolism and disposition. *J. Pharmacol. Toxicol. Methods* 74: 80–92.

Eichstadt, L.R. and Davidson, G.S. (2014). To compound or not to compound: a veterinary transdermal discussion. *Int. J. Pharm. Compd.* 18 (5): 366–369.

Ford, M.M., Dubielziq, R.R., Giuliano, E.A. et al. (2007). Ocular and systemic manifestations after oral administration of a high dose of enrofloxacin in cats. *Am. J. Vet. Res.* 68 (2): 190–202.

Gehring, R., Haskell, S.R., Payne, M.A. et al. (2005). Aminoglycoside residues in food of animal origin. *J. Am. Vet. Med. Assoc.* 227 (1): 63–66.

Grime, K. and Paine, S.W. (2013). Species differences in biliary clearance and possible relevance of hepatic uptake and efflux transporters involvement. *Drug Metab. Dispos.* 41: 372–378.

Honda, K., Komatsu, T., Koyama, F. et al. (2011). Expression of two novel cytochrome P450 3A131 and 3A132 in liver and small intenstine of domestic cats. *J. Vet. Med. Sci.* 73 (11): 1489–1492.

Kosa, T., Maruyama, T., and Otagiri, M. (1997). Species differences of serum albumins: I. Drug binding sties. *Pharm. Res.* 14 (11): 1607–1612.

Lee, D.D., Papich, M.G., and Hardie, E.M. (2000). Comparison of pharmacokinetics of fentanyl after intravenous and transdermal administration in cats. *Am. J. Vet. Res.* 61 (6): 672–677.

Lennard, L., Van Loon, J.A., and Weinshilboum, R.M. (1989). Pharmacogenetics of acute azathioprine toxicity. Relationship to thiopurine methyltransferase genetic polymorphism. *Clin. Pharmacol. Ther.* 46: 149–154.

Mahnke, H., Ballent, M., Baumann, S. et al. (2016). The ABCG2 efflux transporter in the mammary gland mediates veterinary drug secretion across the blood-milk barrier into milk of dairy cows. *Drug Metab. Dispos.* 44 (5): 700–708.

Martinez, M.N., Antonovic, L., Court, M. et al. (2013). Challenges in exploring the cytochrome P450 system as a source of variation in canine drug pharmacokinetics. *Drug Metab. Rev.* 45 (2): 218–230.

McConkey, S.E., Grant, D.M., and Cribb, A.E. (2009). The role of para-aminophenol in acetaminophen-induced methemoglobinemia in dogs and cats. *J. Vet. Pharmacol. Ther.* 32 (6): 585–595.

Mealey, K.L., Greene, S., and Bagley, R. (2008). P-glycoprotein contributes to the blood-brain but not blood-crebrospinal fluid barrier in a spontaneous canine P-glycoprotein knockout model. *Drug Metab. Dispos.* 36 (6): 1073–1079.

Mealey, K.L., Peck, K.E., Bennett, B.S. et al. (2004). Systemic absorption of amitriptyline and buspirone after oral and transdermal administration to heathy cats. *J. Vet. Intern. Med.* 18 (1): 43–46.

Miller, R., Schick, A.E., Boothe, D.M. et al. (2014). Absorption of transdermal and oral cyclosporine in sick healthy cats. *J. Am. Anim. Hosp. Assoc.* 50 (1): 36–41.

Mills, P.C. and Cross, S.E. (2006). Transdermal drug delivery: basic principles for the veterinarian. *Vet. J.* 172: 218–233.

Musther, H., Olivares-Morales, A., Hatley, O.J.D. et al. (2014). Animal versus human oral drug bioavailability: do they correlate? *Eur. J. Pharm. Sci.* 57: 280–291.

Nagahisa, A. and Okumura, T. (2017). Pharmacology of grapiprant, a novel EP4 antagonist: receptor binding, efficacy in a rodent postoperative pain model, and a dose estimation for controlling pain in dogs. *J. Vet. Pharmacol. Ther.* 40 (3): 285–292. doi: 10.1111/jvp.12349.

Ndong, C., O'Donnel, D., Ahmad, S. et al. (2011). Cloning and pharmacological characterization of the dog cannabinoid CB2 receptor. *Eur. J. Pharmacol.* 669 (1–3): 24–31.

Okamatsu, G., Kawakami, K., Komatsu, T. et al. (2017). Functional expression and comparative characterization of four feline P450 cytochromes using fluorescent substrates. *Xenobiotica* 47 (11): 1–11. doi: 10.1080/00498254.2016. 1257172.

Preuss, H., Ghorai, P., Kraus, A. et al. (2007). Constitutive activity and ligand selectivity of human, Guinea pig, rat, and canine histamine H2 receptors. *J. Pharmacol. Exp. Ther.* 321 (3): 983–995.

Pulido, M.M., Molina, A.J., Merino, G. et al. (2006). Interaction of enrofloxacin with breast cancer resistance protein (BCRP/ABCG2): influence of flavonoids and role in milk secretion in sheep. *J. Vet. Pharmacol. Ther.* 29 (4): 279–287.

Ramirez, C.J., Minch, J.D., Gay, J.M. et al. (2011). Molecular genetic basis for fluoroquinolone-induced retinal degeneration in cats. *Pharmacogenet. Genomics* 21 (2): 66–75.

Riviere, J.E. (2009). Absorption, distribution, metabolism and elimination. In: *Veterinary Pharmacology & Therapeutics*, 9e (ed. J.E. Riviere and M.G. Papich), 5–46. Ames, IA: Wiley-Blackwell.

Robinson, D. and Williams, R.T. (1958). Do cats form glucuronides? *Biochem. J.* 68: 23–24.

Roden, D.M. and Dan, M. (2014). Principles of clinical pharmacology. In: *Harrison's Principles of Internal Medicine*, 19e (ed. D. Kasper) Chap. 5. New York, NY: McGraw-Hill.

Salavaggione, O.E., Kidd, L., Prondzinski, J.L. et al. (2002). Canine red blood cell thiopruine S-methyltransferase: companion animal pharmacogenetics. *Pharmacogenetics* 12: 713–724.

Sartor, L.L., Trepanier, L.A., Kroll, M.M. et al. (2004). Efficacy and safety of transdermal methimazole in the treatment of cats with hyperthyroidism. *J. Vet. Intern. Med.* 18 (5): 651–655.

Shrestha, B., Reed, J.M., Starks, P.T. et al. (2011). Evolution of a major drug metabolizing defect in the domestic cat and other felidae: phylogenetic timing and the role of hypercarnivory. *PLoS One* 6 (3): e18046. doi: 10.1371/journal.pone.0018046.

Toniti, W., Suthiyotha, N., Puchadapirom, P. et al. (2011). Binding capacity of ER-a ligands and SERMs: comparison of the human, dog and cat. *Asian Pac. J. Cancer Prev.* 12 (11): 2875–2879.

Trepanier, L.A., Ray, K., Winand, N.J. et al. (1997). Cytosolic arylamine N-acetyltransferase (NAT) deficiency in the dog and other canids due to an absence of NAT genes. *Biochem. Pharmacol.* 54: 73–80.

Vamathevan, J.J., Hall, M.D., Jasan, S. et al. (2013). Minipin and beagle animal model genomes aid species selection in pharmaceutical discovery and development. *Toxicol. Appl. Pharmcol.* 270 (2): 149–157.

Wellman, M., DiBartola, S.P., and Kohn, C.W. (2012). Applied physiology of body fluids in dogs and cats. In: *Fluid, Electrolyte and Acid-Base Disorders in Small Animal Practice*, 4e (ed. S.P. DiBartola), 2–25. St. Louis, MO: Elsevier Saunders.

White, S.D., Rosychuk, R.A., Outerbridge, C.A. et al. (2000). Thiopruine methyltransferase in red blood cells of dogs, cats and horses. *J. Vet. Intern. Med.* 14: 552–554.

Yeap, Y.Y., Trevaskis, N.L., Quach, T. et al. (2013). Intestinal bile secretion promotes drug absorption from lipid colloidal phases via induction of supersaturation. *Mol. Pharm.* 10 (5): 1874–1889.

5

Breed Differences and Pharmacogenetics

Katrina L. Mealey

College of Veterinary Medicine, Washington State University, Pullman, WA, USA

Key Points

- Adverse drug reactions can sometimes be associated with certain dog or cat breeds.
- Pharmacogenetic testing is readily available for many drugs used in dogs and cats and is considered the standard of care.

5.1 Introduction

Many human healthcare professionals are surprised to learn that pharmacogenetics is considered the standard of care for treating companion animals with certain drugs. For some drug classes, pharmacogenetic testing is more widely practiced in veterinary medicine than it is in human medicine. Pharmacogenetics involves the study of genetic differences in an individual's response to drugs, whether that individual is a human or veterinary patient. These genetic differences are most often germline (inherited) mutations that affect genes coding for drug-metabolizing enzymes, drug transporters, plasma proteins that are involved in drug binding, or drug receptors. Results of pharmacogenetic testing using DNA extracted from blood or cheek swab samples of dogs and cats are used by the veterinarian to guide appropriate drug selection. In many cases, the veterinarian will use pharmacogenetic testing prior to administering a particular drug to a dog or cat. For example, some antiparasitics, anticancer drugs, and anesthetic agents can cause fatal reactions in dogs or cats carrying a particular genetic mutation, yet the same drugs at the same dose are tolerated well in animals that don't have the genetic mutation. In other circumstances, it is the patient's breed that triggers the veterinarian to perform pharmacogenetic testing because specific mutations are propagated within a narrow group of dog or cat breeds. It is not surprising that some genetic mutations are identified within only a few related breeds when one considers that many purebred dogs and cats are the products of inbreeding. The physical attributes that define a breed are the result of genetic traits selected for over time that are unique to a given breed. In some breeds, a pharmacogenetic mutation has been carried along inadvertently on the same region of DNA as a particular trait. Some reported breed-related adverse drug reactions are listed in Table 5.1. The pharmacogenetic mechanisms for breed-related drug sensitivities have been worked out for some, but not all, of these sensitivities.

Pharmacotherapeutics for Veterinary Dispensing, First Edition. Edited by Katrina L. Mealey.
© 2019 John Wiley & Sons, Inc. Published 2019 by John Wiley & Sons, Inc.

Table 5.1 Examples of breed-associated adverse drug reactions in dogs and cats.

Dogs		
Breed(s)	**Drug(s)**	**Adverse reaction(s)**
Herding breeds (Collie, Australian Shepherd, Border Collie, Old English Sheepdog, German Shepherd, etc.)	Macrocyclic lactones (ivermectin, milbemycin, moxidectin, selamectin, etc.) Loperamide Acepromazine	Sensitivity to central nervous system depression
Doberman Pinscher	Sulfonamides	Immune-mediated reactions involving skin, liver, joints, and lacrimal glands
Greyhounds and other sighthounds	Propofol, thiopental	Prolonged recovery
Boxers	Acepromazine	Hypotension, bradycardia, profound sedation
Cats		
Breed(s)	**Drug(s)**	**Adverse reaction**
Maine Coon	Spironolactone	Facial pruritus

Pharmacogenetic differences between individuals can alter the pharmacokinetics (i.e. absorption, distribution, metabolism, and excretion) or pharmacodynamics (i.e. binding to targets or receptors) of an administered drug. Additionally, the polymorphism (a rarer form of the gene) may affect drug efficacy or drug safety. Therefore, pharmacogenetic testing may enable the veterinarian to predict those patients at high risk for developing drug toxicity. These patients may, for example, be polymorphic for a drug-metabolizing enzyme such that drug clearance is decreased. In these patients, decreasing the drug dose, increasing the dosing interval, or selecting a drug cleared by another mechanism are possible therapeutic options. Other polymorphisms may also allow the veterinarian to identify patients that are most likely to benefit from a particular drug either because of appropriate receptor binding or because a mutation has activated a particular oncogene (Robat et al. 2011). Patients with mutations in drug receptors may respond poorly to certain

pharmaceutical agents. Rather than selecting drugs using a trial-and-error approach, a veterinarian can use pharmacogenetic testing to select the drug most likely to produce the desired pharmacological response and get it right the first time. This chapter describes veterinary pharmacogenetic tests that are commercially available and routinely used by veterinarians, as well as some examples of pharmacogenetic discoveries that are likely to be commercially available in the near future.

5.1.1 P-Glycoprotein Polymorphisms

Polymorphisms in P-glycoprotein cause life-threatening adverse drug reactions in affected dogs and cats. Hence, it is important for pharmacists to understand P-glycoprotein's role in drug disposition and the nature of the canine and feline polymorphisms. P-glycoprotein, the product of the ABCB1 (formerly MDR1) gene, is an energy-dependent efflux transporter that is a member of the ABC (ATP [adenosine triphosphate] binding cassette) superfamily. ABC transporters harness energy from ATP to transport substrates, including many drugs used in veterinary and human medicine, against large concentration gradients. In mammals, P-glycoprotein functions in a protective capacity by minimizing an animal's exposure to potentially toxic drugs. P-glycoprotein is normally expressed on enterocytes, bile canaliculi, renal tubular epithelial cells, the placenta, and brain capillary endothelial cells as part of the blood–brain barrier (Thiebaut et al. 1987; Ginn 1996). Strategically positioned at these tissue barriers, P-glycoprotein effluxes substrate drugs out of the body (into the bile, urine, or intestinal lumen) or away from protected sites (e.g. brain tissue or a fetus). Consequently, it is not surprising that defective P-glycoprotein resulting from ABCB1 polymorphisms can dramatically alter the disposition of P-glycoprotein substrates. Dogs and cats with P-glycoprotein dysfunction have exquisite sensitivity to adverse effects of P-glycoprotein substrate drugs. The fact that dozens of drugs used in veterinary medicine are P-glycoprotein substrates (Table 5.2) broadens the pharmacist's responsibility in preventing adverse drug reactions in affected dogs or cats.

The P-glycoprotein polymorphism in dogs consists of a four base-pair deletion mutation in the ABCB1 gene designated ABCB1-1Δ (Mealey et al. 2001). ABCB1-1Δ results in a frameshift such that several premature stop codons are generated very early in the translation process. Less than 10% of the protein product is synthesized. Dogs with two mutant alleles are essentially P-glycoprotein "knockouts," which makes them phenotypically similar to abcb1 (mdr1) (−/−) knockout mice (Schinkel et al. 1995). Their designated genotype is MDR1 mutant/mutant. Heterozygotes, dogs with one mutant allele and one wildtype allele (MDR1 mutant/normal), have an intermediate phenotype in terms of drug sensitivity. While the overall frequency of the MDR1 mutation (ABCB1-1Δ) in all dogs is approximately 1%, the frequency in some breeds is as high as 75% (Table 5.3). Herding breeds, some sighthound breeds, and mixed-breed dogs of herding or sighthound ancestry are the dogs most likely to be affected by the MDR1 mutation. The MDR1 mutation is distributed worldwide in these dog breeds, with reported breed frequencies similar in the United States (Neff et al. 2004; Mealey and Meurs 2008), Europe (Hugnet et al. 2004; Geyer et al., 2005), Japan (Kawabata et al. 2005), and Australia

Table 5.2 P-glycoprotein substrate drugs that can cause adverse effects in dogs with the MDR1 mutation.

Anticancer agents
Doxorubicin
Docetaxel
Vincristine
Vinblastine
Vinorelbine

Antiparasitics
Macrocyclic lactones (ivermectin, milbemycin, moxidectin, selamectin, etc.)
Emodepside

Opioids
Butorphanol
Loperamide

Miscellaneous
Ondansetron
Acepromazine

Table 5.3 Percentage of dogs affected by the MDR1 mutation (heterozygous and homozygous), by breed.

Breed	Approximate %
Australian Shepherd	50
Border Collie	5
Collie	75
English Shepherd	15
German Shepherd	10
Herding breed mix	10
Longhaired Whippet (Windsprite)	50
Miniature Australian Shepherd	45
Mixed breed	<5
Old English Sheepdog	5
Shetland Sheepdog	10
Silken Windhound	30

(Mealey et al. 2005). Thus, it is imperative that pharmacists understand the propensity of P-glycoprotein substrate drugs, including over-the-counter products, to cause serious adverse drug reactions in dogs with the MDR1 mutation. Prior to dispensing P-glycoprotein drugs, the pharmacist should ensure that the dog has been genotyped for the MDR1 mutation. Based on the MDR1 genotype, an alternative drug may need to be selected, or the drug dose may need to be decreased in accordance with the MDR1 genotype. MDR1 genotyping information, including recommended dose reductions, can be found at https://vcpl.vetmed.wsu.edu.

The discovery of the canine MDR1 mutation was first published in 2001 (Mealey et al. 2001), and since then several hundred journal articles, book chapters, and proceedings articles have been published that address the potential adverse drug effects that can occur in affected dogs. Most veterinarians are well aware of the clinical consequences of the MDR1 mutation in dogs. The feline MDR1 mutation, however, was only recently discovered, with the first publication appearing in 2015 (Mealey and Burke 2015). Approximately 4% of cats harbor a two base-pair deletion mutation (ABCB11930_1931del TC) that generates a number of premature stop codons. The protein product is truncated after only 50% of the protein is synthesized. Like dogs, cats with the feline MDR1 mutation have dysfunctional P-glycoprotein and are expected to experience the same sensitivity to P-glycoprotein substrate drugs that dogs do (Table 5.2). A number of ongoing research projects are investigating drug susceptibility in cats with the MDR1 mutation. In contrast to the canine MDR1 mutation, most veterinarians are not yet aware of the feline MDR1 mutation. Pharmacists can play a key role in preventing adverse drug reactions in cats by recommending MDR1 genotyping of cats prior to dispensing P-glycoprotein substrate drugs.

5.1.2 Pharmacogenetics of Oral Drug Absorption

Contrary to what appears to be the case in other species (humans and rodents) with P-glycoprotein variants, there is currently no evidence of a pharmacogenetic difference in oral drug absorption in either dogs or cats. There were no differences in oral bioavailability of five P-glycoprotein substrate drugs in MDR1 mutant/mutant dogs compared to MDR1 normal/normal dogs (Kitamura et al. 2008; Mealey et al. 2010). Explanations for the apparent discordance between dogs, humans, and mice include the fact that many P-glycoprotein substrates are also cytochrome P450 (CYP) substrates. Variable CYP metabolism between species might obscure differences in P-glycoprotein-mediated drug absorption. Additionally, it is likely that there are species differences in P-glycoprotein substrate binding and/or efflux kinetics such that oral absorption is impacted in one species with dysfunctional P-glycoprotein but not in another. For example, dogs have only one gene that encodes P-glycoprotein (ABCB1), while rodents have two (*abcb*1a and *abcb*1b). Lastly, canine P-glycoprotein is likely saturated at concentrations of drug achieved in the intestine after oral drug administration, blunting a measurable effect of P-glycoprotein dysfunction on oral bioavailability.

5.1.3 Pharmacogenetics of Drug Distribution

Pharmacogenetic differences in dogs and cats can lead to tremendous variations in drug distribution that impact drug safety and efficacy. In particular, the presence of the MDR1 mutation in a dog or cat dictates whether or not life-threatening neurotoxicity will occur with customary doses of certain drugs. P-glycoprotein plays a key role in maintaining the blood–brain barrier, particularly when it comes to limiting access of drugs to sensitive brain tissues. P-glycoprotein substrate drugs distribute to brain tissues at much higher concentrations in dogs and cats with the MDR1 mutation than in MDR1 normal/normal animals (Mealey et al., 2008b). For example, MDR1 mutant/mutant dogs experience adverse neurological effects after even one dose of the antiparasitic drug ivermectin (120 microgram/kg), while MDR1 normal/normal dogs can tolerate ivermectin doses of 600 microgram/kg daily for weeks without demonstrating signs of neurological toxicity. Ivermectin and other macrocyclic lactone antiparasitics, including milbemycin, selamectin, and moxidectin, achieve brain concentrations 30–90 times higher in animals with P-glycoprotein dysfunction compared to normal animals (Pulliam et al. 1985; Geyer and Janko 2012). See Chapter 7 for more information about macrocyclic lactones.

Macrocyclic lactones are not the only drugs that accumulate in brain tissue of dogs or cats with MDR1 truncation mutations. The over-the-counter antidiarrheal agent loperamide (Imodium®) is an opioid that is generally devoid of central nervous system (CNS) activity because it is excluded from the brain by P-glycoprotein (Wandel et al., 2002). Clinical cases and research studies have documented that MDR1 mutant/mutant dogs experience marked CNS depression after loperamide administration, whereas MDR1 normal/normal dogs do not (Mealey et al. 2008b; Sartor et al. 2004). The tranquilizer acepromazine has also been documented to cause more profound and prolonged sedation in MDR1 mutant/mutant dogs compared to normal dogs (Deshpande et al. 2016). Similarly, the antineoplastic drug vincristine, which is a P-glycoprotein substrate, has been reported to cause central neurotoxicity in an MDR1 mutant/mutant dog, suggesting increased brain penetration (Krugman et al. 2012). The magnitude of P-glycoprotein's influence on the blood–brain barrier can be illustrated using a radiolabeled P-glycoprotein substrate (^{99m}Tc-sestamibi). MDR1 mutant/mutant and MDR1 normal/normal dogs received a single intravenous dose of ^{99m}Tc-sestamibi and were imaged using nuclear scintigraphy. Minimal uptake of ^{99m}Tc-sestamibi radioactivity was detected in the brain of MDR1 normal/normal dogs, while uptake of ^{99m}Tc-sestamibi in the brain of MDR1 mutant/mutant dogs was indistinguishable from that in surrounding tissues (Figure 4.2).

P-glycoprotein is also presumed to limit distribution of substrate drugs to the testes and fetus in humans (Choo et al. 2000). Whether or not the P-glycoprotein polymorphism in dogs or cats alters drug distribution to these sites has not been investigated.

Another important drug transporter, ABCG2, was discussed extensively in Chapter 4. As the reader may recall, ABCG2 is a critical component of the blood–retina barrier, thereby limiting drug distribution to retinal tissue. The entire feline species has defective ABCG2 function that results in a peculiar but devastating susceptibility to fluoroquinolone-induced retinal toxicity. Individual ABCG2 polymorphisms have been described in cattle. One particular polymorphism, ABCG2 Tyr581Ser, increases secretion of the fluoroquinolone danofloxacin into milk (Otero et al. 2013). The area under the curve (AUC) and maximum concentration (C_{max}) of danofloxacin in milk were twofold lower in cattle with the wildtype ABCG2 genotype compared to cattle with the ABCG2 polymorphism. Similar results have been described for other ABCG2 substrates in cattle with the ABCG2 Tyr581Ser polymorphism, including other fluoroquinolones and benzimidazole anthelmintics (Mahnke et al. 2016). Thus, this polymorphism has implications for drug residues in dairy milk as well as for the treatment of mastitis, a common disease in dairy cattle.

In addition to drug transporters, another factor that affects drug distribution is the degree of plasma protein binding. The major plasma proteins that are involved in plasma protein binding of drugs are albumin (weak acids), alpha-1 acid glycoprotein (weak bases), and lipoproteins. However, since albumin is the most abundant protein in plasma, it is usually considered the most important in terms of overall contribution to plasma protein binding. Because only unbound drug is pharmacologically active, changes in protein binding can alter the efficacy and toxicity of highly protein-bound drugs. In many instances, only unbound drug is available for metabolism and/or excretion; therefore, clearance of a highly protein-bound drug may be different between individuals if the unbound drug fraction in those individuals is different. Situations that can alter protein binding of a drug for an individual patient include drug interactions (concurrent administration of two highly protein-bound drugs) and changes in plasma albumin concentration (e.g. due to diseases associated with hypoalbuminemia, or rapid increases in plasma albumin after administration of albumin-containing fluids). Additionally, genetic differences in albumin structure between patients may account for differences in protein binding between patients.

In dogs, two linked single-nucleotide polymorphisms (SNPs; G1075T and A1422T) have been identified in the canine albumin gene, resulting in amino acid changes in the albumin molecule (Ala335Ser and Glu450Asp). Compared to dogs with wildtype albumin, dogs with the variant form have altered protein binding and clearance of an investigational drug (Takashi et al. 2009). The investigational drug was >99% protein bound in all canine study subjects, with the mean unbound fraction in wildtype beagles (0.014%) significantly lower than in variant beagles (0.053%). Clearance of the drug was significantly greater in variant beagles (3.66 ml/min/kg) than in wildtype beagles (1.97 ml/min/kg). The prevalence of the variant allele in the research beagle colony was 40% ($n = 47$). The variant allele has been identified in many other breeds as well. Further investigation is necessary to determine if the variant affects highly protein-bound drugs that are commonly used to treat dogs, such as nonsteroidal anti-inflammatory drugs (NSAIDs).

5.1.4 Pharmacogenetics of Drug Metabolism

Polymorphisms in drug-metabolizing enzymes are the most common pharmacogenetic tests ordered by physicians for human patients (Relling and Klein 2011). Pharmacogenetic variation in either phase I or phase II metabolic enzymes can affect drug disposition and therefore drug efficacy and toxicity. Currently, only a few polymorphisms in drug-metabolizing enzymes have been described in dogs and cats, although there are several under active investigation. Some of the polymorphisms that have been described in dogs have no known clinical relevance. For example, a mutation (c1117C > T) in the coding region of CYP1A2 that generates a premature stop codon results in a complete lack of hepatic CYP1A2 protein expression and enzymatic function (Mise et al., 2004; Tenmizu et al. 2004). This mutation was identified in approximately 15% of the beagle colony in a pharmaceutical company. Although there were significant differences in plasma concentrations of investigational drugs (up to 17 times greater in dogs with deficient CYP1A2), there are no known canine therapeutics that rely on CYP1A2 metabolism.

Polymorphisms in CYP2B11 in Greyhounds and other sighthound breeds are thought to be responsible for a phenotype involving anesthetic sensitivity. The phenotype involves prolonged recovery from the injectable anesthetic agents thiopental and propofol. Specifically, Greyhounds take nearly twice as long to stand up without assistance after propofol anesthesia compared to mixed-breed dogs (Court 2013). Plasma clearance of propofol in these breeds is decreased, but the effect is reversible when dogs are pretreated with the CYP inducer phenobarbital. Using canine hepatic microsomes, researchers identified CYP2B11 as the primary enzyme responsible for CYP-dependent clearance of propofol (Court et al. 1999; Hay Kraus et al. 2000). The molecular mechanism has recently been determined (M.H. Court, personal communication), so I am optimistic that a genetic test will be commercially available shortly.

A number of other polymorphisms have been reported for canine CYP2C41, CYP2D15, CYP2E1, and CYP3A12, and feline CYP2E, but the potential impact these variants might have on drug disposition is unknown (Court 2013). Polymorphisms have also been reported in drug-metabolizing enzymes in cattle, but their role in drug metabolism has not been investigated. Instead, these polymorphisms likely serve as genetic markers of productivity (improved feed efficiency, better milk production, etc.).

An important polymorphism in a phase II enzyme in dogs is similar to what is often described as the first pharmacogenetic screening tests in people. Deficient thiopurine methyltransferase (TPMT) activity in a proportion of the human population limits their ability to metabolize 6-mercaptopurine and azathioprine to inactive metabolites (Salavaggione et al. 2005). A ninefold range in TMPT activity exists in dogs, and the enzyme activity level appears to be related to breed. Giant Schnauzers had low TPMT activity, while Alaskan Malamutes had high TMT activity (Kidd et al. 2004). Decreased TPMT activity has been documented to be associated with increased susceptibility to azathioprine-induced bone marrow suppression in both dogs and people.

5.1.5 Pharmacogenetics of Drug Excretion

Drugs are eliminated from the body either as the parent compound or as metabolites. The two most important excretory pathways for exogenous drugs are renal and biliary. Renal excretion is generally responsible for clearance of water-soluble drugs and metabolites. The characteristics that influence whether or not a drug undergoes biliary excretion are more complex, probably because specific active transport processes are involved. Genetic variation in biliary transporters can cause tremendous variation in biliary drug excretion, because these transporters are capable of transporting drugs against large concentration gradients. P-glycoprotein is one of those transporters.

Although P-glycoprotein is expressed on both renal tubular epithelial cells and biliary canalicular cells, genetic defects that cause P-glycoprotein dysfunction seem to impact only biliary drug excretion. The MDR1 mutation in dogs has been shown to radically restrict biliary excretion of substrate drugs. Studies using the radiolabeled P-glycoprotein substrate ^{99m}Tc-sestamibi illustrate that P-glycoprotein function is essential for biliary excretion of substrate drugs (Figure 5.1). Nuclear imaging of treated dogs shows no biliary excretion of ^{99m}Tc-sestamibi in MDR1 mutant/mutant dogs, while the gallbladder of MDR1 normal/normal dogs "lights up" with excreted ^{99m}Tc-sestamibi (Coehlo et al., 2009). MDR1 mutant/normal dogs have an intermediate phenotype. As a consequence of impaired P-glycoprotein excretory activity, plasma and tissue concentrations of P-glycoprotein substrate drugs persist longer in MDR1 mutant/mutant dogs compared to MDR1 normal/normal dogs, resulting in greater overall drug exposure. Severe adverse drug reactions will occur in dogs with the MDR1 mutation if doses of some P-glycoprotein substrate drugs are not decreased. This is the case with anticancer drugs, including *Vinca* alkaloids (vincristine, vinblastine, etc.), doxorubicin, and paclitaxel, since these drugs rely on P-glycoprotein-mediated biliary excretion.

Vincristine-induced myelosuppression was studied prospectively in dogs with lymphoma (Figure 5.1). Dogs with the MDR1 mutation were significantly more likely to develop neutropenia and thrombocytopenia than wildtype dogs (Mealey et al. 2008a). Additionally, I have received separate reports from several veterinarians treating MDR1 mutant/mutant Collies that died from complications of sepsis after receiving the customary dose of doxorubicin (30 mg m^{-2}). These dogs experienced severe gastrointestinal (GI) toxicity within the first few days and severe neutropenia within 10 days of receiving doxorubicin. Dogs for

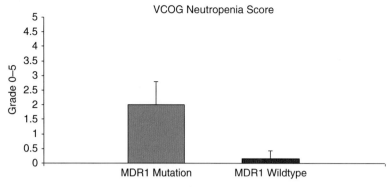

Figure 5.1 Mean neutropenia score for dogs with lymphoma treated with vincristine. Dogs with the MDR1 mutation (*n* = 8) had more severe neutropenia than MDR1 wildtype dogs (*N* = 34).

which chemotherapy is being considered should undergo MDR1 genotyping prior to treatment to determine if dose reductions should be made. The Veterinary Clinical Pharmacology Laboratory at Washington State University can be contacted for dose recommendations based on MDR1 genotype (www.vcpl.vetmed.wsu.edu).

5.1.6 Pharmacogenetics of Renal Excretion

The solute carrier (SLC) superfamily of transporters are integral membrane proteins that function as uptake or efflux transporters that transport substrates into cells or out of cells, respectively. Dozens of endogenous and exogenous compounds are substrates for these SLC transporters (Roth et al. 2012). In humans, rodents, and likely dogs, cats, and other veterinary species, SLC transporters are highly expressed by renal tubular epithelial cells, where they modulate excretion of substrate drugs. SLC transporter polymorphisms identified in people can alter drug excretion and therefore change C_{max} and AUC. The most well-known example in people involves the drug metformin, which relies exclusively on renal excretion (Chen et al. 2013). I am not aware of genetic variants in the canine or feline SLC superfamily that have been associated with changes in drug disposition.

5.1.7 Pharmacogenetics of Drug Receptors and Targets

Genetic polymorphisms can alter the structure and function of drug receptors and effector proteins. Polymorphisms in genes encoding human angiotensin-converting enzyme (ACE), beta-adrenergic receptors, the dopamine receptor, the estrogen receptor, and others are associated with altered function of those proteins (Tribut et al. 2002). A particular polymorphism in the ACE gene has implications in renal and cardiovascular disease as well as success of transplantation of either of those organs (Gard 2010). Depending on the specific polymorphism, human beta-1-adrenergic receptor (ADRB1) variants have either enhanced or suppressed effects on adenylyl cyclase when activated by a ligand. Pharmacogenetic testing for ADRB1 polymorphisms in humans has been proposed but has not been adopted into clinical cardiology practice.

In dogs, ADRB1 polymorphisms have also been identified (Maran et al. 2013). Dogs with the variant alleles are less responsive to the effects of the beta-adrenergic antagonist atenolol. These polymorphisms have been identified in a number of canine breeds. Polymorphisms of feline ADRB1 have also been described, but their functional significance is not yet known (Maran et al. 2012).

A polymorphism in canine phosphodiesterase 5A (PDE5A), the target of vasodilators such as nitric oxide and sildenafil, has recently been described (Stern et al. 2014). Dogs with the polymorphism have significantly lower plasma concentrations of cyclic guanosine monophosphate (cGMP) compared to wildtype dogs. Studies are underway to determine whether or not affected dogs respond differently to nitric oxide or sildenafil. A breed predilection for this polymorphism has not yet been described.

5.1.8 Pharmacogenetics and Idiosyncratic Reactions

Initial research in pharmacogenetics involved type A adverse drug reactions (i.e. predictable, and tend to correlate with plasma drug concentration). However, pharmacogenetic differences can also affect type B adverse drug reactions (idiosyncratic). Idiosyncratic adverse drug reactions are sometimes called hypersensitivity reactions, but this term is misleading because these reactions do not always involve an adaptive immune response. Sulfonamides are a classic example of a drug class that is associated with idiosyncratic adverse reactions – this is the case in both dogs and people. Sulfonamide "hypersensitivity" reactions can be characterized by fever, arthropathy, blood dyscrasias (neutropenia, thrombocytopenia, or hemolytic anemia), cholestasis, hepatic necrosis, skin eruptions, uveitis, or keratoconjunctivitis sicca (Trepanier 2004). In people, slow acetylation by the enzyme NAT2 is considered a risk factor for sulfonamide hypersensitivity reactions. It has been proposed that alternative metabolic pathways in slow NAT2 acetylators produce reactive metabolites. These reactive metabolites covalently bind to cell macromolecules, causing cytotoxicity and generating immune responses to neoantigens. In dogs, there are specific breeds that are predisposed to sulfonamide hypersensitivity reactions (Doberman Pinschers and Rottweilers), which strongly suggests a genetic cause. Although the genetic cause of sulfonamide hypersensitivity in dogs has not been determined, a recent study ruled out the sulfonamide detoxification genes NAT2, CYB5A, and CYP5R3 (Sacco et al. 2012).

5.1.9 Phenoconversion

Phenoconversion is just a fancy way of referring to a drug–drug interaction (most commonly) or another extrinsic factor that modifies a particular patient's response to a drug. Specifically, phenoconversion occurs when a patient with a genotype that corresponds to full enzymatic activity (metabolism or drug transport) behaves phenotypically like a poor metabolizer or poor transporter. In people, the phenomenon of phenoconversion has created clinically relevant problems involving drugs metabolized by CYP2D6, CYP2C19, and TPMT, and it has been reviewed recently (Shah and Smith 2015).

In veterinary medicine, phenoconversion involving the MDR1 gene product P-glycoprotein has been reported in dogs, although it likely occurs in cats also. Numerous drugs inhibit P-glycoprotein function and, when co-administered with a P-glycoprotein substrate, can cause serious adverse effects identical to those seen in dogs with the MDR1 mutation. A Boston Terrier mixed-breed dog (MDR1 normal/normal) suffered fatal GI and bone marrow complications after being treated concurrently with vinblastine (a P-glycoprotein substrate) and ketoconazole (a P-glycoprotein inhibitor) (Mealey and Fidel 2015). While most veterinarians are aware that MDR1 genotyping should precede administration of anticancer drugs that are P-glycoprotein substrates, they are less aware of potential drug–drug interactions. The pharmacist can play a key role in preventing serious drug–drug interactions in veterinary patients by preventing co-administration of P-glycoprotein substrates and inhibitors.

I have referred to this particular MDR1-related phenoconversion as a "Colliemorphism" since 75% of Collies are affected by the MDR1 mutation, establishing the breed as the poster child for P-glycoprotein dysfunction (Figure 5.2). Essentially, a dog of any breed that typically does not have the

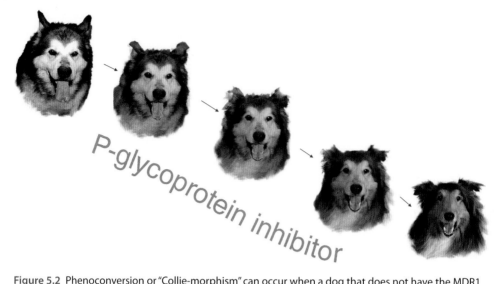

Figure 5.2 Phenoconversion or "Collie-morphism" can occur when a dog that does not have the MDR1 mutation is treated with a drug that inhibits P-glycoprotein. That dog is susceptible to toxicity caused by drugs that are P-glycoprotein substrates (as would be expected in most Collies).

MDR1 mutation can be morphed into a Collie (with respect to susceptibility to adverse drug reactions) simply by administering a drug that inhibits P-glycoprotein.

5.1.10 Veterinary Pharmacogenetic Testing

For dogs and cats, a commercial veterinary pharmacogenetics laboratory (Veterinary Clinical Pharmacology Laboratory, Washington State University; http://www.vcpl.vetmed.wsu.edu) offers MDR1 genotyping combined with pharmacogenetic counseling ($60 per dog). MDR1 genotyping is considered standard-of-care for canine patients that will be treated with vincristine, vinblastine, doxorubicin, loperamide, or ivermectin (extralabel dose for treating mange), and MDR1 genotyping of cats is not far behind. Because the MDR1 mutation in dogs has a very high allelic frequency in many breeds (Collies, Longhaired Whippets, and Australian Shepherds in particular) and because the polymorphism is highly predictive for serious adverse drug events, including death, pharmacogenetic testing in dogs has been readily accepted by veterinarians.

Although MDR1 genotyping is the only veterinary pharmacogenetic test offered commercially at this time, the author is aware of several others that will be available in the near future. Since pharmacogenetic testing has already made an impact on drug safety and efficacy in dogs, newly introduced pharmacogenetic tests are likely to be received enthusiastically by veterinarians. Pharmacists, therefore, should be familiar with pharmacogenetic testing in dogs and cats and be able to serve as a resource for determining dose adjustments for patients based on their particular genotype(s).

Abbreviations

ABCG2	ATP binding cassette transporter family G subfamily 2		C_{max}	Maximum plasma drug concentration
ACE	Angiotensin-converting enzyme		CYP	Cytochrome P450
ATP	Adenosine triphosphate		NAT2	N-acetyl transferase subfamily 2
AUC	Area under the curve		SLC	Solute carrier (family of transporters)
			TPMT	Thiopurine methyltransferase

References

Chen, S., Zhou, J., Xi, M. et al. (2013). Pharmacogenetic variation and metformin response. *Curr. Drug Metab.* 14 (10): 1070–1082.

Choo, E.F., Leake, B., Wandel, C. et al. (2000). Pharmacological inhibition of P-glycoprotein transport enhances the distribution of HIV-1 protease inhibitors into brain and testes. *Drug Metab. Dispos.* 28: 655–660.

Coelho, J.C., Tucker, R., Mattoon, J. et al. (2009). Biliary excretion of technetium-99m-sestamibi in wild-type dogs and in dogs with intrinsic (ABCB1-1Delta mutation) and extrinsic (ketoconazole treated) P-glycoprotein deficiency. *J. Vet. Pharmacol. Ther.* 32 (5): 417–421.

Court, M.H. (2013). Canine cytochrome P450 pharmacogenetics. *Vet. Clin. N. Am.* 43 (5): 1027–1038.

Court, M.H., Hay-Kraus, B.L., Hill, D.W. et al. (1999). Propofol hydroxylation by dog liver microsomes: assay development and dog breed differences. *Drug Metab. Dispos.* 27: 1293–1299.

Deshpande, D., Hill, K.E., Mealey, K.L. et al. (2016). The effect of the canine ABCB1-1Δ mutation on sedation after intravenous administration of acepromazine. *J. Vet. Intern. Med.* 30 (2): 636–641.

Gard, P.R. (2010). Implications of the angiotensin converting enzyme gene insertion/deletion polymorphism in health and disease: a snapshot review. *Int. J. Mol. Epidemiol. Genet.* 1 (2): 145–157.

Geyer, J., Doring, B., Godoy, J.R. et al. (2005). Frequency of the nt230 (del4) MDR1 mutation in collies and related dog breeds in Germany. *J. Vet. Pharmacol. Ther.* 28 (6): 545–551.

Geyer, J. and Janko, C. (2012). Treatment of MDR1 mutant dogs with macrocyclic lactones. *Curr. Pharm. Biotechnol.* 13: 969–986.

Ginn, P.E. (1996). Immunohistochemical detection of P-glycoprotein in formalin-fixed and paraffin-embedded normal and neoplastic canine tissues. *Vet. Pathol.* 33: 533–541.

Hay Kraus, B.L., Greenblatt, D.J., Venkatakrishnan, K. et al. (2000). Evidence for propofol hydroxylation by cytochrome P4502B11 in canine liver microsomes: breed and gender differences. *Xenobiotica* 30: 575–588.

Hugnet, C., Bentjen, S.A., and Mealey, K.L. (2004). Frequency of the mutant MDR1 allele associated with multidrug sensitivity in a sample of collies from France. *J. Vet. Pharmacol. Ther.* 27 (4): 227–229.

Kawabata, A., Momooi, Y., Inoue-Murayama, M. et al. (2005). Canine mdr1 mutation in Japan. *J. Vet. Med. Sci.* 67 (11): 1103–1107.

Kidd, L.B., Salavaggione, O.E., Szumlanski, C.L. et al. (2004). Thiopurine methyltransferase activity in red blood cells of dogs. *J. Vet. Intern. Med.* 18: 214–218.

Kitamura, Y., Koto, H., Matsuura, S. et al. (2008). Modest effect of impaired P-glycoprotein on the plasma concentrations of fexofenadine, quinidine and loperamide following oral administration in collies. *Drug Metab. Dispos.* 36 (5): 807–810.

Krugman, L., Bryan, J.N., Mealey, K.L. et al. (2012). Vincristine-induced central neurotoxicity in a collie homozygous for the ABCB1-1Δ mutation. *J. Small Anim. Pract.* 53 (3): 185–187.

Mahnke, H., Ballent, M., Baumann, S. et al. (2016). The ABCG2 efflux transporter in the mammary gland mediates veterinary drug secretion across the blood-milk barrier into milk of dairy cows. *Drug Metab. Dispos.* 44 (5): 700–708.

Maran, B.A., Mealey, K.L., Lahmers, S.M. et al. (2013). Identification of DNA variants in the canine beta-1 adrenergic receptor gene. *Res. Vet. Sci.* 95: 238–240.

Maran, B.A., Meurs, K.M., Lahmers, S.M. et al. (2012). Identification of beta-1 adrenergic receptor polymorphisms in cats. *Res. Vet. Sci.* 93: 210–212.

Mealey, K.L., Bentjen, S.A., Gay, J.M. et al. (2001). Ivermectin sensitivity in collies is associated with a deletion mutation of the mdr1 gene. *Pharmacogenetics* 11: 727–733.

Mealey, K.L. and Burke, N.S. (2015). Identification of a nonsense mutation in feline ABCB1. *J. Vet. Pharmacol. Ther.* 38 (5): 429–433.

Mealey, K.L. and Fidel, J. (2015). P-glycoprotein mediated drug interactions in animals and humans with cancer. *J. Vet. Intern. Med.* 29 (1): 1–6.

Mealey, K.L., Fidel, J., Gay, J.M. et al. (2008a). ABCB1-1delta polymorphism can predict hematologic toxicity in dogs treated with vincristine. *J. Vet. Intern. Med.* 22: 996–1000.

Mealey, K.L., Greene, S., Bagley, R. et al. (2008b). P-glycoprotein contributes to the blood-brain but not blood-cerebrospinal fluid barrier in a spontaneous canine p-glycoprotein knockout model. *Drug Metab. Dispos.* 36 (6): 1073–1079.

Mealey, K.L. and Meurs, K.M. (2008). Breed distribution of the ABCB1-1delta (multidrug sensitivity) polymorphism among dogs undergoing ABCB1 genotyping. *J. Am. Vet. Med. Assoc.* 233 (6): 921–924.

Mealey, K.L., Munyard, K.A., and Bentjen, S.A. (2005). Frequency of the mutant MDR1 allele associated with multidrug sensitivity in a sample of herding breed dogs living in Australia. *Vet. Parasitol.* 131 (3–4): 193–196.

Mealey, K.L., Waiting, D., Raunig, D.L. et al. (2010). Oral bioavailability of P-glycoprotein substrate drugs do not differ between ABCB1-1D and ABCB1 wildtype dogs. *J. Vet. Pharmacol. Ther.* 33 (5): 453–460.

Mise, M., Yadera, S., Matsuda, M. et al. (2004). Polymorphic expression of CYP1A2 leading to interindividual variability in metabolism of a novel benzodiazepine receptor partial inverse agonist in dogs. *Drug Metab. Dispos.* 32: 240–245.

Neff, M.W., Robertson, K.R., Wong, A.K. et al. (2004). Breed distribution and history of canine mdr1-1Delta, a pharmacogenetic mutation that marks the emergence of breeds from the collie lineage. *Proc. Natl. Acad. Sci. USA.* 101 (32): 11725–11730.

Otero, J.A., Real, R., de la Fuente, A. et al. (2013). The bovine ATP-binding cassette transporter ABCG2 Tyr581Ser single-nucleotide polymorphism increases milk secretion of the fluoroquinolone danofloxacin. *Drug Metab. Dispos.* 41: 546–549.

Pulliam, J.D., Seward, R.L., Henry, R.T. et al. (1985). Investigating ivermectin toxicity in collies. *Vet. Med.* 80: 33–40.

Relling, M.V. and Klein, T.E. (2011). CPIC: Clinical pharmacogenetics implementation consortium of the pharmacogenomics research network. *Clin. Pharmacol. Ther.* 89 (3): 464–467.

Robat, C., London, C., Bunting, L. et al. (2011). Safety evaluation of combination vinblastine and toceranib phosphate (Palladia®) in dogs: a phase I dose-finding study. *Vet. Comp. Oncol.* 10 (3): 174–183.

Roth, M., Obaidat, A., and Hagenbuch, B. (2012). OATPs, OATs, and OCTs: the organic anion and cation transporters of the SLCO and SLC22A gene superfamilies. *Br. J. Pharmacol.* 165 (5): 1260–1287.

Sacco, J.C., Abouraya, M., Motsinger-Reif, A. et al. (2012). Evaluation of polymorphisms in the sulfonamide detoxification genes NAT2, CYP5A and CYB5R3 in patients with sulfonamide hypersensitivity. *Pharmacogenet. Genomics* 22: 733–740.

Salavaggione, O.E., Wang, L., Wiepert, M. et al. (2005). Thioprine S-methyltransferase pharmacogenetics: variant allele functional and comparative genomics. *Pharmacogenet. Genomics* 15 (11): 801–815.

Sartor, L.L., Bentjen, S.A., Trepanier, L. et al. (2004). Loperamide toxicity in a collie with the MDR1 mutation associated with ivermectin sensitivity. *J. Vet. Intern. Med.* 18 (1): 117–118.

Schinkel, A.H., Wagenaar, E., van Deemter, L. et al. (1995). Absence of the Mdr1a P-glycoprotein in mice affects tissue distribution and pharmacokinetics of dexamethasone, digoxin, and cyclosporin A. *J. Clin. Invest.* 96: 1698–1705.

Shah, R.R. and Smith, R.L. (2015). Addressing phenoconversion: the Achilles' heel of personalized medicine. *Br. J. Clin. Pharmacol.* 79 (2): 222–240.

Stern, J.A., Reina-Dorests, Y., Chdid, L. et al. (2014). A polymorphism in the canine phosphodiesterase 5A gene affecting basal cGMP concentrations of healthy dogs. *J. Vet. Intern. Med.* 28: 78–83.

Takashi, I., Takahashi, M., Sudo, K. et al. (2009). Interindividual pharmacokinetics variability of the a4b1 integrin antagonist 4-[1-[3-Chloro-4-[N0-(2-methylphenyl) ureido]phenylacetyl]-(4S)-fluoro-(2S)-pyrrolidine-2-yl]methoxybenzoic acid (D01-4582), in beagles is associated with albumin genetic polymorphisms. *J. Pharm. Sci.* 98: 1545–1555.

Tenmizu, D., Endo, Y., Noguchi, K. et al. (2004). Identification of the novel canine CYP1A2 1117 C>T SNP causing protein deletion. *Xenobiotica* 34: 835–846.

Thiebaut, F., Tsuruo, T., Hamada, H. et al. (1987). Cellular localization of the multidrug-resistance gene product P-glycoprotein in normal human tissues. *Proc. Natl. Acad. Sci. USA.* 84: 7735–7738.

Trepanier, L.A. (2004). Idiosyncratic toxicity associated with potentiated sulfonamides in the dog. *J. Vet. Pharmacol. Ther.* 27: 129–138.

Tribut, O., Lessard, Y., Reymann, J.M. et al. (2002). Pharmacogenomics. *Med. Sci. Monit.* 8: RA152–RA163.

Wandel, C., Kim, R., Wood, M. et al. (2002). Interaction of morphine, fentanyl, sufentanil, alfentanil, and loperamide with the efflux drug transporter P-glycoprotein. *Anesthesiology* 96: 913–920.

6

Human Over-the-Counter (OTC) Products

Precautions for Veterinary Patients

Patricia A. Talcott[1] and Katrina L. Mealey[2]

[1] Integrative Physiology and Neuroscience and Washington Animal Disease Diagnostic Laboratory, College of Veterinary Medicine, Washington State University, Pullman, WA, USA
[2] College of Veterinary Medicine, Washington State University, Pullman, WA, USA

Key Points

- Many human over-the-counter (OTC) drug products are potentially toxic to dogs and/or cats, even at low doses, owing to species differences in drug disposition.
- With few exceptions, human OTC analgesics should not be used in dogs or cats.
- The artificial sweetener xylitol, used in human OTC and prescription drug products, is highly toxic to dogs.

Pharmacists play a key role in maintaining healthy communities by providing their expertise to assist people purchasing over-the-counter (OTC) drug products and nutritional supplements. By helping individuals select a safe and effective OTC product to treat pain, symptoms of upper respiratory infections, or gastrointestinal discomfort, for example, pharmacists serve as an integral member of the human healthcare team. The wide variety of competing products that are sold OTC in pharmacy sections of stores can be overwhelming. For example, if someone is seeking a product useful for general pain or allergy relief, there are dozens of products to choose from, and it is often too much for the average consumer to comprehend. With the pharmacist's expertise, the patient can select the most appropriate product for their particular needs, making sure to avoid ingredients that may interact with prescription drugs the patient may be taking. Equally important, pharmacists are trained to identify conditions for which the human patient should see a healthcare provider. Unfortunately, most pharmacists have not received sufficient education to provide that same level of expertise for veterinary patients.

More importantly, pharmacists should be aware of federal laws regarding extra-label drug use in animals. The key point is that federal law allows extra-label drug use only on the lawful order of a licensed veterinarian in the context of a valid veterinarian–client–patient relationship (see Chapter 1 for legal restrictions to extra-label drug use in veterinary species).

Dramatic difference

Because there is not an exception made for OTC human drugs, then, by law, pharmacists cannot independently (without a lawful order by a licensed veterinarian) recommend use

Pharmacotherapeutics for Veterinary Dispensing, First Edition. Edited by Katrina L. Mealey.
© 2019 John Wiley & Sons, Inc. Published 2019 by John Wiley & Sons, Inc.

of OTC products for veterinary patients. This is in striking contrast to the laws pertaining to pharmacists recommending OTC drugs for human patients. Pharmacists can still perform an important role with regard to OTC drug use in veterinary species – and that is to prevent pet owners from inadvertently poisoning their pet by treating their pet with an inappropriate and potentially toxic human OTC product.

It is our experience that pet owners tend to assume that if a product is sold OTC, it must be "safe," even for dogs and cats. Pharmacists can be instrumental in preventing unintentional poisoning of animals by their owners by providing counseling on which OTC products should never be administered to dogs, cats, or other veterinary patients. Many products available OTC, including products that are considered "safe" for humans, are often not safe for companion animals. As pharmacists know, OTC products may contain drugs that are safe for human patients at the label dose but can cause severe adverse effects if consumed in excess amounts. What pharmacists have not been taught is that these drugs can cause adverse effects in companion animals even at doses that are adjusted for body weight differences (i.e. equivalent mg/kg doses). The goal of this chapter is to enable pharmacists to recognize some of the risks that some OTC drugs pose to companion animals as well as recognize which OTC drugs are relatively safe.

6.1 Analgesics

For information regarding therapeutic use of analgesics in veterinary patients, see Chapter 8.

6.1.1 Acetaminophen

Even though acetaminophen displays some anti-inflammatory properties, this drug is discussed separately from the nonsteroidal anti-inflammatory drugs (NSAIDs) because acetaminophen's toxic effects in veterinary species are quite different from those associated with NSAIDs. The amount of acetaminophen contained in most OTC products is either 325 or 500 mg per dose. One 325 mg tablet can be fatal to an average 10-pound cat. Two 325-mg tablets or capsules can cause serious toxicity in a 20-pound dog. Most pet poisonings associated with acetaminophen occur as a result of accidental ingestion – pets chewing their way into childproof containers (Figure 6.1) or finding those few pills that have fallen to the floor when adult humans are struggling to open childproof containers. Cats are uniquely susceptible to acetaminophen, given their unusual metabolism of this compound.

In human beings, acetaminophen is metabolized to nontoxic metabolites via glucuronidation and sulfation pathways with the conjugates, then excreted into the bile and/or urine. This is the primary route of acetaminophen metabolism for dogs as well. Acetaminophen can also be metabolized via cytochrome P450 (CYP) enzymes, which generates a toxic metabolite, N-acetyl benzoquinonemine (NAPQI). In most species, the CYP pathway is minor, generating minute concentrations of NAPQI that are easily detoxified by glutathione (Sellon 2006). Cats, however, have an unusual combination of metabolic deficiencies (Figure 6.2) that not only result in the production of NAPQI as a primary metabolite, but have feeble mechanisms for NAPQI detoxification as well. Specifically, cats lack the appropriate UDP glucuronyltransferase isoenzyme and are deficient in sulfation relative to dogs and humans (see Chapter 4 for additional information), so acetaminophen is metabolized by CYP as the primary pathway, producing the toxic metabolite NAPQI. Relative to dogs and humans, cats are deficient in glutathione, which is important for detoxifying NAPQI. NAPQI is a powerful oxidant and electrophile, causing oxidative damage to cellular membranes and binding to sulfhydryl-containing amino acids in proteins. In cats, the hemoglobin molecule is particularly sus-

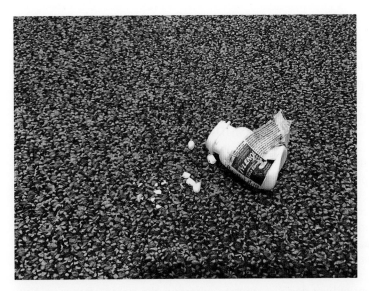

Figure 6.1 A childproof container of acetaminophen is no match for the jaws of a dog ("childproof" is not the same as "dog-proof").

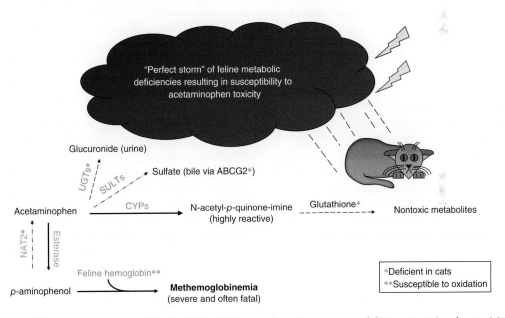

Figure 6.2 Perfect storm of metabolic deficiencies in cats that enhance susceptibility to acetaminophen toxicity.

ceptible to NAPQI-induced oxidation because it contains eight sulfhydryl-containing amino acids compared to four in dogs and humans. Thus, cats (wild felids as well as domestic cats) have the perfect storm of metabolic deficiencies that generate extreme susceptibility to acetaminophen toxicity.

The major target organs of acetaminophen toxicity in dogs and cats are red blood cells (cats > dogs) and the liver (dogs > cats). Within 60 minutes of a toxic dose of acetaminophen, NAPQI will oxidize susceptible amino acid residues of feline hemoglobin, converting it rapidly to methemoglobin that imparts a "chocolate-brown" discoloration to the blood. Methemoglobin has a higher affinity for oxygen than hemoglobin, so oxygen is not released from red blood cells to tissues, resulting in tissue hypoxia. Animals that are suffering from this malady experience respiratory distress and weakness. Damaged hemoglobin begins to accumulate in red blood cells in the form of "Heinz bodies." If the animal survives the acute tissue hypoxic event, a second hypoxic event can occur. The spleen recognizes the Heinz bodies as abnormal red blood cells and subsequently destroys them, leading to severe anemia and further hypoxia. If an affected patient is able to survive this second period of tissue hypoxia, NAPQI will eventually cause liver damage. The extent of liver damage is directly related to prognosis. For unknown reasons, male cats appear to be more sensitive to the hepatotoxic effects of NAPQI than females. Dogs seem to be more sensitive to the hepatotoxic effects of acetaminophen, whereas cats often succumb to methemoglobinemia before signs of hepatotoxicity occur.

Treatment options for the exposed patient may include decontamination procedures (see Section 6.11, "Decontamination Procedures"), if appropriate, along with N-acetylcysteine, which acts by replenishing glutathione, which binds to NAPQI enhancing its urinary excretion. Other supportive care measures may include intravenous fluid therapy, blood transfusions, oxygen therapy, and antioxidants.

6.1.2 Nonsteroidal Anti-Inflammatory Drugs

One of the most common classes of OTC drugs that is found in pharmacies, grocery and department stores, and convenience stores is the NSAIDs. Despite the fact that there are hundreds of different brand names of products that contain these drugs, there are only a handful of individual drug ingredients that are commercially available – common ones include aspirin (acetylsalicylic acid), ibuprofen, and naproxen. These drugs, which are indicated to reduce fever, relieve mild aches and pains, and reduce inflammation, are abundantly available in most households where pets reside. Pharmacists should never recommend a human NSAID drug product for a companion animal without first consulting with a veterinarian. There are many NSAIDs that have been tested for safety and efficacy in dogs, cats, and horses and are US Food and Drug Administration (FDA) approved specifically for these species. These veterinary NSAIDs should be used instead of human products.

Because most households have at least one container of an NSAID-containing product, companion animals often have access to NSAIDs. If an exposure occurs, it is important to ascertain the name of the product, because many NSAIDs are combined with cough suppressants, decongestants, and/or antihistamines that can potentially alter the clinical progression of the toxicity. Most poisonings that occur in companion animals are due to unintentional consumption of the drugs by curious dogs or cats, although there are cases where owners intentionally administer the NSAID to their pets, with the belief that what works for them must work for their pet. And, unbeknownst to many pet owners, it does not take a high dose to poison pets. For example, a single dose of as few as four 200-mg ibuprofen tablets are enough to cause serious gastrointestinal signs in a 30-pound dog (Talcott and Gwaltney-Brant 2013). Cats are considered to be approximately twice as sensitive as dogs to the toxic effects of ibuprofen – one 200-mg tablet can cause gastrointestinal problems (e.g. vomiting and abdominal pain) in the average-sized house cat. A veterinarian or animal poison control hotline (Table 6.1) should be consulted immediately when any pet exposure to NSAIDs occurs.

NSAIDs inhibit the cyclooxygenase (COX, or prostaglandin synthetase) enzyme system in humans and other mammals. Individual NSAIDs have varying degrees of affinity to the constitutive COX1 enzyme versus the inducible COX2 enzyme. It is generally

Table 6.1 Resources for potential poisonings in companion animals.

Organization name Website	Phone number	Comments
ASPCA Animal Poison Control Center aspca.org/pet-care/poison-control	888-426-4435	Fee applies 24-hour service
Pet Poison Helpline petpoisonhelpline.com	800-213-6680	Fee applies 24-hour service
FDA Center for Veterinary Medicine	888-332-8387	No fee Business hours (Eastern Time)
National Pesticide Information Center* npic.orst.edu	800-858-7378	8am to 12 pm (Pacific Time)

accepted that COX1 catalyzes formation of prostaglandins involved in normal physiological functions, while COX2 catalyzes formation of prostaglandins involved in inflammatory processes, although some crossover exists. Some NSAIDs preferentially inhibit COX2 to a greater extent than COX1, which is thought to decrease the risk of gastrointestinal adverse effects compared to NSAIDS that are nonselective COX inhibitors or COX1-selective inhibitors.

Dramatic difference

It is important for pharmacists to know that the relative COX2 selectivity of each NSAID can vary greatly between species. For example, the veterinary NSAID carprofen is COX2 selective in dogs, but not in cats or horses; meloxicam is COX2 selective in humans and dogs, but not cats; and piroxicam shows COX2 selectivity in dogs, but not humans. Thus, COX2 selectivity of NSAIDs is a species-dependent phenomenon that thus far is not predictable based on drug class or structure.

Another important species difference with regard to NSAIDs is drug disposition. NSAID metabolism in cats and dogs can vary widely relative to that of humans, depending on the particular drug. In general, cats are thought to metabolize NSAIDs more slowly than dogs or humans, necessitating longer dosing intervals. For example, the elimination half-life of aspirin in cats is 22 hours, approximately 10 times longer than in humans

(2.3 hours) and five times longer than in dogs (4.5 hours). Thus, *the dosing interval for aspirin in cats is 72 hours.* For meloxicam, the half-lives are similar (approximately 20–24 hours) for all three species. For piroxicam, the situation is reversed. Cats eliminate the drug most rapidly (elimination half-life of 11 hours), which is roughly four times faster than dogs (40 hours) and humans (47 hours). More detailed information about therapeutic use of NSAIDs in veterinary patients can be found in Chapter 8.

In overdose situations, even COX2-selective NSAIDs inhibit COX1, decreasing the production of prostaglandins that augment blood flow to the gastric mucosa. Adequate blood circulation to the gastric mucosa is necessary to maintain mucus and bicarbonate production and epithelial cell turnover and restitution, which protect the stomach from gastric acid. When this normal blood flow is disrupted, mucosal erosion and/or ulceration occurs. Initial clinical signs of acute NSAID poisoning include vomiting (with or without blood), loss of appetite, and hemorrhagic, dark, or black feces (due to the presence of fresh or digested blood).

At higher exposure doses, there is disruption of renal blood flow, leading to acute kidney injury that may resolve or progress to chronic renal failure. Clinical signs associated with renal disease can be very vague and mimic many other diseases – these include loss of appetite, vomiting, diarrhea, abdominal pain, and generally "not doing well." Cats seem to be more sensitive than dogs to NSAID-induced acute kidney injury due to defective function of a renal-protective protein called AIM (apoptosis inhibitor of macrophages). Even after a single label dose of NSAIDs, some cats can develop acute renal failure. This is particularly true if the cat is dehydrated or hypotensive (anesthetic events).

It has also been reported that some dogs and cats exposed to extremely high doses of NSAIDs may exhibit an acute onset of neurologic signs, which include tremors, seizures, and even coma. The pathophysiology of these NSAID-induced neurological signs is currently unknown.

The "antiplatelet" effects of NSAIDs are of limited clinical significance unless the patient is undergoing surgery.

Treatment plans for patients exposed to toxic doses of NSAIDs may include the use of appropriate decontamination measures (see the "Decontamination Procedures" section), sucralfate, parenteral fluids to promote renal blood flow, misoprostol (a prostaglandin E_1 analog) to promote gastric mucosal blood flow, and general symptomatic and supportive care.

6.1.3 Phenazopyridine (Urinary Analgesic)

Phenazopyridine is a urinary anesthetic/analgesic used by human patients for symptomatic relief of pain associated with urinary tract infections or interstitial cystitis. Some cats experience a disease similar to interstitial cystitis in humans in which they suffer from hematuria, stranguria, pollakiuria, and/or dysuria with no apparent cause identified (e.g. infection, uroliths, or urothelial neoplasia). Affected cats often appear to be in distress, presumably due to urogenital pain. Cat owners familiar with this drug may be tempted to use this drug to alleviate their cat's apparent lower urinary tract discomfort. However, this drug causes severe, even fatal, methemoglobinemia and hemolysis in cats (Harvey and Kornick 1976). As was discussed in Section 6.1.1 ("Acetaminophen"), the amino acid composition of feline hemoglobin makes it highly susceptible to oxidative damage compared to that of canine and human hemoglobin. That,

coupled with the fact that felines have limited erythrocyte glutathione stores relative to other species, renders them ill-equipped to handle oxidative injury. A safe dose of phenazopyridine for cats has not yet been established; therefore, its use is contraindicated in cats.

6.2 Allergy, Cough, Cold, and Flu Medications

There are perhaps hundreds of different cough, cold, and flu medications that can be found on pharmacy shelves, with some products containing only one active ingredient (e.g. an antihistamine), while others may contain combinations of multiple drugs (e.g. antihistamine, decongestant, analgesic, and cough suppressant). These OTC combination products should be avoided in veterinary patients for several reasons. First, the dose ratios were designed to meet the general pharmacokinetic and pharmacodynamic needs of human patients, which are quite different from those in other species (see Chapters 4 and 5 for more details). Second, the therapeutic window for many of the individual drugs in these combination products is very narrow (or nonexistent) for dogs, cats, or other veterinary species. Last, there are many FDA-approved veterinary drugs in the same therapeutic classes that are more effective and have greater safety profiles than human OTC drug products. The FDA limits extra-label use of human drug products in veterinary patients to a limited number of circumstances (see Chapter 2 for more detailed information). Briefly, extra-label use of human drugs is permitted if there are no FDA-approved veterinary drugs that can be used to treat the condition or if the FDA-approved veterinary drug(s) have been determined to be ineffective.

6.2.1 Antihistamines (H_1 Receptor Antagonists)

There are several OTC antihistamines that can be used therapeutically in both humans and veterinary patients. For example, Chapter 18 describes their use for symptomatic relief of pruritus in canine atopy. First-generation antihistamines (e.g. brompheniramine, chlorpheniramine, dimenhydrinate, diphen-hydramine, and doxylamine) have been used more frequently than second-generation antihistamines in veterinary patients because they tend to be less expensive and have been more widely available. The fact that they cross the blood–brain barrier and can cause sedation and drowsiness is generally considered an advantage rather than disadvantage in veterinary patients, particularly for pruritic pets. Second-generation OTC antihistamines, such as cetirizine, fexofenadine, and loratadine, are intended to provide allergy relief without causing the drowsiness. This is because they are substrates for the drug transporter P-glycoprotein, which is a component of the blood–brain barrier. As discussed in the pharmacogenetics chapter (Chapter 5), approximately 1% of dogs and 4% of cats have a polymorphism in the ABCB1 gene resulting in P-glycoprotein dysfunction. These animals would be expected to experience drowsiness with second-generation antihistamines. Otherwise, these drugs are well tolerated in

veterinary patients with dose ranges for dogs and cats actually exceeding those for humans on a mg per kg basis. For example, a 25 mg diphenhydramine tablet would be an appropriate dose for a 15–20-pound dog or cat as well as an adult human. Additional dosing information is provided further in this chapter. Antihistamines can be used by owners to treat potential allergic or anaphylactic reactions either at home (for minor allergic reactions) or en route to the veterinary hospital (for anaphylactic reactions). Figure 6.3 shows a dog that suffered from an acute allergic reaction that responded to home treatment with diphenhydramine.

Diphenhydramine is one of the most common toxicities reported in dogs, most often related to unintended consumption of large quantities when the drug container is within a "muzzle's reach." Pharmacologic effects of antihistamines are widely distributed throughout the body, and in overdose scenarios, adverse effects can involve the cardiovascular, gastrointestinal, and nervous systems (Worth

(a)

(b)

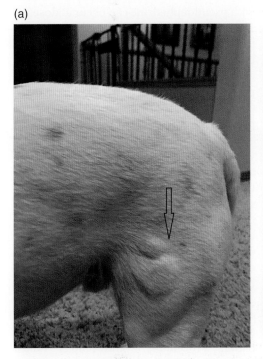 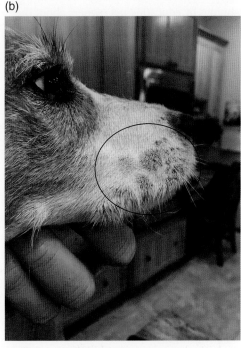

Figure 6.3 A 21-pound dog that experienced an acute allergic reaction as demonstrated by the presence of wheals (a) and angioedema (b). The dog was treated with a 25 mg diphenhydramine tablet and monitored closely by the veterinarian and owner of the dog.

et al. 2016). Nervous system signs may include lethargy, hyperactivity, agitation, hyperthermia, ataxia, tremors, and muscle fasciculations, while the most common cardiovascular system abnormality is tachycardia. Pets ingesting diphenhydramine-containing creams can exhibit vomiting and diarrhea, in addition to the cardiovascular and neurologic signs, most likely due to the vehicle. Clinical signs of illness with diphenhydramine in dogs are generally not observed until exposure doses exceed 13 mg/kg body weight (Worth et al. 2016) – which would equate to a 25 mg tablet consumed by a 5-pound Toy Poodle or 12 tablets (a blister-pack box) consumed by a 50-pound Basset Hound.

While antihistamines themselves have a relatively high therapeutic index in dogs and cats, they are commonly found in combination with other ingredients (e.g. NSAIDs, acetaminophen, decongestants, and cough suppressants) in many OTC products. Because many of these other ingredients have a low safety profile in veterinary patients, combination products should be avoided. Pharmacists can play a key role in preventing accidental pet poisonings by educating pet owners about the potential toxicity of many OTC human drug products. In the event of antihistamine overdoses, treatment options for exposed dogs and cats include decontamination procedures (see Section 6.11, "Decontamination Procedures") and strategies aimed to treat the observed clinical signs.

6.2.1.1 Antihistamine Doses for Veterinary Patients
Cetirizine:

Dogs: 5–10 mg PER DOG PO every 12 hours (maximum dose 2 mg/kg)
Cats: 5 mg PER CAT PO every 24 hours

Chlorpheniramine:

Dogs: 2–8 mg PER DOG PO every 8–12 hours
Cats: 1–2 mg PER CAT PO every 8–12 hours

Diphenhydramine:
Dogs and cats: 2–4 mg/kg PO every 8–12 hours

6.2.2 Decongestants

Decongestants such as pseudoephedrine and phenylephrine, which are common ingredients in many OTC human products (cough and cold remedies, allergy medications, nasal sprays and drops, and hemorrhoid preparations), do not enjoy the wide safety margin that antihistamines do in veterinary patients (Hovda et al. 2016). As sympathomimetic agents, pseudoephedrine and phenylephrine cause stimulation of both the nervous and cardiovascular systems in veterinary species as well as humans. Pseudoephedrine is sometimes used in dogs with urethral sphincter incompetence (urinary incontinence) at low oral doses (Chapter 11). It has a narrow therapeutic index and should not be used in dogs with conditions that might be exacerbated by increased sympathetic drive. Phenylephrine-containing nasal drops are sometimes used in cats with rhinitis. Neither pseudoephedrine nor phenylephrine should be used systemically in cats.

Decongestants have a narrow therapeutic index in dogs and cats. Toxicity associated with pseudoephedrine can occur at doses of 1–2 mg/kg body weight in dogs (Hovda et al. 2016). This means that a single 30 mg tablet of pseudoephedrine is likely to cause signs of toxicity in animals up to 65 pounds (a Labrador Retriever–sized dog)! Commonly reported clinical signs of pseudoephedrine (or other decongestant) overdoses in veterinary species include vomiting, lethargy, diarrhea, restlessness, agitation, hyperactivity, tachycardia, and tremors (Hovda et al. 2016). The onset of signs post exposure will often depend on the formulation of the drug – whether it is a liquid formulation such as nasal drops or sprays (within 30–60 minutes) or an extended-release product (three to six hours or longer).

Treatment of affected patients involves decontamination procedures if deemed appropriate (see Section 6.11, "Decontamination Procedures"), intravenous fluids, tranquilizers to control agitation and hyperexcitability, beta-adrenergic antagonists to manage tachycardia, and anticonvulsants to control seizures.

6.2.2.1 Decongestant Doses for Veterinary Patients
Pseudoephedrine:

Dogs: 0.2–0.4 mg/kg PO every 8–12 hours (for urinary incontinence)
Cats: Do not use in cats.

Phenylephrine pediatric nasal solution:
Cats: 1–2 drops intranasally every 12–24 hours. Do not use adult formulations.

6.3 Cough Suppressants

The most common cough suppressant sold OTC is dextromethorphan. While it has a relatively high margin of safety, it is not considered efficacious in veterinary species. Instead, an opioid antitussive, butorphanol, is FDA approved for relieving cough in dogs and is the drug of choice. Dextromethorphan is not found in any FDA-approved veterinary drug products. Some human OTC products contain dextromethorphan as the sole active ingredient, but it is more commonly found in multi-ingredient cough and cold preparations that contain various combinations of acetaminophen, NSAIDs, guaifenesin, antihistamines, and/or decongestants. Dextromethorphan overdoses can cause signs of toxicity within a few hours post exposure, including vomiting, diarrhea, ataxia, agitation, tremors, and seizures. *Reportedly, some patients may exhibit a pattern of signs consistent with serotonin syndrome*, characterized by muscle tremors, agitation, disorientation, excessive salivation, and seizure activity. Treatment options for poisoned patients may include decontamination measures (see Section 6.11, "Decontamination Procedures"), intravenous fluid therapy, diazepam to control tremors and agitation (unless serotonin syndrome is diagnosed, in which case cyproheptadine should be considered), anticonvulsant medication for seizure control, and general supportive care.

6.4 Gastrointestinal Medications

6.4.1 Antacids

Antacids (aluminum hydroxide, calcium carbonate, and magnesium hydroxide) generally have a wide safety margin in veterinary patients. They are prescribed as phosphate binders for dogs or cats with hyperphosphatemia secondary to renal failure (Chapter 13) more often than they are prescribed to neutralize gastric acid. The histamine-2 receptor antagonists and proton pump inhibitors are more effective in combating gastric acid, and they do not have to be administered as frequently as antacids. Aluminum hydroxide tends to be prescribed most often, since veterinary patients do not appear to be at risk for aluminum toxicity. Magnesium hydroxide is a laxative and cathartic agent. Because it is contraindicated in patients that might have gastrointestinal obstruction, it should not be administered to veterinary patients unless specifically prescribed by a veterinarian. Calcium carbonate should not be used in patients with renal disease that could have either hypercalcemia or hyperphosphatemia.
Aluminum hydroxide:

Dogs: 5–10 mL PER DOG PO every 6–12 hours (lower dose range for smaller dogs)
Cats: 1–3 mL PER CAT PO every 6–12 hours

Calcium carbonate:

Dogs: 1–4 Grams PER DOG PO divided over 24 hours (lower dose range for smaller dogs)
Cats: 0.5–2 Grams PER CAT PO divided over 24 hours

6.4.2 Histamine-2 Receptor Antagonists

Histamine-2 receptor antagonists (H2RAs) tend to be overused by veterinarians. They are frequently prescribed or administered parenterally to any vomiting patient, even though gastric hyperacidity is rarely a cause of vomiting in dogs or cats (Chapter 12).

The reason for this is that H2RAs have a wide safety margin and perhaps satisfy the owner's need to do something for their pet. However, for at-home use (not supervised by a veterinarian), famotidine is the H2RA least likely to cause an adverse event because it does not have prokinetic actions (ranitidine and nizatidine are prokinetics), nor does it inhibit cytochrome P450 enzymes (cimetidine does), so drug–drug interactions are not a concern. Prokinetics are contraindicated for patients with gastrointestinal obstruction, which is always a potential cause of vomiting, lack of appetite, or abdominal pain in a dog or cat.

Famotidine:

Dogs: 0.5–1 mg/kg PO every 12–24 hours
Cats: 0.5 mg/kg PO every 24 hours

6.4.3 Proton Pump Inhibitors

Proton pump inhibitors (PPIs) are highly effective at inhibiting gastric acid production in dogs and cats (Chapter 12). Pharmacists should discourage pet owners from administering PPIs to their pets unless specifically prescribed by a veterinarian because of the potential for secondary complications. Two different formulations of omeprazole paste are FDA approved for use to prevent (lower dose) and treat (higher dose) stress-induced gastric ulcers in horses. Oral bioavailability of omeprazole is low in horses, so the FDA-approved products have been specially formulated for horses. Human products are not bioavailable in horses, so pharmacists should counsel horse owners not to use human formulations of omeprazole.

6.4.4 Antidiarrheals

Pharmacists may be surprised by the fact that serious adverse events can occur if some OTC antidiarrheal drugs are administered to certain veterinary patients. For example, bismuth subsalicylate is metabolized differently in dogs and cats, resulting in longer elimination half-lives relative to human beings. Pharmacists are accustomed to selling products containing bismuth subsalicylate OTC for human use, since there is a low risk of toxicity. Pharmacists should discourage owners from administering bismuth subsalicylate to veterinary patients unless a veterinarian has specifically prescribed it.

Loperamide can pose high risk of neurological toxicity in dogs or cats with polymorphisms of the MDR1 (ABCB1) gene (described in more detail in Chapter 5). The MDR1 gene encodes P-glycoprotein, a key component of the blood–brain barrier. Loperamide is an opioid that does not cause central nervous system (CNS) effects typical of most opioids because P-glycoprotein prevents its entry into the CNS. Dogs and cats with MDR1 polymorphisms either do not express P-glycoprotein (if homozygous for the MDR1 mutation) or express low levels of P-glycoprotein (if heterozygous for the MDR1 mutation) at the blood–brain barrier; therefore, they will experience CNS sedation and even stupor at standard antidiarrheal doses of loperamide. MDR1 genotyping is available for both dogs and cats (Appendix F).

Loperamide:

Dogs: (MDR1 normal/normal genotype only) 0.1 to 0.2 mg/kg PO every 8–12 hours
Cats: (MDR1 normal/normal genotype only) 0.1 to 0.15 mg/kg PO every 12 hours

Other antidiarrheals that are available OTC include products containing the adsorbents kaolin and pectin. Other than potentially interfering with oral absorption of other drugs, these products pose little risk to veterinary patients.

6.5 Vitamin and Mineral Supplements

There are hundreds of OTC products marketed to provide nutritional support for infants, adolescents, teens, adults, and seniors. Most households have at least one type of nutritional supplement that can pose risks to pets. Many products, particularly those marketed for children, are flavored and chewable, which seems to make them particularly attractive to pets. Fortunately, among all the vitamins and minerals present in these products, only a few pose any significant risk when ingested by companion animals.

6.5.1 Iron

The oral bioavailability of iron, an essential element, is directly related to the form that the iron is in – whether elemental iron (insoluble in water), or one of the ferrous and ferric salts (water soluble). In general, ferrous forms of iron appear to be more readily absorbed across the gastrointestinal tract. However, there are natural defense mechanisms that regulates oral iron absorption. An important component of that system is the ability of gastric mucosal cells to sequester iron as ferritin and slowly transport it into the systemic circulation, transferring only the amount that is needed. In instances of excessive ingestion, gastric mucosal cells become saturated, allowing large amounts of iron to enter the systemic circulation. In these situations, pets can quickly succumb to iron's toxic effects due to the inability of the body to adequately eliminate excess iron that is absorbed over a short time period.

Toxic doses, at least in dogs, are based on the amount of elemental iron ingested per kilograms of body weight – so some mathematical calculations must be done to take into account the percentage of elemental iron in whatever form the iron is in. For example, ferrous gluconate is 12% elemental iron, while ferrous sulfate is 37% elemental iron. At exposure doses of elemental iron less than 20 mg/kg, body weight evidence of toxicity would not be expected. Exposures between 20 and 60 mg/kg body weight may cause mild intoxications, which can result in vomiting (with or without blood), gastrointestinal discomfort, and lack of appetite. Exposure doses in dogs that exceed 60 mg elemental iron per kilogram body weight can cause serious gastrointestinal problems, as well as liver and cardiovascular abnormalities (Albretsen 2006). A popular multivitamin contains 27 mg of ferrous sulfate (~10 mg elemental iron) per tablet. As an example, if the owner spills the contents of the container on the floor, a 20-pound Jack Russell Terrier would have to consume 26 tablets to be considered at risk for developing clinical signs of iron toxicity.

Treatment for iron intoxication consists of implementing decontamination procedures in the asymptomatic, acutely exposed patients; symptomatic and supportive care; and sometimes an iron chelator.

6.5.2 Vitamin D

Ingestion of calcium supplements rarely causes hypercalcemia in dogs or cats due to its low intrinsic oral bioavailability. However, vitamin D ingestion can cause severe hypercalcemia in pets through its ability to enhance intestinal calcium absorption. Supplements containing vitamin D_2 (ergocholecalciferol) and vitamin D_3 (cholecalciferol) are readily available OTC. Because these OTC products contain large quantities of vitamin D, toxicity is likely to result if pets ingest them, with the severity of adverse effects dependent upon which form of vitamin D is ingested (D_2 or D_3). With respect to their ability to enhance intestinal absorption of calcium, vitamin D_3 is 10 times more potent than vitamin D_2. Because pharmacists might be the first resource a pet owner turns to when their dog consumes vitamin D–containing supplements, it is essential that pharmacists are able to determine an accurate exposure dose. Some OTC products list vitamin D contents as International Units (IU) per tablet/capsule, while others list the content of vitamin D on a milligram (mg) basis. An exposure dose of 0.1 mg/kg vitamin D_3 (4000 IU/kg) can lead to mild hypercalcemia, while an exposure dose greater than 0.5 mg/kg vitamin D_3 (20 000 IU/kg) can cause severe hypercalcemia (Rumbeiha 2006). For mathematical conversions, one IU of vitamin D_3 is equivalent to 0.000025 mg of vitamin D_3. A popular daily multivitamin supplement

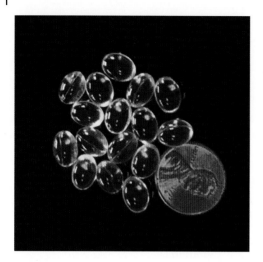

Figure 6.4 It would be relatively easy for a dog to ingest enough vitamin D_3 gel-containing capsules to cause toxicity. The amount shown would be enough to be toxic to a 20-pound dog (penny shown for comparison).

contains 1000 IU vitamin D_3 per tablet, while an OTC pure vitamin D_3 supplement contains 2000 IU vitamin D_3 per capsule. For a 20-pound dog, ingesting sixteen 2000 IU capsules constitutes a toxic dose. While this may seem like a lot of capsules to ingest, the total volume of 16 capsules is about half of a tablespoon (Figure 6.4). Calcitriol, available by prescription only, is 1000 times more potent than vitamin D3, so it has great potential for causing toxicity.

Excess biologically active vitamin D greatly enhances calcium and phosphorus absorption from the gastrointestinal tract (predominant action), increases calcium and phosphorus reabsorption by the kidney, and enhances calcium and phosphorus release from bone. Collectively, these actions lead to hypercalcemia, which is often accompanied by hyperphosphatemia. Hypercalcemia can wreak havoc on the kidneys, muscles, cardiovascular system, and nervous system. Persistent hypercalcemia and hyperphosphatemia can also result in metastatic mineral deposition in soft tissues of many organs. Severe hypercalcemia is a medical emergency and can cause multiple organ failure if it is not immediately recognized and corrected.

Appropriate treatment for exposed patients includes decontamination procedures if the exposure is recent, followed by therapies intended to lower serum calcium and phosphorus concentrations and prevent soft tissue calcification. If the pharmacist suspects that a toxic dose may have been consumed by a dog or cat, the pharmacist should refer the patient to a veterinarian. Treatment options, in order of preference, include parenteral 0.9% NaCl fluid therapy, furosemide, corticosteroids, and possibly bisphosphonates if other options have not been successful.

6.6 Xylitol-Containing Products

Xylitol is one of the newer sugar substitutes and artificial sweeteners that has gained popular use, particularly by people with diabetes. Because of its antibacterial and anticariogenic properties, xylitol is not only found in food products (including candy, gum, and mints) but also in many OTC products found in pharmacies. Xylitol can be found in toothpaste, mouthwash, breath fresheners, dental floss, personal lubricants, lotions, nasal sprays and drops, cosmetics, *gummy* forms of vitamin supplements, and many other items. A careful examination of the label ingredients is warranted whenever a dog ingests any type of OTC product. Since some of these products can contain very high concentrations of xylitol (some dental breath-freshener mints contain 100% xylitol), dogs may be given a lethal dose of what the owner thinks is a very safe product.

Dogs are the only known species to date that are susceptible to toxic effects of xylitol. Other sugar alcohols, like sorbitol, mannitol, erythritol, maltitol, and isomalt, only cause gastrointestinal upset in companion animals even when large amounts are ingested.

Dramatic difference
In canines, xylitol causes an immediate release of insulin from the pancreas, which can lead to profound and potentially

life-threatening hypoglycemia. This can occur as rapidly as 60 minutes after ingestion or it can be delayed for several hours, depending on the exposure dose as well as the form (liquid, "gummy," or tablet) of the material ingested.

Clinical signs of hypoglycemia can be quite vague and nonspecific (e.g. lethargy or being "quiet"), and many dog owners may miss this clinical sign, thinking that their dog is just "tuckered out." In some cases, hypoglycemia can be severe enough to cause seizures. Oral sources of glucose (i.e. Karo syrup) can be administered if the dog is able to swallow, but if obtunded or seizuring, intravenous dextrose solutions are required. Affected patients should be evaluated by a veterinarian to assess liver enzymes, as delayed hepatotoxicity can be caused by xylitol.

Practiced but not proven

Veterinarians may prescribe S-adenosyl methionine to "protect" the liver to dogs that have ingested xylitol, but there are no data to support its efficacy.

6.7 Diaper Rash Creams

Although zinc intoxication in companion animals, particularly dogs, is not an uncommon phenomenon, the source of the zinc is rarely diaper rash ointment. Most zinc poisonings in companion animals are due to ingestion of zinc-containing pennies, minted after 1982; less commonly, poisonings can occur following ingestion of a wide variety of miscellaneous items, including jewelry, galvanized items, bra clasps, pens, zippers, and miscellaneous trinkets. Zinc toxicity in dogs manifests primarily as hemolysis.

It is important to recognize that some diaper rash creams, like the OTC Desitin® ointments, commonly contain between 20% and 40% zinc oxide, which is a form of zinc that is not readily absorbed by the gastrointestinal tract relative to elemental zinc. Pets that do

ingest zinc oxide–containing ointments as a one-time event may experience mild gastrointestinal upset, with vomiting being the most commonly reported clinical sign. Diarrhea has been rarely reported. Treatment procedures rarely require more than parenteral fluid therapy to keep the patient well hydrated and/or an anti-emetic drug (Cerenia® is FDA approved for dogs and cats). There is a report describing a case of zinc toxicity that resulted in hemolysis following *chronic* ingestion of zinc oxide ointment. A determined Sheltie dog, over a period of four days, ingested up to three-quarters of a pound of 40% zinc oxide ointment after it was repeatedly applied to a postsurgical incision near the dog's anus (Breitschwerdt et al. 1986).

6.8 Nicotine-Containing Medications

Transdermal nicotine patches and nicotine gum may also be found in the pharmacy area of stores. Transdermal nicotine patches can contain more than 100 mg of nicotine per patch; and discarded used patches retain enough residual nicotine to pose a risk to pets that have access to them. Nicotine gum typically contains between 2 and 4 mg of nicotine per piece. Xylitol may also be found in gum, so careful evaluation of the ingredient list is warranted when dogs inadvertently ingest gum. Nicotine can also be found in some OTC lozenges, inhalers, and nasal sprays at varying concentrations.

Clinical signs of nicotine toxicity in companion animals often begin at exposure doses of approximately 1 mg/kg body weight. Nicotine is very slowly absorbed in the stomach, but it is rapidly absorbed in the intestine. Clinical signs can occur as soon as 15 minutes to 1 hour after ingestion, depending on the form of nicotine ingested, and the signs can persist anywhere from one to two hours or as long as 24 hours in high-exposure scenarios. Initially, clinical signs of toxicity include CNS stimulation (e.g. tremors and seizures), which can later lead to CNS depression (e.g. lethargy, weakness, and paralysis). Death can occur as a result of respiratory depression. Poisoned patients often vomit prior to the onset of neurological signs, and diarrhea has also been reported.

Treatment options are directed toward the clinical signs the patient is experiencing, and they may include general decontamination procedures (e.g. emetic, activated charcoal, and cathartic), intravenous fluid therapy, anticonvulsants for seizures, sedatives for agitation, and general supportive care.

6.9 Sleep Aids

Some OTC sleep aids contain diphenhydramine, which was discussed under Section 6.2.1 ("Antihistamines"), and others contain melatonin. Some of the melatonin-containing sleep aids also can contain xylitol, which is specifically toxic to dogs as discussed in this chapter. Melatonin is thought to have a wide margin of safety in dogs and cats. However, in overdose situations, melatonin can cause vomiting, diarrhea, and abdominal pain, along with sedation.

6.10 Miscellaneous Products

6.10.1 5-Hydroxytryptophan

L-5-hydroxytryptophan (5-HTP), sometimes referred to as *Griffonia* seed extract, can be found as an OTC dietary supplement in products claiming to provide relief from depression, insomnia, and headaches, as well as promoting weight loss. 5-Hydroxytryptophan is rapidly absorbed from the gastrointestinal tract, and clinical signs in dogs can appear as quickly as 10 minutes post exposure, and persist up to 36 hours. The most common clinical signs in poisoned animals are reported to be associated with the nervous system (e.g. seizures, depression, tremors, hyperesthesia, and ataxia) and the gastrointestinal tract (e.g. vomiting, diarrhea, abdominal pain, and hypersalivation) (Gwaltney-Brant et al. 2000).

Hyperthermia and blindness were less commonly reported, and deaths have been reported, possibly as a result of serotonin syndrome. Adverse effects were reported at exposure doses of 24 mg/kg body weight (Gwaltney-Brant et al. 2000). Treatment recommendations consist of appropriate decontamination procedures, seizure control, cardiovascular support, maintaining normal body temperature, and other basic supportive-care measures.

6.10.2 Caffeine (Guarana)

Caffeine-containing supplements are commonly found in pharmacies, sold as stimulants that provide energy-enhanced mental alertness and weight loss, and as an analgesic aid for certain types of headaches. Some formulations can contain up to 200 mg, if not more, of caffeine per dose. Clinical signs of toxicity typically occur within one to two hours of ingestion, and may include restlessness, agitation, anxiety, muscle tremors, seizures, and death. Caffeine-containing products are often advertised as "safe" because they are "natural" compounds derived from the guarana plant (*Paullinia cupana*). As pharmacists know well, "natural" does not imply "safe." Dogs and cats are thought to be more sensitive to caffeine and other methylxanthines (i.e. theobromine found in chocolate) than humans. This may be because the elimination half-life of methylxanthines is prolonged in dogs and cats relative to humans.

6.10.3 Methionine

Dietary OTC supplements containing methionine can be found in pharmacies, touted to help reduce urinary tract infections by acidifying urine. It is also the active ingredient in products sold in the lawn and garden section of stores that are intended to mitigate the damage of dog urine on grass. Vomiting and ataxia are the most commonly reported clinical signs based on information from over 1500 dogs suffering from methionine overexposures. Clinical signs reported less frequently include lethargy, diarrhea, abnormal posture, weakness, tremors, and lack of appetite (Hickey et al. 2015). Treatment is aimed at alleviating clinical signs (i.e. anti-emetics, and fluid therapy to prevent dehydration). The prognosis for methionine exposed patients is excellent. Clinical signs usually resolve within 48 hours.

6.10.4 Tea Tree Oil

Tea tree oil, also known as Australian tree tea oil or melaleuca oil, is an OTC product touted as possessing powerful bactericidal and fungicidal properties, and it is sold to be used topically for a wide variety of skin disorders. Oral and even topical exposures to concentrated tea tree oil compounds have resulted in systemic signs of toxicity, including lethargy, hind limb weakness, ataxia, tremors, vomiting, and coma in dogs. In one report, eight drops of oil applied dermally along the back of two dogs as a "natural" flea repellant resulted in partial paralysis, CNS depression, and ataxia within 12 hours of application. These signs resolved approximately 24 hours after decontamination (bathing). In cats, excessive drooling, ataxia, lethargy, coma, tremors, and hypothermia have been reported (Khan et al. 2014). Young and smaller cats appear to be more sensitive to the toxic effects of the constituents of this oil. One of three cats treated with tea tree oil topically for "natural" flea control died as a result of exposure despite decontamination and supportive care. Hepatotoxicity is also a potential risk for exposed patients (Khan et al. 2014).

6.10.5 Topical and Local Anesthetics

Gels, liquids, and sprays containing up to 20% benzocaine can be found OTC, in products intended to be applied topically, both orally (to treat "cold sores" and relieve teething pain in infants) and dermally (to relieve insect stings, hemorrhoid pain, and minor abrasions). Toxicities can occur in dogs and cats whether these products are inadvertently ingested or intentionally applied to the pet by the owner in an effort to treat the animal. Pet owners should be discouraged from using these products on pets. Cats and dogs will lick foreign material off of their skin or fur (and may lick foreign material off other animal's skin/fur), essentially ingesting the product or allowing the product to have access to mucous membranes where it may be absorbed into the systemic circulation.

Benzocaine, a local anesthetic, can cause adverse effects in dogs and cats following oral or topical exposures. Clinical signs of toxicity may include vomiting, depression, cardiac abnormalities, and dyspnea (more likely in cats than dogs). Benzocaine can cause oxidative damage to hemoglobin and, as discussed in Section 6.1.1 ("Acetaminophen"), feline hemoglobin is readily converted to methemoglobin because of its unique amino acid structure. Methemoglobin formation in cats often results in Heinz body hemolytic anemia. Cats are also more sensitive to local anesthetic-induced seizures than dogs or humans. Another potential problem associated with oral ingestion is dysphagia. Since benzocaine is a topical anesthetic, swallowing the product can anesthetize the pharynx putting the patient at risk of aspiration pneumonia. Treatment of affected animals may include supplemental oxygen, intravenous fluid therapy, anticonvulsants, methylene blue to combat methemoglobinemia, red blood cell or whole blood transfusions, and intravenous lipid emulsion therapy as is used in human patients who have received overdoses of local anesthetics.

6.10.6 Eye Drops and Nasal Sprays

The imidazoline decongestants – such as naphazoline, oxymetazoline, tetrahydrozoline, tolazoline, and xylometazoline – are commonly found in OTC nasal sprays and eye drops. These compounds have a narrow margin of safety when ingested by pets. Clinical signs can occur within 15 minutes of exposure and can last up to 36 hours. Commonly reported clinical signs include vomiting, lethargy, and cardiovascular collapse (hypertension early, hypotension later, and bradycardia). These exposures are considered to be medical emergencies, and immediate treatment by a veterinarian is absolutely necessary to ensure a successful outcome. Since these compounds are alpha-2-adrenergic receptor agonists, the alpha-2 adrenergic antagonist atipamezole can be employed as an emergency treatment measure, along with atropine, vasopressors, intravenous fluid therapy, and anticonvulsants. Pharmacists can encourage pet owners to keep these medications tucked away in drawers or cabinets, and not on countertops where dogs and cats can reach them.

6.10.7 Thermometers – Batteries

Ingestion of some of the newer thermometers pose little toxicological risk to dogs and cats, other than perhaps acting as a foreign body in the gastrointestinal tract. Those that contain button lithium batteries can cause caustic and corrosive effects on the mucosal lining of the gastrointestinal tract. Once ingested, the veterinarian can take serial abdominal radiographs to monitor the movement of the batteries. If the battery has not been eliminated through the feces by 36 hours after ingestion or if there is a high index of suspicion that the battery has been chewed on (is not intact) and abdominal discomfort is present, surgical removal of the battery is advised.

Once trapped within the gastrointestinal tract, button batteries can actually produce a charge that disrupts the integrity of the gastrointestinal mucosa. Nonbutton lithium batteries, if not chewed, should pass uneventfully out through the feces. But if chewed (not intact), the extreme pH of compounds within the batteries can damage tissues. The risk of batteries releasing heavy metals, such as lead or cadmium, is low, since most batteries no longer contain heavy metals.

In addition to monitoring the transit of batteries through the gastrointestinal tract through serial radiographs, gastrointestinal protectants, including demulcents, can be used to help protect the gastrointestinal mucosa. Other supportive care measure may include intravenous fluid therapy, bulk cathartics, and analgesics.

6.10.8 Thermometers – Mercury

Occasionally, pets ingest the older mercury-containing glass thermometers. The biggest risk to pets who ingest them is the damage that the sharp glass edges can do to gastrointestinal mucosa. Efforts to protect the gastrointestinal tract include bulking up the diet with bread or pumpkin, a short course of sucralfate, or a demulcent. Veterinarians can use serial radiographs to monitor the movement of the mercury thermometer through the gastrointestinal tract. On rare occasions, surgical removal is necessary.

The mercury, interestingly enough, poses very little risk to the patient. Mercury in thermometers is elemental mercury, which is poorly absorbed across the gastrointestinal mucosa. Enhancing gastrointestinal transit time with bulk cathartics is recommended.

6.11 Decontamination Procedures

One of the first steps taken in the event an animal or human patient is exposed to a toxicant is decontamination. The goal of decontamination is to prevent or minimize further toxicant absorption and enhance excretion or elimination of the toxicant. Depending on the route of exposure, decontamination might include dermal, inhalation, ocular, gastrointestinal, diuresis, or surgical means of removing the toxicant from the patient. In most instances, decontamination is best performed at a veterinary hospital for the safety of the owner and for the best outcome for the patient. Most households are not equipped with the basic equipment (large/deep bathing sink, protective gloves and aprons, fluids/syringes for ocular lavage in the event of ocular exposure, etc.) necessary for safely performing decontamination procedures for dogs and cats. Furthermore, many dogs and cats will require restraint or sedatives to undergo these procedures.

6.11.1 Dermal Exposures

Owners should be advised to wear gloves, at minimum, to protect themselves from contact with the toxicant while bathing the animal. Liquid dish soap (not dishwasher soap) and copious amounts of water/rinsing are required, but scrubbing and high-pressure spraying should be avoided. Owners should ensure that the water is body temperature, to avoid scalding the patient or creating hypothermia.

6.11.2 Ocular Exposures

For ocular exposures to a corrosive agent, pet owners should be instructed to gently flush the affected eye(s) with sterile physiologic saline (contact lens wearers may have this on hand) or tap water for 15 minutes before taking their pet to a veterinary hospital. Even if the pet appears to be fine after flushing, the pet's eye should be examined by a veterinarian. Owners should not allow the pet to rub its eyes, nor should the owners instill or apply any type of eye drops or ointments to the eye before seeking veterinary care.

6.11.3 Inhalant Exposures

The most important action is to remove the patient from the source of the inhalant toxicant to an appropriately ventilated area. The patient should be evaluated by a veterinarian to determine if supplemental oxygen therapy is needed.

6.11.4 Exposure by Oral Ingestion

Similar to human infants and toddlers, animals explore the world with their noses and mouths, but unlike their human counterparts, most animals do not outgrow this behavior. This makes dogs, cats, and other household pets highly susceptible to ingested toxicants. Dogs are more likely than cats to ingest toxicants because of their "eat it before someone else does" approach to objects that might be food. For these reasons, gastrointestinal decontamination (including induction of emesis, gastric lavage, and administration of activated charcoal and/or cathartics) is performed frequently in companion animal veterinary hospitals. Contraindications for inducing emesis in veterinary patients are the same as those for inducing emesis in poisoned human patients (e.g. caustic agents, or if the patient is unconscious or stuporous). Although the emetics of choice for dogs and cats are prescription drugs (Table 6.2), some at-home emetic agents to consider will be described further in this section. Equally important, there are OTC emetics that should be avoided.

6.11.4.1 Syrup of Ipecac

Commonly found in pharmacy aisles, syrup of ipecac has been promoted in the past as a highly effective emetic in humans. However, its

Table 6.2 Emetic agents for dogs and cats.

Proposed emetic agent(s)	Species	Comments
Apomorphine	Dogs	Most effective emetic for dogs; prescription drug administered by veterinarian only
α_2 adrenergic receptor agonists	Cats	Most effective emetics for cats; prescription drug(s) administered by veterinarian only; not effective for dogs
3% Hydrogen peroxide	Dogs	Only household antiemetic that is effective; DO NOT USE IN CATS (causes esophagitis and gastritis).
Syrup of ipecac	None	Not effective in dogs or cats, and potentially toxic
Miscellaneous household items: salts, soap, and mustards	None	Not consistently effective

use in humans is now questionable and rarely encouraged by physicians. But this does not seem to prevent many parents from keeping a bottle in the bathroom medicine cabinet. Although one can find doses for syrup of ipecac intended to cause vomiting in dogs and cats, the use of this emetic is ***not*** recommended due to lack of efficacy and risk of cardiotoxicity.

6.11.4.2   Hydrogen Peroxide (3%)

Hydrogen peroxide, 3%, is a common product in pharmacies and grocery stores. It is interesting to note that, in dogs, hydrogen peroxide is an effective oral emetic at a dose of 1 ml per pound of body weight. However, recent evidence suggests oral administration of 3% hydrogen peroxide can cause inflammation of the esophagus, stomach, and intestine that can persist for several days (Niedzwecki et al. 2017). Because cats are highly susceptible to hydrogen peroxide–induced esophagitis and gastritis (Figure 6.2), it should ***not*** be used to induce emesis in cats.

References

Albretsen J. (2006). Toxicology brief: the toxicity of iron, an essential element. Vet. Med. 82–90.

Breitschwerdt, E.B., Armstrong, P.J., and Robinette, C.L. (1986). Three cases of acute zinc toxicosis in dogs. *Vet. Hum. Toxicol.* 28: 109–117.

Gwaltney-Brant, S.M., Albretsen, J.C., and Khan, S.A. (2000). 5-Hydroxytryptophan toxicosis in dogs: 21 cases (1989–1999). *J. Am. Vet. Med. Assoc.* 216 (12): 1937–1940.

Harvey, J.W. and Kornick, H.P. (1976). Phenazopyridine toxicosis in the cat. *J. Am. Vet. Med. Assoc.* 169 (3): 327–331.

Hickey, M.C., Son, T.T., and Wismer, T. (2015). Retrospective evaluation of methionine intoxication associated with urinary acifying products in dogs: 1,525 cases (2001–2012). *J. Vet. Emerg. Crit. Care* 25 (5): 640–645.

Hovda, L.R., Brutlag, A.G., Poppenga, R.H. et al. (2016). Decongestants (pseudoephedrine, phenylephrine). In: *Blackwell's Five-Minute Veterinary Consult Clinical Companion: Small Animal Toxicology*, 2e, 327–338. Hoboken, NJ: Wiley-Blackwell.

Khan, S.A., McLean, M.K., and Slater, M.R. (2014). Concentrated tea tree oil toxicosis in dogs and cats: 443 cases (2002-2012). *J. Am. Vet. Med. Assoc.* 244 (1): 95–99.

Niedzwecki, A.H., Book, B.P., Lewis, K.M. et al. (2017). Effects of oral 3% hydrogen peroxide used as an emetic on the gastroduodenal mucosa of health dogs. *J. Vet. Emerg. Crit. Care* 27 (2): 178–184.

Rumbeiha, W.K. (2006). Cholecalciferol. In: *Small Animal Toxicology*, 2e (ed. M.E. Peterson and P.A. Talcott), 489–498. St. Louis, MO: Elsevier Saunders.

Sellon, R.K. (2006). Acetaminophen. In: *Small Animal Toxicology*, 2e (ed. M.E. Peterson and P.A. Talcott), 550–558. St. Louis, MO: Elsevier Saunders.

Talcott, P.A. and Gwaltney-Brant, S.M. (2013). Nonsteroidal antiinflammatories. In: *Small Animal Toxicology*, 3e (ed. M.E. Peterson and P.A. Talcott), 687–708. St. Louis, MO: Elsevier Saunders.

Worth, A.C., Wismer, T.A., and Dorman, D.C. (2016). Diphenhydramine exposure in dogs: 621 cases (2008–2013). *J. Am. Vet. Med. Assoc.* 249 (1): 77–82.

7

Pharmacotherapy of Parasitic Disease

Cory Langston and Andrea S. Varela-Stokes

Department of Clinical Sciences, College of Veterinary Medicine, Mississippi State University, Mississippi State, MS, USA

Key Points

- Unlike in human medicine, where parasite problems are relatively uncommon in developed countries, both internal and external parasite control are a routine part of small animal health care.
- A great many antiparasitic drugs used in veterinary medicine are not used in humans.
- *Zoonotic risks:* Although relatively rare, some small animal parasites carry zoonotic potential.
- *Roundworms:* Ingestion of roundworm infective forms can cause visceral/ocular larva migrans.
- *Hookworms:* Skin penetration by hookworm larvae can lead to cutaneous larva migrans.
- *Tapeworms:* Ingestion of eggs from *Echinococcus* tapeworms of dogs can cause cystic or alveolar hydatid disease, which can be severe and may be untreatable. Other tapeworm species of significant public health concern include *Taenia saginata* and *Taenia solium*, which are parasites of neither domestic cats nor dogs, but rather infect humans via the ingestion of cysticerci (larvae) found in beef or pork, respectively.
- *Pinworms:* Despite common misconceptions, humans cannot contract pinworms from animals.
- *Mange:* Sarcoptic mange is transmissible between animals and humans, although there is also a human variant.
- *Ticks:* Ticks are common ectoparasites of both humans and animals.
- Due to the hypobiosis phenomenon in the dam, transplacental and transmammary infection of puppies with roundworms and hookworms, respectively, is always presumed. Early infections of kittens with hookworms and roundworms are also commonplace, but transmission is via environmental contamination. Thus, all puppies and kittens should be dewormed against these parasites starting at two weeks of age, and repeated every two to three weeks until eight weeks of age.
- Heartworm disease is now so widespread that all dogs, and arguably all cats, should receive heartworm preventative year-round.
- Fleas may not be a problem in arid regions, but for most of the USA, flea control is almost a necessity, particularly in the southeastern USA. In severe infestations, exsanguination can occur, especially in cats and small dogs. Flea infestations can cause general dermatitis and pruritus, "flea allergy dermatitis" in susceptible dogs and cats (Chapter 18), and disease transmission (i.e. plague) to humans and pets.
- Ticks occur in all geographic locations of the Americas and are vectors of several diseases of importance to humans and pets. Pets with outside access usually warrant the use of tick

---

Pharmacotherapeutics for Veterinary Dispensing, First Edition. Edited by Katrina L. Mealey.

control products, as ticks brought in on pets may be transferred to humans. As with fleas, severe infestation can cause death by exsanguination.

- Lice are uncommon parasites of small animals and are species-specific.
- In individual animals, mite infestations can be a problem, although most mites do not survive long off of animals. Common mites include ear mites, sarcoptic mange mites, and demodectic mange mites.

- Most protozoan parasites cause gastrointestinal disease, and they include the coccidia and flagellates like *Giardia*. Others are vector-borne and may lead to diseases that affect various organs, including the muscle, liver, and skin. Various protozoa, including *Giardia, Cryptosporidium*, and vector-borne protozoa, can be zoonotic. The protozoa are covered in Chapter 9.

7.1 Comparative Aspects of Parasitic Infections

Parasitic infections are most common in human populations in low-income countries, but they also occur in developed countries. However, it is surprisingly difficult to find incidence data for human parasitic infections in the USA and Canada. The few studies that exist tend to rely heavily on serology, a methodology where it is difficult to separate active infection from exposure. The US Centers for Disease Control and Prevention (CDC) has identified one nematode infection (toxocariasis) and one cestode infection (cysticercosis) as being neglected parasitic (helminth) infections deserving of further study. While not diminishing the importance of these infections in humans in the USA, their comparative incidence is small versus that found in companion animals, horses (Chapter 21), and food animals (Chapter 22).

The prevalence of parasite infections in dogs and cats depends in large part on whether they receive regular veterinary care. The infection rates of dogs and cats presented for veterinary care in the USA were under 1.5% for both hookworms and roundworms (Banfield Pet Hospital 2017). However, in shelter animal populations, 33.9% of dogs and 31.8% of cats tested positive for at least one parasite (Villenueve et al. 2015). Heartworm disease, once confined to the

southeastern USA, has been reported in all 50 states and Canada, and is now established in regions of all states except Alaska. All dogs, and arguably all cats, should receive heartworm preventative. In general, prevalence in susceptible cats is approximately 10% of that for susceptible dogs in a given area, and indoor cats are not without risk of infection with this mosquito-borne disease. Humans can be rare accidental hosts for canine heartworms, with 81 cases reported since 1941. Signs in humans primarily involve the lungs, but aberrant migrations of adult worms have occurred in the brain, eye, and testicle (CDC 2012).

Ticks are found throughout the USA, including in colder regions of North America such as Alaska. In addition to the blood loss and the suffering that ticks produce directly, tick-borne diseases in animals and humans are increasing in prevalence and are accompanied by reports of emerging tick-borne diseases. Flea infestation, by contrast, depends on the humidity in that geographic region. Fleas are ubiquitous in the southeastern USA but uncommon in arid regions where the relative humidity is less than 50%. Mange mites (sarcoptic and demodectic) and ear mite infestations are geographically widespread but less common than fleas or ticks. Louse infestations are relatively uncommon in small animals. Lice are species-specific, are more common in large animals, and are not a zoonotic risk.

Because parasites are a significant source of economic loss in large animals and small animals, parasite control products represent a sizeable consumer market, and antiparasitic drugs are a major focus area by pharmaceutical companies involved in animal care. Many of these compounds are unique to veterinary medicine. For pharmacists, this means that currently available software designed to provide patient safety information or drug-interaction alerts lacks any information regarding these drugs. Among the antiparasitics approved for humans, many were first developed for animal use.

There are also regulatory differences in approval and jurisdiction of antiparasitics in animals versus humans. Although drugs approved for ectoparasite control in humans are regulated by the US Food and Drug Administration (FDA), jurisdiction is split for veterinary products. If the drug is absorbed systemically and the parasite is affected after feeding on the host, then the drug is regulated by the FDA. If the drug, however, works through contact after topical application, then the drug is regulated by the US Environmental Protection Agency (EPA). Extra-label drug use in animals is regulated by the Animal Medicinal Drug Use Clarification Act (AMDUCA) through the FDA and does not apply to EPA-registered products; as such, extra-label use of an EPA pesticide is prohibited.

7.2 Diagnostic Testing

7.2.1 Internal Parasites

With the exception of heartworms, the vast majority of internal helminth parasites are gastrointestinal (GI) worms. These spend at least a portion of their life cycle in the GI tract, and examination of the feces for eggs or larvae is the most common diagnostic approach. Although a direct microscopic examination of a fecal sample can be helpful, fecal flotation examination for helminth eggs using a hypertonic salt or sugar solution is the standard diagnostic test for most intestinal parasites. The premise of the test is that the specific gravity of the solution is greater than the parasite egg, allowing it to float and adhere to a microscope slide on top of the test container. It has a high sensitivity for detecting hookworms and roundworms. Whipworm eggs may also be detected in this manner, but infections can be missed. Because of the prepatent period (the time from initial infection until the adult worms produce eggs), it is possible for very young puppies and kittens to be infected with roundworms and hookworms but have no parasite eggs evident on a fecal exam. Various flotation solutions exist and vary slightly in specific gravity. The most commonly used solutions, in order of decreasing specific gravity, are Sheather's sugar solution, sodium nitrate, and zinc sulfate. Still, some especially dense parasite eggs require other fecal examination techniques, such as the use of fecal sedimentation for the heavy eggs of many fluke species. Fecal antigen tests are also available to detect roundworm, hookworm, and whipworm infections. These tests detect antigen from immature and adult nematodes, and they can be useful when disease precedes evidence of eggs or in single-sex infections where eggs would not be produced.

Tapeworm eggs can also be found using fecal flotation, but it is not a very sensitive method because most tapeworm eggs remain in the proglottids (tapeworm segment) and can only be found if the sample that is processed contains the proglottid. Often, visualization of the tapeworm proglottid in the feces is the only indication of infection (Figure 7.1).

The Baermann fecal sedimentation test is used when larval forms must be detected for diagnosis, such as for some lungworm infections. Examination of the urine sediment is performed to diagnose kidney and bladder worms. Cytological examination of bronchial washings may be used along with fecal examination to diagnose lungworm or lung fluke infections.

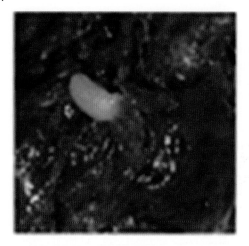 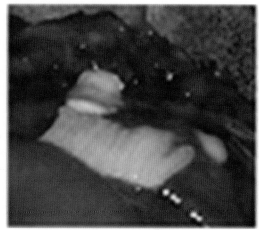

Figure 7.1 Left, *Dipylidium caninum* tapeworm proglottids in feces; oblong "grain of rice" in size. Right, *Taenia* sp. intact tapeworm in feces with multiple proglottids still attached. Individually, the proglottids are rectangular. *Source (left figure):* Courtesy of Thomas Nolan, Laboratory of Parasitology, University of Pennsylvania School of Veterinary Medicine.

Testing for heartworm infections in dogs is accomplished using an immunoassay that detects antigen from female heartworms in the dog's blood. It is typically quite sensitive, although false negatives can occur in dogs with low heartworm numbers or with high antibody concentrations that neutralize the antigen. As such, the American Heartworm Society recommends that the animal also be tested for blood microfilariae using a method that concentrates the microfilariae, such as the Knott's test or a blood filtration test. This test is also used to assess whether microfilaricidal treatment is needed during adulticidal treatment of an infected dog. Radiographs and ultrasound examinations are also useful, particularly in staging the disease.

Testing of cats for heartworms is more problematic. Most infected cats have very low numbers of adult heartworms, and thus low levels of detectable antigen; they are also rarely microfilaremic. A serology test for antibodies to heartworms can help confirm a diagnosis, but a positive result may only mean prior exposure to the heartworm and not necessarily active infection. Diagnosis of heartworm disease in cats is often based on clinical signs, exclusion of other causes, along with a positive antibody test. Observation of heartworms using echocardiography (ultrasound) is most definitive.

7.2.2 External Parasites

Flea infestations are usually readily apparent on close examination of the skin. "Flea dirt," the dark-colored feces of the flea, can often be found when the flea itself may not be. To differentiate flea dirt from other debris, if the material is applied to moistened filter paper or paper towel, a reddish color will appear, derived from the digested blood meal. Animals with flea-bite hypersensitivity can have pruritic dermatitis from even a single flea bite. Although the pruritus may be generalized, it is often associated with the tail-base area in dogs or the neck area of cats. Use of a "flea comb" is beneficial in diagnosing a low-number infestation, as may be an intradermal flea antigen hypersensitivity test for flea allergy. Tick infestations are seen grossly, with the ears, abdomen, groin, and between the shoulder blades being common sites of attachment. Lice or their eggs (nits) may be seen on direct examination of the skin and hair, although they can be easily mistaken for dirt by owners. Microscopic examination will confirm the diagnosis as well as identify whether it is a biting (chewing) or sucking louse.

There are four main types of mite infestations in small animals. Ear mites are common in both dogs and cats. Microscopic examination of the exudate will show the mite, although they can also sometimes be seen grossly as tiny spots on a swab of ear exudate. Hair-clasping mites (*Cheyletiella*), also known as "walking dandruff," can be seen grossly as small moving particulates and confirmed on microscopy often with adhesive cellophane tape preparations. Diagnosis of sarcoptic and demodectic mange requires microscopic examination of skin scrapings, as mites burrow under the skin or may be found in hair follicles and glands, respectively. Mosquito bite hypersensitivity is diagnosed by exclusion of other causes, in conjunction with exposure and a characteristic skin lesion distribution pattern.

7.3 Treatment Considerations for Common Internal Parasitic Diseases

The common internal parasites of small animals are helminths, which include nematodes, cestodes, and trematodes; the latter two are sometimes referred to as flatworms. Often, there are multiple genera and species that comprise each group; however, helminths within a particular group usually respond to the same antiparasitic drugs. Conversely, drugs that are effective for one group (e.g. nematodes) are generally not effective for other helminth groups (cestodes or trematodes), and vice versa. To better match the lay terms that pharmacists are likely to encounter, this chapter will refer to cestodes and trematodes as tapeworms and flukes, respectively. Nematodes will be divided into roundworms, hookworms, whipworms, and heartworms. Many less common parasites exist and are mentioned in Table 7.1, which provides the scientific names, site of infection, and method of transmission of most small animal internal parasites.

The term "anthelmintic" refers to the drugs used to treat or prevent helminth infections. Few drugs, however, have a broad enough spectrum of activity to kill nematodes, tapeworms, and flukes. So, in an effort to provide a single product to the consumer, formulations often contain multiple antiparasitic drugs. Tables 7.2 and 7.3 list the various drugs and drug combinations available, their spectrum, and recommended dosages.

The efforts by drug companies to provide broad-spectrum coverage on a monthly basis by using a single product (e.g. nematocide and cestocide combined with flea or tick products) have raised concern as to whether this promotes parasite drug resistance. The strategy of this approach is to improve owner compliance by marketing a "one product treats all" approach for dogs and cats. It also has been advocated on the basis of decreasing the veterinarian's liability should owners develop zoonotic infections from their pets. However, similarly aggressive (broad-spectrum and frequent) deworming practices in large animals (sheep, goats, horses, and cattle) have led to alarming resistance rates in some parasites. In extreme cases, complete resistance to all available anthelmintics exists in certain livestock populations and geographic regions. Aggressive deworming practices originally developed to eradicate parasites in small ruminants and horses actually selected for parasite populations with mutations that conferred drug resistance. These practices have been replaced with selective deworming of only the most severely affected individuals. The premise here is that the presence of a small population of drug-susceptible parasites (called "refugia") in the population decreases the selection pressure for genetically resistant

Table 7.1 Common and scientific names of small animal internal parasites.

Common name	Scientific name	Location	Transmission	Common treatment
Bladder worm	*Pearsonema* sp. (= *Capillaria* sp.) (dog, cat)	Bladder	Ingestion of intermediate or paratenic host (e.g. earthworms)	fenbendazole, ivermectin
Esophageal worm	*Spirocerca lupi* (dog)	Esophageal, gastric, and aortic walls	Ingestion of intermediate or paratenic host (e.g. beetles and rodents)	difficult to treat, some benefit from macrocyclic lactones
Heartworm	*Dirofilaria immitis* (dog, cat)	Heart	Bite from infected mosquito	tx = melarsomine; see Table 7.2 and text preventatives = multiple; see Tables 7.2 and 7.3
Hookworm	*Ancylostoma caninum* (dog) *Ancylostoma tubaeforme* (cat) *Uncinaria stenocephala* (dog, cat)	GI tract (small intestine)	Larvae from egg are ingested or penetrate skin; paratenic hosts (e.g. rodents); transmammary (*A. caninum*)	multiple tx; see Tables 7.2 and 7.3
Kidney worm	*Dictophymae renale* (dog)	Kidney	Ingestion of intermediate or paratenic host (e.g. oligochaetes and frogs)	surgical removal
Lung fluke	*Paragonimus kellicotti* (dog, cat)	Lung	Ingestion of intermediate host (crayfish)	praziquantel, fenbendazole
Lung worms	*Aelurostrongylus abstrusus* (cat) *Oslerus* (Filaroides) *osleri* (dog) *Eucoleus* (Capillaria) spp. (dog, cat)	Respiratory tract	Ingestion of intermediate or paratenic host	fenbendazole, ivermectin
Roundworm	*Toxascaris leonina* (dog, cat) *Toxocara canis* (dog) *Toxocara cati* (cat)	GI tract (small intestine)	Fecal-oral egg ingestion; paratenic hosts (e.g., earthworms, rodents); transplacental and transmammary (*T. canis*)	multiple tx; see Tables 7.2 and 7.3
Stomach worm	*Physaloptera* spp. (dog, cat)	GI tract (stomach)	Ingestion of intermediate host (beetle)	fenbendazole, pyrantel pamoate, ivermectin
Tapeworm	*Dipylidium caninum* (dog, cat) *Taenia pisiformis* (dog) *Taenia taeniaeformis* (cat) *Echinococcus granulosus* (dog) *Echinococcus multilocularis* (dog, cat) *Spirometra* sp. (dog, cat)	GI tract (small intestine)	Ingestion of intermediate host (varies; e.g. flea for D. caninum, various mammals for others)	praziquantel; see text regarding Spirometra
Whipworm	*Trichuris vulpis* (dog)	GI tract (large intestine)	Fecal-oral egg ingestion	multiple tx; see Tables 7.2 and 7.3

tx, Treatment; multiple tx, several treatments exist – see Tables 7.2 and 7.3.

Table 7.2 Dosing information for most antiparasitic drugs used in small animals.

Trade name	Drug(s)	Species	Minimum age/ body weight	Dose and route frequency (see table legend)	Comments
Acarexx®	Ivermectin	Cats	4 weeks	0.05 mg (one ampule)/ear otic	
Activyl Spot-On® for Cats and Kittens	Indoxacarb	Cats	8 weeks/2 lbs.	WBSO monthly	
Activyl Spot-On for Dogs and Puppies	Indoxacarb	Dogs	8 weeks/4 lbs.	WBSO monthly	
Activyl® Tickplus for Dogs and Puppies	Indoxacarb Permethrin	Dogs	8 weeks/4 lbs.	WBSO monthly	Do NOT use in cats
Adams™ d-Limonene Flea & Tick Shampoo	Limonene	Dogs Cats	12 weeks	shampoo weekly	
Advantage II for Cats®	Imidacloprid Pyriproxyfen	Cats	8 weeks	WBSO monthly	
Advantage II for Dogs®	Imidacloprid Pyriproxyfen	Dogs	7 weeks	WBSO monthly	
Advantage Multi Topical Solution for Cats®	Moxidectin Imidacloprid	Cats	9 weeks/2 lbs.	WBSO monthly	
Advantage Multi Topical Solution for Dogs®	Moxidectin Imidacloprid	Dogs	7 weeks/3 lbs.	WBSO monthly	
Bio Spot Active Care Flea & Tick Spot On® for Cats	Etofenprox Methoprene	Cats	12 weeks	WBSO monthly	Repels mosquitoes
Bio Spot Active Care Flea & Tick Spot On® for Dogs	Etofenprox Methoprene Pyriproxyfen	Dogs	12 weeks	WBSO monthly	Repels mosquitoes
Bravecto Chews for Dogs™	Fluralaner	Dogs	6 months/4.4 lbs.	25 mg/kg po WBO 3 months	Caution in seizure-prone animals Administer with food

(Continued)

Table 7.2 (Continued)

Trade name	Drug(s)	Species	Minimum age/body weight	Dose and route frequency (see table legend)	Comments
Bravecto Topical Solution for Cats®	Fluralaner	Cats	6 months/2.6 lbs.	40 mg/kg topical WBSO 3 months	
Bravecto Topical Solution for Dogs®	Fluralaner	Dogs	6 months/4.4 lbs.	25 mg/kg topical WBSO 3 months	
Capstar®	Nitenpyram	Dogs Cats	4 weeks/2 lbs.	1.0 mg/kg q24h prn	Safe for pregnant or nursing dogs and cats
Catego for Cats®	Dinotefuran Fipronil Pyriproxyfen	Cats	8 weeks/1.5 lbs.	WBSO monthly	
Certifect for Dogs®	Fipronil Methoprene Amitraz	Dogs	8 weeks	WBSO monthly	Approved for use in pregnant or nursing bitches
Cestex®	Epsiprantel	Dogs Cats	7 weeks	dog 5 mg/kg po cat 2.5 mg/kg po	
Cheristin for Cats™	Spinetoram	Cats	8 weeks	WBSO monthly	
Comfortis Chewable Tablets for Cats®	Spinosad	Cats	14 weeks/2 lbs.	50 mg/kg po monthly	
Comfortis Chewable Tablets for Dogs®	Spinosad	Dogs	14 weeks/3.3 lbs.	30 mg/kg po monthly	
Credelio™	Lotilaner	Dogs	8 weeks/4.4 lbs.	20 mg/kg po monthly	Caution in seizure-prone animals Administer with food
Droncit Canine Tablets®	Praziquantel	Dogs	4 weeks	see label directions (varies by wt.) po	

Product	Active Ingredients	Species	Age	Directions	Comments
Droncit Feline Tablets®	Praziquantel	Cats	6 weeks	see label directions (varies by wt.) po	
Droncit Injectable for Dogs and Cats®	Praziquantel	Dogs Cats	dog 4 weeks cat 6 weeks	see directions (varies by wt.) im or sc	
Drontal® for Cats	Praziquantel Pyrantel pamoate	Cats	2 months/2lbs.	WBO	
Drontal® Plus for Dogs	Febantel Praziquantel Pyrantel pamoate	Dogs	3 weeks/2lbs.	WBO	Avoid during pregnancy or with preexisting kidney or liver disease
Drs. Foster & Smith ProWormer-2® Nemex-2®	Pyrantel pamoate	Dogs Cats	2 weeks	dog 5 mg/kg po cat 20 mg/kg po	Dogs weighing <5 lbs. receive 10 mg/kg po
Frontline Gold for Cats®	Fipronil Methoprene Pyriproxyfen	Cats	8 weeks	WBSO monthly	
Frontline Gold for Dogs®	Fipronil Methoprene Pyriproxyfen	Dogs	8 weeks	WBSO monthly	
Frontline Plus for Cats and Kittens® (spot on)	Fipronil Methoprene	Cats	8 weeks/3lbs.	WBSO monthly	
Frontline Plus for Dogs and Puppies® (spot on)	Fipronil Methoprene	Dogs	8 weeks	WBSO monthly	
Frontline Spray for Cats and Dogs®	Fipronil	Dogs Cats	8 weeks	WBSO monthly	
Frontline Tritak for Cats®	Fipronil Etofenprox Methoprene	Cats	12 weeks	WBSO monthly	
Frontline Tritak for Dogs®	Fipronil Cyphenothrin Methoprene	Dogs	12 weeks	WBSO monthly	

(Continued)

Table 7.2 (Continued)

Trade name	Drug(s)	Species	Minimum age/ body weight	Dose and route frequency (see table legend)	Comments
Milbemite® Otic Solution	Milbemycin	Cats	4 weeks	0.25 mg (one ampule)/ear otic	
Nexgard for Dogs®	Afoxolaner	Dogs	8 weeks/4 lbs.	2.5 mg/kg po WBO monthly	Caution in seizure-prone animals
Panacur-C® SafeGuard®	Fenbendazole	Dogs Cats	dog 6 weeks cat extra-label	50 m/kg po	
Preventic Tick Collar for Dogs®	Amitraz	Dogs	12 weeks	collar 3 months	Do NOT use in cats
Program Flavor Tabs for Dogs and Cats®	Lufenuron	Dogs Cats	4 weeks	dog 10 mg/kg po cat 30 mg/kg po monthly	
Program Injectable for Cats®	Lufenuron	Cats	cat six weeks	10 mg/kg sc 6 months	
Program Suspension for Cats®	Lufenuron	Cats	cat 6 weeks	30 mg/kg po monthly	
Proheart 6 for Dogs®	Moxidectin	Dogs	6 months	0.17 mg/kg sc 6 months	
Revolution®	Selamectin	Dogs Cats	dog 6 weeks cat 8 weeks	6 mg/kg topical WBSO monthly	
Scalibor Protector Band (Collar) for Dogs®	Deltamethrin	Dogs	12 weeks	collar 6 months	Do NOT use in cats
Sentinel for Dogs®	Milbemycin Lufenuron	Dogs	4 weeks/2 lbs.	WBO monthly	
Sentinel Spectrum® for Dogs	Milbemycin Lufenuron Praziquantel	Dogs	6 weeks/2 lbs.	WBO monthly	

Product	Active ingredient(s)	Species	Age	Route/dose	Comments
Goodwinol ointment®	Rotenone Benzocaine	Dogs	not stated	topical	Label indication is only for "nonspecific skin irritations of dogs"; questionable efficacy against demodicosis; benzocaine toxic if ingested, especially in cats
Hartz Advanced Care Liquid Wormer® Sergeants Worm Away®	Piperazine salts	Dogs Cats	6 weeks	44–66 mg/kg po	Some formularies recommend 110–200 mg/kg po
Heartgard for Cats®	Ivermectin	Cats	6 weeks	24 µg/kg po WBO	
Heartgard for Dogs®	Ivermectin (low dose for hwp)	Dogs	6 weeks	6 µg/kg po WBO	
Heartgard Plus for Dogs® Tri-Heart Plus for Dogs® Iverhart Plus for Dogs®	Ivermectin Pyrantel pamoate	Dogs	6 weeks	WBO	
Immiticide®	Melarsomine	Dogs	adult dog	2.5 mg/kg deep im epaxials (see Figure 3)	Heartworm adulticide
Interceptor®	Milbemycin	Dogs Cats	dog 4 weeks/2 lbs. cat 6 weeks/1.5 lbs.	dog 0.5 mg/kg po cat 2 mg/kg po WBO	
Iverhart MAX®	Ivermectin Pyrantel pamoate Praziquantel	Dogs	8 weeks	WBO	
K9 Advantix II®	Imidacloprid Permethrin Pyriproxyfen	Dogs	7 weeks	WBSO	Do NOT use in cats; repels mosquitoes and biting flies
Lime Sulfur Dip Concentrate™	Sulfurated lime solution	Dogs Cats	no age specified	dilute for dip/sponge-on q5–7d	Dilute before use as necessary; label indication "parasites responsive to lime sulfur"; used mostly for sarcoptic mange, Cheyletiella (walking dandruff), or dermatophytes

(Continued)

Table 7.2 (Continued)

Trade name	Drug(s)	Species	Minimum age/body weight	Dose and route frequency (see table legend)	Comments
Seresto Cat Collar™	Imidacloprid Flumethrin	Cats	10 weeks	collar 8 months	
Seresto Dog Collar™	Imidacloprid Flumethrin	Dogs	7 weeks/18 lbs.	collar 8 months	8-month duration flea and ticks; labeled for one month duration for lice
Simparica for Dogs™	Sarolaner	Dogs	6 months	2 mg/kg po WBO monthly	Caution in seizure-prone animals
Trifexis for Dogs®	Milbemycin Spinosad	Dogs	8 weeks/5 lbs.	WBO monthly	Caution in seizure-prone animals
Vectra 3D for Dogs®	Dinotefuran Pyriproxyfen Permethrin	Dogs	7 weeks	WBSO monthly	Do NOT use in cats; also effective against *Cheyletiella* (walking dandruff); repels mosquitoes and biting flies
Vectra for Cats and Kittens®	Dinotefuran Pyriproxyfen	Cats	8 weeks	WBSO monthly	
Vectra for Cats®	Dinotefuran Pyriproxyfen	Cats	9 lbs.	WBSO monthly	
Vectra for Dogs and Puppies®	Dinotefuran Pyriproxyfen	Dogs	8 weeks	WBSO monthly	
Virbantel for Dogs®	Pyrantel pamoate Praziquantel	Dogs	12 weeks	WBO	

WBSO = weight-based spot-on topical formulation, see label; WBO = weight-based oral formulation, see label (usually flavored chew or tablet).
Note: See the "Unique Aspect of Parasiticide Dosing" section.

Table 7.3 Antiparasitic activity of most commercial products used in small animals.

Trade name	Drug(s)	HWP	HWA	H-dog	R-dog	W	H-cat	R-cat	TT	DT	ET	F	IGR	T	L	EM	SM	DM
Acarexx®	Ivermectin															+		
Activyl Spot-On for Cats and Kittens®	Indoxacarb											+						
Activyl Spot-On for Dogs and Puppies®	Indoxacarb											+						
Activyl Tick Plus for Dogs and Puppies®	Indoxacarb Permethrin											+		+				
Adams™ D-Limonene Flea & Tick Shampoo®	Limonene											+		+				
Advantage II for Cats®	Imidacloprid Pyriproxyfen											+	+		B			
Advantage II for Dogs®	Imidacloprid Pyriproxyfen											+	+		B			
Advantage Multi Topical Solution for Cats® Advantage Multi Topical Solution for Dogs®	Moxidectin Imidacloprid	+		+	+	+	+	+				+				+		
Bio Spot Active Care Flea & Tick Spot On® for Cats	Etofenprox Methoprene											+	±	+				
Bio Spot Active Care Flea & Tick Spot On® for Dogs	Etofenprox Methoprene Pyriproxyfen											+	±	+				
Bravecto Chews for Dogs™	Fluralaner											+		+		+	+	+
Bravecto Topical Solution for Cats® Bravecto Topical Solution for Dogs®	Fluralaner											+		+		+	+	+
Capstar®	Nitenpyram											+						
Catego for Cats®	Dinotefuran Fipronil pyriproxyfen											+	+	+				

(Continued)

Table 7.3 (Continued)

Trade name	Drug(s)	HWP	HWA	H-dog	R-dog	W	H-cat	R-cat	TT	DT	ET	F	IGR	T	L	EM	SM	DM
Certifect for Dogs®	Fipronil Methoprene Amitraz											+	±	+	B		$	
Cestex®	Epsiprantel								+	+								
Cheristin for Cats™	Spinetoram											+						
Combiva II for Cats® Combiva II for Dogs®	Imidacloprid Pyriproxyfen											+	+					
Credelio™	Lotilaner											±		±				+
Comfortis Chewable Tablets for Dogs®	Spinosad											+						
Droncit Canine Tablets®	Praziquantel								+	+	+							
Droncit Feline Tablets®	Praziquantel								+	+	+							
Droncit Injectable for Dogs and Cats®	Praziquantel								+	+	+							
Drontal for Cats®	Praziquantel Pyrantel pamoate						+	+	+	+	+							
Drontal Plus for Dogs®	Febantel Praziquantel Pyrantel pamoate			+	+	+			+	+	+							
Drs. Foster & Smith ProWormer-2® Nemex-2®	Pyrantel pamoate			+	+		+	+										
Frontline Gold for Cats® Frontline Gold for Dogs®	Fipronil Methoprene Pyriproxyfen											+	±	+				
Frontline Plus for Cats and Kittens® (spot on) Frontline Plus for Dogs and Puppies® (spot on)	Fipronil Methoprene											+	±	+	B		$	
Frontline Spray for Cats and Dogs®	Fipronil											+	+	+	B		$	
Frontline Tritak for Cats®	Fipronil Etofenprox Methoprene											+	±	+	B			

Product	Active Ingredient(s)													
Frontline Tritak for Dogs®	Fipronil Cyphenothrin Methoprene						+	+	±	+	B	+	$	±
Goodwinol ointment®	Rotenone Benzocaine													±
Hartz Advanced Care Liquid Wormer® Sergeants Worm Away®	Piperazine salts			+		+								
Heartgard for Cats®	Ivermectin	+					+							
Heartgard for Dogs®	Ivermectin (low dose for hwp)	+												
Heartgard Plus for Dogs® Tri-Heart Plus for Dogs® Iverhart Plus for Dogs®	Ivermectin Pyrantel pamoate	+		+	+	+								
Immiticide®	Melarsomine		+											
Interceptor®	Milbemycin	+		+	+	+					+	+	+	+
Iverhart MAX®	Ivermectin Pyrantel pamoate Praziquantel	+		+	+	+	+	+						
K9 Advantix II®	Imidacloprid Permethrin Pyriproxyfen						+	+	+	B				
Lime Sulfur Dip Concentrate®	Sulfurated lime solution									+			$	+
Milbemite® Otic Solution	Milbemycin										+			
Nexgard for Dogs®	Afoxolaner						+	+			+	+	+	+
Panacur-C® SafeGuard®	Fenbendazole			+	+	+	+							
Preventic Tick Collar for Dogs®	Amitraz								+					
Program Flavor Tabs for Dogs and Cats®	Lufenuron							+						
Program Injectable for Cats®	Lufenuron						+							

(Continued)

Table 7.3 (Continued)

Trade name	Drug(s)	HWP	HWA	H-dog	R-dog	W	H-cat	R-cat	TT	DT	ET	F	IGR	T	L	EM	SM	DM
Program Suspension for Cats®	Lufenuron												+					
Proheart 6 for Dogs®	Moxidectin	+		+														
Revolution®	Selamectin	+			+		+	+				+		±		+	+	
Scalibor Protector Band (Collar) for Dogs®	Deltamethrin											+		+				
Sentinel for Dogs®	Milbemycin Lufenuron	+		+	+	+							+			+	+	
Sentinel Spectrum® for Dogs	Milbemycin Lufenuron Praziquantel	+		+	+	+										+	+	
Seresto Cat Collar™	Imidacloprid Flumethrin											+		+				
Seresto Dog Collar™	Imidacloprid Flumethrin											+		+	B	+	§	
Simparica for Dogs™	Sarolaner											+		+		+	+	+
Trifexis for Dogs®	Milbemycin Spinosad	+		+	+	+						+/−				+	+	
Vectra 3D for Dogs®	Dinotefuran Pyriproxyfen Permethrin											+	+	+	S,B			
Vectra for Cats® Vectra for Cats and Kittens® Vectra for Dogs and Puppies®	Dinotefuran Pyriproxyfen											+	+					
Virbantel for Dogs®	Pyrantel pamoate Praziquantel			+	+		+	+	+	+	+							

+ = Label indication, † = extra-label indication, ± = limited usefulness, better products exist, § = aids in control, HWP = heartworm preventative, HWA = heartworm adulticide, H-dog = hookworms dog, R-dog = roundworms dog, W = whipworms dog, H-cat = hookworms cat, R-cat = roundworms cat, TT = Taenia tapeworms, DT = Dipylidium tapeworms, ET = Echinococcus tapeworms, F = fleas, IGR = insect growth regulator (immature fleas/flea eggs), T = ticks (see label insert for activity by tick species), L = lice, B = biting (chewing) lice, S = sucking lice, EM = ear mites (Otodectes), SM = sarcoptic mange, DM = demodectic mange.

parasites. Whether or not anthelmintic resistance is a threat in pet populations remains unresolved, although there are early indications of anthelmintic resistance in some strains (or populations) of heartworms.

The remainder of this section provides pertinent information about common parasites that infect dogs and cats, including the pathophysiology of the body system(s) affected by the parasite. Additionally, zoonotic potential is noted as well as the presence of parasite life cycle stages that abrogate susceptibility to antiparasitic drugs.

It is logical that a pharmacist would want to know the treatment options for a disease and their merits. Accordingly, drugs across different antiparasitic families are discussed in this section on internal parasites. Please refer to the "Classes of Antiparasitic Drugs Used in Small Animals" section for a more detailed explanation of the pharmacology of the drug family and individual agents.

7.3.1 Roundworms

The entire nematode class of parasites is sometimes referred to collectively as "roundworms." However, by common convention, the term is more correctly used to refer to ascarids. In this chapter, we will use the term roundworms for the ascarid group of nematodes. These are large worms found primarily in the small intestine, although it is not uncommon to find them throughout the GI tract, and some adult worms may occasionally pass into the feces or be contained in vomitus of heavily infected patients. Roundworm eggs are extremely resistant to the environment and disinfectants and can remain viable for years. Roundworms do not feed on the host directly, but rather compete for nutrients within the GI tract and account for malnutrition and a general failure to thrive. Large masses of roundworms can occasionally cause GI obstruction, which can be fatal. Roundworm infections are particularly problematic in young animals.

A complete discussion of the roundworm life cycle is beyond the scope of this text,

but a few points are clinically pertinent. Roundworm larvae often migrate through tissue before maturing into adult intestinal worms. In adult dogs or cats, many migrating larvae become dormant in tissues in a process called hypobiosis. When pregnancy occurs, these dormant forms are activated and migrate via either the transplacental or transmammary route to infect the fetus and newborn. This occurs with the common ascarid of dogs, but not cats, although transmammary transmission may be possible. Encysted larval forms in pregnant animals are not susceptible to anthelmintics commonly used in small animals, so even if the dam tests negative for parasites, it does not preclude infection of her puppies. Hypobiosis and transmammary infection also occur with hookworms in dogs. Kittens are typically exposed immediately after birth, from environmental exposure to infective hookworm larvae and ingestion of larvated roundworm eggs. As such, all puppies and kittens should routinely be treated with an anthelmintic with efficacy against roundworms and hookworms beginning at two weeks of age and then every two weeks until eight weeks old. Thereafter, a monthly preventative that includes anthelmintic control of these GI nematodes should be initiated. Early evidence suggests that selamectin (a topical anthelmintic; Revolution©) applied to dogs during pregnancy and lactation significantly reduced roundworm fecal egg counts in treated dams and their pups (Payne-Johnson et al. 2000). Daily use of fenbendazole during pregnancy or high-dose ivermectin during pregnancy has also been suggested as effective in decreasing roundworm transmission to puppies, although neither protocol is in widespread use (Burke 1983; Shoop et al. 1988).

A variety of products are available to treat roundworm infections. In young puppies and kittens, pyrantel pamoate is most frequently employed due to its high therapeutic index even in very young animals and its additional activity against hookworms. The liquid formulation and palatability of pyrantel pamoate also make for straightforward administration. Piperazine is marketed as an over-the-counter (OTC) dewormer, but it is rarely recommended as it has no activity against hookworms, a highly prevalent and serious infection of puppies and kittens. Pharmacists can play an important role in educating pet owners about the importance of using the appropriate anthelmintic for deworming dogs and cats. Benzimidazole dewormers such as fenbendazole are also effective but more typically used when a patient is concurrently infected with whipworms. Depending on the product, some heartworm preventatives are also effective against roundworms. For example, Heartgard Plus®, which contains a low dose of ivermectin for heartworm prevention, also contains pyrantel pamoate to treat roundworms and hookworms because the dose of ivermectin is too low to treat other nematodes. All other macrocyclic lactone heartworm preventatives are formulated with doses that effectively treat a wider spectrum of nematodes. An exception is sustained-released moxidectin injection in dogs (Proheart-6®), which is ineffective against roundworms (FDA 2001). When an adult animal is not receiving heartworm preventative effective against roundworms, the deworming is typically repeated in two to three weeks to ensure that all parasites are killed, particularly worms that were in a larval stage of development during the first treatment. See Tables 7.2 and 7.3 for a list of other effective products and dosages.

7.3.2 Hookworms

Hookworms are one of the most common GI parasites of small animals. Adult hookworms reside in the small intestine, where they attach to the mucosa and actively feed on blood. Thus, in additional to general ill health, anemia is common with hookworm infections and can be life-threatening, especially in young animals.

Adult hookworms in the intestine pass eggs in the feces, which hatch and develop into infective larvae in the environment. Larvae may live for several months, although they are susceptible to freezing temperatures. Larvae can be ingested directly or through paratenic hosts, but they usually penetrate intact skin and migrate via lymphatics to the blood and lungs. Paratenic hosts are also called transport hosts in that the parasite neither dies nor matures, but remains infectious to the final definitive host. Once in the lungs, the parasites continue to mature, then migrate up the trachea to be swallowed and complete their maturation to adults in the small intestine. The migratory route of larvae can cause transient skin rashes and lung disease in dogs and cats. Hookworms that infect small animals can be zoonotic, causing cutaneous larva migrans in humans.

As with roundworms, hookworms can undergo hypobiosis, entering a dormant state in tissues of adult animals. Pregnancy can reactivate these dormant larvae, where they migrate into the milk of the lactating bitch and infect nursing puppies. (This transmammary infection is not seen in cats.) Because hypobiotic larvae in tissues are not affected by routine anthelmintics, the dam testing negative on fecal examination does not mean that offspring will not be infected. All puppies and kittens should be presumed to be infected with hookworms and therefore treated with an appropriate anthelmintic beginning at two weeks of age and every two weeks until they are eight weeks old. Thereafter, they should be treated with a monthly preventative. A variety of products noted in Table 7.2 are effective against hookworms. Because of its wide safety margin, pyrantel pamoate is, however, often used in puppies, kittens, or debilitated adults for hookworm treatment. All of the approved heartworm preventatives that contain pyrantel, or that use a macrocyclic lactone other than ivermectin, are effective against hookworms. At the heartworm prevention dose, ivermectin is ineffective for hookworm treatment. As described for roundworms, if an adult animal is not receiving monthly treatment for hookworms (i.e. a heartworm preventative that is also indicated for hookworms), a single administration of an anthelmintic is insufficient. The deworming treatment should be repeated in two weeks to kill worms that may have been in a larval stage at the time of the first treatment.

7.3.3 Whipworms

Whipworms are less ubiquitous than roundworms or hookworms but nevertheless are a common GI parasite in dogs. A feline whipworm exists but is rare in North America. Adult whipworms reside in the cecum and large colon attached to the mucosa, feeding off of mucosal cells and blood. Many infections are subclinical, but intermittent diarrhea that often has increased mucous and streaks of blood can occur. Whipworms are not avid blood feeders, but anemia may be present, especially during large infections.

Female whipworms in the large intestine lay eggs that pass in the feces. In the environment, the eggs become larvated and can remain infective for years. Dogs become infected by ingesting the larvated eggs that hatch in the intestine and develop into adult worms. Although eggs are detectable by fecal flotation testing, eggs are heavy, production is erratic, and infections can be missed. Therefore, many veterinarians treat patients for whipworms despite a negative fecal flotation test. As with roundworms and hookworms, fecal antigen tests may be helpful in diagnosis of whipworms. Because of the long development period of whipworms, infected puppies and kittens would not be diagnosed until around three months of age.

Benzimidazole dewormers such as fenbendazole, febantel, and mebendazole are commonly used to treat whipworm infections. A repeat deworming at three weeks and at one to three months is recommended due to likely re-exposure. The macrocyclic lactones are also effective, depending on dose. The heartworm preventatives containing moxidectin (as a topical product; e.g. Advantage Multi® for Dogs) or milbemycin are macrocyclic lactones that include label indications for treating whipworm infections. Many veterinarians initially prescribe a benzimidazole, and then a monthly heartworm preventative that is effective against whipworms.

7.3.4 Heartworms

Heartworm disease is caused by *Dirofilaria immitis*, a nematode parasite of dogs where large adult worms lodge in the right ventricle and pulmonary artery and in severe cases extend into the vena cava (Figure 7.2). Adult worms produce microfilariae (pre-L1 larvae) that circulate in the blood and are ingested by mosquitoes, the intermediate host and vector. Within the mosquito, the larva molts to the infective L3 form that enters the dog or cat when the mosquito bites. The L3 form migrates through the tissue and molts into L4, then finally enters the vasculature about two months after initial infection as L5 (young adult) heartworms. Heartworms are fully mature about six to seven months after infection, and then live five to seven years, with microfilariae surviving one to two years in the bloodstream.

Dogs infected with a small number of adult worms may be asymptomatic, but as the worm burden increases, the dog will develop cough, exercise intolerance, and respiratory signs. Sedentary dogs are less likely to show clinical signs than active animals. Dogs infected with large numbers of heartworms can develop cor pulmonale with right-sided heart failure. "Caval syndrome," which occurs when worms in the right ventricle, right atrium, and vena cava obstruct valve function and blood flow, leading to hemolysis, liver and kidney dysfunction, and heart failure, is more likely in dogs infected with more than 40 adult heartworms (Nelson et al. 2014). Antigen–antibody complexes may also result in kidney injury, as well as confound diagnostic assays that detect antigen.

Although large burdens of heartworms can mechanically cause injury, primary lung pathology associated with the inflammatory reaction generated by the worms' presence is

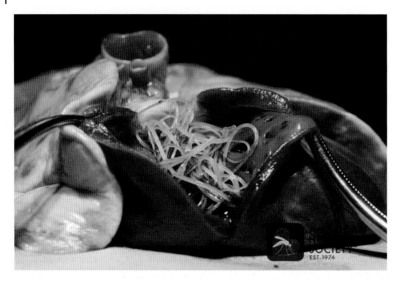

Figure 7.2 Adult heartworms seen in the right ventricle of a dog's heart. *Source:* Courtesy of the American Heartworm Society, https://heartwormsociety.org/veterinary-resources/practice-tools/heartworm-images.

perhaps more important. This is especially true in cats infected with heartworm infection. Adult heartworms also harbor endosymbiotic bacteria belonging to the genus *Wolbachia* (Rickettsiales). These bacteria are believed to exacerbate the host's inflammatory response to adult worms (Nelson et al. 2014).

Cats are not the natural host of the parasite, but heartworm disease does occur in this species, particularly in areas with heavy mosquito burdens. Even indoor cats are at risk. Relatively small numbers of adult worms usually mature in cats, but immature and adult heartworms, as well as dying mature heartworms, will cause an exaggerated inflammatory response compared to dogs, demonstrated by changes in pulmonary vasculature and general lung damage. Although less common in cats, heartworm disease is often severe and life-threatening; hence, many veterinarians prescribe monthly heartworm preventatives for cats.

7.3.4.1 Preventatives

Once restricted to the southeastern USA, heartworm disease now exists throughout the Americas, including Canada. All dogs, and arguably all cats, should be treated with a heartworm preventative. Year-round administration of preventatives is now generally recommended, in part to ensure compliance and thus decrease the risk of resistance, and to provide protection when environmental changes (i.e. warmer winters) allow mosquitos to transmit the parasite "off-season." Seasonal treatment, however, is reasonable in northern areas as long as preventatives are started no later than one month after mosquitoes emerge. Because preventatives have, on rare occasion, caused severe reactions when given to dogs with circulating microfilariae, dogs should test negative for microfilariae before reinstituting preventatives each year. Treatment is continued for at least one month past the seasonal disappearance of mosquitoes due to cold weather. In the southern USA, where mosquitoes are ubiquitous year-round, animals should be treated with heartworm preventative continuously.

The elimination half-life varies for each preventative, but for most of the monthly preventatives, "therapeutic concentrations" are maintained for only a few days. The reason that once-monthly treatment is effective is due to "reach back"; that is, the preventative kills developing L3 and L4 larvae that have infected the animal since the previous dose, although efficacy generally decreases as the heartworms mature. Many owners worry about missing a dose of heartworm preventative, and indeed lack of owner compliance is a major reason for infection. If the dose is only a few weeks late, "reach back" is often still effective at preventing new infections, but compliance with monthly administration is optimal. Pharmacists can play an important role in educating pet owners on the importance of heartworm preventatives in their geographical area.

7.3.4.2 Adulticide (Drugs Used to Kill Adult Worms): Recommended Protocol for Dogs

Once a dog is infected, the heartworms continuously damage the lungs, potentially causing permanent fibrosis. Thus, adulticide treatment is warranted. Melarsomine, an injectable arsenical, is the core drug in adulticidal therapy. The drug label offers two protocols for melarsomine use: (i) A standard protocol in dogs with lower grade disease uses two daily injections; and (ii) a "split protocol" is recommended for more severely affected dogs, where one injection of melarsomine is given to kill a portion of adult heartworms, then one month later two daily injections are administered to complete adulticidal treatment. However, the American Heartworm Society recommends the split protocol for all dogs due to greater efficacy and lower risk. It also recommends that several ancillary therapies be included in the treatment protocol.

The complete American Heartworm Society protocol is outlined in Figure 7.3. The protocol and its rationale will be briefly described. Because young adult worms are less susceptible to melarsomine, heartworm preventative is started two months prior to melarsomine injection. This kills developing larvae and allows young adults (that are not susceptible to the preventatives) to mature, developing susceptibility to melarsomine. Because many heartworm preventatives also have microfilaricidal activity, dogs that harbor microfilariae should be monitored for allergic reactions

secondary to antigen release by dying microfilariae. This is most likely to occur during the first eight hours after the first preventative dose. Pretreatment with histamine-1 receptor antagonists may be warranted prior to preventative administration in dogs with high microfilaria burdens. Doxycycline (or minocycline) is initiated prior to melarsomine administration to decrease the inflammatory response associated with *Wolbachia* organisms that are symbiotic with adult heartworms. For dogs that are symptomatic, a glucocorticoid is initiated simultaneously, then tapered over four weeks. Sixty days after starting the protocol, the first melarsomine injection is administered by a veterinarian according to label instructions. The tapering glucocorticoid regimen is given. Strict exercise restriction is absolutely essential to minimize the risk of adulticide complications. One month later, melarsomine is administered on two consecutive days, and the glucocorticoid regimen is repeated for an additional four weeks. Exercise restriction continues for another six to eight weeks. Thirty days after the last dose of melarsomine, the dog is tested for microfilaremia, and a microfilaricide is administered if needed. Historically, a wide variety of macrocyclic lactones have been used for this purpose, although moxidectin topical (Advantage Multi for Dogs) is the only product that is FDA approved for this indication.

7.3.4.3 Adulticide: Alternative Protocol for Dogs and Cats

Heartworm preventative medications were historically viewed as having no efficacy against adult heartworms. However, newer data indicate that monthly preventatives shorten the lifespan of adult heartworms in dogs from about five years to approximately 9 to 30 months (McCall 2005). This approach has been referred to as the "slow-kill" or "trickle-kill" protocol.

Since young heartworms are more susceptible to this approach, the earlier the treatment is initiated after heartworms are diagnosed, the shorter their survival time. Among FDA-approved heartworm preventatives, those

Day	Treatment
Day 0	Dog diagnosed and verified as heartworm positive: • Positive antigen (Ag) test verified with microfilaria (MF) test. • If no microfilariae are detected, confirm with second Ag test from a different manufacturer Begin exercise restriction. • The more pronounced the signs, the stricter the exercise restriction. If the dog is symptomatic: • Stabilize with appropriate therapy and nursing care. • Prednisone prescribed at 0.5 mg/kg BID first week, 0.5 mg/kg SID second week, 0.5 mg/kg EOD third and fourth weeks.
Day 1	Administer heartworm preventive. • If microfilariae are detected, pretreat with antihistamine and glucocorticosteroid, if not already on prednisone, to reduce risk of anaphylaxis. • Observe for at least 8 hours for signs of reaction.
Days 1–28	Administer doxycycline 10 mg/kg BID for 4 weeks. • Reduces pathology associated with dead heartworms. • Disrupts heartworm transmission.
Day 30	Administer heartworm preventive.
Day 60	Administer heartworm preventive. First melarsomine injection 2.5 mg/kg intramuscularly (IM) Prescribe prednisone 0.5 mg/kg BID first week, 0.5 mg/kg SID second week, 0.5 mg/kg EOD third and fourth weeks. Decrease activity level even further. • Cage restriction/on leash when using yard.
Day 90	Administer heartworm preventive. Second melarsomine injection 2.5 mg/kg IM.
Day 91	Third melarsomine injection 2.5 mg/kg IM Prescribe prednisone 0.5 mg/kg BID first week, 0.5 mg/kg SID second week, 0.5 mg/kg EOD third and fourth weeks. Continue exercise restriction for 6 to 8 weeks following last melarsomine injections.
Day 120	Test for presence of microfilariae. • If positive, treat with a microfilaricide and retest in 4 weeks. Establish year-round heartworm prevention.
Day 271	Antigen test 6 months after completion; screen for microfilariae.

Figure 7.3 Heartworm adulticide treatment protocol recommended by the American Heartworm Society. *Source:* Courtesy of the American Heartworm Society, https://heartwormsociety.org.

containing ivermectin or topical moxidectin have the greatest efficacy, followed by selamectin and injectable moxidectin, with milbemycin being least effective. The use of slow-kill protocols is controversial and not recommended by the American Heartworm Society because the presence of heartworms continues to induce inflammation in the host and may promote resistance to the macrocyclic lactones. In situations where melarsomine therapy is not possible or is contraindicated, the slow-kill protocol is preferable to no treatment. As recommended in the standard adulticide protocol, a course of doxycycline is often prescribed to address the *Wolbachia* component of the disease.

Cats with heartworm do not tolerate melarsomine adulticide treatment due to the severe, life-threatening inflammatory response. Its use is contraindicated in cats. Recommended treatment of cats with heartworm disease is similar to the slow-kill protocol in dogs. Cats that are symptomatic or have radiographic abnormalities of the lung may benefit from tapering doses of prednisolone. Nonsteroidal anti-inflammatory drugs (NSAIDs) have failed to demonstrate a benefit and actually may worsen parenchymal lung damage (Jones et al. 2014). Whether cats would benefit from doxycycline therapy is undetermined, although its use has been suggested based on the benefit seen in canine heartworm disease treatment (Jung and Dillon 2016).

Dramatic difference

If doxycycline is used in cats, the suspension is preferred because tablets or capsules can cause esophageal ulcers due to delayed esophageal transit. Studies have indicated a rapid loss of stability beyond seven days for compounded doxycycline suspensions, so appropriately timed refills are necessary to ensure adequate potency (Papich et al. 2013).

7.3.4.4 Surgical Removal of Adult Worms

Dogs with pre-caval syndrome may be in such dire condition that surgical removal of heartworms (debulking by snare introduced through the external jugular vein) may be warranted. After several weeks of recovery, adulticide therapy should be considered (Nelson et al. 2014). Surgical removal has also been suggested for severely affected cats, but it is more difficult since there are fewer worms and anatomical differences limit access to the right ventricle (Jones et al. 2014).

7.3.5 Tapeworms

The three most common tapeworms in dogs and cats are *Dipylidium*, *Taenia*, and *Echinococcus*. The first two occur throughout the USA, while *Echinococcus* is more limited in its distribution and is primarily a dog tapeworm. Dogs and cats become infected by ingesting intermediate hosts containing the larval form of the tapeworm. Because fleas are the intermediate hosts for *Dipylidium*, it is the most commonly encountered tapeworm. Both *Taenia* and *Echinococcus* use mammals as intermediate hosts; these are often species that serve as prey for dogs and cats, such as rabbits and rodents, respectively.

Adult tapeworms attach to the intestine and most shed gravid (egg-laden) proglottids. Although parasite eggs may be found on fecal flotation, the method is not highly sensitive as proglottids are not evenly distributed and may not be present in the fecal sample. The infection is frequently discovered by owners, who are repulsed by the sight of proglottid segments in the feces or around the anus. *Dipylidium* proglottids resemble grains of rice, while *Taenia* tend to be square segments. For the tiny tapeworm *Echinococcus*, the small proglottids disintegrate in feces or are simply too small to be visualized grossly.

Adult tapeworms typically reside in the small intestine, where they absorb nutrients but are otherwise generally well tolerated unless large numbers cause intestinal obstruction, a possibility for the larger *Dipylidium* and *Taenia* species. The tapeworm *Spirometra*, which is more common in dogs and cats in the southern USA, can cause vomiting, diarrhea, and other GI signs on its own, but it is more of an exception. Treatment of tapeworms is primarily for aesthetic and zoonotic reasons.

Relative to zoonotic risks, human cysticercosis is due to the larval stages of *T. solium*, a species that normally uses swine as an intermediate host. Adult *T. solium* as well as the beef tapeworm, *T. saginata*, can be found in human intestines; neither tapeworm uses dogs or cats in their life cycle. Ingestion of fleas can cause *Dipylidium* infection in humans, particularly in younger children who have a knack for placing things in their mouths. Although *Dipylidium* proglottids are obviously distressing to pet owners, the *Dipylidium* itself causes few problems for the pet. The zoonotic infections of most significant concern in the USA are cystic echinococcosis (unilocular hydatid disease, due to *Echinococcus granulosus*) and alveolar echinococcosis (multilocular hydatid disease, due to *Echinococcus multilocularis*) when humans become the accidental intermediate host. The cysts and granulomatous lesions of these diseases occur primarily in the liver and lung, although central nervous system (CNS) infections are particularly serious. Albendazole is the treatment of choice in humans for tissue forms of tapeworm infections. Surgical removal, or a process of aspirating the cyst "prior to and after injection of a chemotherapeutic" (PAIR), is possible for *E. granulosis* cysts, but due to the rapid growth and invasive nature of the alveolar cyst, treatment is more challenging.

The drugs most commonly used to treat tapeworms in dogs and cats are the isoquinolines praziquantel and epsiprantel. Praziquantel is effective against *Taenia, Dipylidium*, and *Echinococcus*. Some countries require deworming of pets with this drug prior to importation to avoid bringing *Echinococcus* into the country. This is true for importation of pets into the UK, as it is presently free of *E. multilocularis*. Epsiprantel is likewise effective against *Taenia* and *Dipylidium*, but it is not labeled for use against *Echinococcus. Spirometra* can also be successfully treated with praziquantel using a higher, off-label dose. The need for repeated treatment is based on reinfection by ingestion of the intermediate host.

7.3.6 Miscellaneous

Numerous other parasites affect dogs and cats, but they are less common and beyond the scope of this chapter. Table 7.1 lists these parasites and the drugs used in their treatment.

7.4 Treatment Considerations for Common External Parasitic Diseases

The external parasites of small animals belong to the phylum Arthropoda, which is divided by class into either insect (fleas, flies, lice, and mosquitoes) or arachnid families (ticks and mites). Insects are treated by insecticides or insect growth regulators (IGRs), while arachnids are treated with acaracides. Drugs used to treat external parasites in companion animals have a broad spectrum of activity, but none are universally effective against all of these parasites. Indeed, even within a parasite family, some drugs are effective against one member but ineffective against another (e.g. sarcoptic versus demodectic mange.)

Pharmacists should be aware of the interpretation of drug labels relative to the drug's efficacy against specific parasites and the safety of the drug in young animals. Fleas are the most ubiquitous of external pet parasites, and the activity of most products is well established and clearly indicated on the label. Conversely, a drug's activity against a particular species of tick is not consistently indicated on the label. The tick species is actually quite important because only certain tick species serve as disease vectors. Examples include the deer tick (*Ixodes scapularis*), which transmits Lyme disease; the lone star tick (*Amblyomma americanum*), which is the primary vector for cytauxzoonosis in cats; the brown dog tick (*Rhipicephalus sanguineus*), which transmits *Ehrlichia canis* to dogs; and the American dog tick (*Dermacentor variabilis*), which is the primary vector for Rocky Mountain spotted fever. The product label often simply includes the statement "effective against most ticks," leaving the burden on the pharmacist or veterinarian to explore more definitive resources (e.g. https://www.capcvet.org/parasite-product-applications) if more detailed information on efficacy is desired.

There are also limitations in labeling relative to the age at which a patient should be treated with the drug. A common phrase is: "for control of [X parasite(s)] in [animal species] over [Y] weeks of age." Sometimes, the age limit represents a true risk of toxicity in younger animals, but another possibility is that the manufacturer did not test animals younger than that age, often for economic reasons (limited potential sales) or an inability to recruit adequate patient numbers. The same is true regarding use of these products in pregnant and lactating animals. As pharmacists know, drug use involves weighing risks versus benefits, and since the risks associated with external parasites are generally not high, it is best to err on the side of caution.

With regard to other external parasites, there are a limited number of FDA-approved products to treat certain mite infestations, particularly demodectic mange, as well as lice and mosquitoes. Therefore, extra-label use is common in these situations.

To enhance the spectrum of activity and provide a one-drug-treats-all solution, many manufacturers combine several drugs into one product that has activity against both internal and external parasites. See Tables 7.2 and 7.3 for a listing of common formulations, their spectrum, and dosages.

This section's following discussion on external parasitic diseases is intended to provide pharmacists with a broad overview of treatment considerations for external parasites and compare treatment options across drug families. Please refer to the "Classes of Antiparasitic Drugs Used in Small Animals" section for a more detailed explanation of the pharmacology of the drug family and individual agents.

7.4.1 Fleas

The impact of fleas on pets varies geographically in the USA. They are especially common in the southeastern portion of the country, while pets in the cooler and more arid regions such as the Northern Plains or desert Southwest may have few flea problems. It is essential for pharmacists to understand that during infestations, large reservoirs of fleas exist off of the animal. In such infestations, it is important that fleas in the home and the outdoor environment be addressed because medication of the animal alone will not provide adequate control.

Adult fleas feed exclusively on the blood of their host. Fleas have a host preference, but if deprived of their preferred host (e.g. if the dog is boarding), fleas will also bite humans. The most common flea in small animals, the cat flea (*Ctenocephalides felis*), prefers cats but readily bites dogs and other hosts, including wildlife and humans. A large flea infestation on an animal can cause severe anemia, as well as causing extreme misery in the form of pruritic dermatitis. Flea allergy dermatitis can be an especially miserable skin disease and is caused by hypersensitivity to antigens in the saliva of fleas, where even very small numbers of fleas (e.g. a single flea) can trigger a reaction in sensitive animals (see Chapter 18 for more detailed information).

Fleas also carry a variety of diseases, including *Mycoplasma haemofelis* (formerly *Haemobartonella felis*) and zoonotic diseases, including cat scratch fever (*Bartonella henselae*), murine typhus (*Rickettsia typhi*), flea-borne typhus (*Rickettsia felis*), and tapeworms (*Dipylidium caninum*). Regarding the latter parasite, ingestion of an infected flea, which is the intermediate host for that tapeworm, has resulted in development of adult *D. caninum* (tapeworms) in human pediatric patients. Rodent fleas acquired by dogs and cats in the southern Rocky Mountain states and southwestern states may be vectors for bubonic plague (*Yersinia pestis*) when the fleas leave the host to bite humans (Companion Animal Parasite Council 2017).

A variety of topical and oral ectoparasiticides are available to control fleas on dogs and cats. IGRs supplement the activity of many of the topical products. Lufenuron is a monthly oral (dog and cat) and injectable (cat) IGR also used to control fleas. See Table 7.3 for a listing of products and their activities.

Practiced but not proven

Nutritional supplements including brewer's yeast or garlic have been recommended to control fleas in dogs and cats. A study, however, failed to show any benefit from brewer's yeast. Garlic may cause Heinz body anemia in small animals, and its use is discouraged (Baker and Farver 1983).

7.4.2 Ticks

Ticks are arachnids found throughout North America. Ticks infect all species, including dogs and cats, although the latter are less commonly affected. Among the two main tick groups, hard (Ixodid) and soft (Argasid), the hard ticks are more widely distributed in North America, more commonly found attached to animals due to their feeding behavior, and more often associated with pathogen transmission (i.e. they serve as vectors). While all ticks are typically small and flat when unfed, their size increases after a blood meal. This is particularly evident in female ticks, whose hard scutum covers only a small portion of the body (unlike male ticks, which are completely covered). The remainder of the female tick's body is soft integument, allowing them to expand as much as 100-fold after feeding on host blood, whereas the size increase in male ticks is not apparent. Thus, large engorged ticks found on the animal are typically females; immature ticks will also engorge but are smaller in size overall. The life cycle of the tick after egg hatching includes larva, nymph, and adult, with each stage requiring a blood meal to continue its development. So-called "seed ticks" are usually the larval stage and are so named because their size resembles a small seed or pinhead. The larval stage has six legs, while nymphs and adults have the eight legs characteristic of arachnids.

Ticks can attach to any part of an animal's skin to feed on blood but are usually found in and around the ears, in the groin area, on the abdomen, and between the shoulder blades. They cause a focal dermatitis as well as blood loss. In animals with severe tick infestations, death can occur from exsanguination. As described for flea infestations, the home and yard may need environmental treatment in combination with treatment of the animal in order to control the infestation. Monthly tick preventatives, including orally and topically administered products as well as collars, can be quite efficacious when used judiciously.

Ticks carry a variety of serious and potentially zoonotic pathogens that cause diseases, including Rocky Mountain spotted fever, ehrlichiosis, Lyme disease, anaplasmosis, babesiosis, tularaemia, hepatozoonosis, and cytauxzoonosis. Usually, a particular tick species is the vector for a specific disease agent. Table 7.3 lists treatment and preventative options for tick control.

7.4.3 Mites

The four most common mites affecting dogs and cats are ear mites, sarcoptic mange mites, demodectic mange mites, and to a lesser extent *Cheyletiella* (hair-clasping mite, or "walking dandruff").

7.4.3.1 Ear Mites

Although not nearly as common as flea and tick problems, ear mites (*Otodectes cynotis*) are nevertheless important parasites afflicting both dogs and cats. They cause a severe inflammatory reaction in the external ear canal, usually in conjunction with a bacterial or yeast infection. A very common sequela of ear mites in dogs is an aural hematoma (hematoma of the ear pinna) that results from vigorous headshaking. Ear mites are easily transmitted by casual contact and can cross species. Diagnosing ear mites in one pet in a household warrants screening the other pets for infection. Human infestations can occur through close contact, although this is extremely rare.

A variety of products are available to treat ear mites. These include topical pyrethroids and thiabendazole, but topical macrocyclic lactones are more commonly used. Many systemic therapies, both approved and extra-label, are also effective; see Table 7.3.

7.4.3.2 Sarcoptic Mange

Sarcoptic mange (scabies) is caused by burrowing mites: *Sarcoptes scabiei* in dogs, humans, and other hosts, or *Notoedres cati* in cats. Infestations are intensely pruritic and typically affect the ears, face, elbows, and hocks of dogs, or the face of cats. It causes extreme discomfort to affected individuals. Zoonotic transmission is possible. The disease can be difficult to diagnose, so a trial therapy against scabies is sometimes prescribed.

Organophosphate and pyrethroid dips are still available but have largely been replaced by other treatments that are more efficacious, are safer, and involve more straightforward administration. An exception is the use of lime sulfur dip, which is a good option for very young puppies and kittens due to its extremely high therapeutic index. Lime sulfur has an odor (rotten egg) that is disagreeable to pet owners and can stain furniture or carpet, especially if the animal is not thoroughly dried after its treatment. Amitraz topical, as a dip or sponge-on, is a highly effective extra-label treatment for the control of *Sarcoptes* mites. Amitraz is a monoamine oxidase inhibitor, which, as pharmacists know, can cause serious drug–drug interactions. Although not a curative treatment, topical fipronil and selamectin can aid in the control of sarcoptic mange.

For years, the standard treatment for sarcoptic mange has been the macrocyclic lactones, which are extremely efficacious and well tolerated. (See, in Chapter 5, the exception of ivermectin toxicity in certain breeds with the ABCB1-1Δ gene defect.) Although a single treatment usually brings relief of signs, a repeat treatment is recommended for a complete cure. Extra-label use of the isoxazolines is also gaining popularity due to their ease of use and high owner compliance, especially with fluralaner (Bravecto®).

7.4.3.3 Demodectic Mange

Demodex canis is an obligate parasite of dogs believed to exist as normal flora in healthy dogs, albeit at low numbers. However, some *Demodex* species (e.g. *Demodex cornei* in dogs and *Demodex gatoi* in cats) may cause disease with initial infestations and are considered primary pathogens. The development of cutaneous disease due to *Demodex* results from an underlying immunodeficiency involving T-cell function. Demodicosis in puppies can manifest as a localized

dermatitis involving one or more focal lesions. Depending on immune system development and possible breed predilections, this may be self-resolving or develop into generalized demodicosis. Adult-onset demodectic mange is usually generalized and caused by an underlying immunosuppressive disorder such as hyperadrenocorticism (Cushing's disease), hypothyroidism, glucocorticoid or other immunosuppressive treatments, or neoplasia. Demodicosis in either its localized or generalized form is surprisingly nonpruritic unless a secondary pyoderma exists.

Localized demodicosis in the puppy typically does not require treatment and will either self-resolve or progress to generalized demodicosis based on immune development in the puppy. Veterinarians will sometimes dispense topical antibiotics or antiseptics to suppress secondary bacterial or fungal infections at the lesions, although their necessity is debatable.

Practiced but not proven

One older treatment still employed by some veterinarians for local demodicosis is Goodwinol® ointment, a combination of rotenone and benzocaine. The effectiveness of Goodwinol has never been established, and some view its use as simply palliating the owner. If used, a word of caution is appropriate. If the animal ingests the ointment (e.g. due to grooming), the benzocaine can cause methemoglobinemia, particularly in secondary exposures to cats.

Generalized demodicosis in dogs is one of the most difficult parasite infestations to cure. Throughout most of the twentieth century, it equated to an eventual death sentence for the dog. Although effective treatment still remains a challenge today, there are now several therapies that are highly effective.

A breakthrough in treatment of generalized demodectic mange came with the introduction of amitraz topical solution

(Mitaban®). It remains the only FDA-approved treatment for the disease and is typically highly effective. Initial studies showed an efficacy of approximately 92% (Mueller 2004). Extra-label use of more concentrated solutions or shorter dosing intervals have been advocated, though, as refractory cases and poorer success rates have been reported. See further in this chapter for a discussion on its pharmacology, adverse effects, and drug interactions.

Alternatives to amitraz have been sought because of resistance to the drug and its cumbersome and labor-intensive method of application. While the macrocyclic lactones were initially thought to be ineffective against demodectic mites, studies eventually discovered that high-dose daily treatments could be effective. A variety of macrocyclic lactones have been used in an extra-label manner for treating demodicosis, including ivermectin, milbemycin, moxidectin, and doramectin. Although generally well tolerated if dosed correctly, adverse events have occurred with overdose, when administered to dogs with the ABCB1-1Δ gene defect (MDR1, or "ivermectin-sensitive breeds"), or when P-glycoprotein pump inhibitors are concomitantly given (e.g. spinosad, ketoconazole, and cyclosporine). Screening in susceptible breeds for the gene defect along with gradual dose escalation are prudent with macrocyclic lactone treatment for demodicosis. See the "Macrocyclic Lactones" section for further information on pharmacology, adverse effects, and drug interactions.

An increasingly popular treatment for demodicosis are the isoxazoline products afoxolaner (Nexgard®), fluralaner (Bravecto), sarolaner (Simparica™), and lotilaner (Credelio™). Although their use for demodicosis is extra-label and still relatively new, the dose and frequency for their labeled use in flea and tick control appear effective against demodicosis.

Demodectic mange occurs less commonly in cats than in dogs and is often associated with the related "normal flora" mite, *Demodex cati*. There are no FDA-approved products for use in cats, but lime sulfur dips and doramectin weekly injections have been used successfully (Medleau and Willemse 1995; Mueller 2004).

7.4.3.4 Walking Dandruff (*Cheyletiella* sp.)

Cheyletiellosis (walking dandruff) affects dogs, cats, and other animals. The mites are nonburrowing but feed on skin keratin, leading to sloughing from the epidermis and visible skin flakes. Mites can be transmitted on shared objects (fomites) such as bedding and may cause transient human infestations. Pruritus is variable, and lesions typically occur on the dorsum and are mildly erythematous with excessive scaling. In cats, papulocrustous lesions (miliary dermatitis) may develop; in dogs, pyotraumatic dermatitis may occur. There are no FDA-approved treatments in the USA, but cheyletiellosis is responsive to a wide variety of parasiticides, including lime sulfur dip, macrocyclic lactones, amitraz, pyrethrins, fipronil, organophosphates, and carbamate topicals.

7.4.4 Miscellaneous External Parasites

Mosquitoes carry a variety of diseases transmissible to humans and are the vector for heartworm disease in dogs, cats, and ferrets. Their bite does not produce a severe reaction in dogs and cats unless a hypersensitivity to the saliva develops. The latter unfortunately does occur, particularly in cats. While permethrin has a repellent action against mosquitoes in dogs, it is too toxic for use in cats.

Lice are infrequent external parasites of dogs and cats. They are host-specific, so zoonotic transfer is not a concern, although on rare occasion the incidental human louse has been found on pets through contact with an infected human owner. Although it is likely that most products with activity against fleas would likewise be effective against lice, these are often not tested in small animals for economic reasons. Table 7.3 indicates those products where activity against lice has been demonstrated.

7.5 Classes of Antiparasitic Drugs Used in Small Animals

Traditionally, antiparasitic agents were organized by whether their action was directed against internal versus external parasites. However, many newer compounds are "endectocides," which have activities against both internal and external parasites. As such, this section is not necessarily divided into internal versus external parasite control products. See Table 7.3 for information on the spectrum of commercial products.

7.5.1 Amitraz

Arachnids, such as mites and ticks, use octopamine as a neurotransmitter rather than the mammalian neurotransmitter norepinephrine. Amitraz acts as an agonist at the octopamine receptor, resulting in overexcitation and consequently paralysis and death of the parasite. It is not active against fleas. It is the only FDA-approved treatment for demodectic mange in the USA and is sometimes used in an extra-label manner for sarcoptic mange. There is also an FDA-approved amitraz-impregnated collar for tick control. Both products are labeled for dogs only. Use in cats is not recommended.

Amitraz as a diluted dip (Mitaban; sponge-on) is applied per label instructions every 14 days for three to six treatments. At this dosage, initial studies indicated a 92% improvement and an 80% cure rate for demodicosis (Folz et al. 1984). Poorer performance and relapses have been described in other studies, with response rates in the 50% to 65% range (Medleau and Willemse 1995). More concentrated solutions or more frequent applications have been used in an extra-label manner for refractory cases.

Amitraz is also the active ingredient of a very effective slow-release collar for dogs (Preventic®) to control ticks. It is used frequently for hunting dogs and dogs with outside access in regions where Lyme disease (transmitted by the deer tick) is prevalent. It does not have cidal action against the tick,

but rather prevents it from biting and attaching. The collar's duration of activity is approximately three months if kept dry. Much of the amitraz in the collar can be lost if the dog swims. It is also available in combination with fipronil and methoprene as a topical spot-on product, Cetifect®.

After topical application of the sponge-on product, systemic absorption can be sufficient to cause adverse effects, the most common of which is sedation occurring in about 8% of dogs receiving the label treatment. Sedation usually occurs within eight hours and can last 72 hours, although most animals recover within 24 hours (Pharmacia and Upjohn Company 1998; Page 2008). Sedation is thought to be mediated by alpha-2 adrenergic agonist activity, since it can be reversed by atipamezole or other alpha-2 adrenergic antagonists. Pruritus, erythema, and transient hyperglycemia are also sometimes noted.

Oral ingestion of the impregnated collar, which dogs may do, can be particularly serious depending on the amount ingested. In an oral acute toxicity study, two dogs given a single dose of 100 mg/kg developed CNS depression, ataxia, hypothermia, bradycardia, muscular weakness, emesis, uncontrolled vocal spasm, and micturition. Clinical laboratory data indicated hemoconcentration and transient elevations in blood glucose, blood urea nitrogen, and serum potassium. One of the two dogs died. Dogs given 20 mg/kg had similar but less severe signs that resolved within three days. At 4 mg/kg, dogs were minimally affected, with only mild drops in rectal temperature that returned to normal within 24 hours (Pharmacia and Upjohn Company 1998).

Amitraz is a potent monoamine oxidase inhibitor in mammals and, as such, can cause drug interactions. In veterinary medicine, this is most likely an issue with drugs working through serotonergic or adrenergic mechanisms such as fluoxetine, clomipramine (or other tricyclic antidepressants), trazodone, and tramadol. Amitraz is typically applied by the veterinarian, and the animal is allowed to dry before returning home. Should the solution be dispensed for owner use, care to avoid contact with the solution or the wet dog is prudent.

7.5.2 Benzimidazoles

The benzimidazole class of drugs includes some of the most widely used antiparasitics in large and small animals. They bind to tubulin to disrupt cell division and inhibit fumarate reductase to block mitochondrial function in the parasite. Fenbendazole is the most commonly used drug in this family and is FDA approved for use in not only dogs, horses, goats, sheep, and cattle but also a surprising number of zoo and exotic animal species. It is even approved for use during pregnancy in dogs. Oddly, it is not approved in the USA for cats, although it is commonly used in an extra-label manner in Felidae and is effective against some of the same parasite groups as those it is labeled for in dogs. Fenbendazole is effective against hookworms, roundworms, and *Taenia* tapeworms (but not *Dipylidium* or *Echinococcus*) in dogs and cats (Roberson and Burke 1980). It is also effective against canine whipworms, lungworms, and lung flukes. It was serendipitously found to be quite effective in treating *Giardia* in dogs and cats.

Dramatic difference

Due to its high therapeutic index, low incidence of side effects, and shorter treatment duration, fenbendazole has largely replaced metronidazole as the treatment of choice in dogs and cats for the protozoan parasite *Giardia*.

Fenbendazole has a very high therapeutic index and is generally well tolerated. The activity of fenbendazole is attributed to two active metabolites. While single doses are effective in large animals, three daily dosings are required in dogs and cats, as they are less efficient at producing these metabolites. (In severe infections, five daily dosings are sometimes advocated.)

Febantel is a prodrug that is metabolized to fenbendazole and oxfendazole, the latter a benzimidazole that is labeled for use in cattle. It is similar to fenbendazole with the exception that single doses may be effective against whipworms. The reason for this difference is unknown. Also, two adverse events were found in the approval studies for febantel that are not known to occur with fenbendazole. First, deaths occurred in cats with preexisting liver and/or kidney dysfunction treated at high doses; therefore, its use is discouraged in patients with either condition. Also, a warning exists for use in pregnancy, as six days of a 3× dose in early gestation resulted in an increased incidence of abortion and fetal abnormalities (FDA 1991).

Mebendazole is similar in activity and is an approved oral product for dogs. It is, however, used much less frequently in practice than fenbendazole.

Albendazole is a unique benzimidazole for having activity not only against flukes but also against the tissue phases of larval *Echinococcus* and *Taenia*, where it is used in human patients to treat hydatid cyst disease and cysticercosis, respectively. However, it is teratogenic and can cause bone marrow suppression in dogs. As such, albendazole should not be used in dogs and cats.

7.5.3 DEET

DEET (N,N-diethyl-meta-toluamide) is one of the most common insect and tick repellents used in humans. Its safety and efficacy in pets, however, remain largely undetermined. A product containing 8.55% DEET and fenvalerate, Hartz Blockade® for cats and dogs, was sold in the late 1980s and early 1990s. Although the product was widely used safely in most dogs and cats, some serious adverse events, including death, were reported in both species (Streitfeld 1991). The clinical signs included vomiting, tremors, excitation, ataxia, and seizures (Dorman 1990). Whether DEET, fenvalerate, or the combination were the cause for these adverse events was never determined. It was conjectured but not proven that overzealous administration by owners may have contributed to the toxic risk.

Oddly, DEET appears to have a high margin of safety in dogs based on pesticide safety studies. In a chronic (one-year) oral toxicity test in dogs, the no observable effect level (NOEL) for DEET was 100 mg/kg per day, and the lowest effect level (LEL) was 400 mg/kg per day. Clinical signs at the LEL dose were excess salivation and a decreased appetite. Two dogs had tremors (US Environmental Protection Agency. Reregistration Eligibility Decision DEET. Regist Eligibility Decis. 1998;(September):9–13. doi:EPA738-R-98-010). In another study, dogs given 0.1–0.3 ml/kg per day of 95% DEET orally for 13 weeks displayed tremors and hyperactivity following each dose (Dorman 1990). Similar data are not available for cats, which many veterinarians believe to be more sensitive.

The role of DEET as a flea, fly, mosquito, and tick repellent for dogs and cats remains unclear. Anecdotally, veterinarians have recommended use of the lowest available concentration of DEET (for children) sparingly in dogs for mosquito repellence. It is generally avoided in cats.

7.5.4 Docusate

Docusate (dioctyl sodium sulfosuccinate, or DSS) is well known to pharmacists as a stool softener. It is also an ingredient in an EPA-registered flea shampoo and spray containing 2.1% docusate and 0.5% undecylenic acid. At least some of these products are labeled to "control fleas, ticks, and lice on dogs, cats and other nursing animals" (EPA 1995b). The species indicated on the label include dogs, cats, puppies, kittens, and reptiles (EPA 2010). Information on the mechanism of action, safety, and efficacy could not be found, although the EPA registration refers to submission of evidence for efficacy against fleas (EPA 1995a). The product is said to have a rapid knock-down effect but no residual activity.

7.5.5 Emodepside

Emodepside is an octadepsipeptide that binds to presynaptic latrophilin receptors and SLO-potassium channels, causing flaccid paralysis and death of the parasite (Holden-Dye et al. 2012). Emodepside is effective against roundworms and hookworms. It is approved in combination with praziquantel (Profender®) as a systemically absorbed spot-on topical for cats. In target animal safety studies of this product, two of eight cats receiving a 10× dose developed self-limiting hypersalivation, tremors, and lethargy. A 1× oral dose (to mimic accidental ingestion) of emodepside/praziquantel topical solution caused salivation and vomiting with transient decreased food consumption and weight loss (FDA 2007). Topical repeated treatment at 3× the therapeutic dose was tolerated in pregnant and lactating bitches/queens and their offspring, and it is believed safe at the recommended treatment dose in pregnant cats. This information is part of the European approval documentation; however, the label specifically states that use in pregnant cats has not been evaluated for approval in the USA (Epe and Kaminsky 2013).

Mandatory monitoring

Emodepside interfered with fetal development in rats and rabbits and, as such, carries a label warning that the product should not be handled by women who are pregnant or may become pregnant (Bayer HealthCare 2010). Pharmacists should ensure that women of childbearing age receive appropriate counseling before this product is dispensed.

7.5.6 Fipronil

Fipronil is a topical insecticide formulated as either a ready-to-use spray or a concentrated spot-on product for use in dogs and cats. It likely affects GABA-gated and glutamate-gated chloride channels of the insect nervous system. It is effective against fleas, ticks, some mites, and biting lice. It may help control, but will not cure, sarcoptic mange. Most fipronil-containing spot-on products have added IGRs (Frontline Plus® with methoprene and Frontline Gold® with methoprene and pyriproxyfen) to help break the flea life cycle and decrease the development of resistance to fipronil. Fipronil is promoted as being able to prevent the spread of tick-borne diseases because of its rapid cidal effect on some ticks (Jacobson et al. 2004).

Spray products are applied over the major portions of the body, while spot-on products spread from a local application over the body through the oils of the skin. The product label claims resistance to rain, swimming, and routine bathing. As with most spot-on products, veterinarians usually recommend that baths be avoided for two to three days before and after product application. Fipronil is stored in sebaceous glands and hair follicles of the dog or cat, enabling a long duration of action. Although some products claim a 90-day duration against fleas, some resistance has developed, and better flea control is achieved with monthly applications. Fipronil-containing products may cause focal dermatitis after topical administration, but this is rare. Accidental oral ingestion of the veterinary products has caused hypersalivation, gagging, and vomiting, perhaps more as a result of the vehicle than the pesticide. Fipronil is relatively nontoxic to most mammals. The LD_{50} for oral fipronil in rats and mice is 97 and 95 mg/kg, respectively (Wismer and Means 2012). There are no acute toxicity studies in dogs or cats, but an oral subchronic toxicity study in dogs dosed orally at 10 mg/kg per day for 13 weeks showed GI and CNS signs (Australian Authority Pesticides and Veterinary Medicines 2011). In those studies, a NOEL of 0.5 mg/kg per day and a LEL of 2.0 mg/kg per day were reported (EPA 1996). Rabbits seem uniquely sensitive to even topical application of dog products, with CNS signs, including seizures, seen even several days after exposure (Stern et al. 2015).

7.5.7 Insect Growth Regulators

IGRs do not kill adult fleas or other insects. Instead, they interfere with the maturation process, preventing the emergence of adults by inhibiting chitin production, mimicking juvenile hormones in the insect, or disrupting molting. The latter method is used by the compound cyromazine, which specifically targets fly pests of agricultural animals and is not used in small animals.

7.5.7.1 Lufenuron

Lufenuron (Program®) is a chitin biosynthesis inhibitor used in flea control. It has no action on adult fleas but rather is ovicidal and larvicidal, helping to break the flea life cycle. There is insufficient chitin in the cuticle of ticks for the product to be effective against this parasite (Page 2008). The oral tablet for dogs and cats and the oral suspension for cats are both administered once monthly. A repository injectable formulation lasting six months is approved for cats, where the lipophilic formulation is slowly released from fat stores. Combination products with other agents are also marketed. All pets in the household must be concurrently treated with lufenuron for it to be effective. Concomitant use of an agent effective against adult fleas is usually recommended.

Because mammals do not produce chitin, lufenuron has a very high therapeutic index. In acute toxicity studies where dogs and cats received 20× and 10× the label dose, respectively, no adverse events were evident. This was also true for multiple chronic and subchronic toxicity studies (EPA 1994, 1995a).

In the acute toxicity study of the sustained-release injection for cats at 10× the label dose (in divided injection sites), some discomfort at administration sites was reported. Four of six cats developed firm injection site swelling, with evidence of inflammation detected histopathologically (Novartis Animal Health US 1998). There is a concern among veterinarians that repeated injections of inflammation-inducing medications in cats may initiate fibrosarcoma development. This has been most closely linked to certain feline vaccines (see Chapter 20 for additional information on feline injection site sarcomas). Some feline practitioners avoid injecting anything that stimulates inflammation at the injection site, although there is no evidence to either confirm or refute this concern for the injectable form of lufenuron.

7.5.7.2 Methoprene and Pyriproxyfen

In insects, juvenile hormone (JH) refers to a group of hormones that allow growth of the larva while preventing metamorphosis. As long as there is sufficient JH, larva-to-larva molts occur, but with lower concentrations of JH, pupation occurs. A complete absence of JH is necessary for development to the adult stage. Both methoprene and pyriproxyfen mimic JH, preventing the insect from completing its life cycle. Although mainly used in flea control, there is evidence that pyriproxyfen may also impair the reproductive ability of ticks (Estrada-Peña and Rème 2005). Pyriproxyfen is the more stable of the two compounds, as methoprene is susceptible to degradation by UV light. The products can be found in a variety of formulations, including premise sprays and topical products for dogs and cats, often in combination with adulticides active against fleas and ticks. Sometimes, the two IGRs are used in the same product for an additive effect.

Methoprene is considered of low toxic risk in mammals, with an acute oral LD_{50} in the dog of greater than 5000 mg/kg.

7.5.8 Isoquinolines

Praziquantel and epsiprantel, the primary tapeworm treatments for small animals, affect voltage-gated calcium channels, leading to paralysis of the tapeworm. After oral administration, praziquantel is absorbed, enters the bile, and is excreted into the intestine where it affects the tapeworm (Bayer HealthCare 2003). Epsiprantel is poorly absorbed orally, simply remaining in the GI tract (Pfizer Animal Health 2007). These isoquinolines cause both spastic and tetanic muscular contractions and rapid vacuolization of the tegument, exposing tapeworm antigens that stimulate the host's immune system to target the parasite. Tapeworm segments are usually digested prior to fecal passage, such that owners will not see evidence of tapeworms. Praziquantel (Droncit) has the majority of the market and is available as a tablet (also in combination with other antiparasitic drugs) or subcutaneous injection; it is also available as a combination product applied topically for systemic absorption (Profender). Epsiprantel (Cestex®) is available as a tablet.

Praziquantel is effective against all tapeworms of dogs and cats, including *Taenia*, *Dipylidium*, and *Echinococcus*. Some countries require treatment with praziquantel as an import requirement for pets to prevent entry of the *Echinococcus* tapeworm into the country. Extra-label administration of praziquantel at about two to five times the label dose for up to three days has been used to treat some tapeworms (e.g. *Spirometra*) and lung flukes (*Paragonimus*) in small animals. Epsiprantel is also effective against *Taenia* and *Dipylidium*, but it is not approved to treat *Echinococcus* infections, although some data suggest it is effective (Page 2008).

As stand-alone products, both praziquantel and epsiquantel are labeled for use in young puppies and kittens four to seven weeks of age, depending on the product. Food has no effect on oral absorption of either drug. The injectable product may cause transient pain when given subcutaneously, with some injection site swelling reported. Both pioneer drugs have been shown to be safe in pregnant and breeding animals. The products seem exceedingly safe, with daily 5× label dosing of praziquantel for 14 days producing no adverse effects in either dogs or cats. Symptoms of overdose with praziquantel, including vomiting, excessive salivation, and depression, were seen at 33× to 40× doses. Epsiprantel has a similar safety margin. Deaths occurred in five of eight cats treated subcutaneously and in all eight cats injected intramuscularly, but only at doses 20× the label dose for injectable praziquantel (Pfizer Animal Health 2007). Efficacy studies for transdermal praziquantel combination products support its transdermal absorption.

7.5.9 Isoxazoline Ectoparasiticides

A relatively recent addition to the ectoparasiticides is the isoxazoline family. These are potent inhibitors of gamma-aminobutyric acid (GABA)-gated chloride channels (GABACls) and l-glutamate-gated chloride channels (GluCls), leading to membrane hyperpolarization, inhibition of postsynaptic potential, and decreasing neuron firing (Gassel et al. 2014). They are highly selective for insect and arachnid versus mammalian channels (European Medicines Agency Committee 2014).

The isoxazolines approved in the USA for oral use (soft chews and chewable tablets) in dogs include afoxolaner (Nexgard®), fluralaner (Bravecto®), sarolaner (Simparica®), and lotilaner (Credelio®). Fluralaner is also approved as a topical formulation for use in dogs and cats. All products are effective against fleas and typically have good activity against ticks. One important difference between these agents is that the elimination half-life of afoxolaner, sarolaner, and lotilaner allows for once-a-month dosing, while that of fluralaner allows for dosing once every three months.

While research indicates that isoxazolines may have a broad spectrum of activity against insects and arachnids, their utility against many companion animal ectoparasites remains to be determined. One extra-label use of considerable importance is in the treatment of generalized demodectic mange. This is one of the more difficult ectoparasite infestations to cure, perhaps owing to a T-cell deficiency in affected dogs. With few other treatment options available (see the amitraz and macrocyclic lactones sections of this chapter), isoxazolines are an appealing alternative. All have shown efficacy in extra-label studies against demodicosis (Fourie

et al. 2015; Beugnet et al. 2016a; Six et al. 2016; Snyder et al. 2017). Afoxolaner, fluralaner, and sarolaner also have supporting studies for extra-label use against sarcoptic mange and *Otodectes* (ear) mites (Becskei et al. 2016; Beugnet et al. 2016b; Carithers et al. 2016; Taenzler et al. 2016, 2017). It is likely that lotilaner may likewise be effective, but so far confirmatory studies are lacking.

There are a few differences in the four drugs (formulations and dosing frequency have already been described). Fluralaner and lotilaner should be administered with food, whereas food is optional with the other two products. Afoxolaner and lotilaner are labeled for use in puppies beginning at two months of age, whereas the other two products restrict use to dogs six months of age or older.

Mandatory monitoring

The risk of seizures was a concern in the approval studies for afoxolaner, fluralaner, sarolaner, and lotilaner. For afoxolaner, two dogs with a history of seizures that were in the clinical trial experienced seizures after dosing, with one having another seizure after the second dosing (FDA 2013).

For sarolaner, CNS signs, sometimes with seizures, were observed in puppies at 3× and 5× overdoses given over a 10-month period. CNS signs were not seen in dogs older than 6 months of age (FDA 2016b). Seizures and CNS signs were seen in a small number of animals included in target animal safety or field studies for oral and topical flurolaner (FDA 2014, 2016a). For lotilaner, in one field study, a dog with a history of seizures experienced seizure activity six days after receiving the drug but recovered without treatment and completed the study (FDA 2018). These products should be used cautiously in animals prone to seizures. Pharmacists should counsel pet owners to monitor their animal closely for signs of seizure activity and report such activity to their veterinarian before administering another dose.

Among the isoxazolines, fluralaner is the only drug that was tested in pregnant dogs. A teratogenic effect was seen when three or four doses were administered at eight-week intervals at a 3× label dose. Limb deformities, enlarged heart, enlarged spleen, and cleft palate were observed in puppies. The teratogenic risk at the label dose is unknown. Based on similar mechanisms of action, use of these compounds during pregnancy is best avoided.

Other than the CNS effects just described, fluralaner topical was well tolerated at 1×, 3×, and 5× in dogs. Three applications in kittens 78–91 days of age resulted in an increased incidence of renal tubular degeneration/regeneration in the 3× and 5× dosing, although the clinical significance of this was undetermined. Oral dosing of the topical product at the label dose to mimic accidental ingestion showed short-term salivation, coughing, and mild GI signs (FDA 2016a). As with all newly released products, less common adverse reactions may yet occur, but based on available evidence, all four drugs seem otherwise generally well tolerated at label doses, except as stated in this chapter.

7.5.10   Levamisole

Levamisole is the active L-form of racemic tetramisole and acts as a nicotinic agonist. It was once a widely used anthelmintic in cattle, where it still is occasionally utilized. It is no longer used in small animals due to its narrow therapeutic index and the emergence of newer and better products. It has received some interest as an immune stimulant, although it has never been widely employed for this purpose.

If toxic exposure occurs, the signs seem related to cholinergic stimulation, perhaps due to its structural similarity to nicotine. In one case report of toxicity in a dog, the adverse signs included bradycardia, panting, ataxia, stupor, diarrhea, and miosis. Treatment included atropine or glycopyrrolate to control the bradycardia and general

supportive measures. The dog recovered after approximately three days of hospitalization (Montgomery and Pidgeon 1986).

7.5.11   Lime Sulfur

Lime sulfur topical solution (sulfurated lime solution) is one of the oldest ectoparasiticides still in use. It contains calcium polysulfides formed by reacting calcium hydroxide with sulfur. Often sold as a concentrate, it should be diluted to a 2–3% solution before being used as a dip/sponge-on. Its main use is in the control of sarcoptic mange or dermatophytosis, although it has been recommended for a variety of other ectoparasites, including *D. cati*, *Cheyletiella*, and lice. Lime sulfur has also been used for nonspecific dermatitis due to its antibacterial, keratolytic, and supposed antipruritic properties.

Lime sulfur solutions are especially useful in young puppies and kittens because of its wide safety margin when used properly. Contact with eyes should be avoided, but if this occurs, the eyes should be rinsed gently but thoroughly. Oral ingestion can sometimes cause stomatitis or mouth ulcers, especially in cats. Elizabethan collars may need to be applied while the fur is still wet to prevent cats from licking the solution. Skin irritation may also occur. The main drawback of lime sulfur for both owners and veterinarians is the "rotten egg" odor. It will also stain furniture, clothing, and jewelry if contact is made while the animal is still wet.

Although the diluted product is considered extremely safe, lime sulfur is typically sold as a concentrated solution intended for dilution. The concentrate is very caustic with a pH of 11.5. Accidental use of the undiluted product on an animal can be fatal, especially if ingestion occurs where lime sulfur combined with gastric acid produces hydrogen sulfide. Animals exposed to the undiluted concentrate should have their eyes and skin thoroughly rinsed and treated for caustic burns as warranted. If the concentrate is ingested, vomiting should *not* be instituted, but rather egg white or cream (or milk if nothing else is available) should be administered. Treatment for hydrogen sulfide poisoning along with supportive care is warranted (Davis 2008).

7.5.12 Limonene

Limonene (D-limonene) is an essential oil terpene derived from citrus fruit peels. It is sometimes sought by owners wanting a "natural" flea control product. Efficacy is not well documented, but it is touted as being effective against fleas, ticks, and lice. The potential mechanism of limonene as an ectoparasiticide is not defined. Although it has been suggested that it disrupts the outer covering of the insect, leading to desiccation, this has not been established. It may act as a neurotoxin to the arthropod, as supported by a synergy with piperonyl butoxide. Limonene is an ingredient in various pet sprays, shampoos, and dips/sponge-ons. It has a relatively rapid knock-down but little residual activity.

In most mammals, including the dog, limonene is considered nontoxic with very high LD$_{50}$s. Cats, however, appear more sensitive, and systemic toxicity has been reported. At the approved concentration, cats usually do well, although there are reports of transient hypersalivation, ataxia, and dermatitis (Texas A&M AgriLife Extension n.d.). More commonly, toxicity is seen when the concentrate is mixed incorrectly. It may be a skin irritant at high concentrations. In one study, using 5× the recommended concentration, cats showed mild hypersalivation, ataxia, and muscle tremors. At 15× the recommended concentration, clinical signs included hypersalivation for 15 to 30 minutes, moderate to severe ataxia lasting one to five hours, muscle tremors lasting one to four hours, and severe hypothermia lasting five hours. All animals recovered, even at the highest dose rate (Hooser et al. 1986). A rare but serious immune-mediated dermatopathy has been reported (Rosenbaum and Kerlin 1995; Lee et al. 2002).

7.5.13 Macrocyclic Lactones

The macrocyclic lactone family, originally developed for agricultural animal use, includes two major groups, the avermectins and milbemycins. From a clinical perspective, there are no important differences between the groups, with both having broad-spectrum activity against nematodes and many ectoparasites. The are not effective however against tapeworms or flukes.

Macrocyclic lactones bind to glutamate receptors and cause an influx of chloride ion, resulting in hyperpolarization of neurons and paralysis and death of the parasite. These channels play fundamental roles in the systemic nervous system of nematodes and insects. Selective toxicity to parasites is a function of the inability of macrocyclic lactones to gain access to mammalian glutamate receptors, which are located exclusively within the CNS. Macrocyclic lactones are substrates for P-glycoprotein, a key component of the mammalian blood–brain barrier. The P-glycoprotein efflux pump removes macrocyclic lactones faster than they diffuse into the brain. Accidental overdoses can occur if dogs ingest highly potent large-animal macrocyclic lactone dewormers, overwhelming this removal mechanism and allowing access to the CNS. Clinical signs of macrocyclic lactone toxicity include transient blindness, seizures, and other CNS effects, including respiratory paralysis and death. Intravenous lipid therapy is indicated in such cases to hasten recovery.

Macrocyclic lactones have a high margin of safety in man and are used globally to treat and prevent many human parasites. In fact, it is predicted that over 200 million people will be treated annually with macrocyclic lactones in an effort to eradicate devastating parasitic diseases. This is a testament to the safety of macrocyclic lactones in humans. In the treatment of "river blindness" (onchocerciasis), human patients may however experience reactions to the dying parasites.

Dramatic difference

Pharmacogenetics plays a key role in the safety profile of macrocyclic lactones in both dogs and cats. A fraction of dogs and cats have a mutation in the ABCB1 (MDR1) gene that results in defective P-glycoprotein function (Chapters 4 and 5 provide more detailed information).

There is a breed predilection for the defect in dogs, with Collies and Australian Shepherds being particularly overrepresented, although other breeds are also affected (see Table 7.4). Although heartworm preventive doses are safe even for animals with defective P-glycoprotein function, toxicity becomes an issue when extra-label doses are used (e.g. for the treatment of mange) or in overdose situations. Macrocyclic lactone toxicity in these individuals is less responsive to intravenous lipid rescue therapy. Pharmacogenetic testing

Table 7.4 Approximate frequency of the ABCB1-1Δ (MDR1) gene defect in dogs.

Breed	Approximate percentage
Australian Shepherd	50%
Australian Shepherd, Mini	50%
Border Collie	<5%
Chinook	25%
Collie	70%
English Shepherd	15%
German Shepherd	10%
Herding Breed Cross	10%
Long-Haired Whippet	50%
McNab	30%
Mixed Breed	5%
Old English Sheepdog	5%
Shetland Sheepdog	15%
Silken Windhound	30%

"Mealey KL. Breeds affected by the MDR1 mutation. 2017:1." http://vcpl.vetmed.wsu.edu/affected-breeds. Accessed November 28, 2017

is readily available for dogs and cats (Appendix F). There are no known genetic mutations that predispose to macrocyclic lactone sensitivity in humans, horses, or ruminants.

Toxicity to these agents can also occur if an animal is concomitantly receiving a P-glycoprotein pump inhibitor, regardless of whether it has the gene defect. In veterinary medicine, this has been documented with the flea control product spinosad (Comfortis®), ketoconazole, and cyclosporine.

As a family, the macrocyclic lactones are used as heartworm preventatives but also treat hookworms, roundworms, most mites, and lice. Many of these indications beyond heartworm prevention are, however, extra-label, and the dosages required to achieve efficacy against the different parasites vary.

Selamectin differs from other macrocyclic lactones, as it also has activity against fleas. It is a poor choice for ticks, although it carries a label claim against one tick species. Selamectin is approved for use in cats to treat roundworm and hookworm infections. In dogs, it treats roundworms (extra-label) but is rather ineffective against hookworms and whipworms.

In addition to activity against adult parasites, the macrocyclic lactone family is unique in that it has activity against many immature larval nematodes during the tissue migration portion of their life cycle. Macrocyclic lactones are given to dogs and cats mainly for heartworm prevention. Indeed, all currently marketed heartworm preventatives in the USA are in this family. Most products also carry additional indications beyond heartworm prevention.

Ivermectin was the first macrocyclic lactone dewormer marketed for horses and cattle. It is FDA approved as a small animal heartworm preventative product requiring an exceedingly low dose (6 micrograms per kg) orally once monthly. This dose of ivermectin is safe in all breeds of dogs, including the ivermectin-sensitive breeds. However, this low dose is not effective against other nematodes, so it is also marketed in combination with pyrantel pamoate. It is approved in cats at 24 micrograms/kg orally once monthly, a dosage also labeled for control of adult and immature feline hookworms.

Historically, diethylcarbamazine was used daily as a heartworm preventative. This drug is no longer marketed in the USA and has long since been replaced by members of the macrocyclic lactone family that work by killing the immature tissue-migrating larvae. This includes the L3 stage deposited by the mosquito and the subsequent L4 larval stage. This ability to kill immature migrating nematodes, although not totally unique, is an uncommon attribute among anthelmintics.

The macrocyclic lactones approved in the USA for heartworm prevention include ivermectin (Heartgard®; oral), milbemycin (Interceptor®; oral), selamectin (Revolution®; transdermal topical), and moxidectin (Proheart®; sustained-release injectable and transdermal topical). Although the dose of macrocyclic lactones required to prevent heartworm disease is amazingly low, the manufacturers have opted for higher doses in some products to include label claims for other parasites. The macrocyclic lactones are typically highly effective as heartworm preventatives; however, heartworm resistance has been detected in the Mississippi Delta area. It is believed these resistant strains have mutations of the parasite's P-glycoprotein ortholog, thereby providing more efficient removal of the macrocyclic lactones. Some disease models using laboratory strains of the resistant strain, MP3, suggest moxidectin may be effective as a preventative due to its longer duration in the animal, but this remains unproven clinically (Blagburn et al. 2016). Milbemycin activity against the MP3 strain has shown contradictory results in two studies, one where three consecutive months of treatment were quite effective and another where it failed to prevent development of all adults (Snyder et al. 2011; Blagburn et al. 2016). There is a suggestion that the number of L3 larvae used in the challenge tests play a role, implying large exposures may overwhelm protection.

Ivermectin is approved in humans for systemic use to treat strongyloidiasis and onchocerciasis (river blindness). It has also been used in humans to treat lymphatic filariasis (elephantiasis). Oral ivermectin is also used extra-label in humans for *Sarcoptes*. Its topical use is approved in humans for head lice and for inflammatory lesions of rosacea, with the mechanism of action in the latter disease unknown.

7.5.14 Neonicotinoids

The neonicotinoids act by displacing acetylcholine from its nicotinic receptor. Their selective toxicity to insects is due to a higher affinity for insect receptors versus mammalian receptors. They are effective against fleas and lice, but lack activity against ticks and mites. Five neonicotinoid insecticides are used in small animals: nitenpyram (Capstar®; oral), spinosad (Comfortis®; oral), dinotefuran (Vectra®; topical spot-on), imidacloprid (Advantage®; topical spot-on), and spinetoram (a derivative of spinosad and considered its toxicological equivalent, it was recently released as a topical spot-on product for cats, Cheristin for Cats™).

7.5.14.1 Nitenpyram

Nitenpyram (Capstar®) is an oral tablet approved for use in dogs and cats for flea control. It has a rapid onset at around 30 minutes and is >98% effective at four hours, providing a quick knock-down of adult fleas on the animal. It has a short half-life with no residual activity. As such, it is primarily used by veterinarians to rid animals of fleas prior to boarding or hospitalization. The drug seems quite safe, with target animal safety studies showing no adverse effects at 3× the label dose in four-week-old puppies or at 10× the label dose in seven-month-old dogs and cats.

7.5.14.2 Spinosad

Spinosad (Comfortis®) is also an oral tablet approved for use in dogs and cats for flea control. It has a rapid onset like nitenpyram but a long duration, with 96% efficacy at 30 days. Food enhances absorption, and it is recommended that the drug be administered with a meal.

In a target animal safety study, for six dogs receiving 10× the label dose for 10 days, the drug caused few adverse events beyond vomiting. The label for the dog oral product warns against use in dogs with epilepsy. This is perhaps based on a clinical trial where two dogs with a history of seizure activity had at least one seizure within a week of dosing. Four dogs with preexisting seizure conditions did not experience any seizure activity during the study. How much of a risk the drug poses in lowering the seizure threshold is unknown, but some veterinarians prefer to avoid spinosad in epileptic patients.

Spinosad is a potent inhibitor of P-glycoprotein. As such, dogs treated with the drug will be predisposed to the same adverse drug events as dogs with the ABCB1-1Δ (MDR1) gene defect seen in the "ivermectin-sensitive breeds." Because the P-glycoprotein pump is an important part of the blood–brain barrier, toxic signs are predominantly CNS-related; see the "Macrocyclic Lactones" section. The dose of ivermectin in heartworm preventative products is safe to use with spinosad, as are all other FDA-approved heartworm preventative products if administered at the label dose.

It is unknown at this time whether the closely related drug spinetoram is also a P-glycoprotein inhibitor. Based on its similar structure to spinosad, caution is advised until more information is available.

7.5.14.3 Imidacloprid and Dinotefuran

Imidacloprid (Advantage) and dinotefuran (Vectra) are both topical spot-on products. They are known for their rapid onset of flea kill, and each lasts approximately one month after application. Since they are not appreciably absorbed transdermally, they are quite safe aside from occasional local skin reactions. Both insecticides exist as formulations with other drugs that enhance their spectrum.

Dramatic difference

The combination formulations with neonicotinoids in dogs often include permethrin to provide tick control. The concentrated permethrin in these products, while quite safe for dogs, is extremely toxic to cats. Use of flea and tick preventives that are not FDA approved for cats is contraindicated.

7.5.15 Organophosphates and Carbamates

Organophosphate (OP) and carbamate compounds have been used in animals for control of both helminths and ectoparasites. As acetylcholinesterase inhibitors, they cause acetylcholine to accumulate at muscarinic and nicotinic receptors, thereby overstimulating the nervous system.

Organophosphates and carbamates were once the primary ingredient in ectoparasite products for both large and small animals. One of the more ubiquitous products was carbaryl (Sevin®). At one time, it was common in shampoos and flea collars. As of 2009, registration for use of carbaryl products on animals was canceled by the EPA. The powder may still be encountered in an extra-label manner, applied either directly to the animal or to its environment. Resistance in fleas is, however, extremely common. Cythioate (Proban®) tablet and fenthion transdermal (Pro-Spot®) are approved OPs for systemic absorption that kill fleas after feeding. Other products intended for external application to kill fleas, ticks, and lice by contact are numerous and include diazinon, coumaphos, malathion, and phosmet.

The use of organophosphates and carbamates in pets is highly discouraged, and few products are still available in the USA because safer and more effective products now exist. Exposure of dogs and cats to organophosphates and carbamates is therefore likely to be accidental or malicious. Greyhounds and whippets may be more sensitive to acetylcholinesterase inhibitor poisoning than other dog breeds, and cats are more sensitive than dogs. Toxic signs are associated with overstimulation of the parasympathetic nervous system resulting in excess salivation, lacrimation, urination, and defecation (SLUD), often with muscle tremors from stimulation of the nicotinic receptors at the neuromuscular junction.

Decontamination after toxic exposure is the same as for any poisoning (see Chapter 6). The oxime pralidoxime (2-PAM) will reverse the acetylcholinesterase inhibition of an

OP but not a carbamate. Atropine may be administered to reverse the muscarinic signs (SLUD, bradycardia, and respiratory distress). Diphenhydramine is surprisingly effective as a mild nicotinic antagonist at decreasing the severity of the muscle tremors.

7.5.16 Piperazine

Piperazine is a heterocyclic compound that is one of the oldest anthelmintics still marketed. It has been used in all major species, including pets. While extremely safe, its activity is limited to roundworms. Because of this limited spectrum, it is no longer used by veterinarians. Products containing piperazine are still available OTC in retail stores, often labeled as "puppy dewormer." While likely effective against the roundworms of puppies, the pharmacist should realize the product has no activity against hookworms, a more serious and common parasite of puppies and kittens. Owners may make a false assumption when using the piperazine product that they are providing the necessary deworming of their puppy or kitten, only to have it subsequently die from hookworm anemia. Pharmacists can play a key role in appropriate education of pet owners about the spectrum of piperazine.

7.5.17 Pyrethrins and Synthetic Pyrethroids

Both natural pyrethrins and synthetic pyrethroids are used extensively as topical products for ectoparasites in dogs and cats. They work by disrupting sodium ion transport, thereby poisoning neurotransmission. They are very effectively hydrolyzed to inert products by mammalian liver enzymes (Roberts and Reigart 2013).

Natural pyrethrins are extracts from the chrysanthemum flower and are nearly always combined with piperonyl butoxide, a synergist that inhibits the insect's detoxification enzymes. Natural pyrethrins are known for their rapid cidal activity ("quick knockdown") of most insects and acarides. The compounds have little residual effect. They are found primarily in premise sprays and topical animal sprays, shampoos, and dips/sponge-ons where a rapid kill is desired.

The synthetic pyrethroids were developed to provide a more persistent action and enhanced potency. These have been divided by some authors into "generations," with first generations largely being synthetic versions of natural pyrethrins, through fifth-generation pyrethroids with the greatest duration and potency. (The newer generations do, however, have a slower kill by comparison to the natural pyrethrins.) Other classification schemes are based on the presence of a cyano group on the molecule, which causes a longer duration of the sodium current in the axon and slightly different toxicity signs in mammals, as noted further in this chapter. Common type I pyrethroids include permethrin and resmethrin, while common type II products include cypermethrin, deltamethrin, fenvalerate, flumethrin, and tetramethrin. Etofenprox is unique structurally and is classified as a pseudopyrethroid that is claimed to be less toxic to environmental aquatic organisms and mammals while maintaining good activity against insects.

There are a number of different products marketed, especially as premise sprays and to a lesser degree in shampoos. For spot-on animal use, permethrin is most commonly used, but other compounds such as deltamethrin and flumethrin are incorporated into pet collars for a sustained release. Although pyrethroids have activity against fleas and lice, they are more commonly added to other products to provide activity against ticks. They are one of the few effective insect and tick repellents for dogs.

Natural pyrethrins are very safe and can be used in all mammal species. The risk of synthetic pyrethroids is much harder to assess, as there is a surprising paucity of acute toxicity data in dogs and cats. This may be because the EPA requires limited acute toxicity trial data in the target species for pesticide approval. It is important for pharmacists to know that cats are at much greater risk of toxicity than dogs to the synthetic pyrethrins. Cats are well known for their limited amount of glucuronyl transferase (Chapter 4) that subsequently limits their ability to detoxify many compounds into glucuronide conjugates. This may be an underlying reason for their sensitivity to synthetic pyrethrins. This is not universal as some products such as the Seresto™ collar containing sustained-released flumethrin (and imidacloprid) are approved for use on cats.

> **Dramatic difference**
>
> Permethrin products administered to cats are one of the top 10 most common toxicities reported by the ASPCA Animal Poison Control Hotline. This usually occurs when an owner mistakenly treats their cat with a concentrated permethrin spot-on product intended for dogs. Second-hand toxicity can occur when cats interact with dogs recently treated with these products.

Cats begin to experience clinical signs about 2 hours post exposure, although this may be delayed for up to 10 hours. The signs include tremors/muscle fasciculations (86%), twitches (41%), hyperesthesia (41%), hyperthermia (29%), seizures (33%), and a variety of other CNS signs, including temporary blindness (12%). Permethrin poisoning in cats is a medical emergency that should be treated by a veterinarian; however, it may be helpful for owners to decontaminate the skin of the cat by bathing with a dish soap (e.g. Dawn®, not dishwasher detergent) prior to taking their cat to the veterinarian for oral exposure decontamination and treatment (see Chapter 6 for more information about decontamination procedures). Reported mortality rates have ranged from 2% to 37% (Boland and Angles 2010).

At high doses, other species can obviously experience toxicity. Type I pyrethroids will cause similar signs as permethrin. Type II pyrethroids cause depolarizing conduction blocks, with weakness and paralysis being common. Again, decontamination and supportive therapy are used in managing these toxicities. Paresthesias are common in humans following dermal application of pyrethroids. Since animals cannot describe this sensation, it is presumed that ear twitching, paw flicking, and/or tail flicking are clinical signs caused by the animal experiencing paresthesia (Wismer and Means 2012).

7.5.18 Rotenone

Rotenone is extracted from the roots of several South American plants, the most common of which is cube root. It has been used by indigenous peoples for centuries to harvest fish by mixing the pulverized root into the water, after which the fish would float to the top for harvest. When ingested, rotenone undergoes such a high first-pass detoxification that the fish are safe for human consumption. As a piscicide, it is still used in fish management to reclaim lakes for game fishing.

Rotenone is a potent inhibitor of the NADH dehydrogenase system interfering with electron transport. It may be the active ingredient in products to treat ear mites and in topical Goodwinol ointment for treating local demodectic mange. However, the efficacy of the latter is questionable given the recalcitrant nature of demodectic mange. It is sometimes combined with piperonyl butoxide as a synergist or with other insecticides.

In crop agriculture, inhalation of rotenone powder has resulted in poisoning. Due to the limited use of diluted topical solutions and ointments and a strong first-pass detoxification, the risk to pets from rotenone parasiticides is considered low. It is worth mentioning that Goodwinol ointment also contains benzocaine, which can cause methemoglobinemia when ingested, such as through grooming behavior of cats.

7.5.19 Tetrahydropyrimidines (Pyrantel)

Pyrantel is a nicotinic agonist causing depolarizing neuromuscular blockade, and subsequent tonic paralysis and death of the parasite. It is effectively used against roundworms and hookworms as an FDA-approved product for dogs, and it is frequently used in an extra-label manner in cats. It is not consistently effective against whipworms, *Strongyloides*, tapeworms, or flukes.

Pyrantel is available as oral suspensions of either a pamoate (embonate) or a tartrate salt. The pamoate salt is poorly absorbed from the GI tract, providing a very safe product for use in young or debilitated animals. The oral LD_{50} in dogs is reported to be >2000 mg/kg (European Agency for the Evaluation of Medicinal Products Committee 1998). Its activity is primarily limited to the GI tract, which may explain its limited benefit against parasites in other parts of the body. The tartrate salt, FDA approved for use in horses, has greater oral bioavailability and hence has a greater risk of toxicity. As such, it is not recommended for use in small animals. Pyrantel pamoate suspension is often the preferred anthelmintic in many veterinary practices for routine treatment of roundworm and hookworm infections, particularly in puppies and kittens (e.g. Nemex®). It is often combined with other parasiticides for products with broad-spectrum label claims. The products that contain pyrantel as a sole ingredient are used in an extra-label manner in cats; however, some combination products containing the drug are FDA approved in this species.

7.6 Unique Aspect of Parasiticide Dosing

Baths and dips were once the standard "administration" methods used for external parasite treatment. The term "dip" is still used in describing many topical treatments, although it really infers pouring the solution over the animal so that it soaks the hair over the entire body. More correctly, these are now referred to as "sponge-ons." In large part, however, dips have been supplemented and often replaced by topical "spot-on" products.

These concentrated formulations, such as fipronil and imidacloprid, are applied to one spot on the skin of the animal, often between the shoulder blades, and rapidly spread over the entire skin through the normal sebaceous secretions and movement of the pet. There may nevertheless be distal areas of the body with less coverage that are more prone to infestation (e.g. between the toes). Most of these products move into the sebaceous glands of the skin, where the oils serve as a drug reservoir providing longer duration of activity. Bathing a few days before or after application may limit their effectiveness by stripping oils from the skin. This is a key client education message that pharmacists should include when counseling pet owners. Other spot-on products such as selamectin are designed to be absorbed transdermally to affect the flea (and other susceptible parasites) when they feed on the pet.

Several oral products such as nitenpyram, spinosad, sarolaner, fluralaner, and afoxolaner affect external parasites as they feed. They have become very popular due to their efficacy, long duration, and dosing convenience.

Table 7.2 lists dosing information for most commercially available products. The pharmacist may, however, find antiparasitics dosing expressed differently than for other classes of drugs. This is because of peculiarities unique to the marketing of parasiticides in veterinary medicine. Most of the EPA-approved ectoparasiticide products are intended for owner administration and are not dosed on a standard mg/kg of body weight basis. Instead, they are typically dosed with a volume of a stated concentration to be applied based on the weight of the animal within a specified, but fairly broad, range. For example, Advantage II® is sold in different-sized vials for dogs of four weight ranges (<10, 11–20, 21–55, and >55 lbs.) and for cats of three weight ranges (<5, 5–9, and >9 lbs.). The acronym "WBSO" used in Table 7.2 corresponds to "weight-based spot-on" topical formulation. This is to alert the pharmacist that different products exist for that species based on their weight, and it also indicates that the method of application is to be topical "spot-on."

In contrast to EPA-regulated pesticides, FDA-approved antiparasitic products typically require a dose given in mg/kg of body weight as part of the approval process. For formulations in Table 7.2 that contain only one drug, a dose in mg per kg of body weight is indicated. Many products, however, contain multiple drugs, again complicating the usual process of stating a single dose. The acronym "WBO" corresponds to "weight-based oral," alerting the pharmacist that again different products exist based on body weight

and that they are intended for oral administration, typically as flavored chews or tablets.

Many parasiticides are intended for one-time use to cure an infection and therefore have no dosing interval per se. The pharmacist should refer to the sections of this chapter regarding each parasite for information on the need for repeat treatments. For the drugs that are intended to provide continuous control of a parasite, the recommended interval for that product is stated in Table 7.2 (e.g. monthly).

References

Australian Authority Pesticides and Veterinary Medicines. (2011). Safety of fipronil in dogs and cats: a review of literature. https://apvma.gov.au/sites/default/files/publication/15191-fipronil-prf-vol2-animal-safety-literature_0.pdf.

Baker, N.F. and Farver, T.B. (1983). Failure of brewer's yeast as a repellent to fleas on dogs. *J. Am. Vet. Med. Assoc.* 183 (2): 212–214.

Banfield Pet Hospital. (2017). State of pet health report. https://www.banfield.com/state-of-pet-health.

Bayer HealthCare LLC Animal Health Division (2003). *Droncit® injectable for dogs and cats label*, 1–4. Shawnee Mission, KS: Bayer HealthCare.

Bayer HealthCare LLC Animal Health Division (2010). *Profender FDA label*. Shawnee Mission, KS: Bayer HealthCare.

Becskei, C., De Bock, F., Illambas, J. et al. (2016). Efficacy and safety of a novel oral isoxazoline, sarolaner (SimparicaTM), for the treatment of sarcoptic mange in dogs. *Vet. Parasitol.* 222: 56–61.

Beugnet, F., Halos, L., Larsen, D. et al. (2016a). Efficacy of oral afoxolaner for the treatment of canine generalised demodicosis. *Parasite* 23: 14.

Beugnet, F., de Vos, C., Liebenberg, J. et al. (2016b). Efficacy of afoxolaner in a clinical field study in dogs naturally infested with *Sarcoptes scabiei. Parasite* 23: 26.

Blagburn, B.L., Dillon, A.R., Arther, R.G. et al. (2016). Comparative efficacy of four commercially available heartworm preventive

products against the MP3 laboratory strain of *Dirofilaria immitis. Parasit. Vectors* 9 (1): 191–197.

Boland, L.A. and Angles, J.M. (2010). Feline permethrin toxicity: retrospective study of 42 cases. *J. Feline Med. Surg.* 12 (2): 61–71.

Burke, T.M. (1983). Fenbendazole treatment of pregnant bitches to reduce prenatal and lactogenic infections of *Toxocara canis* and *Ancylostoma caninum* in pups. *J. Am. Vet. Med. Assoc.* 9: 987–990.

Carithers, D., Crawford, J., De Vos, C. et al. (2016). Assessment of afoxolaner efficacy against *Otodectes cynotis* infestations of dogs. *Parasites and Vectors* 9 (1): 1–5.

Centers for Disease Control and Prevention (CDC). (2012). Dirofilariasis FAQs, pp. 1–5. http://www.cdc.gov/parasites/dirofilariasis/faqs.html.

Companion Animal Parasite Council. (2017). Fleas: CAPC guidelines, pp. 6–9. https://www.capcvet.org/guidelines/fleas.

Dorman, D. (1990). Diethyltoluamide (DEET) insect repellent toxicosis. *Vet. Clin N. Am Sm. Anim. Pract.* 20 (2): 387–391.

Environmental Protection Agency (EPA). (1995a). De Flea Shampoo: EPA efficacy review, p. 1. https://www3.epa.gov/pesticides/chem_search/cleared_reviews/csr_PC-079027_21-Jul-95_001b.pdf.

Environmental Protection Agency (EPA) (1995b). Safe and Sure Products: approval of a pesticide product registration. *Fed. Regist.* 60 (177): 47575.

Environmental Protection Agency (EPA). (1996). Fipronil new pesticide fact sheet. https://nepis.epa.gov/Exe/ZyPURL. cgi?Dockey=P1001KCY.txt.

Environmental Protection Agency (EPA). (2010). De Flea Pet Shampoo (EPA Reg. No. 45729, EPA Label Notif. Pestic. Regist. Not. 98–10), pp. 1–6. https:// www3.epa.gov/pesticides/chem_search/ ppls/045729-00004-20100511.pdf.

Epe, C. and Kaminsky, R. (2013). New advancement in anthelmintic drugs in veterinary medicine. *Trends Parasitol.* 29 (3): 129–134. doi:10.1016/j.pt.2013.01.001.

Estrada-Peña, A. and Rème, C. (2005). Efficacy of a collar impregnated with amitraz and pyriproxyfen for prevention of experimental tick infestations by *Rhipicephalus sanguineus, Ixodes ricinus*, and *Ixodes scapularis* in dogs. *J. Am. Vet. Med. Assoc.* 226 (2): 221–224.

European Agency for the Evaluation of Medicinal Products Committee for Veterinary Medicinal Products. (1998). Summary report for pyrantel embonate. http://www.ema.europa.eu/docs/ en_GB/document_library/Maximum_Residue_ Limits_-_Report/2009/11/WC500015797.pdf.

European Medicines Agency Committee for Medicinal Products for Veterinary Use (2014). *CVMP assessment report for NexGard.* London: European Medicines Agency Committee http://www.ema.europa.eu.

Folz, S.D., Kakuk, T.J., and Henke, C.L.D. (1984). Clinical evaluation of Amitraz as a treatment for canine demodicosis. *Vet. Parasitol.* 16: 335–341.

Food and Drug Administration (FDA). (1991). Freedom of information summary: RINTAL TABLETS, pp. 1–15. https:// animaldrugsatfda.fda.gov/adafda/app/ search/public/document/downloadFoi/526.

Food and Drug Administration (FDA). (1994). Freedom of information summary; PROGRAM TABLETS IN DOGS, pp. 1–38. https://animaldrugsatfda.fda.gov/adafda/ app/search/public/document/ downloadFoi/567.

Food and Drug Administration (FDA). (1995). Freedom of information summary: PROGRAM SUSPENSION IN CATS, pp. 1–32. https://animaldrugsatfda.fda.gov/

adafda/app/search/public/document/ downloadFoi/561.

Food and Drug Administration (FDA). (2001). Freedom of information summary: PROHEART-6 IN DOGS, pp. 1–21.

Food and Drug Administration (FDA). (2007). Freedom of information summary: PROFENDER topical solution. https:// animaldrugsatfda.fda.gov/adafda/app/ search/public/document/downloadFoi/834.

Food and Drug Administration (FDA). (2013). Freedom of Information Summary NEXGARD TABLET IN DOGS, pp. 1–22.

Food and Drug Administration (FDA) (2014). *FDA-Label. Bravecto Flavored Chews for Dogs*, 1. Washington, DC: FDA.

Food and Drug Administration (FDA) (2016a). *Freedom of Information Summary BRAVECTO TOPICAL SOLUTION DOGS AND CATS*, 1–66. Washington, DC: FDA.

Food and Drug Administration (FDA) (2016b). *Freedom of Information Summary SIMPARICA TABLETS IN DOGS*, 1–42. Washington, DC: FDA.

Food and Drug Administration (FDA). (2018). Freedom of information summary: CredelioTM chewable tablets for dogs, pp. 1–44. https://animaldrugsatfda.fda.gov/ adafda/app/search/public/document/ downloadFoi/3101.

Fourie, J.J., Liebenberg, J.E., Horak, I.G. et al. (2015). Efficacy of orally administered fluralaner (BravectoTM) or topically applied imidacloprid/moxidectin (Advocate®) against generalized demodicosis in dogs. *Parasit. Vectors* 8 (1): 1–7.

Gassel, M., Wolf, C., Noack, S. et al. (2014). The novel isoxazoline ectoparasiticide fluralaner: selective inhibition of arthropod gamma-aminobutyric acid- and l-glutamate-gated chloride channels and insecticidal/ acaricidal activity. *Insect Biochem. Mol. Biol.* 45 (1): 111–124.

Holden-Dye, L., Crisford, A., Welz, C. et al. (2012). Worms take to the slo lane: a perspective on the mode of action of emodepside. *Invertebr. Neurosci.* 12 (1): 29–36.

Hooser, S.B., Beasley, V.R., and Everitt, J.I. (1986). Effects of an insecticidal dip containing d-limonene in the cat. *J. Am. Vet. Med. Assoc.* 189 (8): 905–908.

Jacobson, R., McCall, J., Hunter, J. et al. (2004). The ability of fipronil to prevent transmission of *Borrelia burgdorferi*, the causative agent of Lyme disease to dogs. *J. Appl. Res. Vet. Med.* 2 (1): 39–45.

Jones, S., Graham, W., von Simson, C. et al. (2014). Current feline guidelines for the prevention, diagnosis, and management of heartworm (*Dirofilaria immitis*) infection in cats. *Am. Heart Soc.* 1–20.

Jung, S. and Dillon, R. (2016). Feline heartworm disease. In: *August's Consultations in Feline Internal Medicine*, vol. 7 (ed. S.E. Little), 433–438. Philadelphia: Saunders.

Lee, J.A., Budgin, J.B., and Mauldin, E.A. (2002). Acute necrotizing dermatitis and septicemia after application of a d-limonene-based insecticidal shampoo in a cat. *J. Am. Vet. Med. Assoc.* 221 (2): 258–262.

McCall, J.W. (2005). The safety-net story about macrocyclic lactone heartworm preventives: a review, an update, and recommendations. *Vet. Parasitol.* 133 (2–3): 197–206. doi:10.1016/j.vetpar.2005.04.005.

Mealey, K.L. Breeds affected by the MDR1 mutation. 2017:1. http://vcpl.vetmed.wsu.edu/affected-breeds. Accessed November 28, 2017.

Medleau, L. and Willemse, T. (1995). Efficacy of daily amitraz therapy for refractory, generalized demodicosis in dogs: two independent studies. *J. Am. Anim. Hosp. Assoc.* 31 (3): 246–249.

Montgomery, R.D. and Pidgeon, G.L. (1986). Levamisole toxicosis in a dog. *J. Am. Vet. Med. Assoc.* 189 (6): 684–685.

Mueller, R.S. (2004). Treatment protocols for demodicosis: an evidence-based review. *Vet. Dermatol.* 15 (2): 75–89.

Nelson CT, McCall JW, Carithers D. (2014). Current canine guidelines for the prevention, diagnosis, and management of heartworm (*Dirofilaria immitis*) infection in dogs. https://www.heartwormsociety.org/images/pdf/Canine-Guidelines-Summary.pdf.

Novartis Animal Health US (1998). *Program® six month injectable label*. Greensboro, NC: Novartis.

Page, S.W. (2008). *Antiparasitic Drugs*, 2e, vol. 334 (ed. J. Maddison, S. Page and D. Church). Amsterdam: Elsevier.

Papich, M.G., Davidson, G.S., and Fortier, L.A. (2013). Doxycycline concentration over time after storage in a compounded veterinary preparation. *J. Am. Vet. Med. Assoc.* 242 (12): 1674–1678. doi:10.2460/javma.242.12.1674.

Payne-Johnson, M., Maitland, T.P., Sherington, J. et al. (2000). Efficacy of selamectin administered topically to pregnant and lactating female dogs in the treatment and prevention of adult roundworm (*Toxocara canis*) infections and flea (*Ctenocephalides felis felis*) infestations in the dams and their pups. *Vet. Parasitol.* 91 (3–4): 347–358.

Pfizer Animal Health (2007). *Cestex® for dogs and cats label*, 1–3. Parsippany, NJ: Pfizer Animal Health.

Pharmacia and Upjohn Company (1998). *Mitaban FDA label*, 1–6. London: Pharmacia and Upjohn Company.

Roberson, E.L. and Burke, T.M. (1980). Evaluation of granulated fenbendazole (22.2%) against induced and naturally occurring helminth infections in cats. *Am. J. Vet. Res.* 41 (9): 1499–1502.

Roberts, J.R. and Reigart, J.R. (2013). Pyrethrins and pyrethroids. In: *Recognition and Management of Pesticide Poisonings*, 6e (ed. J.R. Roberts and J.R. Reigart), 38–42. Washington, DC: US Environmental Protection Agency.

Rosenbaum, M. and Kerlin, R. (1995). Erythema multiforme major and disseminated intravascular coagulation in a dog following application of a d-limonene-based insecticidal dip. *J. Am. Vet. Med. Assoc.* 207 (10): 1315–1319.

Shoop, W., Egerton, J., Eary, C. et al. (1988). Control of *Toxocara canis* transmission from bitch to offspring with ivermectin. Program and Abstracts. *Am. Soc. Parasitol.* 53(Abstract 143: 59–60.

Six, R.H., Becskei, C., Mazaleski, M.M. et al. (2016). Efficacy of sarolaner, a novel oral isoxazoline, against two common mite infestations in dogs: *Demodex* spp. and

Otodectes cynotis. Vet. Parasitol. 222: 62–66.

Snyder, D.E., Wiseman, S., Bowman, D.D. et al. (2011). Assessment of the effectiveness of a combination product of spinosad and milbemycin oxime on the prophylaxis of canine heartworm infection. *Vet. Parasitol.* 180 (3–4): 262–266.

Snyder, D.E., Wiseman, S., and Liebenberg, J.E. (2017). Efficacy of lotilaner (CredelioTM), a novel oral isoxazoline against naturally occurring mange mite infestations in dogs caused by *Demodex* spp. *Parasit. Vectors* 10 (1): 1–7.

Stern, B.L.A., Animal, A., Control, P. et al. (2015). Fipronil toxicosis in rabbits. *DVM 360*: 6–10.

Streitfeld D. (1991). Blockade: the beef goes on. Washington Post, February 5, p. c05.

Taenzler, J., Liebenberg, J., Roepke, R.K.A. et al. (2016). Efficacy of fluralaner administered either orally or topically for the treatment of naturally acquired *Sarcoptes scabiei* var. canis infestation in dogs. *Parasit. Vectors* 9 (1): 1–5.

Taenzler, J., De Vos, C., Roepke, R.K.A. et al. (2017). Efficacy of fluralaner against *Otodectes cynotis* infestations in dogs and cats. *Parasit. Vectors* 10 (1): 8–13.

Texas A&M University AgriLife Extention. (n.d.). Botanical insecticides. https://landscapeipm.tamu.edu/types-of-pest-control/chemical-control/organic/botanical.

Villeneuve, A., Polley, L., Jenkins, E. et al. (2015). Parasite prevalence in fecal samples from shelter dogs and cats across the Canadian provinces. *Parasit. Vectors* 8 (1): 281. doi:10.1186/s13071-015-0870-x.

Wismer, T. and Means, C. (2012). Toxicology of newer insecticides in small animals. *Vet. Clin. North Am. Small Anim. Pract.* 42 (2): 335–347. doi:10.1016/j.cvsm.2011.12.004.

8

Pain Management in Veterinary Species

Butch Kukanich

Department of Anatomy and Physiology, College of Veterinary Medicine, Kansas State University, Manhattan, KS, USA

Key Points

- Dogs and cats are more sensitive to gastro-intestinal and renal adverse effects of non-steroidal anti-inflammatory drugs (NSAIDs) than are humans and should never be treated with ibuprofen or naproxen.
- Over-the-counter (OTC) gastric acid suppres-sants such as omeprazole or famotidine (often called "gastroprotectants" by veterinarians) may decrease the severity and frequency of gastrointestinal adverse effects of prescrip-tion veterinary NSAIDs in dogs and cats.
- Acetaminophen is inherently toxic to cats and should never be administered to cats.

- Acetaminophen can be administered to dogs, but it has low efficacy and a short half-life (30–60 minutes) relative to that in humans (2–3 hours).
- Compared to human patients, opioids pro-duce minimal respiratory depression in otherwise healthy, opioid-naïve dogs, and cats.
- Opioids have low and variable oral bioavail-ability in animals, so they are infrequently prescribed. When they are, higher doses are required compared to opioid-naïve humans.

8.1 Comparative Aspects of Pain

The physiology of pain in animals and humans is very similar. Ascending pathways propagate or enhance pain transmission, while descending pathways can modulate pain. Opioid receptor agonists, NSAID (non-steroidal anti-inflammatory drug) cyclooxy-genase (COX) inhibitors, alpha-2 agonists, serotoninergic drugs such as tricyclic antide-pressants and tramadol, gabapentinoids, and local anesthetics may provide analgesia for specific types of pain. Alpha-2 adrenergic

agonists are used frequently for surgical procedures in many veterinary species but will not be covered here, as they are paren-teral drugs that would not be dispensed to pet owners by community pharmacies.

Managing pain in animals extends beyond prescribing drugs. As with humans, weight loss and maintaining ideal body weight decrease the risk of developing intervertebral disc disease (IVDD) in predisposed dog breeds and the development and progression of osteoarthritis (Frye et al. 2016). A species-appropriate, well-balanced diet fed to achieve the appropriate caloric and nutrition profile

Pharmacotherapeutics for Veterinary Dispensing, First Edition. Edited by Katrina L. Mealey.
© 2019 John Wiley & Sons, Inc. Published 2019 by John Wiley & Sons, Inc.

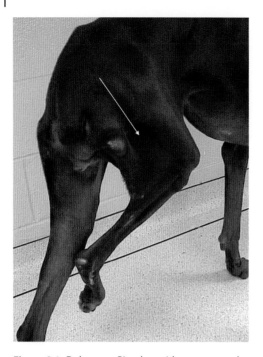

Figure 8.1 Doberman Pinscher with severe muscle atrophy as a result of complications from a femur fracture. Muscles surrounding the femur have atrophied (arrow), so that the outline of the femur is visible. Normally, the outline of the femur is not visible in dogs. *Source:* Photo courtesy of Dr. James K Roush, Kansas State University.

little data from controlled clinical trials in dogs and cats. Home or lifestyle modification can dramatically improve quality of life by taking steps to minimize pain-inducing behaviors with adjustments such as elevating food and water bowls, using ramps or platforms to minimize jumping, using softer bedding, and placing rugs on slippery floors as appropriate. There are few data supporting use of acupuncture as a treatment modality for pain in dogs and cats (Rose et al. 2017); however, that does not mean it is ineffective, just unknown. There are even fewer data on chiropractic use and massage therapy in dogs and cats. True homeopathic remedies have essentially been discredited and are therefore not recommended (Epstein et al. 2015).

Accurately assessing pain in animals is one of the most difficult aspects of veterinary medicine. It is even more difficult than assessing pain in human infants because of instinctual survival behaviors in animals. There is no universal technique or approach to diagnosing pain in animals. For example, if a dog or cat tries to escape or vocalizes when the veterinarian or owner is palpating the animal during a physical examination, that response may be an indicator of pain or it may just be a behavioral response such as anxiety. Many pet owners believe that if their dog is whining, then the dog must be in pain. While whining could be due to pain, it could also be caused by anxiety, excitement, or dysphoria. Lameness could be due to pain, but could also be an indicator of neurologic dysfunction or mechanical dysfunction (e.g. long toenails and anatomic deformities). Even more objective measures are not always reliable indicators of pain. An elevated heart rate could be due to pain, or could be due to excitement, stress, anxiety, or cardiovascular disease. Pain may also be manifested as decreased activity levels, but other disease states such as renal, hepatic, and cardiovascular disease, among others, need to be ruled out. Even aggression can be associated with pain, especially if it is new-onset aggression; but new-onset aggression can also be due to

is the primary driver to maintaining or achieving an ideal body weight in dogs and cats. Muscle atrophy (Figure 8.1) is often present in animals with osteoarthritis, degenerative joint disease, and IVDD, and regular, controlled exercise increases the muscle mass necessary to support the joints. Exercise also facilitates weight loss or maintenance of ideal body weight. Application of heat (warm packs) or cold therapy (ice) to an affected joint may be beneficial for localized pain, but care must be taken not to cause temperature-associated damage to the skin and underlying tissues. Physical therapy is often recommended to increase the range of motion of affected joints; increase the strength of supporting structures, such as tendons, ligaments, and muscles; and minimize joint pain (Dycus et al. 2017). Most of these recommendations are based on extrapolation from humans, since there are neoplasia (especially intracranial), renal or liver disease, or other changes such as a new pet or children in the household, or visitors, or it could be a developing behavioral issue (Chapter 16) such as food, treat, or toy aggression.

Sometimes, response to analgesic treatment is used as a diagnostic tool for pain in animals. However, it is important to note that the placebo effect can occur when pet owners and veterinarians assess treatment effects in animals. In a double-blinded placebo-controlled study assessing dogs with osteoarthritis treated with NSAIDs, 39–40% of the dogs in the placebo group were being judged as having improved compared to 65–70% of dogs in the NSAID-treated group being judged as having improved, based on the owner's assessment of the dog's quality of life, lameness, and overall activity level (US Food and Drug Administration 1996, 2002). Since these were placebo-controlled studies, an even higher placebo response rate would be expected if the owner had not been informed that their dog may be receiving a placebo. Although it seems counterintuitive that an animal would have a placebo response, several factors might contribute to this. For example, many painful conditions have a waxing and waning disease course, and the treatment may have been administered just as the waning phase of the disease began. Another factor contributing to a placebo response in animals is bias of the human evaluator, whether owner or veterinarian. This phenomenon is called the "caregiver effect" (Gruen et al. 2017). Additionally, improvement in the disease itself (e.g. as a fracture or surgical site heals, the pain generally diminishes) may be the true cause of pain relief for the animal, even if the owner perceives it was a treatment response. Finally, a veterinarian or pharmacist may lose follow-up on a patient and assume the animal's pain resolved with treatment since the patient did not return. However, this assumption may or may not be correct.

Monitoring animals for pain, as discussed here, is difficult. Although there are many "pain scales" suggested for animals, most are not sufficiently sensitive to distinguish a true effect from a placebo effect. The pain scales/assessments include, among others, the client-specific outcome measures, Canine Brief Pain Inventory, Helsinki Chronic Pain Index, activity levels, and lameness assessments. These are often confounded, producing inaccurate results. There have been no validated grimace scales for dogs or cats, but there have been some published for other species such as rats, rabbits, and ferrets. The American Animal Hospital Association (AAHA) has handouts for pet owners describing "how to tell if your dog or cat is in pain," but these are essentially a compilation of other subjective scales and have their limitations as described here (AAHA 2007).

As can be appreciated, something that seems as straightforward as assessing an animal for pain can be quite difficult. To complicate matters further, each species has adapted to pain in a different manner such that pain indicators that are valid in one species may be less so in a different species. Due to the serious nature of diseases that may directly cause pain or diseases that could be mistaken for pain, symptomatic analgesic treatment of animals by pet owners is not recommended. Animals that are displaying signs of pain should be thoroughly evaluated by a veterinarian to ensure that an accurate diagnosis is made so that specific treatment for the underlying cause of the animal's pain is adequately addressed. Pharmacists can play a key role in educating pet owners to seek veterinary care for their pet rather than treat with analgesics without establishing a diagnosis. Symptomatic analgesic treatment without diagnosing the underlying cause may result in prolonged pain or increase the risk of morbidity or mortality due to progression of an underlying disease.

As is the case with human patients, there are many reasons analgesics may be prescribed for a veterinary patient. Postoperative analgesics are commonly administered both in the hospital and as outpatient treatments. Osteoarthritis, degenerative joint diseases, and congenital orthopedic diseases are common conditions in dogs and cats that require pain management. Pain due to trauma, neoplastic pain, and IVDD and other causes of neuropathic pain, as well as inflammatory pain, also occur in dogs and cats.

8.2 Diagnostic Testing

An accurate history and physical exam are crucial to diagnosing the cause of pain in dogs and cats. Lameness, crepitus, pain on palpation, and a neurologic exam can be useful for ruling in or ruling out specific diseases. Fever may accompany some infectious, inflammatory, autoimmune, or neoplastic diseases. The normal rectal temperature of dogs and cats (100–102 °F) is higher than that of humans, and temperatures 103 °F or above are considered fevers (Appendix C). It is important to note that exercise, excitement, or elevated environmental temperatures can easily increase a dog's body temperature to 104 °F or higher (hyperthermia vs. fever). Radiographs can help diagnose or confirm musculoskeletal defects, osteoarthritis, neoplasia, and traumatic injury. Advanced imaging procedures including ultrasound, computed tomography, and magnetic resonance imaging may be required for certain diseases, such as abdominal neoplasia, IVDD, or intracranial neoplasia. A complete blood count, serum chemistry profile, and urinalysis may help with diagnoses, but it can also serve as a screening tool for health status to ensure a selected analgesic is safe for administration. Infectious disease testing can also help rule in and out infectious diseases that may cause pain (e.g. Rickettsial diseases, septic arthritis, and others).

Common diagnostic procedures:

- History and physical exam
- Neurologic exam
- Radiographic exam
- Complete blood count, serum chemistry profile, and urinalysis
- Infectious disease testing (bacterial culture and susceptibility, serology, and molecular diagnostic techniques)
- Advanced imaging (ultrasound, computed tomography, and magnetic resonance imaging).

8.3 Pharmacological Treatment of Pain

8.3.1 NSAIDs and Acetaminophen

NSAIDs are commonly used in dogs to treat a variety of painful conditions, but are less commonly used in cats as some cats seem more sensitive to the renal adverse effects of NSAIDs. Some cats have a variant form of a normally renoprotective protein that may explain this susceptibility to acute kidney injury (Sugisawa et al. 2016). NSAIDs are prescribed for conditions suspected to cause mild to moderate pain, while moderate to severe pain is better managed by parenteral opioids (Epstein et al. 2015).

NSAIDs that are US Food and Drug Administration (FDA) approved for companion veterinary species include carprofen, deracoxib, firocoxib, meloxicam, and robenacoxib. Each of these veterinary NSAIDS requires a prescription. The FDA-approved meloxicam tablets for humans (7.5 and 15 mg) are too large to be safely used in cats and nearly all dogs, as the dose of meloxicam is 0.05–0.1 mg/kg once daily (i.e. a 7.5 mg tablet would treat a 75 kg, 165-pound dog). Since these tablets are not scored, tablet splitting is not recommended. The FDA-approved NSAIDs for dogs and cats are cyclooxygenase-2 (COX2) preferential or selective. This is preferred to nonselective COX inhibitors (many human NSAIDs) due to the enhanced sensitivity of the canine and feline gastrointestinal (GI) tracts to NSAID-induced adverse effects. It is interesting to note that COX selectivity of an NSAID is species specific and may be vastly different between species. For example, carprofen in humans inhibits COX1 to a greater degree than COX2, but in dogs carprofen inhibits COX2 to a greater extent than COX1 and consequently has a relatively greater GI safety profile in dogs than humans (Warner et al. 1999; Streppa et al. 2002).

Aspirin was used relative frequently in dogs prior to the development of canine and feline FDA-approved COX2 preferential or selective NSAIDs. Due to the high risk of GI adverse effects, aspirin is no longer recommended for use as an analgesic in dogs or cats because there are so many safer options available.

The human NSAID piroxicam is occasionally used to minimize clinical signs associated with transitional cell carcinoma in dogs or as an adjunctive therapy for certain neoplasias (Chapter 20). Due to the frequency and severity of GI adverse effects of this drug, it should always be administered with either omeprazole or misoprostol.

The oral bioavailability of FDA-approved NSAIDs in dogs and cats is typically high, and the duration of effect is 12–24 hours depending on the specific drug and dose. NSAIDs are primarily eliminated by hepatic mechanisms, including phase I metabolism (deracoxib, firocoxib, meloxicam, and potentially robenacoxib), phase II metabolism (carprofen), and biliary excretion. The extensive phase I metabolism of deracoxib and robenacoxib (potentially) could be affected by significant drug interactions with cytochrome P450 (CYP) inhibitors such as ketoconazole, itraconazole, fluconazole, chloramphenicol, cimetidine, and fluoxetine, resulting in decreased elimination. However, specific interactions have not been documented. The metabolism of meloxicam may be more affected by CYP inducers, resulting in increased elimination and loss of therapeutic efficacy, since it has a low hepatic clearance. Firocoxib is an intermediate-extraction drug and as such could be affected by both CYP inducers and inhibitors. However, no drug–drug metabolism interactions studies have been published. Only a small amount of each NSAID is eliminated by renal mechanisms.

Although acetaminophen is not an NSAID, it is often included with NSAIDs when discussing analgesics. Acetaminophen does not inhibit COX-like NSAIDs, but appears to act through serotonin receptors and transient receptor potential cation channel subfamily V member 1 (TRPV1). As such, acetaminophen is not associated with GI or renal adverse effects at clinically appropriate dosages. Acetaminophen has a moderate oral bioavailability in dogs, but a short half-life of 30–60 minutes (Neirinckx et al. 2010; KuKanich 2016). It is rarely used as a sole analgesic in dogs due to its short half-life, but is more commonly used in combination with opioids in products such as acetaminophen with codeine or hydrocodone. Acetaminophen is inherently toxic to cats (Chapter 4) and should never be administered to cats, even in combination products. Therefore, if presented with a prescription for codeine for a cat, the pharmacist must not substitute an acetaminophen-combination product for the sole ingredient product.

8.3.2 Opioids

Opioids are effective for treating mild to severe pain when sufficient systemic drug exposure occurs. In dogs and cats, parenteral administration is often required to achieve clinical analgesia, since the oral bioavailability of most opioids is low, resulting in highly variable clinical efficacy. Additionally, the durations of action are short due to rapid elimination (KuKanich 2013). There are currently no FDA-approved oral formulations of opioids that are indicated for pain in dogs or cats. Butorphanol is FDA approved for dogs in tablet form, but the label indication is for cough suppression.

Because morphine, oxycodone, and butorphanol have very low oral bioavailability (<10%) and short elimination half-lives (one to two hours), they are rarely prescribed for oral administration to dogs and cats to control pain. Buprenorphine has a very low oral bioavailability in dogs and cats as well (<10%), but some absorption can occur through the oral mucous membranes if it remains in contact for a sufficient time period and the drug is not immediately swallowed. The oral bioavailability of methadone in dogs is very poor (<10%) and has not been studied in cats. The oral bioavailability of hydrocodone has not been reported in cats, but in dogs it is poor (<10–40%), but enough systemic exposure may occur to provide some analgesic effect in some animals. Hydrocodone is most often used as an antitussive, rather than as an analgesic, in dogs. The oral bioavailability of codeine is low (~4%) in both dogs and cats, and neither species metabolizes codeine to morphine efficiently, but analgesia may occur due to other codeine metabolites, including codeine-6-glucuronide in dogs and norcodeine in cats (Figure 8.2).

Opioids are considered a very safe drug class for use in animals because lethal doses are substantially higher than clinically effective doses (Table 8.1). In contrast to humans, opioids produce only mild respiratory depression in animals, which is considered a clinically relevant problem only in select circumstances such as head trauma, underlying respiratory disease, or co-administration of other respiratory-depressant drugs such as anesthetic agents. Dependence on opioids has been well described in dogs, with opioid antagonists or abrupt discontinuation capable of eliciting signs of acute withdrawal (Martin and Eades 1964). Defecation, salivation, urination, mydriasis, rhinorrhea, lacrimation, tachycardia, tremors, restlessness, whining, and gnawing and biting at surroundings have been observed with acute withdrawal in dogs precipitated by an opioid antagonist. However, this has not been observed commonly in clinical patients due

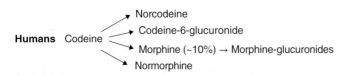

Dogs   Codeine ⟶ Codeine-6-glucuronide

Cats   Codeine ⟶ Norcodeine

Humans   Codeine ⟨ Norcodeine
Codeine-6-glucuronide
Morphine (~10%) → Morphine-glucuronides
Normorphine

Figure 8.2 Codeine metabolism in dogs, cats, and humans. Note that neither dogs nor cats metabolize codeine to morphine, the most pharmacologically active metabolite.

Table 8.1 The clinically effective intravenous (IV) dose, IV lethal dose in 50% of the population (LD_{50}), and ratio of the LD_{50} to effective dose of selected opioids in healthy, opioid-naive dogs.

Drug	IV effective dose (mg/kg)	IV LD_{50} (mg/kg)	Ratio (LD_{50}/effective dose)
Morphine	0.5	175	350
Fentanyl	0.005	14	2800
Methadone	0.5	29	58
Codeine	2.5	98	39.2
Buprenorphine	0.02	79	3950
Butorphanol	0.4	10	25
Nalbuphine	0.5	140	280

Note: A high ratio illustrates the safety of these opioids in healthy dogs.

to the short durations of parenteral opioid treatment and poor bioavailability of oral opioids. However, withdrawal has occurred when an antagonist (butorphanol) was administered after a week of IV morphine administration (B. KuKanich, personal observation). Due to the low oral bioavailability and short durations of effect, simple discontinuation of oral opioid therapy presents a low risk for eliciting withdrawal responses in dogs.

Dogs	Tramadol ⟶ M2 ⟶ M5
Cats	Tramadol ⟶ M1
Humans	Tramadol ⟶ M1 ↘ M2 ⟶ M5

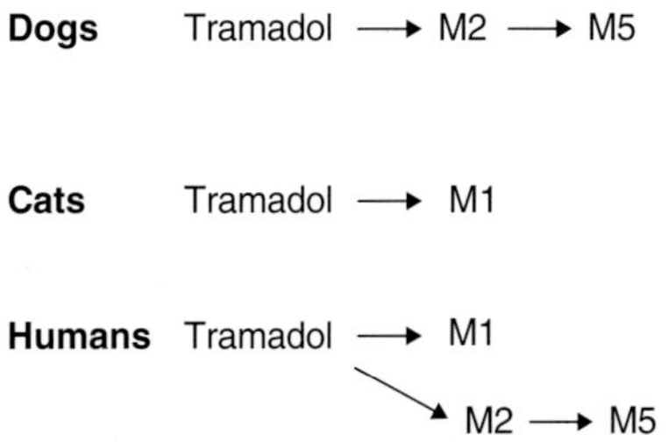

Figure 8.3 Primary pathways of tramadol metabolism in dogs, cats, and humans. M1, Active opioid metabolite; M2, M5, inactive metabolites. Note that dogs do not produce the active metabolite.

Practiced but not proven

Codeine is probably the most common opioid administered orally to dogs. There is debate as to whether oral codeine produces analgesic effects in dogs. Even if the analgesic effects of codeine are marginal in dogs, combining codeine with an NSAID may result in better clinical analgesia than an NSAID alone through additive effects. For example, oral codeine administered with carprofen seems to have higher efficacy than carprofen alone, even if codeine administered alone does not produce an analgesic effect.

8.3.3 Tramadol

Tramadol is a centrally acting analgesic that is FDA approved for use in humans but is prescribed frequently for extra-label use in dogs. Tramadol acts primarily as a serotonin/norepinephrine reuptake inhibitor, but an active metabolite of tramadol can produce mu opioid effects in some species. Most dogs do not produce sufficient quantities of the active metabolite (Figure 8.3) and do not exhibit opioid effects after tramadol administration (KuKanich 2013). Thus, tramadol does not provide sufficient analgesia for most dogs (Budsberg et al. 2018), which is an important problem because the drug is routinely prescribed by veterinarians. Another problem with tramadol's use in dogs is that first-pass metabolism is induced (presumably by intestinal CYP3A isoforms) by about 300% within the first week of treatment, with

plasma drug exposure dropping to approximately one-third of the original concentration without changes in elimination half-life. To my knowledge, this has been documented only in dogs. The reasons for this canine-specific phenomenon are unknown. Another reason for tramadol's lack of efficacy in most dogs is that its elimination half-life is short (one to two hours in dogs, compared to about seven hours in humans). Consequently, the dose of tramadol for dogs must be high (up to 15 mg/kg PO every six to eight hours; a 50 mg tablet for an 8-pound dog) to achieve targeted tramadol drug concentrations with subacute to chronic administration, but even those doses will not achieve opioid effects due to the inability of most dogs to produce the active metabolite – similar to humans with the poor-metabolizer phenotype. Tramadol has a longer elimination half-life in cats (three to four hours) relative to dogs, and cats metabolize tramadol in a manner that produces a large amount of the active opioid metabolite, which has a half-life of four to five hours, similar to humans with the ultra-metabolizer phenotype (Figure 8.3). Thus, cats have profound opioid effects after oral tramadol administration. As a result, the dose of tramadol in cats is much lower than in dogs, 1–2 mg/kg PO every 12 hours (5–10 mg per cat every 12 hours). Multiple-dose pharmacokinetics have not been reported in cats; therefore, it is unknown if metabolism changes over time in cats, as it does for dogs.

Practiced but not proven

Although tramadol is commonly used in dogs, evidence of its efficacy is lacking. Based on single doses, some experimental models have demonstrated efficacy, whereas others have not. No clinical trials in dogs have demonstrated efficacy. However, it is commonly prescribed to dogs, because it is inexpensive and adverse effects in dogs are rare.

Pharmacists can play a key role in educating veterinarians about tramadol's lack of therapeutic efficacy for most canine patients. Dog owners should be counseled to contact their veterinarian if pain control is inadequate, so that an alternate, or additional, analgesic can be prescribed. Tramadol is not commonly used in cats since the dosage needed, 5–10 mg total dose per cat, is hard to achieve with commercially available FDA-approved tablet strengths. The bitter taste of tramadol typically makes administration of split tablets nearly impossible in cats, and most suspensions and solutions are also difficult to administer to cats.

8.3.4 Amantadine

Amantadine was originally developed as an antiviral drug, but additional pharmacological effects including dopamine agonistic and NMDA (N-methyl D-aspartate) antagonistic effects have been described. The NMDA antagonistic effects of amantadine may have some utility in animals with subacute and chronic pain when central sensitization (i.e. "wind-up") has occurred. A clinical trial in osteoarthritic dogs that were refractory to NSAIDs demonstrated that concurrent administration of amantadine improved indices of analgesia. It is important to note that the benefit was delayed, occurring about six weeks after initiation of amantadine. However, the delay may have been due to the fact that amantadine had been administered only once daily (Lascelles et al. 2008). Subsequent pharmacokinetic studies have identified that amantadine has a short half-life in dogs (5 hours) compared to that in humans (17 hours), suggesting that twice-daily dosing may provide more rapid and improved pain control (Norkus et al. 2015). Based on the pharmacokinetics studies, a dose of 3 mg/kg PO every 12 hours is suggested for dogs, typically combined with an NSAID.

The pharmacokinetics of amantadine have been described in healthy research cats, for which the drug has an elimination half-life intermediate to that of dogs and humans (five to six hours) (Siao et al. 2011). Clinical trials assessing the efficacy of amantadine in cats have not been reported. Based on pharmacokinetics studies, a dose of 3 mg/kg PO every 12 hours has been suggested for cats.

8.3.5 Gabapentinoids

Although gabapentin and pregabalin are not FDA approved for any veterinary species, gabapentin is prescribed more frequently than pregabalin for dogs and cats primarily due to cost differences. Clinical trials detailing analgesic efficacy for either drug are lacking in dogs and cats. Gabapentin is sometimes prescribed for behavioral problems in dogs and cats, including various phobias and anxieties (Chapter 16). As with people, the analgesic efficacy of gabapentin is probably greatest for neuropathic pain, such as IVDD, cervical spinal pain, or other neuropathic pain conditions in dogs and cats. The pharmacokinetics of gabapentin indicate dosing at a rate of 10–20 mg/kg PO every eight hours in dogs and cats to maintain drug exposure, but optimal dosing has not been adequately described. The pharmacokinetics of pregabalin suggest a dosing rate of 4 mg/kg PO every 12 hours in dogs, but no clinical efficacy data are available. There are no published data on pharmacokinetics of pregabalin in cats.

Dramatic difference

Gabapentin oral solution, the FDA-approved human formulation, contains xylitol at a concentration of 300 mg/mL. Xylitol is highly toxic to dogs and can result in severe hypoglycemia and liver failure. This formulation of gabapentin should not be dispensed to dogs.

8.3.6 Tricyclic Antidepressants

Tricyclic antidepressants (TCAs) are serotonin and norepinephrine reuptake inhibitors and are considered among the most effective drugs for managing neuropathic pain in humans, but adverse effects are common (antimuscarinic, antihistaminic, and alpha-1 adrenergic antagonistic) and sometimes limit their use. In contrast, TCAs are well tolerated in veterinary patients but are not commonly used as analgesics. There are no clinical studies that have assessed the efficacy of TCAs for analgesic effects in dogs and cats. Clomipramine is approved for use in dogs for the management of separation anxiety in combination with behavioral training (Chapter 16). A few case reports have suggested that amitriptyline may be an effective analgesic in dogs. Recent pharmacokinetic studies involving oral amitriptyline in dogs indicate that their dose requirement may be much higher than that in humans, with dogs requiring up to 8 mg/kg PO every 12 hours to achieve targeted plasma concentrations. The higher required dosage is due to a lower oral bioavailability in dogs (approximately 6%) compared to that in humans (30–60%) (Norkus et al. 2015). Vomiting was noted when higher doses were administered to fasted dogs, but not fed dogs. Unless additional evidence becomes available, TCAs are expected to be used infrequently as analgesics for veterinary patients. Amitriptyline may have a better pharmacokinetics profile in cats after oral administration, but more studies, particularly multiple-dose studies, are needed to confirm the pharmacokinetics of amitriptyline (Mealey et al. 2004).

8.3.7 Local Anesthetics

Local anesthetics such as lidocaine are available as both over-the-counter (OTC) and prescription topical products, but only topical formulations with tetracaine are approved for dermatologic use in dogs and cats. It is important for pharmacists to know that dogs and cats are likely to ingest topically applied drugs, including local anesthetics. Grooming (licking the skin or haircoat) is a normal behavior for most veterinary patients. Grooming becomes more frequent and vigorous near areas that are painful or if the animal detects a foreign material on their skin or fur. Therefore, the pharmacist and pet owner should assume that oral ingestion will occur if local anesthetic ointments, sprays, or creams are applied topically to a veterinary patient unless an Elizabethan collar, also called an E-collar or "cone of shame," is used (Figure 8.4). Even low-dose benzocaine (8.1 mg total dose) has been associated with toxicity in cats when used as a topical anesthetic spray for the larynx to facilitate intubation (see Chapter 6). Excessive doses or inadvertent ingestion of lidocaine in cats can result in decreased cardiac output. In both dogs and cats, lidocaine can cause cardiac and central nervous system (CNS) toxicity, including arrhythmias, sedation, ataxia, and incoordination, which can progress to seizures. Dibucaine is available OTC in 0.5% and 1% formulations, and it has been reported to cause local anesthetic toxicity when ingested. Because of its greater potency than lidocaine, accidental ingestion by dogs or cats may be more likely to result in fatal arrhythmias in addition to the neurologic signs (Welch 2000). Pharmacists should counsel pet owners not to use topical local anesthetics on their animal without consulting a veterinarian.

(a)

(b)

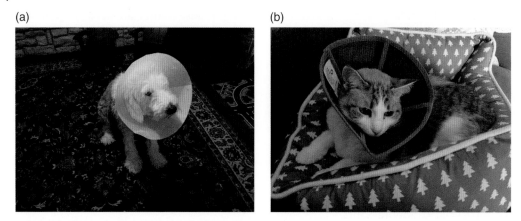

Figure 8.4 A dog (a) and cat (b) with an Elizabethan collar (or "E-collar") to prevent self-trauma. *Source:* Photos courtesy of Dr. Kate KuKanich, Kansas State University.

8.4 Adverse Effects in Veterinary Species

8.4.1 NSAIDs and Acetaminophen

The most common class of drugs reported to the FDA for adverse effects in animals are NSAIDs. The majority of adverse effects are thought to be directly related to inhibition of prostanoids such as prostaglandin E2 (PGE), prostaglandin I2 (aka prostacyclin, or PGI), and thromboxane A2 (TXA), among others. Both PGE and PGI produce gastroprotective effects by increasing mucus production in the GI tract, decreasing acid secretion, enhancing bicarbonate secretion, and enhancing blood flow to the mucosa via vasodilation. These beneficial physiologic effects are probably most important in the stomach and duodenum, where mucus creates a physical barrier between gastric acid and the gastric/duodenal mucosa (epithelial cells lining the stomach), and bicarbonate secretion forms a layer between the mucosa and the mucus layer that neutralizes any acid that penetrates the mucous layer. Vasodilation enhances nutrient delivery and waste product removal from GI epithelial cells. Because of the rapid turnover rate of gastric epithelial cells, this tissue has a high metabolic rate that requires constant delivery of oxygen and nutrients. Upregulation of COX2 occurs in

healing GI lesions (erosions, ulcerations, and surgical incisions) to enhance healing through increased production of PGE and PGI. In the kidney, PGE and PGI production and upregulation are required to maintain localized vasodilation and renal perfusion in physiologic states of increased vascular tone, dehydration, hypotension, or hemorrhage. Shunting of the arachidonic acid pathway to production of leukotrienes, which is a result of some NSAID treatments, results in enhanced gastric acid secretion and vasoconstriction. This effect may contribute to the adverse effects of NSAIDs.

Both dogs and cats are more sensitive to the GI adverse effects of NSAIDs than humans. NSAIDs can result in kidney and liver failure as well. Pet owners should be instructed to monitor for signs of lethargy, anorexia, vomiting, diarrhea, black and tar-like stools, changes in mucous membrane or eye color (icterus), or changes in the amount (increased or decreased) of water consumed or urination (increased or decreased amount of urine), and immediately contact their veterinarian if observed. Due to the severity of GI adverse effects from the human OTC NSAIDs ibuprofen and naproxen, they should never be administered to dogs and cats. Aspirin should only be administered to dogs and cats if specifically directed by a veterinarian. Aspirin is much more likely to cause GI, and potentially renal, adverse effects than the prescription NSAIDs that are FDA approved for veterinary patients. Ingestion of OTC "human" NSAIDs and acetaminophen are among the most common toxicities in dogs and cats.

Hepatotoxicity from NSAIDs, including formulations approved for veterinary patients, can occur through dose-dependent toxicity, but can also be idiosyncratic (dose-independent). There are no identified risk factors for idiosyncratic toxicity other than a previous episode of idiosyncratic toxicity. In rare cases, NSAIDs have caused acute fatal hepatic necrosis in dogs. Although some sources state Labrador Retrievers are at an increased risk as a breed (numerous sites on the internet are dedicated to this topic), this has not been identified as a risk factor. Labrador Retrievers are the most common dog breed in the USA and are popular worldwide. The breed typically has a high prevalence of orthopedic diseases, such as hip dysplasia, elbow dysplasia, cranial cruciate ligament injuries, degenerative joint disease, and osteoarthritis. Labradors are a large breed; therefore, they are more likely to show overt clinical signs related to musculoskeletal pain, since larger dogs have a greater than proportional force applied to the joints per pound of body weight compared to smaller breed dogs. As such, Labradors represent a large portion of the canine population that are treated with NSAIDs relative to other dog breeds. Accounting for these factors, Labradors are not at a higher risk for idiosyncratic toxicity than other dog breeds.

> **Practiced, but not proven**
>
> In humans, co-administration of drugs that suppress gastric acid production, such as proton pump inhibitors (e.g. omeprazole) and histamine 2 (H2) receptor antagonists (e.g. famotidine) or other "gastroprotective" drugs, including sucralfate and misoprostol, decreases the prevalence of GI adverse effects of NSAIDs. Experimental data in dogs suggest similar beneficial effects, but clinical trials demonstrating decreased GI adverse effects have not been reported.

Drug interactions with NSAIDs can result in decreased efficacy or increased risk of adverse effects (Table 8.2). Furosemide and angiotensin-converting enzyme (ACE) inhibitors increase the risk of renal adverse effects of NSAIDs by generating subclinical dehydration and hyponatremia (furosemide) or renal hypotension (ACE inhibitors). Concurrent administration of multiple NSAIDs or NSAIDs and glucocorticoids greatly increases the risk of GI adverse effects in dogs and cats and is generally contraindicated. Concurrent use of serotonergic drugs

Table 8.2 Drug interactions that can increase the risk of NSAID adverse effects.

Drug	Adverse effect system	Strength of evidence
Glucocorticoids	Gastrointestinal	High
Concurrent NSAIDs	Gastrointestinal	High
Bismuth subsalicylate	Gastrointestinal	Low
Tramadol	Gastrointestinal	Low
Serotonergic drugs (SSRIs, SNRIs)	Gastrointestinal	Low
ACE inhibitors (enalapril, benazepril)	Renal	Low
Diuretics (furosemide)	Renal	Moderate

ACE, Angiotensin-converting enzyme; NSAID, nonsteroidal anti-inflammatory drug; SSRI, selective serotonin reuptake inhibitor; SNRI, serotonin–norepinephrine reuptake inhibitor.

such as fluoxetine and potentially tramadol may increase the risk of GI adverse effects. Conversely, NSAIDs decrease the efficacy of both furosemide and ACE inhibitors by inhibition of prostaglandin-mediated actions of these drugs. Therefore, NSAIDs could cause acute exacerbation of cardiovascular disease by inhibiting the effects of furosemide and ACE inhibitors in addition to enhancing sodium, and therefore water, retention.

Life-threatening acetaminophen toxicity occurs at essentially any dose in cats and can occur with excessive doses in dogs. Cats lack the enzymes to form glucuronide conjugates of acetaminophen, and as a result, cytochrome P450 metabolism of acetaminophen occurs, producing toxic metabolites (see Chapters 4 and 6 for more detailed information). Adverse effects can include Heinz body anemia, methemoglobinemia, and hepatotoxicity. Clinical signs include lethargy, weakness, depression, vomiting, increased respiratory rate, discolored mucous membranes, edema of the paws and face, and death. If a cat ingests acetaminophen, it should be immediately taken to a veterinarian for treatment.

Dramatic difference

Acetaminophen is HIGHLY toxic to cats and should never be administered to cats, even in combination products.

8.4.2 Opioids

In general, opioids are well tolerated in dogs. Respiratory depression can occur with excessive doses, but in otherwise healthy animals even massive overdoses result in a mild to moderate depression that rarely requires treatment. More common adverse effects include sedation, dysphoria/euphoria, and salivation/drooling. In dogs, panting with mild to moderate hypothermia can occur due to activation of hypothalamic opioid receptors. As is the case with humans, nausea, vomiting, and anorexia can occur as well as constipation. It is important to reiterate that opioids in combination with

acetaminophen should never be administered to cats, as acetaminophen is extremely toxic to cats. Pharmacists may find references to "morphine mania" (referring to CNS excitation) with regard to opioid use in cats. However, the initial reports of "morphine mania" were based on cats receiving doses 10–20 times higher than recommended doses. Cats that are treated with appropriate opioid doses are not expected to experience CNS excitation any more than dogs. Cats may exhibit sedation, purring, euphoria/dysphoria, hallucinations, anorexia, and constipation. Opioids have a miotic effect in dogs, presumably through parasympathetic stimulation, but a pronounced mydriatic effect in cats, presumably through sympathetic stimulation.

8.4.3 Tramadol

Tramadol is frequently prescribed as an analgesic for dogs because it is well tolerated. Unfortunately, the reason it is so well tolerated is because the plasma concentrations of tramadol and its opioid metabolite are subtherapeutic, producing little pharmacologic effects (beneficial or adverse) in most dogs. At high doses, or in susceptible dogs, adverse effects of tramadol are very similar to those of TCAs (discussed further in this chapter), since the primary mechanism of action in dogs is mediated via serotonin and norepinephrine reuptake inhibition. Higher doses can cause vomiting, anorexia, mydriasis, and sedation. Overdoses (e.g. if a dog gains access to and consumes the entire vial) can result in seizures, which are responsive to intravenous (IV) diazepam. Often, just a single dose of diazepam is needed. The author has treated a previously well-controlled epileptic dog that presented in status epilepticus within four hours of tramadol administration (appropriate dose). It is unclear if tramadol was the cause of the status epilepticus or if the stress of the previous veterinary visit and injury were contributing factors. Regardless, pharmacists should alert the veterinarian and client about potential risk of tramadol use in animals prone

Table 8.3 Drugs used in veterinary medicine with the potential for causing serotonin syndrome.

Drug class	Drug
Analgesic	Tramadol
Tricyclic antidepressants	Clomipramine
	Amitriptyline
Selective serotonin reuptake inhibitors	Fluoxetine
	Paroxetine
	Sertraline
Antidepressants	Buspirone
	Trazodone
Monoamine oxidase inhibitors	Selegiline
	Amitraz

Note: Concurrent administration of any of these drugs may greatly increase the risk of serotonin syndrome.

to seizures. The bitter taste of tramadol may result in salivation, pawing at the mouth, and vomiting when administered orally to dogs and cats. In cats, tramadol produces prominent opioid effects (similar to ultra-metabolizer humans). Sedation, purring, euphoria/dysphoria, hallucinations (pawing at the air, or appearing to watching objects that are not truly there), mydriasis, anorexia, and constipation may occur in cats. Since tramadol produces effects at least in part through serotonin reuptake, the possibility of serotonin syndrome exists if combined with other drugs affecting serotonin reuptake, such as selective serotonin reuptake inhibitors (fluoxetine is approved for use in dogs for separation anxiety), TCAs (clomipramine is approved for use in dogs for separation anxiety), or serotonin norepinephrine reuptake inhibitors (uncommon use in dogs and cats) (Table 8.3).

8.4.4 Amantadine

Amantadine is not commonly prescribed for dogs and cats; therefore, a complete description of potential adverse effects is not available. Because amantadine is not FDA approved for use in dogs or cats, there are not extensive data available. In preclinical studies for

development of amantadine for human use, amantadine was administered to dogs orally at doses up to 50 mg/kg daily for 30 days (the recommended dog and cat dose based on pharmacokinetic studies is 3–5 mg/kg PO every 12 hours). Overall, it seems to be well tolerated when administered within the recommended dose ranges. Anxiety, tremors, ataxia, salivation, and vomiting have occurred with overdoses due to accidental ingestion. Although data in animals are lacking, amantadine is avoided in animals with congestive heart failure and seizure risks based on extrapolation from human data.

8.4.5 Gabapentinoids

Gabapentin is not FDA approved for use in any veterinary species, but it is prescribed for some patients with refractory pain. Gabapentin seems to be well tolerated in dogs, with lethargy, sedation, and ataxia reported at high doses. To my knowledge, rebound or autonomic seizures have not been reported with abrupt discontinuation of gabapentin, as has been reported in human patients. However, veterinary experts often recommend weaning the dose over the course of a few days to a week out of an abundance of caution, especially for animals receiving high doses or prolonged courses of therapy.

> **Dramatic difference**
>
> The oral solution of gabapentin contains xylitol. Because dogs are uniquely susceptible to xylitol toxicity (see Chapter 6 for more detailed information), the oral solution is not recommended for use in dogs.

Pregabalin is not FDA approved for any veterinary species and is rarely prescribed for dogs and cats. Similar to gabapentin, lethargy, sedation, and ataxia are the most expected adverse effects. Peripheral edema is an adverse effect of pregabalin in humans, but to my knowledge, peripheral edema has

Table 8.4 FDA-approved veterinary drug products with no human drug equivalent.

Brand name	Active ingredient	Drug class	Rationale / notes
Torbutrol	Butorphanol	Mu opioid antagonist/ kappa opioid agonist	Approved for antitussive use only
Deramaxx	Deracoxib	NSAID – coxib	COX2-selective inhibitor
Onsior	Robenacoxib	NSAID – coxib	COX2-selective inhibitor
Previcox	Previcoxib	NSAID – coxib	COX2-selective inhibitor
Rimadyl	Carprofen	NSAID – propionic acid	COX2-preferential inhibitor

not yet been reported in dogs or cats. More adverse effects may become evident if the use of pregabalin increases in veterinary patients.

8.4.6 Tricyclic Antidepressants

In general, antidepressant drugs are well tolerated in dogs and cats. Clomipramine is approved for use in dogs as part of a comprehensive behavioral management program to treat separation anxiety. Lethargy and sedation are among the more common adverse effects; however, in patients with pain, these effects may actually be advantageous under some circumstances. Adverse effects can vary somewhat between different TCAs. For example, high plasma concentrations of amitriptyline have been associated with tachycardia and sedation, whereas clomipramine produces sedation with bradycardia, sinoatrial block, and atrioventricular block. Therefore, pharmacists should counsel pet owners to monitor their animal carefully if cardiac disease is present. Increased risk of seizures is expected with antidepressants that inhibit reuptake of serotonin, so they should be avoided in animals prone to seizures. Acute overdoses of TCAs can also cause seizures, even in animals not predisposed to seizures – this may be due to serotonin syndrome. If vomiting occurs with TCA administration, pharmacists can counsel clients to try administering the drug with food – this seems to decrease vomiting. Cats treated with TCAs may be more prone to

constipation and urinary retention (antimuscarinic effects) than dogs. Because TCAs increase CNS concentrations of serotonin, pharmacists must monitor for drug–drug interactions that might predispose to serotonin syndrome. Pharmacists should familiarize themselves with commonly used veterinary drugs that have serotonergic activity (Table 8.4).

8.5 Nutritional Supplements for Managing Pain

Glucosamine and chondroitin sulfate are marketed to both human and veterinary patients as "chondroprotectives." Glucosamine and chondroitin sulfate are commonly administered to veterinary patients for the management and prevention of osteoarthritis. They tend to be well tolerated with few adverse effects; however, massive ingestion of glucosamine and chondroitin products (20+ tablets) has caused hepatotoxicity. Double-blinded controlled clinical trials in dogs have failed to consistently show improvements in osteoarthritis with glucosamine and chondroitin supplements when measured by a variety of tests, including owner or veterinarian assessments, lameness scores, and ground reaction forces (Bhathal et al. 2017; Scott et al. 2017). Although "clinical impressions" are reported as indicators of efficacy, it is important to remember that placebo effects occur commonly in animals (40%) in controlled clinical studies, and the caregiver effect may result in a nearly 80% placebo effect (Gruen et al. 2017). Therefore, it is not surprising that owners and veterinarians might perceive a benefit in cats and dogs, but a true benefit has not been demonstrated.

A variety of other nutraceuticals have been used for pain management, primarily for osteoarthritis in dogs and cats, but most have not been demonstrated to be effective in controlled clinical trials (Comblain et al. 2016). Avocado–soybean unsaponifiables, curcumin (turmeric), polyunsaturated fatty acids, green-lipped mussel (*Perna canaliculus*), beta 1,3- and 1,6-glucans from yeast (*Saccharomyces cerevisiae*), and *Boswellia* resin (*Boswellia serrata*) have not demonstrated analgesic efficacy in placebo-controlled clinical trials.

Oral administration of undenatured type II collagen was evaluated in a double-blinded placebo-controlled clinical trial in dogs. The commercially available collagen product resulted in significant improvement, compared to placebo, when assessed by lameness scores and physical examinations (D'Altilio et al. 2007). In contrast, glucosamine and chondroitin had no significant effects in the same study. This was a small study with only five dogs per group; therefore, results should be interpreted cautiously.

A double-blinded placebo-controlled clinical trial of a commercially available product containing calcium fructoborate showed some potential improvements in osteoarthritis pain in dogs based on client assessments (Canine Brief Pain Inventory [CBPI]), but there was no effect on peak vertical force from a pressure map (Price et al. 2017). Further studies are needed to assess potential use of orally administered calcium fructoborate in dogs with osteoarthritis.

References

American Animal Hospital Association (AAHA). (2007). Pain management in dogs and cats. https://www.aaha.org/public_documents/professional/guidelines/painmngt_dogcathandouts-web.pdf.

Bhathal, A., Spryszak, M., Louizos, C. et al. (2017). Glucosamine and chondroitin usein canines for osteoarthritis: a review. *Open Vet. J.* 7 (1): 36–49.

Budsberg, S.C., Torres, B.T., Kleine, S.A. et al. (2018). Lack of effectiveness of tramadol hydrochloride for the treatment of pain and joint dysfunction in dogs with chronic osteoarthritis. *J. Am. Vet. Med. Assoc.* 252 (4): 427–432.

Comblain, F., Serisier, S., Barthelemy, N. et al. (2016). Review of dietary supplements for the management of osteoarthritis in dogs in studies from 2004 to 2014. *J. Vet. Pharmacol. Ther.* 39 (1): 1–15.

D'Altilio, M., Peal, A., Alvey, M. et al. (2007). Therapeutic efficacy and safety of undenatured type II collagen singly or in combination with glucosamine and chondroitin in arthritic dogs. *Toxicol. Mech. Methods* 17 (4): 189–196.

Dycus, D.L., Levine, D., and Marcellin-Little, D.J. (2017). Physical rehabilitation for the management of canine hip dysplasia. *Vet. Clin. North Am. Small Anim. Pract.* 47 (4): 823–850.

Epstein, M., Rodan, I., Griffenhagen, G. et al. (2015). 2015 AAHA/AAFP pain management guidelines for dogs and cats. *J. Am. Anim. Hosp. Assoc.* 51 (2): 67–84.

Frye, C.W., Shmalberg, J.W., and Wakshlag, J.J. (2016). Obesity, exercise and orthopedic disease. *Vet. Clin. North Am. Small Anim. Pract.* 46 (5): 831–841.

Gruen, M.E., Dorman, D.C., and Lascelles, B.D.X. (2017). Caregiver placebo effect in analgesic clinical trials for cats with naturally occurring degenerative joint disease-associated pain. *Vet. Rec.* 180 (19): 473.

KuKanich, B. (2013). Outpatient oral analgesics in dogs and cats beyond nonsteroidal antiinflammatory drugs: an evidence-based approach. *Vet. Clin. North Am. Small Anim. Pract.* 43 (5): 1109–1125.

KuKanich, B. (2016). Pharmacokinetics and pharmacodynamics of oral acetaminophen in combination with codeine in healthy greyhound dogs. *J. Vet. Pharmacol. Ther.* 39 (5): 514–517.

Lascelles, B.D., Gaynor, J.S., Smith, E.S. et al. (2008). Amantadine in a multimodal analgesic regimen for alleviation of refractory osteoarthritis pain in dogs. *J. Vet. Intern. Med.* 22 (1): 53–59.

Martin, W.R. and Eades, C.G. (1964). A comparison between acute and chronic physical dependence in the chronic spinal dog. *J. Pharmacol. Exp. Ther.* 146: 385–394.

Mealey, K.L., Peck, K.E., Bennett, B.S. et al. (2004). Systemic absorption of amitriptyline and buspirone after oral and transdermal administration to healthy cats. *J. Vet. Intern. Med.* 18 (1): 43–46.

Neirinckx, E., Vervaet, C., De Boever, S. et al. (2010). Species comparison of oral bioavailability, first-pass metabolism and pharmacokinetics of acetaminophen. *Res. Vet. Sci.* 89 (1): 113–119.

Norkus, C., Rankin, D., and KuKanich, B. (2015). Pharmacokinetics of intravenous and oral amitriptyline and its active metabolite nortriptyline in greyhound dogs. *Vet. Anaesth. Analg.* 42 (6): 580–589.

Price, A.K., de Godoy, M.R.C., Harper, T.A. et al. (2017). Effects of dietary calcium fructoborate supplementation on joint comfort and flexibility and serum inflammatory markers in dogs with osteoarthritis. *J. Anim. Sci.* 95 (7): 2907–2916.

Rose, W.J., Sargeant, J.M., Hanna, W.J.B. et al. (2017). A scoping review of the evidence for efficacy of acupuncture in companion animals. *Anim. Health Res. Rev.* 11: 1–9.

Scott, R.M., Evans, R., and Conzemius, M.G. (2017). Efficacy of an oral nutraceutical for the treatment of canine osteoarthritis: a double-blind, randomized, placebo-controlled prospective clinical trial. *Vet. Comp. Orthop. Traumatol.* 30 (5): 318–323.

Siao, K.T., Pypendop, B.H., Stanley, S.D. et al. (2011). Pharmacokinetics of amantadine in cats. *J. Vet. Pharmacol. Ther.* 34 (6): 599–604.

Streppa, H.K., Jones, C.J., and Budsberg, S.C. (2002). Cyclooxygenase selectivity of nonsteroidal anti-inflammatory drugs in canine blood. *Am. J. Vet. Res.* 63 (1): 91–94.

Sugisawa, R., Hiramoto, E., Matsuoka, S. et al. (2016). Impact of feline AIM on the susceptibility of cats to renal disease. *Sci. Rep.* 12 (6): art. no. 35251. https://doi.org/10.1038/srep35251.

US Food and Drug Administration (FDA). (1996). Freedom of information summary: NADA 141–053, Rimadyl (carprofen) tablets for dogs. Freedom of Information Office, Center for Veterinary Medicine, FDA, Rockville, MD.

US Food and Drug Administration (FDA). (2002). Freedom of information summary: NADA 141–203, Deramaxx (deracoxib) chewable tablets. Freedom of Information Office, Center for Veterinary Medicine, FDA, Rockville, MD.

Warner, T.D., Giuliano, F., Vojnovic, I. et al. (1999). Nonsteroid drug selectivities for cyclo-oxygenase-1 rather than cyclo-oxygenase-2 areassociated with human gastrointestinal toxicity: a full in vitro analysis. *Proc. Natl. Acad. Sci. USA.* 96 (13): 7563–7568.

Welch SL. (2000). Local anesthetic toxicosis. Veterinary Medicine. https://aspcapro.org/sites/default/files/toxbrief_0900.pdf.

9

Pharmacotherapeutics of Infectious Disease

Mark G. Papich

Clinical Pharmacology, College of Veterinary Medicine, North Carolina State University, Raleigh, NC, USA

Key Points

- Antimicrobial therapy in veterinary patients follows the same principles as those used for treating infections in human patients. However, species differences exist in:
  - Most common pathogens
  - Drug disposition, including oral bioavailability
  - Adverse drug effects
  - Breakpoints for determining antimicrobial susceptibility.

- Pharmacists should be aware that the FDA prohibits use of some antimicrobial drugs in certain species.
- Antimicrobial stewardship guidelines exist with the intent of minimizing antimicrobial resistance.
- Bacterial, viral, fungal, and protozoal infections are common in veterinary species.

9.1 Introduction

The infectious diseases considered for this chapter will be bacterial, fungal, protozoal, and viral. Infections caused by parasites are covered in Chapter 7, so they will not be included here. Bacterial diseases are the most common infections treated and have the most antimicrobial agent approvals for animals. Human-labeled drugs are also prescribed for bacterial infections in veterinary patients. There is only one antifungal drug approved for animals, but other human drugs are used. There are no antiviral agents approved for use in veterinary medicine, but a few human drugs are used. A number of antiprotozoal drugs are approved for use in veterinary species, but human-labeled drugs are also prescribed.

9.2 Comparative Aspects of Infectious Diseases

Bacterial, viral, fungal, and protozoal infections are a common cause of disease in all veterinary species. Pharmacists are likely to be familiar with some of the pathogens that infect veterinary species because these pathogens are also common causes of infection in human patients (e.g. Staphylococci, *Escherichia coli*, Trichophyton, *Giardia*,

---

Pharmacotherapeutics for Veterinary Dispensing, First Edition. Edited by Katrina L. Mealey.
© 2019 John Wiley & Sons, Inc. Published 2019 by John Wiley & Sons, Inc.

and others). However, other pathogens are more common, or exclusively, pathogens of veterinary patients (e.g. *Bordetella bronchiseptica, Rhodococcus equi, Pasteurella multocida,* equine herpes virus, *Hepatozoon canis,* and others). Pharmacists should be aware of which pathogens pose a high risk for zoonotic transmission so that they can provide appropriate counseling to pet owners. A list of zoonotic diseases can be found in Appendix I.

It is important for pharmacists to understand that not all pathogens that cause infections in both veterinary and human patients undergo zoonotic transmission. In some instances, humans and animals can contract the same infection simply because they share the same environment. For example, diagnosis of blastomycosis in a pet dog may be a sentinel for the household. Among households where a dog or person was diagnosed with blastomycosis, another member of that household was diagnosed within a short time period 14% of the time. Similarly, coccidioidomycosis in veterinary patients (dogs and a horse) helped the US Centers of Disease and Prevention (CDC) confirm that the fungus is endemic to parts of Washington State, previously thought to be free of *Coccidioides*.

Box 9.1 Terminology

"Antibiotic" refers to a compound synthesized by microorganisms, whereas "antimicrobial" is a compound that is effective against organisms other than just bacteria. Not all antibacterial drugs are antibiotics, and not all antimicrobials are antibacterial. In this chapter, antibiotic, antimicrobial, and antibacterial will be used interchangeably. Some standard-setting organizations have preferred terminology. For example, the Clinical and Laboratory Standards Institute (CLSI) prefers the term "antimicrobial agent" to refer to these drugs.

There are also important examples of "reverse zoonosis," whereby humans transmit infectious diseases to animals. Bacterial, viral, fungal, and protozoal infections have been spread to animals from people. Understanding this risk is important not only in preventing animal suffering when humans serve as a biological threat to animals, but in some instances the animal can remain a carrier and transmit the pathogen to other humans. This has been the case with *Staphylococcus aureus* (normal flora in people, but not dogs), for example. Pharmacists dispensing antimicrobial drugs to veterinary patients will become a critical link in the One Health strategy working to prevent transmission of disease *between* animals and humans (rather than simply assuming that disease transmission occurs in one direction only: from animals to humans).

9.3 Antibiotics (Antibacterial Agents)

Antibacterial drugs are the most frequently prescribed drugs in veterinary medicine for treating infections. Although many of the older drugs are still useful, some new drugs with better activity and more favorable pharmacokinetics have become available. In animals, we use both veterinary-labeled drugs and human-labeled antimicrobials. Veterinarians can use veterinary-labeled drugs more effectively because we have a database of species-specific pharmacokinetic information, and susceptibility testing standards for antimicrobials used in veterinary medicine. Veterinarians can prescribe more accurately and avoid unnecessary use and misuse thanks to this information. Species-specific drug dose regimens are available in other resources (Papich 2016; Riviere and Papich 2018).

This chapter will review general principles of antibiotic therapy, the major classes of antibiotics, and their use in veterinary medicine. References to specific diseases are also available to consider the rational use of anti-biotics for these conditions and the factors that influence therapy.

One of the growing concerns in veterinary medicine is the emergence of drug-resistant bacteria. Drug-resistant bacteria are increasingly important, and sometimes highly active drugs developed for people are used in animals to treat these infections. Concerns over drug residues in food animals, and the development of bacterial resistance to antibiotics in food animals, have increased public awareness for responsible use of antimicrobials. Because of the risk of drug-resistant bacteria in food animals that may pose a public health threat, risk assessments are performed on new drugs, and some drugs may be restricted for use or even banned for veterinary use.

9.3.1 Important Terminology

9.3.1.1 MIC
Following administration, it is possible to achieve concentrations that either kill or inhibit bacteria. The minimal inhibitory concentration (MIC) is the lowest concentration that inhibits visible bacterial growth in appropriate culture media and testing conditions. Other terms used to define bacterial susceptibility are the MIC_{50} and the MIC_{90}: These values are the *in vitro* concentrations needed to inhibit 50% and 90% of bacterial isolates, respectively. It is sometimes cited in error that the MIC_{50} and MIC_{90} are the concentrations necessary for 50% and 90% efficacy.

9.3.1.2 Bactericidal and Bacteriostatic Antibiotics
Some drugs have been classified as *bactericidal*, others are *bacteriostatic*, and for some drugs it is variable. This classification is entirely determined using laboratory (*in vitro*) testing and often has no relationship to clinical effects.

The clinical importance of bacteriostatic versus bactericidal has been exaggerated. Some drugs produce both effects, depending on the concentration and species of bacteria. It has been assumed that immunosuppressed patients require bactericidal treatment. However, this has not been confirmed in clinical studies. In human medical studies, there was no difference in outcome between bactericidal and bacteriostatic agents, including patients receiving immunosuppressive drugs (anticancer drugs) (Nemeth et al. 2015). Pharmacists should assume that drugs and diseases that can cause immunosuppression in human patients will do so in veterinary patients. Table 9.1 lists causes of immunosuppression in veterinary patients that pharmacists may be unfamiliar with.

Table 9.1 Potential causes of immunosuppression in veterinary species.

Species	Viral	Drugs	Diseases/conditions
Canine	CPV	Cyclosporine (Atopica™) Toceranib (Palladia™) Oclacitinib (Apoquel™) Drugs that are immunosuppressive for human patients	Cancer Diabetes mellitus Hyperadrenocorticism
Feline	FeLV FIV FPV	Drugs that are immunosuppressive for canine and human patients	Cancer Diabetes mellitus
Equine	EIA	Drugs that are immunosuppressive in other species	Failure of passive transfer in foals PPID

CPV, Canine parvovirus; FeLV, feline leukemia virus; FIV, feline immunodeficiency virus; FPV, feline panleukopenia virus; EIA, equine anemia virus (transient immunosuppression); PPID, pituitary pars intermedia dysfunction.

The lines separating bacteriostatic and bactericidal antibiotics are becoming more blurred. Drugs now are usually referred to as time-dependent or concentration-dependent (as discussed further in this chapter). Macrolides, chloramphenicol, and tetracyclines may be more bactericidal than once thought. Some older references have suggested that clinicians should not simultaneously administer drugs that produce *both* a bactericidal and bacteriostatic effect. Does this produce an interaction that will compromise effective therapy? Apparently not. There are no documented situations in veterinary medicine in which these combinations produce a less effective interaction.

9.3.2 Relationship of MIC to Clinical Outcome (Pharmacokinetic-Pharmacodynamic Relationships)

To predict antibacterial efficacy in patients, the concentration of the drug in the blood (or plasma or serum) has been related to clinical outcome by examining the magnitude and duration of the drug concentration above the MIC. Referring to Figure 9.1, the terms most often used are:

- C_{MAX}/MIC: Ratio of the maximum plasma concentration (peak) to the MIC
- *Time above MIC:* Duration (hours) that plasma concentrations remain above MIC during a 24-hour dosing interval. Often abbreviated as T > MIC.
- *AUC/MIC:* A measure of total drug exposure. The AUC is the area under the curve for the time versus concentration profile. The AUC/MIC ratio is the ratio of the total area under the plasma concentration versus time curve (AUC) during a 24-hour interval to the MIC. Sometimes abbreviated as AUC_{24}/MIC.

To achieve a cure, the drug concentration in plasma, serum, or tissue fluid should be maintained above the MIC, or some multiple of the MIC, for at least a portion of the dose interval. When pharmacokinetic data are used with pharmacodynamic information (i.e. MIC data), it is possible to develop more accurate dosing guidelines. Antibacterial dosage regimens are based on this assumption. However, antibacterial drugs vary in the type of exposure needed for a clinical cure. Some drugs achieve a better cure rate with high peak concentrations (C_{MAX}/MIC); other drugs are more effective when there is a longer duration above the MIC (T > MIC). For several drugs,

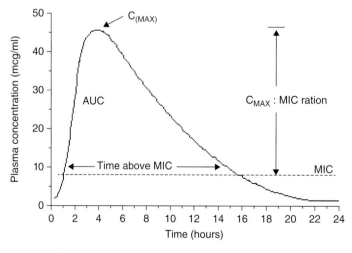

Figure 9.1 Pharmacokinetic-pharmacodynamic (PK-PD) relationships relevant to veterinary antibacterial drugs.

the total exposure – measured as AUC/MIC – is the best way to predict clinical success. Pharmacokinetic-pharmacodynamic (PK-PD) relationships consider how these factors correlate with clinical outcome and how dosage regimens can be formulated that optimize the PK-PD relationships. Some examples of how these relationships affect drug regimens are described throughout the remainder of this section.

9.3.2.1 Beta-Lactam Antibiotics (Time-Dependent)

Beta-lactam antibiotics such as penicillins, potentiated aminopenicillins (amoxicillin-clavulanate), and cephalosporins require exposure over time for the full inhibition of target enzymes, so their concentrations should be kept above the MIC throughout as much of the dosing interval as possible (approximately one-half the interval for most drugs). Dosage regimens for the beta-lactam antibiotics should consider these pharmacodynamic relationships. Therefore, for treating a Gram-negative infection, especially a serious one, it is necessary to administer many of the penicillin derivatives and cephalosporins three to four times per day if they have short half-lives (as is the case in most veterinary species). Long-acting drugs can be used to take advantage of a long half-life and less frequent dosing. For example, some third-generation veterinary cephalosporins have long half-lives (five or six days for cefovecin in dogs and cats, respectively), and less frequent regimens have been used for some of these drugs (e.g. ceftiofur, cefpodoxime proxetil, and cefovecin [Convenia, Zoetis]).

9.3.2.2 Aminoglycosides (Concentration-Dependent)

Aminoglycosides (e.g. gentamicin or amikacin) are more bactericidal when the peak plasma concentration/MIC ratio is high. After attaining this peak, plasma concentrations can fall below the MIC for 8–12 hours and achieve a cure because of a post-antibiotic effect that suppresses bacterial growth.

For example, if a high enough dose is administered once daily, it will produce a peak of 8–10× the MIC (a C_{MAX}/MIC ratio of 8–10). This regimen is at least as effective as, and less nephrotoxic than, lower doses administered more frequently. Most of our clinical regimens in animals employ this strategy. Gentamicin can be administered safely and effectively at a dose of 10–15 mg/kg once-daily intravenously (IV) for dogs and 4–6.8 mg/kg for horses. The corresponding dose for amikacin is 15–30 mg/kg IV for dogs and 7–15 mg/kg for horses.

9.3.2.3 Fluoroquinolones

For the veterinary fluoroquinolone antimicrobials (enrofloxacin, marbofloxacin, danofloxacin, orbifloxacin, and pradofloxacin), either the peak concentration or the area under the plasma concentration curve ratio (AUC) may predict antibacterial success. In addition to higher cure rates, high peak concentration/MIC ratios have been associated with a lower incidence of resistance. A peak concentration that is 8–10× the MIC (C_{MAX}/MIC ratio of 8–10), or a AUC/MIC ratio greater than 100–125, has been associated with the optimum antibacterial effect. For Gram-positive bacteria, a AUC/MIC ratio of 30–50 may be sufficient for some infections. The AUC is measured for an entire 24-hour interval, regardless of the frequency of administration.

To achieve this goal, fluoroquinolones are administered once daily with equal effectiveness as a dose regimen that divides the dose into fractions of two or three doses per day. The magnitude of the dose can be adjusted to account for differences in MIC among bacteria. For bacteria with a high MIC, an increase in the dose will proportionately increase the AUC. For treating susceptible bacteria, the veterinary fluoroquinolones such as enrofloxacin, marbofloxacin, pradofloxacin, and orbifloxacin are usually administered once daily. For food animals, enrofloxacin and danofloxacin administration is effective with administration, either daily at a low dose or given as a single high dose.

9.3.2.4 Other Time-Dependent Antimicrobial Drugs

Drugs that are considered time-dependent include tetracyclines, macrolides (erythromycin), chloramphenicol, trimethoprim–sulfonamides, and clindamycin. These drugs are usually considered bacteriostatic (although this definition is fuzzy, as mentioned in Section 9.3.1.2). For these drugs, drug concentrations should be maintained at the site of infection above the MIC throughout most of the dosing interval. The clinical efficacy is predicted from the time above MIC (T > MIC), or also measured from the AUC/MIC ratio. For macrolide antibiotics that have long persistent effects (e.g. azithromycin, tulathromycin, gamithromycin, and tildipirosin), the AUC/MIC is the best predictor of clinical effect.

9.3.3 Antibacterial Drug Resistance

Antimicrobial drug resistance is an important problem that makes successful therapy more difficult. Resistant bacteria emerge in veterinary patients through horizontal spread, through transfer of genetic elements carrying genes for resistance, and from mutations arising during treatment. An infection typically consists of a mixed population of susceptible wild-type and resistant bacteria. The resistant strains can emerge and become dominant through selection and amplification. Antibiotics administered to dogs and cats do not necessarily *cause* resistance in bacteria. A more accurate description is that antibiotic exposure – if not active enough to eliminate resistant isolates – can select for resistant strains, which then can multiply and flourish. Resistant strains emerge because the competition from more susceptible bacteria is reduced or eliminated during antibiotic administration. The resistant strains can potentially be transferred to other animals, people, and the environment. Inadequate antibiotic treatment consisting of doses too low, infrequent administrations, or selection of a poorly active drug is probably the most common reason for emergence of drug resistance.

Over many years of antibiotic use, resistant strains have been selected that are encountered in veterinary practice. Many of these resistant strains are now common, making it difficult for veterinarians to select effective antibiotics for some patients. Bacteria that cause resistant infections in small animals are (not necessarily in order) *E. coli*, *Pseudomonas aeruginosa*, methicillin-resistant *Staphylococcus* species, and *Enterococcus* species. The extent to which prescribing practices can influence this trend is not straightforward.

Many studies in veterinary and human medicine indicate that antibiotic use increases the risk for emergence of resistant bacteria. Previous antibiotic administration, hospitalization, and prolonged treatment are all risk factors. Because of the co-selection and persistence of resistance genes, it is not entirely clear that a single antibiotic, or antibiotic class, is responsible for the emergence of resistance, and a precise correlation between specific antibiotic class use and resistance is difficult to establish. Infection control for some bacteria may be more important than restrictions on antibiotic use. Pharmacists should counsel pet owners to follow reasonable infection control precautions when antibiotics are dispensed.

9.3.3.1 Antibiotic Stewardship Principles

Antimicrobial stewardship refers to the actions that veterinarians take to preserve the effectiveness and availability of antimicrobial drugs for both human and veterinary patients. Recently, the American Veterinary Medical Association (AVMA) published a Stewardship Definition (see https://www.avma.org/KB/Policies/Pages/Antimicrobial-Stewardship-for-Veterinarians-Defined.aspx). Specifically, the AVMA offers this definition: "Antimicrobial stewardship involves maintaining animal health and welfare by implementing a variety of preventive and management strategies to prevent common diseases; using an evidence-based approach in making decisions to use antimicrobial drugs; and then using antimicrobials judiciously, sparingly, and with continual evaluation of the outcomes of therapy, respecting the client's available resources." Among other core principles, the AVMA recommends antimicrobial judicious use principles and periodic evaluation of antimicrobial prescribing in veterinary hospitals. The AVMA has published several other resources to guide prescribers of antimicrobials. This resource can be found at this web site: https://www.avma.org/KB/Resources/Reference/Pages/Antimicrobial-Use-and-Antimicrobial-Resistance.aspx. Pharmacists can play an important role in implementing and monitoring the stewardship program.

Antibiotic use guidelines have been published by the International Society for Companion Animal Infectious Diseases (ISCAID; www.ISCAID.org), other organizations, and country-specific policies interested in promoting prudent and rational use of antimicrobials (Weese et al. 2011; Beco et al. 2013; Hillier et al. 2014; Lappin et al. 2017). These guidelines stress the importance of a careful diagnosis, and consideration for the most appropriate antimicrobial agent for the condition treated. The guidelines also list antimicrobial agents according to their use as first-tier, second-tier, and third-tier (or similar classification, such as first choice, restricted use, and last-resort use), which guides veterinarians on which drugs to select as empiric agents for treating routine infections compared to the agents reserved for treating resistant infections (Guardabassi and Prescott 2015).

9.3.4 Susceptibility Testing

Bacterial susceptibility testing is essential to good clinical practice. Although many infections can be treated empirically (selecting agents before susceptibility results are available), when treatment is complicated or resistance suspected, susceptibility test results can help guide antibiotic selection.

The most important information for the clinician is simply which drugs have an "S" (susceptible) and which ones have an "R" (resistant). These results then guide treatment. What really goes into this interpretation? The standards for interpretation are available from the Clinical and Laboratory Standards Institute (CLSI; http://www.clsi.org). Not all laboratories use CLSI standards; it is a voluntary program. However, it is the only global organization that develops susceptibility-testing standards for animals. If a laboratory does not adhere to a public standard such as CLSI's, breakpoints may vary, and interpretation may be inconsistent from laboratory to laboratory, or among different regions of the country.

9.3.4.1 Is Susceptibility Interpretation by CLSI Specific for Veterinary Species?

In past years, veterinary diagnostic laboratories had to rely heavily on CLSI interpretation from human standards. There were not enough veterinary-specific interpretive criteria available to establish breakpoints for veterinary drugs and veterinary species. There has been tremendous advancement in this area, and the current edition (published in 2018 and found at www.CLSI.org) of the CLSI standard document for veterinary drugs has tables clearly separated into those drugs with veterinary interpretive categories, and drugs that still rely on human standards for interpretation. In the last several years, CLSI has expanded the list of drugs for which there are veterinary-specific breakpoints. There are now several veterinary-specific breakpoints for human drugs. It should be noted that for most agents that are used in both human and veterinary medicine, the veterinary breakpoint is different – often much lower – than the human breakpoint. Examples of these differences are shown in Table 9.2. As shown in Table 9.2, there can be considerable differences in what is considered "susceptible" between humans and animals, and even between animal species and, for some agents (e.g. cefazolin), the tissue (urine vs. other). Isolates tested using human

Table 9.2 Comparison of susceptible breakpoints for antibiotics used in human and veterinary medicine; these breakpoints represent the limits for the "Susceptible" category.

Drug	Human	Canine	Equine
Amikacin	≤16 mcg/mL	≤4 mcg/mL	≤4 mcg/mL
Ampicillin/amoxicillin	≤8 mcg/mL (Enterobacteriaceae)	≤0.25 mcg/mL	≤0.25 mcg/mL
Amoxicillin–clavulanate	8 mcg/mL	≤0.25 mcg/mL	–
Cephalosporins first generation (cefazolin)	≤2 mcg/mL	≤2 mcg/mL	≤2 mcg/mL
Cephalosporins first generation (cefazolin for urine isolates)	≤16 mcg/mL	≤16 mcg/mL	–
Ciprofloxacin	≤1 mcg/mL	≤0.06 mcg/mL (not official)	–
Doxycycline	≤4 mcg/mL	≤0.12 mcg/mL	≤0.12 mcg/mL
Enrofloxacin	–	≤0.5 mcg/mL	≤0.12 mcg/mL
Minocycline	≤0.4 mcg/mL	≤0.5 mcg/mL	≤0.12 mcg/mL
Penicillin G	≤0.12 mcg/mL	–	≤0.5 mcg/mL

medicine standards might be reported as susceptible, when they are actually resistant if current veterinary standards are used. Until veterinary-specific breakpoints are established for other antibiotics used in companion animals, we will continue to rely on the human breakpoints for drugs such as chloramphenicol, erythromycin, carbapenems (imipenem), some penicillins, sulfonamides, and potentiated sulfonamides. The CLSI committee is working on filling in these gaps (CLSI 2018).

9.4 Overview of Major Antibiotics Classes

(Dosages and information on specific products are located in Papich [2016] and Riviere and Papich [2018].)

9.4.1 Beta-Lactam Antibiotics

The beta-lactams are among the most commonly prescribed antibiotics for veterinary patients. Their usefulness and popularity are related to their safety, efficacy, availability of a variety of dosage forms, and relatively low expense. They consist of the penicillins (natural ones such as penicillin, and semisynthetic ones such as ampicillin and amoxicillin), cephalosporins, and carbapenems (such as imipenem and meropenem). Their mechanism of action against veterinary bacterial pathogens is the same as that for human pathogens.

Important resistance mechanisms include a modified target, the penicillin-binding protein (PBP). Because of changes in this target, *Staphylococcus* species can become resistant. When this form of resistance occurs among *Staphylococcus*, it is referred to as methicillin-resistant *Staphylococcus aureus* (MRSA), which is the most common species of resistant *Staphylococcus* in human medicine. Veterinary strains (non-*aureus*) of *Staphylococcus* are also recognized as carrying this resistance. The most common in small animals

is *Staphylococcus pseudintermedius* (also known as MRSP). When MRSP strains are identified in veterinary infections, they are resistant to all beta-lactam antibiotics and usually carry multidrug resistance to other classes. These strains may require treatment with antimicrobial agents not labeled for or regularly used in veterinary medicine, such as chloramphenicol, rifampin, linezolid, or, occasionally, vancomycin.

Another major resistance mechanism is through production of beta-lactamase enzymes. There are many beta-lactamase enzymes that are capable of hydrolyzing the cyclic amide bond of the beta-lactam structure and inactivating the drug. In some classifications, they have been called penicillinases and cephalosporinases. Investigators have described over 190 unique beta-lactamase proteins that have this ability. *Staphylococcus* species produce these enzymes, which can be overcome by addition of clavulanate (e.g. Augmentin™ for human patients and Clavamox™ for veterinary patients). There are many important gram-negative beta-lactamases. This is a very diverse group that can arise through mutation or via transferable genetic elements (e.g. transposons or plasmids). Among the most serious gram-negative beta-lactamases are the extended-spectrum beta-lactamases (ESBLs). These beta-lactamases will produce resistance to even the most active (extended-spectrum) cephalosporins, as well as penicillins. The ESBL-producing strains of *E. coli* and *Klebsiella pneumoniae* are resistant to all penicillins, most cephalosporins, and other common agents. Often, the only agents active against these strains are carbapenems or aminoglycosides (amikacin).

9.4.1.1 Penicillin G

Penicillin G is historically important because it was the first antibiotic introduced in medicine. Penicillin G is effective primarily against gram-positive bacteria, especially *Streptococcus*, which can cause infections in veterinary species as well as humans. It is also effective against some obligate anaerobes, and the spectrum includes some important gram-negative veterinary pathogens such as *Pasteurella* spp. and *Mannheimia haemolytica*.

Formulations: Penicillin formulations are not practical for veterinary use, except when administered as injections to cattle, pigs, or horses by veterinarians who treat livestock. For small animals, there are very few bacteria susceptible, and the injections are not practical for routine use.

Adverse effects: Like most beta-lactams, adverse effects are rare. Adverse effects that have been reported include: immune-mediated reactions – allergic reactions (Type I hypersensitivity reactions); central nervous system (CNS) reactions – penicillins (and other beta-lactam antibiotics) at high concentrations can inhibit GABA (an inhibitory neurotransmitter) and cause excitement and seizures; and procaine, which is in some injectable preparations, causes excitement in some animals (horses).

9.4.1.2 Aminopenicillins (Amoxicillin and Ampicillin)

The addition of an amino group characterizes these penicillin derivatives as *aminopenicillins*. Amoxicillin and ampicillin are similar chemically and pharmacologically. Aminopenicillins are popular because they have a slightly broader spectrum of activity compared to penicillin G; they can be administered orally, and are relatively inexpensive and safe. Amoxicillin is better absorbed orally than ampicillin by a factor of approximately twofold in most animals.

Formulations: There are several injectable formulations, but their use is limited to in-hospital use, or injections to pigs, cattle, or horses by large animal veterinarians. Oral products that include amoxicillin include tablets, capsules, and oral liquid suspension. These are the same formulations as used in people, but some may have veterinary labels. For these agents, the human oral products can be used interchangeably with the veterinary oral products. However, the flavoring agents used for the human suspensions are often not palatable to veterinary patients.

An important difference between the aminopenicillins and penicillin G is that the aminopenicillins are not inactivated by gastric acid and may be administered orally. Amoxicillin has twice the systemic bioavailability of ampicillin when administered orally in pigs, preruminant calves, and dogs. For example, in dogs, the systemic availability for ampicillin is 30–40%, and for amoxicillin it is approximately 60–80%, but bioavailability may be decreased when administered with food. This group of antibiotics is absorbed poorly in horses and ruminants (except pre-ruminant calves; see Chapter 22) compared to other species following oral administration.

Adverse effects: Adverse effects from semisynthetic penicillins are similar to those from natural penicillins, in that allergy is a possibility. Oral administration of ampicillin, amoxicillin, and similar formulations may cause vomiting at high doses and diarrhea in some animals. Diarrhea is most likely caused by altered intestinal flora.

9.4.1.3 Beta-Lactamase Inhibitor–Penicillin Combinations

The beta-lactamase inhibitors are a specific class of drugs with little antibacterial effects of their own, but they inhibit the beta-lactamase enzyme. They are always combined with another active drug of the beta-lactam class. The primary drugs of this group are clavulanic acid (also called potassium clavulanate), sulbactam, and tazobactam.

The beta-lactamase inhibitors bind to the beta-lactamase enzyme that is produced by gram-negative or gram-positive bacteria. This usually is an irreversible, noncompetitive binding. An inactive enzyme complex is formed so that the co-administered antibiotic (e.g. amoxicillin or ampicillin) can exert its antibacterial effect.

Important examples include amoxicillin–clavulanic acid (Clavamox). This is one of the most popular oral antibiotics used in small animals. Clavamox extends the spectrum of amoxicillin to include many of the beta-lactamase-producing bacteria. There are equivalent drugs used in people (Augmentin and a generic version), which are among the most popular drugs in human medicine. The human formulation of amoxicillin–clavulanate behaves in an identical manner when treating infections in dogs and cats.

Dramatic difference

The human drug Augmentin is not entirely identical to Clavamox because the proportion of amoxicillin/clavulanate may be different. Clavamox has a 4:1 ratio, whereas the Augmentin amoxicillin/clavulanate ratio ranges from a 4:1 ratio to a 7:1 ratio. Despite the difference in ratios, the human product and veterinary product can be used interchangeably.

Two other beta-lactamase inhibitor–penicillin combinations are used in veterinary medicine. Both are injectable human drugs but are used in veterinary hospitals. Sulbactam–ampicillin (Unasyn) is a human drug, but similar veterinary preparations exist in other countries and are available for injection to dogs, horses, and cattle. Piperacillin–tazobactam is popular for in-hospital use in human medicine and also has been used in veterinary medicine. Often called "Pip-Taz," it has broad-spectrum activity that includes streptococci, staphylococci,

P. aeruginosa, and enteric gram-negative bacteria, including some ESBL-producing strains. Because of the requirement for frequent injections, it is not used outside of veterinary hospitals.

9.4.1.4 Cephalosporin Antibiotics

The cephalosporin antibiotics are extremely important in veterinary medicine. They have the same mechanism of action as penicillins but a broader spectrum of activity, and they are more resistant to beta-lactamase enzymes. Although the antibiotic was first isolated from *Cephalosporium acremonium* in 1948, they were not available commercially until 1962. There are now over 30 cephalosporin antibiotics on the market (most on the human pharmaceutical market), but new ones have recently been introduced to the veterinary market (Table 9.3).

The spectrum includes most of the same bacteria that are affected by amoxicillin and ampicillin, but also includes some beta-lactamase-producing bacteria, depending on the specific generation of cephalosporin, and greater activity against gram-negative bacteria. In general (with exceptions noted here), the cephalosporins owe their usefulness to activity against *Staphylococcus* spp. (beta-lactamase positive), but not methicillin-resistant strains, streptococci (but not

Table 9.3 Cephalosporins commonly used in veterinary species (excluding mastitis use in cattle).

Drug	Status	Clinical use
Cephalexin (Keflex, Rilexine)	Human generic form and approved canine tablets	Oral use in dogs, and occasionally other species
Cefadroxil (Cefa-tabs, Cefa-drops)	Veterinary approved and human generic	Oral use in dogs, cats, and occasionally other species
Cefazolin	Human generic	Injectable; widely used in many veterinary species, particularly as a prophylactic antibiotic intravenously at the time of surgery
Cefpodoxime proxetil (Simplicef)	Veterinary approved; human generic also available	Oral tablets approved for dogs (once-daily administration)
Cefovecin (Convenia)	Veterinary approved; no human equivalent	Injectable; approved for dogs and cats (a single injection lasts 7–14 days)
Ceftiofur (Naxcel)	Veterinary approved; no human equivalent	Injectable; approved for cattle, pigs, horses, and dogs (approved for urinary tract infection only)

enterococci), and gram-negative bacteria (except *P. aeruginosa*). However, the activity against gram-negative bacteria of the Enterobacteriaceae is highly dependent on the *generation*, with third-generation drugs being more active than first-generation drugs.

Formulations and routes of administration: The most common oral cephalosporin administered to companion animals is cephalexin. There is a veterinary-specific oral chewable tablet (Rilexine), but the human tablets and capsules can be used interchangeably. Oral cefpodoxime proxetil approved for dogs (Simplicef) is identical to the human formulation (Vantin). Cephalosporins formulated as the sodium salt for injection must be reconstituted before administration. The reconstituted preparations generally have a relatively short shelf life (except for long-acting ceftiofur formulations). Examples include cefazolin sodium and ceftiofur sodium. These are administered parenterally and are impractical for outpatient use, so they are unlikely to be dispensed by pharmacists.

Classification: The cephalosporin classification system (first-, second-, third-, fourth-, and fifth-generation cephalosporins, depending on their activity) does not differ for veterinary drugs compared to human drugs. As shown in Table 9.2, first-generation cephalosporins are used more commonly in veterinary patients than second-generation cephalosporins. Among third-generation cephalosporins, most of the injectable human-labeled drugs are used in veterinary medicine only when resistance has been shown to other drugs. Ceftiofur (Naxcel, Excenel, and Excede), an injectable veterinary third-generation cephalosporin, has been used extensively in cattle, pigs, and horses. Cefpodoxime proxetil is an oral third-generation cephalosporin, first used in human medicine, but now approved for veterinary use in dogs, (Simplicef and generic). Another addition to the veterinary drugs is cefovecin (Convenia), which is an injectable formulation that has an extremely long

half-life compared to other cephalosporins and has a duration of action of approximately two weeks. *Third- and fourth-generation cephalosporins are often called "extended-spectrum cephalosporins."*

Adverse effects: Most cephalosporins have a high therapeutic index and a good safety profile in animals. Some adverse reactions include allergies (although this is less common than for penicillins). Gastrointestinal (GI) problems occur from oral products. Some dogs vomit after receiving oral cephalosporins (e.g. cefadroxil and cephalexin), particularly at high doses. The bleeding disorders that have been reported with some cephalosporins in humans have not been reported to be a clinical problem in veterinary patients, probably because it is associated with only a few specific cephalosporins that are rarely used in animals.

9.4.1.5 Carbapenems

Carbapenems have the broadest antibacterial action of drugs currently in use, even surpassing many third-generation cephalosporins. In veterinary medicine, their use has been limited to serious infections caused by bacteria resistant to other antibiotics. None are approved by the US Food and Drug Administration (FDA) for veterinary use.

Carbapenem use has been limited to serious bacterial infections that are resistant to multiple agents. Other carbapenems are used in human medicine, but meropenem is the most common carbapenem used in veterinary medicine. Because they have the broadest spectrum of any available antibiotic, they are valuable in some patients that have not responded to other drugs. They have also been administered to exotic animals (Chapter 23) and marine mammals for treatment of resistant infections.

9.4.2 Aminoglycosides

The aminoglycosides include gentamicin, tobramycin, kanamycin, dihydrostreptomycin, netilmicin, amikacin, and neomycin.

These are all injectable agents (if intended for systemic use), or are used topically in ophthalmic medications, otic formulations, or other products to treat infections on the surface of the skin (ointments, lotions, or topical solutions). They are rapidly bactericidal and are most valuable for their in-hospital use to treat infections caused by gram-negative bacilli. Their systemic use by IV, subcutaneous (SC), or intramuscular (IM) injection is limited by the potential for toxicity. Adverse effects include nephrotoxicity, ototoxicity, and vestibulotoxicity. Kidney injury is the most common. Ototoxicity in veterinary patients may not be apparent until the animal becomes completely deaf. For this reason, aminoglycosides may not be an appropriate choice for service or performance animals (Chapter 24). Because prescriptions for outpatient use are unusual from a pharmacy, they will not be discussed in further detail in this chapter. Topical uses may be discussed in other sections in the book.

9.4.3 Tetracyclines

The tetracyclines include tetracycline, oxytetracycline, doxycycline, minocycline, and rolitetracycline. Chlortetracycline is the prototype, developed in 1948. Doxycycline and minocycline are the most important drugs in veterinary medicine to treat companion animals, horses, and exotic animals.

Long half-lives for tetracyclines, and persistence in tissues, can contribute to a long exposure and a high AUC/MIC. Long-acting forms of tetracyclines have been developed for large animal use (e.g. oxytetracycline, LA-200) that also extend this time interval. The long-acting injectable products are not used in companion animals.

Clinical use: Tetracyclines are broad spectrum because they are active against gram-negative and gram-positive bacteria, as well as *Chlamydia*, spirochetes, *Mycoplasma*, L-form bacteria, some protozoa (*Plasmodium* and *Entameba*), and

Rickettsiaceae. Protozoal disease treatments are covered later in this chapter. The family Rickettsiaceae includes *Rickettsia* and *Ehrlichia*. Tetracyclines, particularly doxycycline, are considered the first drug of choice for these infections. The rickettsia-like organism found in canine heartworms, *Wolbachia*, is susceptible to tetracyclines, which have been used as adjunctive treatment for heartworm disease and other filarial worms. In birds, doxycycline is the drug of choice for treatment of *Chlamydophila psittaci* (formerly called *Chlamydia psittaci*). Tetracyclines are useful against organisms that lack a cell wall that would ordinarily be resistant to beta-lactam antibiotics, for example *Mycoplasma* respiratory and joint infections. Another important use is for hemoplasmosis caused by hemotropic mycoplasmas (hemoplasmas) such as *Mycoplasma haemofelis* (formerly called *Haemobartonella felis*). Many anaerobic bacteria (70% or more) are susceptible to doxycycline. Tetracyclines are not consistently active against staphylococci and streptococci. The enterococci, *Pseudomonas* spp., and Enterobacteraceae (*E. coli, Klebsiella*, and *Proteus*) are usually resistant.

The oral route is a common method of administration. Oral absorption sometimes is erratic and unpredictable, but it is high enough for oral treatment in most animals. Calcium and other divalent cations will chelate tetracyclines and inhibit oral absorption, although this is less of a problem for doxycycline than for other tetracyclines. Absorption of tetracyclines is best if they are administered on an empty stomach in dogs, cats, and horses.

Formulations used in animals: Although it is not FDA approved for animals, the human form of doxycycline (usually the generic version) is the most common tetracycline used in veterinary medicine. Doxycycline is available in two forms, doxycycline hyclate and doxycycline monohydrate. Doxycycline hyclate (hydrochloride) has been used more commonly, but the monohydrate also is available. There are no reported differences between these two formulations with respect to oral absorption, but the hyclate form is associated with more injury to the esophagus (see "Adverse effects and interactions" below in this section).

The other common form of tetracycline used in animals is minocycline. Minocycline has a similar spectrum as doxycycline, but some *Staphylococcus* may be resistant to doxycycline (mediated by *tet[K]*) but susceptible to minocycline.

Adverse effects and interactions: Calcium-containing products or other di- or trivalent cations (Mg^{++}, Fe^{++}, and Al^{+3}) will chelate with tetracyclines and interfere with GI absorption. Doxycycline is less susceptible to this interaction and can be administered to people (children) even when mixed with milk before oral administration.

Doxycycline entrapped in the esophagus from a broken tablet or incompletely dissolved capsule can cause esophageal injury and stricture. This readily occurs in cats after administration of a capsule or broken tablet; thus, a syringeful of water, or some food should be administered after the doxycycline to ensure it is delivered to the stomach. Pharmacists should caution owners about the risk of esophageal damage with doxycycline. This problem has been primarily associated with doxycycline hyclate (the form most common in the USA), rather than doxycycline monohydrate.

Tetracyclines bind to bone and teeth. They may produce teeth discoloration and inhibit growth of long bones in young animals or the offspring of pregnant animals treated with tetracyclines. The true incidence of this problem is not known in veterinary medicine, but in human medicine, tetracyclines are avoided in children younger than seven years of age. It is prudent to avoid tetracyclines in animals during the time of teeth development. The effects on bones are probably only important with high doses.

Compounded forms: Doxycycline tablets made for people are often not suitable for some animals. Therefore, doxycycline hyclate

has been formulated into aqueous suspensions, sometimes with flavoring added, for oral administration to dogs, cats, horses, and exotic pets. These formulations in aqueous suspensions have been tested and retain nominal strength for only seven days. After that time, the formulation should be discarded and a new formulation prepared. The change was evident by examining a color change at seven days. When formulated in oil, the strength is maintained for the beyond-use date (BUD) allowed by the US Pharmacopeia (USP), which is not later than either six months or the time remaining until the earliest expiration date, whichever is earlier.

9.4.4 Amphenicols

Chloramphenicol is the most familiar and most commonly used drug in this group, but it also includes two drugs that pharmacists are likely not familiar with: thiamfenicol and florfenicol. Chloramphenicol is used in both veterinary medicine and human medicine, but the human use has declined because of the risk of serious adverse effects.

Chloramphenicol has a wide spectrum of activity that includes streptococci, *Histophilus somni* (formerly *Haemophilus*), *Salmonella*, staphylococci, *Pasteurella* spp., *Mycoplasma*, anaerobes (*Bacteroides*), and *Brucella*. The activity against *E. coli*, *Klebsiella*, and *Proteus* is unpredictable, and resistance is common. The activity against *P. aeruginosa* is poor. The activity against bacteria often considered resistant to other drugs – such as methicillin-resistant *Staphylococcus* and *Enterococcus* – has increased its use in small animal patients.

Rickettsia, *Chlamydia*, and *M. haemofelis* (formerly called *Haemobartonella felis*) are susceptible to chloramphenicol. Tetracyclines are usually the drugs of first choice for these infections, and chloramphenicol may be considered as a secondary choice.

Chloramphenicol is absorbed by the oral route in most animals. Injectable or topical products are rarely, if ever, used. Another advantage is the wide volume of distribution, which can be effective for treating infections that are intracellular or in difficult-to-reach sites such as the CNS.

Formulations available: In recent years, the use of chloramphenicol has increased because it is used for resistant infections in animals (non-food animals) when other drugs are ineffective. However, there are only a few preparations of chloramphenicol left on the market. Many human formulations have been voluntarily discontinued by manufacturers. Chloramphenicol tablets and capsules are most often used. The brand of Chloromycetin tablets (100, 250, and 500 mg) is an FDA-approved form for dogs, but it is not actively marketed. Chloramphenicol palmitate is an insoluble ester of chloramphenicol intended for oral administration. It must be hydrolyzed in the gut before it is active. This preparation is absorbed poorly in cats, particularly if they have been fasting (as most sick cats are).

Florfenicol: Florfenicol is a unique animal drug, closely related to chloramphenicol. It is not used in people. Because of a change in structure, it does not pose the risk of aplastic anemia in people and has greater activity against some bacteria. There are no products for oral or injectable use in dogs or cats, but sometimes the cattle products are used. Two topical formulations for treatment of ear infections (common in dogs) are available. The product Osurnia* contains florfenicol combined with terbinafine (an antifungal agent) and betamethasone (a corticosteroid) in a slow-release gel for treatment of ear infections in dogs. The product Claro™ contains florfenicol, terbinafine, and mometasone.

Clinical use: Chloramphenicol is banned for use in food animals because of the risk of residues in treated animals because drug residues may persist in tissue for 42 days after injection (see Table 9.6). But it has been used for a variety of infections in companion animals that are caused by susceptible organisms. It has sometimes been used when resistance has occurred to other drugs, for example multiresistant *Staphylococcus* and *Enterococcus*. It has been a drug of choice for

infections of the CNS and eyes. It also has been used for pneumonia, enteritis caused by *Salmonella* spp., and *E. coli*, as well as intracellular infections, anaerobic infections, pyoderma, and other soft tissue infections. In horses, chloramphenicol is used by veterinarians to treat pneumonia and pleuritis.

Adverse effects and interactions: A decrease in protein synthesis in the bone marrow may be associated with chronic treatment. This effect has been well-documented in cats and can occur after 14 days of therapy with standard dosages. Because of the potential injury to bone marrow cells, pharmacists should ensure that it is not used in neonatal animals or pregnant animals. Idiosyncratic aplastic anemia has been described in humans only. The incidence is rare (1/24 000 to 1/40 000 people who are exposed to chloramphenicol), but the consequences are severe. It is this risk that led to the ban of chloramphenicol use in food animals. Because of this risk, it is *extremely important* to warn animal owners about the risks from human exposure to chloramphenicol. It should be handled carefully (preferably with gloves) and kept away from children and other medications.

Dramatic difference
A unique adverse effect in dogs is a peripheral neuropathy. In dogs, this effect causes signs of ataxia and rear-leg paresis. Dogs usually recover if the medication is discontinued.

Chloramphenicol is a microsomal enzyme inhibitor. It will decrease the clearance of other drugs that are metabolized by the same metabolic enzymes. Drugs known to be affected are barbiturates and some opiates.

9.4.5 Macrolide Antibiotics

The macrolide antibiotics include erythromycin, tylosin, tilmicosin, and tiamulin. Erythromycin was the first of the macrolides, discovered in 1952. Newer derivatives of macrolides labeled for human medicine include clarithromycin and azithromycin. In pets and exotic animals, erythromycin is used rarely (because it is a frequent cause of vomiting in dogs), but azithromycin is in common use. There are newer veterinary forms for cattle and pigs (tilmicosin, gamithromycin, tulathromycin, and tildipirosin), but these are not used in other animals.

The concentration should be maintained above the MIC for a long time to achieve the best effects from these drugs. Fortunately, this can be achieved because of a long half-life for agents such as azithromycin in dogs, cats, and horses, and for the newer agents for cattle and pigs.

Macrolides are limited by their narrow spectrum of activity. The pathogens most often susceptible to macrolides are the respiratory pathogens of various species. Susceptible bacteria include staphylococci (*S. aureus* and *S. pseudintermedius*), streptococci, *Campylobacter jejuni*, *Clostridium* spp., some mycobacteria, *R. equi* (a common cause of pneumonia in foals), and *Mycoplasma* species. Gram-negative bacteria (e.g. *E. coli, Salmonella, Pseudomonas,* etc.) are inherently resistant. Other bacteria can also develop resistance with repeated exposure. For example, staphylococci causing pyoderma in small animals may develop resistance with continued use, and the incidence of resistance may be as high as 12–50%.

Oral absorption of erythromycin is inconsistent in animals because it is not stable in the stomach. Various attempts have been made to improve stability in the stomach, including salts of erythromycin, poorly soluble esters, and enteric coating. Azithromycin is better absorbed but requires some buffering of oral formulations to improve absorption from tablets or solutions.

Distribution of macrolides into cells and tissues is the feature that distinguishes this class from many other antibiotics. These drugs have a very large volume of distribution, which is particularly good in the respiratory tract, making them highly effective for respiratory tract infections. For the newer drugs such as azithromycin, tulathromycin, gamithromycin, tildipirosin, and tilmicosin, high concentrations in tissue persist for much longer than plasma concentrations. The affinity for some tissues (e.g. lungs, leukocytes, liver, etc.) results in concentrations 100-fold higher than plasma concentrations.

Formulations used in animals: Erythromycin oral tablets and capsules are not used much in veterinary medicine. They are not well absorbed and cause frequent vomiting. Pharmacists are likely not familiar with the veterinary product tylosin. Tylosin powder is administered as a feed or water supplement for control of *Mycoplasma* pneumonia in pigs and respiratory infections in poultry, but also it has gained use in dogs to control some forms of chronic diarrhea that have been referred to as "Tylosin-responsive diarrhea in dogs" (Chapter 12). The action responsible for this response is not identified, but it may be via an antibacterial property.

Adverse effects: Diarrhea and vomiting are the adverse effects most often associated with erythromycin. Erythromycin is a common cause of vomiting and regurgitation in small animals. In one study, erythromycin oral administration produced the most frequent adverse effects in comparison to other drugs. Although some nausea from the oral preparations is possible, most of this effect is believed to be related to a drug-induced increase in GI motility.

Dramatic difference

There is a special warning about the use of tilmicosin (Micotil) in people. It is labeled for use as an injectable antibiotic for respiratory infections in cattle. However, it is *very dangerous in people and horses.* Injection in people, either by accident or intentionally, will produce cardiac toxicity and death.

Clinical use of azithromycin (Zithromax®): Azithromycin is a substituted form of erythromycin with activity against gram-positive cocci, *Mycoplasma, Chlamydia, Mycobacteria,* and *Bartonella.* It has a very long half-life in dogs and cats that allows for infrequent administration (e.g. once-daily or once every 48 hours). It is most often used for respiratory infections. Because of its ability to concentrate in leukocytes, azithromycin is used in foals as a treatment for *R. equi* infections. Azithromycin also is used for some protozoal infections, which is covered later in this chapter.

9.4.6 Lincosamides: Clindamycin and Lincomycin

Clindamycin and lincomycin are the most common drugs from this class. They are not related to the macrolides by chemical structure, but there are many overlapping properties such as pharmacokinetics and antimicrobial activity. Lincomycin is the product of microbial fermentation. Clindamycin differs from lincomycin with only the addition of chlorine on the molecule, and it has replaced lincomycin for small animal use.

The lincosamides inhibit bacterial protein synthesis by binding to the 50S ribosomal subunit and interfering with the process of peptide chain elongation. The important feature that distinguishes clindamycin from the macrolides is that it has good activity against most anaerobic bacteria. Other susceptible bacteria include staphylococci (*S. aureus* and *S. pseudintermedius*), streptococci, *C. jejuni*, and *Clostridium* spp. Some human *Mycoplasma* are resistant, but most veterinary *Mycoplasma* are susceptible. There is little activity against most gram-negative organisms, particularly the enteric bacteria (Enterobacteriaceae). Clindamycin may have some activity on protozoa, but, except for *Toxoplasma*, it has not been commonly used for treating these infections. Oral absorption is good in dogs and cats. Clindamycin is absorbed better than lincomycin and is used more often.

Clinical use: Clindamycin is administered to dogs and cats as tablets, capsules, and an oral liquid (clindamycin hydrochloride) form available for small animals (Antirobe˚ and generic); the human formulation is clindamycin palmitate liquid (Cleocin˚), an ester that must be hydrolyzed in the GI tract.

Human formulations and veterinary formulations may be used interchangeably.

In small animals, clindamycin has been used for pyoderma, osteomyelitis, and soft tissue infections. Some veterinarians consider clindamycin a first drug of choice for treating staphylococcal pyoderma. Clindamycin also is useful for infections caused by anaerobic bacteria, such as infections of the oral cavity. After clindamycin became available, lincomycin has become rarely used by small animal veterinarians. When administering clindamycin, because of its narrow spectrum, its use is limited to infections caused by gram-positive bacteria. Clindamycin is used for some protozoal infections, particularly to treat toxoplasmosis (covered further in this chapter).

Adverse effects: The most serious adverse effect is intestinal bacterial overgrowth. Lincomycin and clindamycin have been associated with bacterial overgrowth, especially *Clostridium difficile*, in the colon. These drugs *should not* be administered orally in ruminants or small rodent pets. Serious and fatal diarrhea has been reported in humans, rabbits, ruminants, and horses from oral administration. In people, clindamycin-associated diarrhea is common, and a serious disease known as *pseudomembranous colitis* can occur as a consequence of clindamycin administration. This is an unusual and rare occurrence in dogs and cats.

Clindamycin as the hydrochloride form can be irritating. Like doxycycline hydrochloride, it has been associated with esophageal injury from oral administration to cats.

9.4.7 Oxazolidinones: Linezolid (Zyvox)

Linezolid is the first in the class of oxazolidinones to be used in medicine. It is valuable for treating resistant gram-positive infections caused by enterococci and streptococci in people. It is one of the few oral drugs that is consistently effective against MRSA and drug-resistant *Enterococcus* in people. Because of the increase in the incidence of methicillin-resistant *Staphylococcus* in dogs

Table 9.4 Drugs used for systemic treatment of methicillin-resistant staphylococcus in animals.

Rifampin
Chloramphenicol
Minocycline (confirm first with susceptibility test)
Linezolid (Zyvox and generic)
Vancomycin (injectable only)
Amikacin or gentamicin (best combined with other agents)

and cats (MRSP), linezolid is being prescribed with increasing frequency for animals, even though it is not labeled for veterinary use (Table 9.4).

Linezolid is one of the few drugs with efficacy against multi-drug-resistant bacteria that can be administered orally. Tablets are the most common form administered to dogs and cats. There is another oxazolidinone available for people, tedizolid (Sivextro), which is available in tablet (200 mg) and injectable (IV) formulations. It has properties and clinical indications similar to those of linezolid.

Linezolid is absorbed orally and is available in 600 mg tablets and oral suspension. The tablets are ordinarily very expensive – over $200 per tablet for the brand-name version. But recent availability of a generic version has greatly reduced this cost.

Adverse effects have not been reported from use in dogs in cats. However, because clinical use has been infrequent, there is insufficient experience to document the incidence of adverse events in dogs and cats. In people, nausea and diarrhea can occur. Long-term use can cause bone marrow suppression (e.g. thrombocytopenia) in people, but this has not been reported in dogs or cats.

9.4.8 Potentiated Sulfonamide Combinations

Potentiated sulfonamide combinations for veterinary medicine include trimethoprim and ormetoprim, in combination with one of three different sulfonamides. Potentiated sulfonamides have been used in animals for several decades. The most common forms are trimethoprim combined with sulfadiazine or sulfamethoxazole and ormetoprim (similar to trimethoprim) combined with sulfadimethoxine.

Trimethoprim–sulfonamide combinations are considered broad-spectrum and are active against pathogens in both large and small animals. Bacteria that are consistently susceptible include *Streptococcus* spp. (*Streptococcus equi subsp zooepidemicus* or *S. equi subsp equi* from horses), *Pasteurella* spp., *Proteus* spp., *Salmonella* spp., the protozoa *Toxoplasma*, and coccidia. Bacteria that can be susceptible, but can develop resistance include *Staphylococcus* spp., *Stenotrophoomonas maltophilia*, and *Nocardia asteroides*. The activity of trimethoprim–sulfonamide against anaerobic bacteria is variable. When measured *in vitro*, trimethoprim–sulfonamides have good activity against anaerobic bacteria, but clinical results are not as good because thymidine and para-aminobenzoic acid (PABA) (inhibitors of trimethoprim–sulfonamide activity) may be present in anaerobic infections.

Formulations: Examples of available formulations include trimethoprim and sulfadiazine (Tribrissen*, EQUILSUL-SDZ, Di-Trim*, Tucoprim, and others for horses). Trimethoprim–sulfamethoxazole (Bactrim*, Septra*, and generic) is a human formulation that is frequently prescribed for dogs and cats. Ormetoprim–sulfadimethoxine (Primor) is an approved form only for dogs. There may be differences in pharmacokinetic parameters among the sulfonamides. However, despite these differences, there are no clinical studies that suggest that one trimethoprim–sulfonamide product is therapeutically superior for treating infections caused by susceptible bacteria.

Sulfonamides are absorbed well in all species, including horses. It is one of the few oral antimicrobials that is well-absorbed orally in horses without causing an unacceptable degree of diarrhea. Oral administration to dogs, cats, and horses is the most common route.

Clinical use: Because other oral drugs can cause problems in horses, or they are not well-absorbed, trimethoprim–sulfonamides are sometimes among the few drugs that are inexpensive enough to treat horses. They are commercially available in formulations for horses, including oral paste and oral suspension. A common use is for treatment of respiratory infection caused by *S. equi*, for which it has FDA approval and proven effectiveness. Trimethoprim–sulfonamides have also been prescribed for horses to treat pleuritis, *Salmonella* enteritis, *Actinobacillus* infections, and protozoan encephalitis (often with pyrimethamine).

In dogs and cats, trimethoprim–sulfonamides have been used for pyoderma (staphylococcal), osteomyelitis, prostatitis, pneumonia, tracheobronchitis, and urinary tract infections.

Adverse effects: The list of adverse reactions is longer than that of other antimicrobials covered in this chapter, and dogs are more susceptible than other species. However, the risk of adverse events does not prohibit routine use for common infections. Most animals can be treated without adverse effects, and these drugs have been in use for many years. However, pharmacists can play a role in considering the relative risks of therapy prior to dispensing. There have been several attempts to explain the unique sensitivity of dogs to the adverse effects from sulfonamides. The currently accepted explanation is that canine species do not acetylate drugs. Subsequently, sulfonamides follow alternate metabolic pathways in dogs with a greater risk of producing a cytotoxic hydroxylamine metabolite. There is evidence that Doberman Pinschers are at more risk than other breeds.

Many adverse effects are caused by a reaction to a sulfonamide metabolite that can injure the liver, blood-forming cells, kidney, and skin. Fever and muscle or joint pain is also possible. The reaction is reversible if recognized and the medication discontinued. Pharmacists can play a key role in educating dog owners to monitor for these adverse effects. Another adverse event is keratoconjunctivitis sicca, also known as KCS and "dry eye" (Chapter 19). This reaction is caused by a lacrimotoxic effect in which the sulfonamide drug injures the tear-forming glands of the eye.

Mandatory monitoring

Dogs treated with sulfonamides should have tear production checked periodically during the course of treatment (Chapter 19). Other reactions that are less common are folate deficiency, thyroid dysfunction, and skin eruptions.

9.4.9 Fluoroquinolone Antimicrobials

Enrofloxacin, orbifloxacin, difloxacin, danofloxacin, and marbofloxacin are FDA-approved veterinary quinolones. Human drugs from this class also are used in animals, especially ciprofloxacin and occasionally levofloxacin, because they are available in inexpensive oral forms. Enrofloxacin (Baytril and generic) is the most recognized veterinary preparation, but orbifloxacn (Orbax) and marbofloxacin (Zeniquin) are also approved for treatment of infections in small animals. Pradofloxacin (Veraflox) is the newest drug, and it is approved for dogs and cats in Europe and approved for cats in the USA. Enrofloxacin injection (Baytril-100) is the first fluoroquinolone approved for cattle in the USA; it was approved in June 1998, followed by danofloxacin for cattle (Advocin) approved in October 2002. The FDA considers any use of fluoroquinolones in food-producing animals that is extra-label (an unapproved drug or unapproved dose) illegal (Chapter 22).

The quinolones have a unique mechanism of action. They inhibit two DNA enzymes that are important for DNA replication and function. One enzyme, called DNA gyrase (also called topoisomerase type II), is the dominant target for gram-negative bacteria. The mammalian form of DNA gyrase is resistant to the usual concentrations achieved; therefore, this produces selective inhibition of microorganisms. The other enzyme is topoisomerase IV, which is the primary target for gram-positive bacteria. Different affinity for these targets explains the higher activity for gram-negative bacteria compared to gram-positive bacteria. The advantage of the newer generation drugs (e.g. pradofloxacin in veterinary medicine and moxifloxacin in human medicine) is that they are capable of acting as dual inhibitors and inactivating *both* DNA gyrase and topoisomerase IV.

The quinolones are broad-spectrum drugs. Enrofloxacin, marbofloxacin, orbifloxacin, and ciprofloxacin have excellent activity against most bacteria; they are particularly active against gram-negative bacilli of the family Enterobacteriaceae (*E. coli, Salmonella, Enterobacter,* and *Klebsiella*), including some that are resistant to some aminoglycosides and cephalosporins. In addition, the spectrum may include *P. aeruginosa*, although higher concentrations may be needed. Other susceptible bacteria include *Pasteurella* spp., bovine and swine respiratory pathogens, and staphylococci. Fluoroquinolones have variable activity against streptococci and are not active against enterococci (*Enterococcus faecalis* and *Enterococcus faecium*). The activity against anaerobic bacteria is poor. Exceptions to this list are the human drug moxifloxacin and the veterinary drug pradofloxacin, which have better activity against gram-positive cocci and anaerobic bacteria.

Quinolones are sufficiently lipid soluble that they penetrate animal cells and are active against *Brucella, Legionella, Chlamydophila* (*Chlamydia*), and *Mycobacterium*, but activity against mycobacteria is inconsistent. They may be active against *Mycoplasma*, but this activity can also be inconsistent. The activity against *Mycoplasma hemofelis* in cats produces efficacy for treating feline infectious anemia. They have good *in vitro* activity against *Rickettsia. Actinomyces* and *Nocardia* are not susceptible at the typical concentrations achieved.

The quinolones are considered bactericidal in a concentration-dependent manner. Both the peak concentration (C_{MAX}/MIC) and area under the curve (AUC/MIC) have been used to predict clinical success. The AUC/MIC ratio has been the most consistently used, as it measures total exposure during a 24-hour interval. From clinical and experimental studies, a ratio of AUC to MIC > 100–125 is associated with clinical success. There is evidence that ratios in the range of 40–50 may be effective, particularly in immune-competent animals and to treat infections caused by some gram-positive organisms. To achieve the necessary concentrations for an optimum effect, flexible doses have been employed, so that low doses can be used to treat bacteria with a low MIC, and higher doses used to treat bacteria that have a high MIC. All doses can be administered once daily because the magnitude of the concentration is more important than the duration of activity.

Clinical use: Because of the wide spectrum of activity and clinical experience in many animal species, the fluoroquinolones are prescribed for many infections, including skin and soft tissue, urinary tract infections, pneumonia, and systemic infections. Use of these drugs as a first-line treatment for common, less serious infections when other drugs would be effective is discouraged to avoid promoting resistance. Organisms that have been associated with rapid development of resistance include *E. coli, P. aeruginosa*, and staphylococci. Organisms usually inherently resistant to traditional fluoroquinolones include enterococci (e.g. *E. faecalis*) and anaerobes (*Bacteroides* and *Clostridium*).

Pharmacokinetic properties: An important property of fluoroquinolones is their good oral bioavailability in all animals, including exotic and zoo animal species. This feature provides tremendous versatility to use these agents in many animals. Horses are an exception to this generalization, because the oral absorption of enrofloxacin is moderate, and absorption of ciprofloxacin is low (less than 10%). Therefore, ciprofloxacin is not suitable for oral use in horses, and oral doses of enrofloxacin may need to be higher than in other animals. Another important feature is their elimination by both kidney and liver mechanisms. Impairment of one organ system will not substantially alter the pharmacokinetics. An important metabolism feature is that enrofloxacin is partially converted to the active drug ciprofloxacin in most animals. Therefore, antimicrobial activity is enhanced by the metabolic formation of ciprofloxacin.

Examples of formulations: All currently approved fluoroquinolones have a similar spectrum of activity, although MIC values may vary slightly. There is no clear evidence for an advantage of one veterinary formulation over another for most infections. Against some organisms, ciprofloxacin (licensed for humans) is slightly more active than enrofloxacin, but it is not known if this translates to better clinical response. Pradofloxacin, a new drug for small animals, is more active against some pathogens but has not demonstrated superiority to other drugs in clinical studies. See Table 9.5 for examples of formulations used in animals.

9.4.9.1 Adverse Effects and Interactions

Central nervous system: Fluoroquinolones are generally well-tolerated, but some important adverse effects should be noted. High doses or rapid IV administration can cause CNS toxicity such as excitement, confusion, and seizures. There may be a risk with using these drugs in epileptic patients, but this has not been shown clinically. Headache and mental confusion have been reported in people from administration of fluoroquinolones, but it is not known if this occurs in animals.

Risks in young animals: In young, rapidly growing animals, these drugs can produce cartilage injury (arthropathy). In dogs, the window in which they are most susceptible is between the ages of 8 and 28 weeks. Cats and calves appear more resistant to these effects. Although young foals are susceptible to the adverse effects on joint cartilage, adult horses are resistant. The damage to the joint is related to the drug's ability to bind to and chelate magnesium in developing cartilage. The effects may be reversible if recognized early enough during the course of treatment.

Dramatic Difference

In people the effects on joint and ligaments have been highlighted. The EMA (European agency) has recommended discontinuation of fluoroquinolones in people because of these adverse effects. The most serious problem has been tendinitis, and rupture of tendons (eg, Achilles tendon) after use. This problem has not been identified in veterinary patients.

Ocular safety in cats: The FDA-approved dose for enrofloxacin (Baytril) for use in dogs is a range of 5–20 mg/kg/day. But doses in cats should not exceed 5 mg/kg. At higher doses, ocular lesions were reported in cats, including degenerative lesions in the retina. These lesions seem to be specific to cats. Fluoroquinolone ocular toxicity has reported after intravitreal injection of a compounded moxifloxacin product in people. Besides enrofloxacin, the other fluoroquinolones approved for use in cats are orbifloxacin (Orbax), pradofloxacin (Veraflox), and marbofloxacin (Zeniquin). These drugs have been tested in cats and were safe at 2× the highest label dose of orbifloxacin, 10× the lowest label dose for marbofloxacin, and high doses of pradofloxacin. Pharmacistists can play a role in preventing these reactions in cats by paying particular attention to the dose of enrofloxacin prescribed so that it does not exceed 5 mg/kg per day.

Drug interactions: Di- and trivalent cations (Ca^{++}, Al^{+3}, and Fe^{+3}) may inhibit oral absorption. Drugs containing these cations such as sucralfate, iron supplements, and oral antacids may decrease oral absorption via chelation. Fluoroquinolones may inhibit hepatic metabolism of some drugs. For example, clearance of theophylline is inhibited by co-administration of fluoroquinolones.

Regulatory status: The FDA has prohibited the extra-label use of fluoroquinolones in food-producing animals. Approved use of approved products is still allowed, but extra-label use of fluoroquinolones in food animals is considered illegal by the FDA. The basis of this action is a concern that use of fluoroquinolones in animals may contribute to the development of resistance in bacteria pathogenic to human beings. Other prohibited drugs are shown in Table 9.6.

9.4.10 Metronidazole and Related Nitroimidazoles

Metronidazole (Flagyl® and generic) is the most common drug prescribed from the nitroimidazole group. Tinidazole (Tindamax™) tablets are approved in people

Table 9.5 Fluoroquinolone antimicrobials prescribed for animals.

Drug	Brand name	Formulation	Species	Comments
Enrofloxacin	Baytril and generic	Tablets and 2.27% injection	FDA approved in dogs, and cats. Also used often in horses and many zoo and exotic animal species.	Oral absorption is good in most animal species. Most animals convert partially to ciprofloxacin. Do not give high doses to cats because of risk of blindness.
Enrofloxacin	Baytril-100	100 mg/mL injection	FDA approved for pigs and cattle, and also used in horses and some exotic animals.	This formulation is 100 mg/mL in an arginine base. This formulation has been injected in other species, and occasionally administered orally to horses. However, because of the arginine excipient, it is alkaline and caustic to the oral mucosa and irritating from IM injection.
Ciprofloxacin	Cipro and generic	250, 500, and 750 mg tablets, and 2 and 10 mg/mL injection	Not FDA approved for animals, but is often administered orally to dogs. Oral absorption in other animals is low.	Oral absorption in dogs is low and inconsistent. It is acceptable for oral treatment in dogs only if the organism has been identified and is highly susceptible (MIC less than 0.12 µg/mL).
Orbifloxacin	Orbax	Tablets and oral suspension	FDA approved for dogs and cats. Occasionally used in other animals.	Not as active as other fluoroquinolones but is well absorbed and attains high blood concentrations.
Levofloxacin	Levaquin, and generic	Tablets (250, 500, and 750 mg) and Injection	FDA approved for people, but not animals. Broad spectrum of activity. More active against gram-positive bacteria than others.	Although not FDA-approved for animals, it can be used legally in non-food animals. The oral absorption in dogs is approximately 100% and is conveniently dosed at 250 mg for small dogs, 500 mg for medium dogs, and 750 mg for large dogs.
Marbofloxacin	Zeniquin	Tablets (injectable in some countries)	FDA approved for dogs and cats. Also used in other species.	More active than some of the other fluoroquinolones against some gram-negative bacteria.
Danofloxacin	Advocin	Injection 180 mg/mL	FDA approved for use in cattle as the mesylate salt. Used primarily in cattle, but also has been injected in some zoo animals.	Approved for SC injection in cattle for bovine respiratory disease.
Pradofloxacin	Veraflox	Available as oral 2.5% suspension for cats, and outside the USA as tablets for dogs.	FDA approved only for cats in the USA, but for dogs in other countries. Experience in other animal species is very limited.	Pradofloxacin is one of the newer generation fluoroquinolones, which has broader activity than older drugs. It has better ocular safety in cats than enrofloxacin.

Table 9.6 Antibiotics prohibited from use in food animals by the FDA.

Chloramphenicol
Furazolidone and other nitrofurans
Fluoroquinolones used off-label
Glycopeptides (e.g. vancomycin)
Nitroimidazoles (e.g. metronidazole)
Sulfonamides in lactating cows (except approved drugs)
Cephalosporins: Extra-label doses are prohibited as well as unapproved formulations.

Note: For other prohibited drugs, see Chapters 2 and 22.

for treating *Giardia, Trichomonas*, and entamoeba. Similar drugs, but ones not available presently in the USA, are nimorazole (Naxogin), ornidazole (Tiberal), ronidazole, and benzindazole (Rochagan). Ronidazole is not an approved drug in the USA, but compounded formulations have been used to treat infections caused by intestinal *Trichomonas* in cats.

Metronidazole is a unique antimicrobial in that it has very little effect on aerobic gram-positive and gram-negative organisms, but it is highly effective against *anaerobic* bacteria (*Bacteroides, Fusobacterium, Clostridium, Peptococcus*, and *Peptostreptococcus*). It is not effective against bacteria that may be facultative anaerobes. It has good activity against many protozoa (e.g. *Giardia lamblia, Entameba*, and *Trichomonas*). The use for treating protozoal infections is covered later in this chapter. Metronidazole is rapidly and nearly completely absorbed in small animals and horses. It is also used in exotic and zoo animals, but it is illegal to administer to food-producing animals (Table 9.6).

Adverse effects: The most significant adverse effect is neurotoxicity. The reactions observed appear to be caused by inhibition of the GABA neurotransmitter. At doses exceeding the recommended dose metronidazole has caused ataxia, lethargy, proprioceptive deficits, nystagmus, and seizure-like signs in dogs. Dogs have recovered if drug administration was discontinued, but it may

require one to two weeks. Affected dogs may be treated with diazepam. Neurotoxicosis also has been observed in cats with high doses.

Its unpleasant taste hampers oral administration to small animals and horses. The drug is very bitter, and animals may salivate excessively or refuse oral treatments. This may be alleviated somewhat by using capsules, or using the compounded version of metronidazole benzoate (discussed further in this section).

There has been a concern expressed because metronidazole has been shown in some studies to produce mutations in bacteria. Carcinogenicity also has been expressed in laboratory mice with prolonged exposure, and cell transformations have been documented in cats. At this time, the clinical significance of these reactions is not known, except as it relates to prohibition of its use in food animals (see Chapter 2). Its use in pregnant animals is not contraindicated, but it should be used cautiously.

Formulations and clinical use: Flagyl and generic forms are available in tablets (250 and 500 mg tablets) and injection (500 mg/100 mL). In small animals, another formulation, metronidazole benzoate, is sometimes used. The benzoate ester of metronidazole is not an FDA-approved formulation, but has been used by pharmacists to compound metronidazole for small animal patients. Metronidazole benzoate is less soluble and lacks the bitter taste, which is especially important for treating cats. Because it is an ester, pharmacists must consider the potency when substituting for metronidazole. Metronidazole benzoate is 62% (by weight) metronidazole. Therefore, 20 mg/kg metronidazole benzoate delivers 12.4 mg/kg metronidazole. Oral absorption is good in cats and stable for 90 days when formulated with Ora-Plus and Ora-Sweet excipients.

Metronidazole is prescribed for anaerobic infections in non-food animals. These include oral infections (bacterial stomatitis), osteomyelitis, pneumonia (lung abscesses), and intra-abdominal infections.

Metronidazole also is prescribed for presurgical preparation for a patient undergoing intestinal surgery if a decrease in the anaerobic bacterial population in the intestine is desired. Some patients with idiopathic colitis and diarrhea respond to a trial of metronidazole, although this may not be related to the antibacterial effects (Chapter 12). Metronidazole is commonly used to treat giardiasis caused by *G. lamblia*, which is discussed in more detail later in this chapter.

Clinical use of ronidazole: Although not an FDA-approved drug, ronidazole has been compounded for cats. It is a preferred treatment for intestinal infections in cats caused by the organism *Trichomonas foetus*. It is one of the few drugs effective for eradication of this organism. This agent is covered in more detail with the antiprotozoal drugs later in this chapter.

9.4.11 Rifamycins: Rifampin

Rifampin is one of the group of rifamycins. Rifabutin is a derivative of rifamycin C and used for *Mycobacterium* infections in people. Rifampin is the most commonly used drug of this group in veterinary medicine. In some countries, rifampin is called rifamycin.

Rifampin has activity against gram-positive enteric bacteria, staphylococci, *Corynebacterium* spp., *Clostridium* spp., anaerobes, *Chlamydia*, and *Mycoplasma*. This drug has activity against *R. equi*, for which it has been used to treat infections in horses. In small animals, rifampin has activity against gram-positive bacteria, especially staphylococci, and including many methicillin-resistant isolates (MRSP). It has moderate activity against *Actinobacillus equuli* and *Pasteurella* spp. It has also been used in small animals for treatment of *Bartonella* spp. in combination with azithromycin or other drugs.

The mutation rate is very high among bacteria for rifampin, and resistance develops rapidly. For some bacteria, especially *Mycobacteria*, resistance is less likely if it is administered with another antibiotic; therefore, it is commonly administered concurrently with another drug for *Mycobacteria*. However, the need to administer with another agent has not been established for other bacteria (e.g. *Staphylococcus* species). There is sufficient evidence from human and veterinary studies that rifampin can be administered successfully as a single agent for treatment of infections caused by methicillin-resistant *Staphylococcus* species. Gram-negative bacteria are inherently more resistant by limiting penetrability.

Clinical use: Rifampin is not approved for animals. All use in veterinary species is extralabel using the human formulations. It is an important drug for treating *R. equi* infections in foals. Rifampin also has been used for *Corynebacterium* infections and intracellular *S. aureus* infections (e.g. chronic mastitis). It also has been used to treat Potomac horse fever. Cases of Johne's disease in goats (*Corynebacterium pseudotuberculosis*) have been treated, but the effect was only palliative.

In small animals, rifampin has been prescribed for resistant gram-positive bacterial infections. It has been valuable to treat methicillin-resistant *Staphylococcus* (MRSA and MRSP) that are otherwise multi-drug resistant. It may be useful for treating chronic granulomatous disease, osteomyelitis, septic arthritis, abscesses, and endocarditis. It has also been used in combination with other drugs (e.g. azithromycin) for treatment of *Bartonella* spp. infections. Rifampin has been used against *Brucella*, but this infection is not often treated clinically.

Adverse effects: Dogs are more susceptible to the adverse effects, because this drug reaches higher blood concentrations in dogs than other animals, which may be 10× concentrations achieved in horses at comparable doses. Rifampin increases liver enzyme activity in dogs and horses. In dogs, the most serious adverse effect is liver injury. This reaction has occurred in up to 20–25% of dogs. If liver injury is observed, rifampin should be discontinued immediately.

Owners should be advised that it will cause an orange-red color of the urine, tears, saliva, sweat, and feces (and will stain clothing from spillage of the equine formulations). Many horses develop loose feces when receiving rifampin. Horse owners should be advised to stop treatment if diarrhea develops. In addition, because horses are reluctant to swallow the drug because of bad taste, it may cause anorexia during treatment.

Drug interactions: Rifampin is a potent inducer of hepatic metabolizing enzymes (cytochrome P450 [CYP450]). Subsequently, it may increase clearance of barbiturates, digoxin, anticoagulants, itraconazole, ketoconazole, and steroids when they are administered with rifampin. Rifampin induces its own metabolism in horses, which may persist for days after cessation of therapy.

9.5 Antifungal Drugs

Antifungal drugs are important in all veterinary species: mammals, fish, reptiles, and birds. We rely primarily on just a few of these agents for systemic treatment. For many skin infections, topical treatment also can be used. For a thorough review of these drugs, consult more detailed books that have dosages and other details of the drugs' pharmacology (Papich 2016; Riviere and Papich 2018).

Treating fungal infections has some similarities to antibacterial treatment, but also some differences. There are far fewer drugs to select from for antifungal treatment – most are oral azole antifungal agents. Because fungal organisms grow much more slowly than bacteria, and the drugs are fungistatic, not fungicidal, courses of treatment are much longer than for antibacterial treatment. There are very few antifungal agents approved for veterinary use, and their indications are limited to dermatophytes. Therefore, veterinarians often have to prescribe human drugs. Fortunately, there are pharmacokinetic studies to guide dosing and clinical experience to guide drug selection for fungal diseases.

9.5.1 Griseofulvin

Griseofulvin (Fulvicin) is one of the oldest drugs used when systemic treatment is needed for dermatophyte infections caused by *Microsporum* spp. and *Trichophyton* spp. It is sometimes used in combination with topical therapy. Griseofulvin has a limited spectrum and is not effective for the treatment of yeasts or bacteria.

Because oral absorption is favored in the presence of fat, administration of the drug with a high-fat meal can tremendously enhance the extent of absorption. Administration of a formulation made up of fine particles also will increase absorption. Two formulations are available, microsize and ultramicrosize. Veterinary formulations are generally composed of microsize preparations, and this is reflected in the dosage regimens described further here. If the ultramicrosize preparations are used, the dose should be decreased by one-half.

Griseofulvin is metabolized primarily by the liver to demethylgriseofulvin and the glucuronide.

Dramatic difference
It is metabolized approximately six times faster in animals than in people, which is the reason why animal doses are higher than human doses (a half-life in dogs is reported to be less than 1 hour, as compared to 20 hours in people).

Clinical use: Although griseofulvin has acceptable efficacy, its use has diminished in recent years because of the need for a high dose, the requirement for administration with food, and the long duration of treatment needed. Many veterinary dermatologists prefer to administer an azole drug instead (these agents are discussed further in this chapter).

Griseofulvin has good efficacy for treatment of dermatophyte infections, but long-term therapy often is needed (four weeks or longer). Dosage recommendations have varied, and consulting with specific references should be used for dosing (Papich 2016). Treatment as long as four months may be necessary to treat onychomycosis.

Cats are the species most susceptible to the adverse effects of griseofulvin. The adverse effects may be dose-related, and pharmacists should warn owners of the potential for toxicosis. Do not dispense to pregnant cats, as there is a clear association between griseofulvin therapy and congenital malformations in kittens. Anemia and leukopenia have been observed in cats after griseofulvin treatment, particularly in cats with feline immunodeficiency virus (FIV). Whether this is caused by high doses or is an idiosyncratic reaction is not understood. These effects resolve in cats when treatment is stopped, but irreversible idiosyncratic pancytopenia also has been reported. Other adverse effects that may be seen include anorexia, depression, vomiting, and diarrhea. The dosage should be decreased if these signs occur.

9.5.2 Amphotericin B

Amphotericin B (Fungizone) is an important antifungal agent for serious or life-threatening systemic fungal infections. It is administered by injection, usually by intravenous infusion. Therefore, it is limited to in-hospital use and is not an agent dispensed by community pharmacies. Because of these limitations, the description here is abbreviated.

Amphotericin B is a polyene macrolide antibiotic with antifungal activity. It has no effect on bacteria but is active against some protozoa (*Leishmania*). Although it is a valuable drug for the treatment of serious systemic fungal infections, it is associated with a high incidence of adverse effects, which requires careful administration and patient monitoring.

The spectrum of activity for amphotericin B includes *Blastomyces dermatitidis*, *Histoplasma*, *Cryptococcus*, *Coccidioides*, *Candida*, and *Aspergillus*.

The most common veterinary diseases treated with amphotericin are blastomycosis, histoplasmosis, and coccidioidomycosis.

Ketoconazole and itraconazole have replaced amphotericin B as the sole treatment for some of these infections, because they are easier to administer. *(See the discussions of these drugs in Sections 9.5.3.1 and 9.5.3.2.)* Amphotericin B also has been used to treat canine leishmaniasis.

The most severe adverse effect, which is usually the cause for discontinuing therapy, is kidney injury. Early reversible nephrotoxicosis is seen with each daily dose, but permanent kidney injury is related to the total cumulative dose. Renal function should be carefully monitored throughout treatment. It may become necessary to abandon therapy with amphotericin if azotemia is persistent. Other adverse effects may include vomiting, tremors, pyrexia, and anorexia. These effects may be associated with each daily treatment and are somewhat alleviated with pre-medication with antihistamine drugs, nonsteroidal anti-inflammatory drugs (NSAIDs), and antiemetics. Phlebitis is a problem with IV administration. To avoid phlebitis, alternate catheter sites from one vein to another for administration.

Newer formulations made of lipid complexes are used in people, but use has been limited in veterinary medicine because of the high cost. The main advantage over traditional formulations is that lower toxicity allows administration of higher doses. The lipid formulation most often used in animals is amphotericin B lipid complex (ABLC, Abelcet).

9.5.3 Azole Antifungal Drugs

Azole antifungal drugs are the most important systemic antifungal drugs used in people and animals (Table 9.7). They exert their effects via inhibition of 14-alpha sterol demethylase (CYP450-dependent enzyme), leading to accumulation of methyl sterols, which disrupts phospholipids and inhibits fungal growth.

9.5.3.1 Ketoconazole (Nizoral)

Ketoconazole is one of the oldest in this group that is administered orally. It is still used frequently in veterinary medicine, but

Table 9.7 Azole antifungal drugs used in animals.

Drug	Brand name	Formulation	Use in animals
Ketoconazole	Nizoral and generic	Tablets	Oral administration to dogs and cats for dermatophytes and systemic fungal infections. Drug interactions and adverse effects are common.
Itraconazole	Sporanox (human form) and Itrafungol (veterinary form)	Capsules and oral solution	One of the most common azoles used in veterinary medicine. Active against a wide range of fungi. Oral absorption can be variable, but oral solution is absorbed more consistently than oral capsules. Avoid compounded formulations because they are not well absorbed orally.
Fluconazole	Diflucan and generic	Tablets	Oral use in dogs, cats, horses, and zoo and exotic animal species. Well absorbed and relatively safe, but the limited spectrum of activity limits its usefulness in veterinary medicine.
Posaconazole	Noxafil	Oral suspension and extended-release tablets	Oral suspension is adequately absorbed in dogs and cats. Tablets are better absorbed in dogs than the suspension. Posaconazole is the most active of the azole antifungal agents, with a wide spectrum of activity, but clinical experience has been limited. Human formulations are expensive for animals.
Voriconazole	Vfend	Oral tablets and oral suspension	Highly active azole antifungal agent with good activity against *Aspergillus*. Clinical use has been limited in dogs and cats because of high expense and concern about adverse effects in cats.

the use has diminished in human medicine because of adverse effects and drug interactions. At commonly used doses, ketoconazole is fungistatic. At least 5–10 days of administration are necessary before ketoconazole achieves a significant antifungal effect. Ketoconazole has a wide spectrum of activity that includes yeast (e.g. *Malassezia pachydermatis*), systemic fungi, dermatophytes, and bacteria such as staphylococci.

Ketoconazole is absorbed well after oral administration, but its absorption is favored in an acidic environment (i.e. after feeding). Concurrent use of antacids, H_2 blockers (famotidine or ranitidine), or proton pump inhibitors (omeprazole) will decrease absorption. In horses, unless administered in an acid medium, the oral absorption was nil. Even in an acid environment, oral absorption in horses is only 23%. Therefore, it is not used in horses.

Clinical use: Although ketoconazole is seldom used in people, it is still used in veterinary patients because of the low expense. It is effective for the treatment of yeasts such as *M. pachydermatis* (a common cause of ear infections in dogs) and infections caused by *Histoplasma, Coccidioides*, and *Blastomyces*. It is less effective for *Aspergillus* infections. It has been used alone to treat infections caused by *Coccidioides* and *Histoplasma*, but severe infections caused by *Blastomyces* are more effectively treated with amphotericin B.

Adverse effects: One of the disadvantages of ketoconazole is that it causes more adverse effects than other azole antifungal agents. Nausea, anorexia, and vomiting are the most common adverse effects. They are usually dose-related and may be diminished by decreasing the dose, dividing the total dose into smaller doses, and administering each dose with food. Ketoconazole inhibits the synthesis of steroid hormones (via inhibition of CYP450 enzymes), most notably cortisol and testosterone. Although this may be a side effect of therapy, it has been utilized for the temporary management of hyperadrenocorticism in dogs, and as an anti-androgen treatment. Steroid synthesis inhibition is a temporary effect that persists only during dosing with ketoconazole (e.g. for an eight-hour duration). Ketoconazole will not cause permanent hypoadrenocorticism. Some dogs may have a lightening of the hair coat with ketoconazole therapy. Cats may develop a dry hair coat.

Hepatic enzyme elevation may occur with treatment (especially alkaline phosphatase [ALP] and alanine aminotransferase [ALT]), and hepatotoxicosis is possible. This reaction may be idiosyncratic (unpredictable), but liver toxicosis appears more likely with high doses. Do not dispense to patients with signs of hepatic disease or to pregnant animals because fetal death may occur.

Drug interactions: Ketoconazole is one of the most potent inhibitors of hepatic and intestinal microsomal enzymes (CYP450 enzymes). It may inhibit metabolism and elimination of several other drugs. It also is an inhibitor of the MDR membrane pump known as P-glycoprotein (Pgp), which is involved in drug transport across the intestine, blood–brain barrier, and other tissues. An example of this interaction is seen with cyclosporine (see Chapter 14 for additional information). When ketoconazole is administered orally with cyclosporine, cyclosporine blood concentrations are increased in dogs. This has been used in dogs to lower the required dose (and therefore cost) of cyclosporine. Ketoconazole at 5–10 mg/kg/day will lower the dose of cyclosporine by one-half or more in dogs.

Pharmacists should advise pet owners not to administer with drugs that inhibit stomach acidity, such as antacids, H_2-blockers (cimetidine), or omeprazole. These drugs inhibit oral absorption.

9.5.3.2 Itraconazole

Itraconazole is an azole of the triazole group. Triazoles and imidazoles have similar antifungal mechanisms of action, but triazoles lack affinity for some of the CYP450 enzymes in animals, which results in fewer endocrine effects.

Itraconazole (Sporanox and generic) is one of the most frequently prescribed azole drugs. It has been used successfully to treat both systemic and cutaneous fungal infections in animals. It is considerably more potent than ketoconazole (5–100 times more active) and is associated with fewer adverse effects. Compared to ketoconazole, it has no endocrine effects. Itraconazole is highly protein bound in plasma, and there is strong binding to keratin. This binding produces drug concentrations in skin that persist two to four weeks after cessation of drug therapy. It is also excreted into the sebum, increasing the concentrations in skin. The persistent concentrations in skin allow for pulse-dosing for some diseases, such as dermatophyte treatment in cats in which a one-week-on, one-week-off treatment schedule can be used.

Itraconazole has a spectrum that includes *Histoplasma, Cryptococcus, Coccidioides,* and *Blastomyces. Candida, Aspergillus, Fusarium,* and *Penicillium* are less sensitive. Dermatophytes are also susceptible (e.g. *Microsporum* and *Trichophyton*), as well as cutaneous yeasts (*M. pachydermatis*). Itraconazole has been used to treat infections caused by all these organisms in dogs, cats, exotic animals, and zoo animal species.

Formulations: Itraconazole is insoluble in aqueous solutions. It is a weak base with a pKa of less than 3. Very low pH is needed to maintain solubility. Compounded formulations prepared from bulk powder may not be stable or soluble. The low solubility of compounded products results in poor oral absorption (and therefore low efficacy) in dogs and cats. Sporanox formulations include 100 mg capsules and 10 mg/mL cherry-flavored liquid solubilized by hydroxypropyl-beta-cyclodextrin (400 mg/mL) as a molecular inclusion complex, which is necessary to keep itraconazole in solution, thereby facilitating oral absorption. This liquid formulation has greater oral bioavailability in cats and horses than the capsules. The granules in the capsules or the solution may be added to food for convenience, but granules should not be crushed. The disadvantage of itraconazole human formulations is the cost of treatment.

The only FDA-approved veterinary formulation is Itrafungol, which is identical to Sporanox liquid. It is labeled for treatment of dermatophytosis in cats at a dose of 5 mg/kg once daily on alternating weeks.

Adverse effects: Itraconazole is better tolerated in dogs and cats than ketoconazole, but adverse reactions are still possible. Hepatopathy is not as common as for ketoconazole, but it has been reported to be as high as 10% of treated dogs. Liver enzyme elevations may occur in 10–15% of dogs. Hepatotoxicosis also is possible in cats and may be idiosyncratic. Anorexia may occur as a complication of treatment, especially with high doses and high plasma concentrations. It usually develops in the second month of therapy in dogs. In cats, there are dose-related GI effects of anorexia and vomiting (Mancianti et al. 1998).

Drug interactions: Like ketoconazole, itraconazole oral absorption is decreased when the stomach is less acidic. Oral capsules should be administered with food to increase absorption. The oral solution, on the other hand, can be absorbed on an empty stomach.

Some CYP450 enzyme inhibition occurs, and itraconazole may increase concentrations of cyclosporine, digoxin, and cisapride, when used concurrently. However, enzyme inhibition is less in comparison to ketoconazole. Itraconazole is also a P-gp inhibitor and may increase the concentrations of other drugs via this mechanism.

9.5.3.3 Fluconazole

Fluconazole is commonly prescribed to veterinary patients because it is available as an inexpensive generic drug. Fluconazole (Diflucan) is better tolerated than other azoles, but it is not as active against many fungi. Fluconazole is less active than itraconazole against dermatophytes, *Blastomyces*, and *Histoplasma*, but it has good activity against *Coccidioides* spp. and *Cryptococcus*

neoformans. In animals, it has been prescribed for blastomycosis, dermatophytes, cryptococcal infections, and yeast infections caused by *Malassezia*. It is also active against the yeast *Candida*, but it has weak activity against *Aspergillus* and filamentous fungi.

Fluconazole is more water-soluble than the other azoles, and therefore has different pharmacokinetic characteristics than ketoconazole and itraconazole. It is available in tablets, oral suspension, and IV injection. Fluconazole tablets (Diflucan and generic) and oral suspension 10 mg/mL are absorbed well, and the oral dose is similar to the IV dose. In horses, oral absorption was 100%, compared to low oral absorption for itraconazole and ketoconazole.

Clinical use: For cats with systemic cryptococcosis, clinical studies have shown a benefit from a dose of 100 mg/cat/day in one or two divided doses. It has also been used for blastomycosis and coccidioidomycosis in dogs.

Adverse effects and interactions: Fluconazole has no effect on endocrine activity. It has less of a tendency to cause drug interactions compared to itraconazole. Drug-induced hepatic toxicity is a possibility, but less so than with other azoles. Like other azoles, it should not be used in pregnancy. In people, fluconazole is known as a potent CYP450 inhibitor for some enzymes. Whether or not these enzymes are affected in animals is unknown.

9.5.3.4 Voriconazole (Vfend)

Voriconazole is one of the newer azole drugs. It is a triazole like itraconazole and fluconazole. It has become an important drug for humans, especially to treat disseminated aspergillosis. Its use in animals has been limited at this time, but work is underway to identify appropriate doses for mammals, reptiles, and birds.

Voriconazole has excellent activity against yeasts, dermatophytes, and some filamentous fungi. Voriconazole is similar in structure to fluconazole, but small changes increase the spectrum of activity and potency as well as the fungicidal activity against some species of molds, including *Aspergillus* and *Fusarium* spp. Compared to other azoles, it is the most active against the latter two organisms.

Voriconazole is well-absorbed after oral administration to dogs, cats, and horses. It has a relatively short half-life in dogs, and frequent administration may be necessary, although clinical studies have not been performed. In cats, the opposite effect seems to occur, with longer half-life after repeated dosing, and after oral administration compared to IV. After an IV dose, the half-life was 12.4 hours in cats, but after oral administration it was 43 hours. This may contribute to adverse effects in cats.

Clinical use: At this time, there has been little clinical experience with voriconazole in dogs and cats, primarily because of the high cost of oral medications and lack of clinical studies.

Adverse effects: Adverse effects consisting of CNS reactions and ocular problems have been reported in cats. This may be caused by high levels, as concentrations in people >5.5 mcg/mL are associated with neurotoxicity. Lower doses in cats may need to be evaluated. Voriconazole should not be used in cats until further information is available. Safety has not been established in dogs. However, because hepatotoxicity has been a problem in people, liver enzymes and bilirubin should be monitored in treated dogs. Like other azoles, it should not be used in pregnancy.

9.5.3.5 Posaconazole

Posaconazole (Noxafil) is the newest azole antifungal drug, available as an oral suspension (40 mg/mL), a delayed-release tablet (100 mg), and an injectable solution. It is similar to itraconazole, but it has a slightly different spectrum of activity and is more active (lower MIC values) compared to the other azole antifungal agents. In addition to other fungi in the spectrum of azoles, it is active against *Candida, Aspergillus, Mucorales* (formerly *Zygomycetes*) such as *Mucor* and *Rhizopus*, as well as *Fusarium*.

Clinical use in dogs and cats: At this time, clinical use of posaconazole in animals has been limited to a few case reports in cats because the formulations are expensive. Oral absorption is good enough in dogs and cats to achieve drug concentrations in the effective range with repeated dosing. In dogs, the oral delayed-release tablets were much better absorbed and produced higher plasma drug concentrations than the liquid suspension, and tablets can be administered every 48 hours in dogs. In cats, the oral suspension produced a long enough half-life that effective concentrations can be achieved with a loading dose, followed by every-other-day oral dosing. The limited use in dogs and cats has not revealed any adverse effects.

9.5.4 Terbinafine

Terbinafine (Lamisil) is a highly fungicidal antifungal agent. It is a synthetic drug of the allylamine class. A closely related drug of the same class is naftifine (Naftin), which is used as a topical cream for dermatophyte infections in people. Terbinafine inhibits squalene epoxidase to decrease synthesis of ergosterol. Fungal cell death results from disruption of cell membrane.

Terbinafine is active against yeasts and a wide range of dermatophytes with a low MIC of 0.01 mcg/mL or less. It is fungicidal against *Trichophyton* species, *Microsporum* species, and *Aspergillus* species. It is also active against *B. dermatitidis, C. neoformans, Sporothrix schenckii, Histoplasma capsulatum, Candida*, and *M. pachydermatis* yeast. There may be some activity against protozoa (e.g. *Toxoplasma*).

Oral absorption is moderate in dogs and cats, but low in horses. In people, it has the advantage of high lipophilicity, with high concentrations attained in tissues such as stratum corneum, hair follicles, sebum-rich skin, and nails. In people, after 12 days of therapy, the concentrations in stratum corneum exceed those in plasma by a factor of 75×. In cats after a daily dose of 30–40 mg/ kg, the concentrations in hair may be 10× the serum concentrations and persist for weeks after discontinuation of treatment at 14 days. Interestingly, these tissue concentrations have not been observed in dogs. One study indicated that concentrations in canine skin, subcutaneous tissue, and sebum were not above the concentration needed to inhibit *Malassezia*, and skin concentrations were only 1–2% of serum concentrations. The reason for these species differences is not known.

Clinical use: Since terbinafine has become available as a less expensive generic product, the interest in its use in veterinary medicine has increased.

Dramatic Difference
It should be noted that animal doses are much higher than human doses. Doses in animals are usually 30 mg/kg, but by comparison, doses in people are much lower at 125 mg twice daily (approximately 1.8 mg/kg q12h [every 12 hours]), with pediatric doses in the range of 4–8 mg/kg once a day.

Clinical results have been mixed based on limited studies. Some veterinarians believe it is effective in cats for dermatophytes (30 mg/kg once daily). However, for the treatment of *Malessezia* dermatitis in dogs when given at 30 mg/kg PO, or 30 mg/kg 2× per week for at least three weeks, it produced insufficient resolution and only partial remission.

Adverse effects: In cats, vomiting has been reported after oral administration, and facial dermatitis and pruritus have also been reported. This reaction is a problem because it may be confused with an ongoing dermatophyte infection. In dogs, reports of adverse effects are variable. One study reported GI signs and increased liver enzymes occurring in one-third of treated dogs. Other studies reported ocular problems in some dogs.

9.5.5 Topical Agents for Treating *Malassezia* and Dermatophytes

Topical agents are also used for dermatophytes and *Malassezia* skin infections in dogs, cats, horses, and other species. There are many human-labeled products and some veterinary-labeled products, as well as shampoos and rinses that contain antifungal agents. Some examples are listed in Table 9.8.

Table 9.8 Topical antifungal agents used for animals.

Drug	Example
Miconazole	Conofite cream
Clotrimizole	Lotrimin topical
Nystatin	Mycostatin[*]
Natamycin	Natacyn[*]
Clotrimazole	Mometamax and Otomax ear products (with other agents)
Terbinafine	Osurnia and Claro (with other agents) used for ear infections.

9.6 Antiviral Drugs

Compared to human medicine, antiviral drugs have a much smaller role for treating animals. Except for topical treatments, there are only a few agents used in veterinary medicine. Many of the antiviral agents used in people are designed for specific diseases such as hepatitis C, HIV/AIDS, influenza virus, and herpes virus. However, these human diseases do not occur in animals, or the viruses in animals are sufficiently different that they do not respond to human drugs. Additionally, some relatively nonspecific human antiviral drugs are extremely toxic to cats and cannot be used. For example, acyclovir and ribavirin are toxic to cats (ribavirin causes hemolysis, hepatotoxicity, and myelotoxicity).

Unfortunately, there are no specific antiviral agents approved for animals. Therefore, veterinarians have used human-label drugs, and sometimes experimental drugs, to manage viral infections. Because of the lack of veterinary-specific products available, veterinarians rely on published evidence of efficacy for guidance on safety and dosing.

Table 9.9 Summary of common antiviral drugs used in animals.

Zidovudine (AZT): Has produced some benefit in cats with FIV infection, but it is less effective for cats with FeLV. High doses have caused adverse effects in cats.

Famcyclovir: Has produced improvement when administered to cats with feline herpes virus-1 (FHV1).

Acyclovir: Only used for IV treatment of equine herpes virus-1 (EHV1).

Valacyclovir (Valtrex and generic): Used as oral treatment of EHV1.

These agents have been considered for experimental protocols, but not for clinical use:

Stavudin (D4T)

Didanosine (ddl)

Zalcitabine (ddC)

Lamivudine (3TC)

Suramin

Foscarnet

Ribavirin

Plerixafor

Table 9.10 Examples of topical antiviral agents used in animals (primarily cats).

Disease	Drug name	Clinical Use
Feline herpes virus-1	Idoxuridine	Topical ointment (eyes)
Feline herpes virus-1	Vidarabine	Topical ointment (eyes)
Feline herpes virus-1	Trifluridine	Topical ointment (eyes)
Feline herpes virus-1	Cidofovir	Topical solution (eyes), in compounded formulation

Fortunately, there have been many advances in the last 10 years that have provided much of this needed information (Table 9.9).

The administration of systemic antiviral drugs has been very limited in veterinary medicine (see Table 9.9). The use of antiviral agents has been primarily in the realm of ophthalmology treatment, particularly for feline herpes ocular infections. These treatments usually employ topical ointments (Table 9.10).

9.6.1 Systemic Antiviral Agents

Systemic treatment of viral diseases in dogs and cats is limited to only a few agents and diseases. Many dosing protocols are anecdotal, rather than derived from well-controlled clinical trials. Treatment of most viral diseases in dogs and cats primarily relies on supportive care and prevention and treatment of secondary bacterial infections.

For the agents available, antiviral drugs: (i) prevent entry of virus into host cells, (ii) prevent DNA synthesis in host cells, or (iii) prevent exit to inhibit infecting other cells. Antiviral agents are virustatic. They do not kill viruses and act only on replicating viruses; they do not affect latent virus. *Antiviral chemotherapy does not eliminate the virus in infected dogs and cats.*

9.6.1.1 Acyclovir

Acyclovir (Zovirax and generic brands) is the prototype of other agents used primarily for treatment of herpes virus infections. These drugs all share a similar mechanism of action, but vary in their pharmacokinetics and adverse effects. Acyclovir monophosphate accumulates in cells infected with herpes virus and is converted by guanylate cyclase to acyclovir diphosphate and subsequently to the triphosphate form, which is an inhibitor of viral DNA polymerase. This terminates viral enzyme activity.

For feline herpes virus-1 (FHV1):

Dramatic difference

FHV1 is much less efficient (by a factor of 1000) at converting acyclovir to the monophosphate form than human herpes simplex virus-1 (HSV1). Therefore, it has little efficacy for treating cats with FHV1. In addition, oral absorption is very low, producing ineffective plasma drug concentrations. More importantly, if high concentrations are achieved, toxicity is common in cats.

Equine herpes virus (EHV1) is more responsive to acyclovir than FHV1. Unfortunately, acyclovir is not absorbed orally in horses (less than 3%). The only effective use is from slow IV infusions (a slow infusion is necessary to prevent phlebitis). A typical dose is 10 mg/kg q12h IV infused over one hour.

9.6.1.2 Valacyclovir

Valacyclovir is the L-valine ester prodrug of acyclovir. It is converted to acyclovir and valine by esterases once absorbed, thus improving overall bioavailability. However, because of higher concentrations, the risk of toxicity in cats is high (myelosuppression, hepatotoxicity, and kidney injury). ***Valacyclovir should never be administered to cats.***

Because of poor absorption of acyclovir in horses (as discussed here), valacyclovir has been used to treat EHV1. It is not effective for all cases, because there are differences in activity against various strains of EHV. It has been used successfully in equine outbreaks to prevent severity of EHV infection. Oral absorption of valacyclovir in horses is much

better than that of acyclovir. A typical dose for treating EHV1 is a 27 mg/kg oral loading dose q8h, for two days, followed by a maintenance dose of 18 mg/kg PO q12h for 7–14 days.

9.6.1.3 Penciclovir

Penciclovir is another nucleoside analog with a similar mechanism of action as acyclovir. It also requires cellular phosphorylation by the virus to convert to the monophosphate form. It is highly active against FHV1 and can be useful to treat cats; however, it is not absorbed orally unless administered as a prodrug (see famciclovir in Section 9.6.1.4).

9.6.1.4 Famciclovir

Compared to the other systemic drugs listed in this section, this is the only one that has practical use for oral treatment of cats with FHV1. After oral absorption, it is first converted by di-deacetylation to an intermediate inactive metabolite (BRL 42359), and then through oxidation to the active penciclovir. The problem for cats is that the oxidation step is less efficient than in humans. The metabolite BRL 42359 accumulates to high levels. Fortunately, it is not harmful. There have been multiple studies in cats (summarized by Thomasy and Maggs 2016) that demonstrate that the pharmacokinetics are complex. Effective concentrations of penciclovir can be attained, but it requires higher doses compared to people. Determination of the appropriate dose has been difficult because of the complex pharmacokinetics and discrepancies in results. After studying doses of 20, 30, 40, and 90 mg/kg, given twice or three times daily, it was concluded that an oral dose of 90 mg/kg two or three times per day is the most effective and produces plasma drug concentrations in the desired range. It is available in 125, 250, and 500 mg tablets, and some references have cited a dose of 125 mg per cat three times daily. By comparison, the recommended dosage of famciclovir for the treatment of herpes zoster (shingles) in people is 500 mg per person every eight hours (approximately 7 mg/kg). Like other drugs in this class, adverse effects are possible. To monitor for bone marrow suppression, the patient's complete blood count (CBC) should be checked periodically.

9.6.1.5 Zidovudine (AZT, Retrovir)

Zidovudine, frequently known as AZT, was one of the first antiviral drugs developed to treat HIV in humans. It acts to inhibit the viral enzyme reverse transcriptase that prevents conversion of viral RNA into DNA. Other drugs in this class include lamivudine, didanosine, and zalcitabine, which have not had clinical use in veterinary medicine.

In cats, AZT has been used in experimental infections of feline leukemia virus (FeLV) and feline immunodeficiency virus (FIV). Although it improved some clinical signs in experimental cats, it has not been effective for the naturally occurring disease, and the efficacy in cats has been disappointing. In some cats, it may more helpful for FIV, but more work is needed before recommending clinical use. Adverse effects are common in cats at high doses. Otherwise, it has not been used often in animals; therefore, a full range of potential adverse effects has not been reported.

9.6.1.6 L-Lysine

Pharmacists should be aware that cat owners may find information on the internet promoting the use of L-lysine for cats with conjunctivitis secondary to FHV1. The information here is provided to help pharmacists provide appropriate client education on this nutritional supplement. L-lysine is an amino acid that has been administered to treat or prevent FHV1. The use has been controversial, but experts conclude that it is not helpful, and may actually be harmful to cats with infections. In theory, it competitively interferes with arginine incorporation into viral DNA, and arginine is essential for herpes virus replication.

In experimental cats, administration was associated with less severe conjuncitivitis and reduced viral shedding. But in shelter cats, administration of an oral supplement at 250–500 mg twice daily had no positive effects compared to placebo. In other studies in which the diet was supplemented with L-lysine, there was more severe disease and viral shedding in treated cats compared to a diet not supplemented with L-lysine.

9.6.1.7 Oseltamivir (Tamiflu)

Oseltamivir is a neuraminidase inhibitor used in people to treat influenza. Neuraminidase inhibitors prevent release of virus from the patient's cell. They inhibit virus replication by binding the viral enzyme neuraminidase, a viral surface glycoprotein. They must be started early in the course of the infection. It does not cure influenza, but it may shorten the course of the disease in people. The only drug in this group used in animals has been oseltamivir. Although there are anecdotal reports of improved outcome, the activity of oseltamivir against canine parvovirus is unlikely because canine parvovirus does not possess a neuraminidase. Oseltamivir is prohibited by the FDA for use in poultry.

9.6.1.8 Immune Stimulation and Immunomodulators

For some diseases, such as FeLV, use of acemannan, interferon-omega, bacterins, and other products purported to act as "immune stimulants" has been attempted, with little documented evidence of efficacy. Unfortunately, what constitutes "immunomodulation" or "immune stimulation" is not well defined. There is some evidence that interferon-omega may improve survival in cats infected with FeLV, but other evidence is lacking. The use of drugs to stimulate the immune system may seem counterproductive for some viral diseases (e.g. feline infectious peritonitis), because the clinical signs are a result of an immune-mediated process.

9.6.1.9 Interferons (Interferon-Alpha and Interferon-Omega)

An interferon does not have direct antiviral activity but exerts its effect by inhibiting internal synthesis mechanisms of infected cells. Despite some anecdotal accounts of use for treatment of viral disease in cats, interferons have not shown a clear clinical benefit.

Multiple interferons are available for human use (e.g. treatment of AIDS-related diseases and cancer-associated diseases). These interferons may be alpha-2a, alpha-2b, n-1, and n-3. But interferon types are not interchangeable, and one cannot assume they will be effective in animals. Interferon-alpha has improved clinical signs in some cats with FIV, but the studies are very limited. The limitation for use in cats is that weekly injections eventually become ineffective because cats develop neutralizing antibodies to human interferons. Interferon-alpha has been examined in limited studies for FeLV infection, but the conclusion among experts is that it is not effective.

9.6.1.9.1 Interferon-Omega
The product used in animals (Virbagen omega) is a recombinant form of interferon-omega. It is produced by silkworms previously inoculated with interferon-recombinant baculovirus. Interferon-omega of feline origin, produced by genetic engineering, is a Type 1 interferon closely related to interferon-alpha. *This product is not available in the United States.*

Interferon-omega has been used to stimulate immune cells in dogs with parvovirus and in cats with feline retrovirus (FeLV and FIV). In limited studies, some clinical improvement has been reported in cats treated with interferon-omega, but some of these studies had no control group. It has not been effective for feline infectious peritonitis virus (FIP) in cats. There are no data to support interferon-omega for treating FHV1 infection.

Adverse effects of interferon may include vomiting, nausea, and diarrhea. In some animals, it may induce hyperthermia three to six hours after injection. A slight decrease in white blood cells, platelets, and red blood cells and an increase in the concentration of ALT have been observed. These parameters usually return to normal in the week following the last injection. In cats, it may induce transient fatigue during the treatment.

Clinical use is limited to a small number of reports. Doses and indications for animals are based on extrapolation of human recommendations, experimental studies, or specific studies in cats with viral infections. In dogs, it is administered at a dose of 2.5 million units/kg IV once daily for three consecutive days. For cats with FIV or FeLV infection, the dose is 1 million units/kg of recombinant feline interferon-omega IV or SC once daily for five consecutive days. Three separate five-day treatments are usually performed at day 0, day 14, and day 60.

9.7 Antiprotozoal Drugs

There is a long list of drugs used to suppress or kill protozoal infections in animals. Most of the drugs approved for this indication are used in food-producing animals, primarily poultry, pigs, and cattle. However, protozoal infections also occur in companion animals, and there is a need for antiprotozoals for treatment in dogs, cats, horses, and many zoo and exotic animals. Many of these agents also act on bacteria; therefore, there will be some overlap with their mention here and the discussion earlier in this chapter regarding their use to treat bacterial infections.

Protozoa that cause disease in animals most often are associated with intestinal disease. They cause acute or chronic diarrhea in infected animals. Systemic infections also occur that can affect the CNS (meningitis), lungs, and other organs. Some of these organisms include *G. lamblia, Balantidium coli, Entamoeba histolytica, T. foetus, Pentatrichomonas hominis, Trichomonas gallinae, Histomonas maleagridis,* and *Trypanosomas* spp. Compared to bacterial infection, culture and susceptibility testing is not usually performed for protozoal infections. The diagnosis is often made directly by identifying the organisms in tissue samples, biopsies, or cytological examination. Antibody tests can also detect the presence of protozoa. There are no standards for performing or interpreting susceptibility tests. Therefore, protozoal infections are treated empirically with the agents listed in the remainder of this section, based on demonstrated activity and clinical experience.

Except for their use in poultry and livestock, there are few antiprotozoals approved for use in dogs, cats, and horses. Many human-label drugs or food animal drugs are used in an extra-label manner in other species. Many products are approved exclusively to be added to water or feed for poultry, pigs, and cattle to control protozoal infections, especially intestinal coccidia. Because these are exclusively livestock medications and unlikely to be dispensed from a community pharmacy, they will not be discussed here. Other references have extensive information on these products and their uses (Riviere and Papich 2018).

9.7.1 Nitroimidazoles

Drugs in this class include metronidazole, tinidazole, ronidazole, dimetridazole, ornidazole, carnidazole, benznidazole, ipronidazole, and secnidazole. Metronidazole is easily the most often used in veterinary medicine, even though there are no approved veterinary formulations. The human forms, or compounded versions, are necessary for veterinary use. Occasionally, tinidazole is used, especially for refractory cases of *Giardia*. Many older drugs that were primarily used in poultry have been removed from the market. It is illegal to administer these agents to food-producing animals in the USA.

The mechanism of action of all the drugs in this class is similar. After entry into the protozoa, there is a reductive reaction that produces toxicity to the organism. A detailed review of the mechanism of action and resistance mechanisms can be found in the paper by Dingsdag and Hunter (2017).

9.7.1.1 Metronidazole

Metronidazole (Flagyl and generic) was discussed in Section 9.4.10.

9.7.1.2 Tinidazole

Tinidazole (Tindamax, Simplotan˚, or Fasigyn˚) is a second-generation nitroimidazole that is FDA approved for treating *Trichomonas vaginalis*, *Giardia* spp., and *E. histolytica* infections in people. Use of tinidazole in animals has been infrequent, but it has favorable properties. It is almost completely absorbed after oral administration to dogs, cats, and horses.

Clinical use in dogs and cats: Tinidazole has not been studied in clinical trials in animals. However, because of its effectiveness in people, it is also likely to be useful for *Giardia* infections in dogs and cats. In people, it has been effective at a single dose, but whether or not this would be an effective strategy in animals is undetermined. Use in horses has not been reported.

9.7.1.3 Ronidazole

Ronidazole is not approved for human or veterinary use, so pharmacists may be presented with prescriptions for compounded ronidazole. Experimental studies and clinical results demonstrate that it is one of the few agents effective for treatment of *T. foetus* in cats. It is likely that it would be effective against other intestinal protozoa. It also is effective for treating *Giardia* in dogs, based on limited reports.

In cats, it is rapidly absorbed after oral administration and has a long enough half-life that once-daily treatment can be effective. Adverse effects attributed to CNS toxicity are possible (as described in this chapter for metronidazole; see Section 9.4.10). If these occur, the pet owner should consult with the prescribing veterinarian. Pharmacists should counsel pet owners accordingly.

9.7.2 Pentavalent Antimonials

The agents in this group include sodium stibogluconate and meglumine antimonite. Pentavalent antimonials are used to treat *Leishmania* infections in dogs. This disease is uncommon in the USA, but outbreaks have been described. These agents have a mechanism of action that is unclear. Pharmacokinetics are not well described in animals, and dosing protocols are based on anecdotal accounts and limited clinical experience. Both sodium stibogluconate and meglumine antimonate are administered on the basis of their antimony content.

Sodium stibogluconate (Pentostam˙) is available in the USA from the Centers for Disease Control and Prevention for treatment of leishmaniasis in human beings. Canine leishmaniasis is treated with sodium stibogluconate to deliver 30–50 mg/kg pentavalent antimony. The administration is IV or SC, so it is unlikely that this product would be dispensed from community pharmacies.

Meglumine antimonate (Glucantime˙) may be less likely to cause adverse effects than sodium stibogluconate. It is also administered by injection (either IM or SC) to dogs. Therefore, it would be unusual to dispense this agent from a pharmacy.

9.7.3 Benzimidazoles

Benzimidazoles include albendazole, fenbendazole, and febantel. They are also used as antiparasitic agents, and more details of their use are listed in Chapter 7 of this book. Some drugs in this group have excellent activity against *Giardia* spp. The benzimidazoles bind to beta-tubulin subunits of microtubules and interfere with microtubule polymerization, which leads to structural changes in *Giardia* trophozoites consistent with microtubule damage to the adhesive disk and internal microtubule cytoskeleton but not the external flagella.

Albendazole: Albendazole (Valbazan˙) is the most often used for *Giardia*. It is available in liquid and paste formulations, and has been used in both dogs and cats. Most of the drug is retained in the intestine, but it can also cause adverse effects, including myelosuppression. It is potentially teratogenic, so it should not be given to pregnant animals.

Fenbendazole: Fenbendazole (Panacur˙ and other brands) is available in numerous preparations as a paste, suspension, or granules for large and small animals. It is generally safe but can be associated with vomiting and diarrhea (which are difficult to distinguish from the underlying disease).

Febantel: Febantel (Drontal-Plus˙ and Drontal Flavour Plus˙) is usually used to treat intestinal parasites (Chapter 7). It is available as a combination product with pyrantel pamoate or pyrantel embonate and praziquantel for the treatment of intestinal nematodes and cestodes in dogs and cats. In limited experience, it has been used for treatment of *Giardia* in dogs and cats and has produced clinical improvement and decreased shedding.

9.7.4 Aminoglycosides

The only aminoglycoside used for treatment of protozoa is paromomycin. Other aminoglycosides were discussed in Sections 9.3.2.2 and 9.4.2. Paromomycin has been effective for treatment of *G. lamblia, Leishmania* spp., and *Entamoeba* spp. Paromomycin is used in the treatment of luminal amoebiasis, leishmaniasis, and cryptosporidiosis. It has also been used in humans for the treatment of resistant giardiasis. It is poorly absorbed following oral administration, which leads to high intestinal luminal drug concentrations.

Although little is absorbed from the intestinal tract, enough can be absorbed, especially in animals with a compromised intestinal barrier, that adverse kidney effects can occur. These effects have been described in cats that were treated for *Trichomonas* infection. Some cats have been treated orally for intestinal protozoa infections, but experience is limited.

In dogs, it has been administered IM for treatment of visceral leishmaniasis. Because it is administered either IM or SC, dispensing from a pharmacy is unlikely.

9.7.5 Tetracyclines

The tetracyclines include oxytetracycline, doxycycline, and minocycline. They were covered in Section 9.4.3. However, they are discussed again here, because they also have antiprotozoal activity against amoebae, mucosal flagellates, piroplasms, and ciliates.

A common use of oxytetracycline in cattle and other livestock is to control *Anaplasma* and other protozoa. The use in cattle can be found in other references. It is only used in an injection formulation (IV or IM).

Oral doxycycline is effective at preventing clinical manifestations of *Babesia canis* infection in dogs, but a more common treatment is atovaquone in combination with azithromycin (see Section 9.7.6).

9.7.6 Hydroxyquinolones

Atovaquone: Atovaquone (Mepron® suspension) is a hydroxyquinolone that has broad-spectrum antiprotozoal activity. Atovaquone is supplied as a bright-yellow suspension of microfine particles at a concentration of 150 mg atovaquone/mL. It is administered orally, but should be given with food. In humans, it has been used to treat malaria, but also it is used in small animals because of the activity against *Toxoplasma gondii* and *Babesia* spp. It also has activity against *Eimeria* spp.

In dogs, atovaquone in combination with azithromycin is the treatment of choice for canine babesiosis. It is given concurrently with azithromycin for 10 consecutive days to eliminate *Babesia gibsoni* infection. Dogs with *B. gibsoni* infection are often "fighting" dogs, and breeds such as pit bulls are frequently affected. Because the treatment with atovaquone can be expensive, compounded atovaquone is sometimes prepared by pharmacies for treatment (Kirk et al. 2017). In cats with *Cytauxzoon felis*, atovaquone is administered concurrently with azithromycin for a duration of 10 days.

9.7.7 Thiamine Analogs

Amprolium: Amprolium (Corid® and Amprol®) is the most important drug in this group and is used in a variety of animals to treat intestinal coccidiosis. It is among the most commonly administered anticoccidial agents in veterinary medicine, and it is used primarily for poultry and other livestock. It is structurally related to vitamin B_1 (thiamine), and the antiparasitic activity of the drug is thought to be related to competitive inhibition of active thiamine transport into the parasite. Because of this effect, long-term or high-dose administration of amprolium can lead to clinical thiamine deficiency in animals, resulting in cerebrocortical necrosis (polioencephalomalacia).

For treatment of dogs, it has been administered orally or added to drinking water once a day for 7–12 days. It also has been used in cats for treatment of coccidiosis once a day for 7–12 days.

9.7.8 Triazine Derivatives

Triazines are used commonly in horses, but are also used in small animals, zoo species, and exotic species, for treatment of *Sarcocystis neurona*, coccidiosis, toxoplasmosis, *Neospora caninum*, and *Neospora hughesii*. Triazines include diclazuril, toltrazuril, and ponazuril.

Triazines act on the apicoplast, a plastid obtained by endosymbiosis that exists in apicomplexan parasites but is not present in animals. The exact function of the apicoplast is not known; however, it may play a vital role in biosynthesis of amino acids and fatty acids, assimilation of nitrate and sulfate, and starch storage. Inhibition of apicoplast function results in effective antiprotozoal activity. Triazines have had a good margin of safety, with no serious adverse effects reported.

Diclazuril: Diclazuril (Clinicox® and Protazil®) is a benzene acetonitrile that is usually administered in the feed. Against one of the equine pathogens, *S. neurona*, it inhibits merozoite production. Diclazuril is an FDA-approved treatment for equine protozoal myeloencephalitis (EPM), which is caused by *S. neurona* (Table 9.11). Compared to other dose forms, an alfalfa-based pelleted formulation (Protazil™) facilitates treatment of

Table 9.11 FDA-approved drugs for treating equine protozoal myeloencephalitis (EPM) in horses.

Drug	Brand name	Formulation	Comments
Diclazuril	Protazil	Pellets for feed additive	Administered daily in feed. Also has been used in other animals.
Ponazuril	Marquis	Oral paste	An active metabolite of toltrazuril, another antiprotozoal agent that is not available in the USA.
Sulfadiazine–pyrimethamine	ReBalance	Oral suspension	Can produce adverse effects related to folate deficiency.

horses with diclazuril. Lower doses can be used for disease prevention.

Ponazuril: Ponazuril (Marquis˚), also known as toltrazuril sulfone, is an active metabolite of toltrazuril (toltrazuril is not available in the USA). It is available in a paste formulation for horses. It has activity against *S. neurona, T. gondii, Isospora suis*, and *N. caninum*. In horses, it is FDA approved for treatment of EPM (Table 9.11). Occasionally, the equine form has been administered to zoo and exotic animal species, and dogs and cats (e.g. for toxoplasmosis in cats).

9.7.9 Sulfonamides

There are many sulfonamides used to treat or prevent intestinal coccidiosis in animals, including sulfaguanidine, sulfadiazine, sulfadimethoxine, sulfadoxine, sulfamethazine (also called sulfadimidine), sulfamethoxazole, sulfanitran, and sulfaquinoxaline. They are widely used in poultry, pigs, cattle, and other livestock, usually added to feed and water. Because most of the use is on the farm, they will not be discussed in detail in this chapter.

Sulfonamides are often used in combination with dihydrofolate reductase–thymidylate synthase inhibitors such as trimethoprim, pyrimethamine, or ormetoprim, which are discussed in Section 9.7.9.1 (trimethoprim and pyrimethamine) and Section 9.4.8 (ormetoprim).

Use in dogs and cats: Several agents have been used to treat intestinal coccidiosis in dogs and cats, but only sulfadimethoxine is FDA approved for this use, which is discussed here. Sulfadimethoxine (Albon) is administered orally as tablets or oral suspension. Adverse effects were described in Section 9.4.8.

9.7.9.1 Dihydrofolate Reductase Inhibitors: Trimethoprim and Pyrimethamine

These agents can be used alone but are almost always combined with a sulfonamide. (See use of trimethoprim–sulfonamides in Section 9.4.8.) For protozoa, their spectrum includes intestinal coccidia, *Toxoplasma* spp., *Neospora* spp., *S. neurona*, and *Hepatozoon americanum*. They inhibit dihydrofolate reductase and act synergistically with sulfonamides.

Trimethoprim is available in several formulations both alone and in combination with sulfonamides for oral or parenteral administration. Examples include trimethoprim + sulfadiazine (Tribrissen and Di-Trim) and trimethoprim + sulfamethoxazole (Bactrim, Septra, and human drugs). Both human-labeled and veterinary-labeled drugs are used in dogs, cats, horses, and exotic animals. In addition to their antibacterial use (as discussed previously in this chapter), these agents are used to treat coccidiosis, toxoplasmosis, neosporosis, EPM (see Table 9.10), and malaria. Adverse effects from the sulfonamides are more common in dogs than other species, but other effects are possible, as described in this chapter.

Pyrimethamine has greater affinity for the protozoal dihydrofolate reductase enzyme compared to the bacterial enzyme, which makes this agent more effective for protozoal treatment than for bacterial treatment. Pyrimethamine is available in human-labeled tablet form, but these have become very expensive. This drug has been used to treat protozoal infections such as malaria in people, protozoal infections in horses, and toxoplasmosis in dogs and cats. Pyrimethamine is administered orally and is well-absorbed in dogs, cats, and horses.

Clinical use: In horses, pyrimethamine in combination with sulfadiazine (ReBalance) has been used for treating EPM. The organism *S. neurona* appears to be responsive to this combination and is among the choices for treatment (see Table 9.11, and reference by Reed et al. 2016). The FDA-approved formulation for horses is a suspension of pyrimethamine (12.5 mg/mL) + sulfadiazine (250 mg/mL). This combination is administered to horses once daily for 30 days after clinical improvement has plateaued. Treatment duration is long (12 weeks on average). Relapse is possible if horses are not treated long enough, and reactivation of the infection may occur during periods of unusual stress.

In small animals – particularly cats – it has been used for protozoal infections, such as those caused by *Toxoplasma*, but clinical study results are not available to assess efficacy. In dogs, pyrimethamine and sulfonamide combinations have been used for *N. caninum* infection, but clinical efficacy has not been reported. In people, pyrimethamine has been used with clindamycin for toxoplasmosis. However, the efficacy for treatment of toxoplasmosis when used alone is not very encouraging unless high doses are used.

Adverse effects: The most commonly cited adverse effect from pyrimethamine is anemia secondary to folate deficiency. This is more common with high doses.

Horses should be maintained on feeds or pasture that is high in dietary folacin during

Mandatory monitoring
Patients treated with pyrimethamine should be monitored periodically for anemia and leukopenia (i.e. a CBC every two weeks).

treatment. Use cautiously in pregnant mares because congenital defects, including skin lesions, bone marrow aplasia, and renal dysplasia, have been reported and can occur despite folic acid supplementation to the mare during treatment. If horses are supplemented, folinic acid, not folic acid, is recommended for treatment of folate deficiency.

9.7.10 Lincosamides

Lincosamides were discussed in Section 9.4.6. The most common drug in this group is clindamycin (Antirobe, Cleocin, and generic), but formulations of lincomycin still exist as feed additives for pigs and poultry. (*Note:* They should never be added to feed for cattle, sheep, goats, rabbits, or rodents.)

The most important antiprotozoal indication for lincosamides in dogs and cats is for disseminated toxoplasmosis. Clindamycin is active against tachyzoites of *T. gondii* and is initially coccidiostatic, but it becomes coccidiocidal after a few days of treatment. Usually, dogs and cats are treated with clindamycin twice daily for four weeks. Adverse effects are the same as described in Section 9.4.6 for these agents.

9.7.11 Macrolides

Macrolide antibiotics were discussed in Section 9.4.5 with the antibacterial agents (e.g. see azithromycin). They also have an antiprotozoal spectrum that includes cryptosporidiosis, toxoplasmosis, babesiosis, and cytauxzoonosis. The macrolide used most commonly in dogs, cats, and zoo and exotic animals is azithromycin (Zithromax and generic). This is a human formulation that is not approved for animals, but it is used extra-label.

When used as an antiprotozoal agent, azithromycin is almost always administered concurrently with atovaquone (Section 9.7.6). This combination has been highly effective for *B. gibsoni* infection, even in dogs that had already failed other treatments. In cats, it is used to treat infections caused by *C. felis*, also in combination with atovaquone.

9.7.12 Chloroquine

Chloroquine is an antimalarial drug (*Plasmodium* sp.) that is used in veterinary medicine only for treating avian malaria. The mechanism of action against malarial organisms involves concentration of the drug, which is a weak base, within the acidic food vacuoles of the parasites. This causes rapid clumping of heme pigments by inhibiting plasmodial heme polymerase activity. Heme then accumulates to toxic levels, causing cell death. Its use is described for treatment of birds in captive exhibit facilities (e.g. penguins in zoos).

9.7.13 Diminazene Diaceturate

Diminazene diaceturate (Berenil® and Ganaseg®) has been used to treat piroplasmosis caused by *H. canis* and *Babesia*. It has a very long half-life and is administered only by IM injection. Because it is not commonly used, it would be unlikely to be dispensed from a pharmacy.

In horses, diminazene has been used to treat *Babesia caballi* infections. In dogs, it has been effective against canine babesiosis caused by *B. canis*. In cats, it has been used to treat *Cytauxzoon* infection with two injections, but it was ineffective.

9.7.14 Imidocarb Dipropionate

Imidocarb diproprionate (Imizol®) is one of the treatments of choice for babesial infections in animals. In horses, it has been used to eliminate *B. caballi* from horses, but it must be administered IM for a total of four doses. It may cause hepatotoxicity; therefore, careful monitoring is needed. In dogs, it is administered subcutaneously, and a single dose has been shown to completely clear *B. canis* infections. In cats, it has been used to treat *H. canis* infections with injections (SC or IM) every two weeks. Because this drug is administered only by injection, it is unlikely to be dispensed by a community pharmacy.

9.7.15 Nitazoxanide

Nitazoxanide is from the group of nitrothiazole derivatives with activity against *Giardia, Coccidia, Cryptosporidiosis*, and *S. neurona*. The antiprotozoal action of the nitrothiazole derivatives is thought to be via interference with the pyruvate–ferredoxin oxidoreductase enzyme-dependent electron transfer reaction, which is essential for anaerobic energy metabolism of these protozoa.

The only commercial form used in animals was nitazoxanide (Navigator®), a paste formulation used to treat EPM. The adverse effects in horses became a problem, and they included fatal enterocolitis; therefore, it was voluntarily withdrawn from the market by the sponsor. It had limited use in cats, but it produced adverse effects and so is no longer used.

References

Beco, L., Guaguere, E., Méndez, C.L. et al. (2013). Suggested guidelines for using systemic antimicrobials in bacterial skin infections: part 2 – antimicrobial choice, treatment regimens and compliance. *Vet. Record* 172 (6): 156.

Clinical and Laboratory Standards Institute(CLSI). Performance Standards for Antimicrobial Disk and Dilution Susceptibility Tests for Bacteria Isolated From Animals. 5th ed. CLSI standard VET01. Clinical and Laboratory Standards Institute, 950 West Valley Road, Suite 2500, Wayne, Pennsylvania 19087 USA, 2018.

Clinical and Laboratory Standards Institute(CLSI). Performance Standards for Antimicrobial Disk and Dilution Susceptibility Tests for Bacteria Isolated

From Animals. 4th ed. CLSI supplement VET08. Clinical and Laboratory Standards Institute, 950 West Valley Road, Suite 2500, Wayne, Pennsylvania 19087 USA, 2018.

Dingsdag, S.A. and Hunter, N. (2017). Metronidazole: an update on metabolism, structure–cytotoxicity and resistance mechanisms. *J. Antimicrob. Chemo.* 73 (2): 265–279.

Guardabassi, L. and Prescott, J.F. (2015). Antimicrobial stewardship in small animal veterinary practice: from theory to practice. *Vet. Clin. Small Anim. Pract.* 45 (2): 361–376.

Hillier, A., Lloyd, D.H., Weese, J.S. et al. (2014). Guidelines for the diagnosis and antimicrobial therapy of canine superficial bacterial folliculitis (antimicrobial guidelines working group of the International Society for companion animal infectious diseases). *Vet. Dermatol.* 25 (3): 163.

Kirk, S.K., Levy, J.K., and Crawford, P.C. (2017). Efficacy of azithromycin and compounded atovaquone for treatment of *Babesia gibsoni* in dogs. *J. Vet. Intern. Med.* 31 (4): 1108–1112.

Lappin, M.R., Blondeau, J., Boothe, D. et al. (2017). Antimicrobial use guidelines for treatment of respiratory tract disease in dogs and cats: antimicrobial guidelines working group of the International Society for companion animal infectious diseases. *J. Vet. Intern. Med.* 31 (2): 279–294.

Mancianti, F., Pedonese, F., and Zullino, C. (1998). Efficacy of oral administration of itraconazole to cats with dermatophytosis caused by *Microsporum canis. J. Am. Vet. Med. Assoc.* 213 (7): 993–995.

Nemeth, J., Oesch, G., and Kuster, S.P. (2015). Bacteriostatic versus bactericidal antibiotics for patients with serious bacterial infections: systematic review and meta-analysis. *J. Antimicrob. Chemo.* 70 (2): 382–395.

Papich, M.G. (2016). Handbook of Veterinary Drugs, 4e. Amsterdam: Elsevier.

Reed, S.M., Furr, M., Howe, D.K. et al. (2016). Equine protozoal myeloencephalitis: an updated consensus statement with a focus on parasite biology, diagnosis, treatment, and prevention. *J. Vet. Intern. Med.* 30 (2): 491–502.

Riviere, J.E. and Papich, M.G. (2018). *Veterinary Pharmacology & Therapeutics*, 10e. Hoboken, NJ: Wiley.

Thomasy, S.M. and Maggs, D.J. (2016). A review of antiviral drugs and other compounds with activity against feline herpesvirus type 1. *Vet. Ophthalmol.* 19 (S1): 119–130.

Weese, J.S., Blondeau, J.M., Boothe, D. et al. (2011). Antimicrobial use guidelines for treatment of urinary tract disease in dogs and cats: antimicrobial guidelines working group of the international society for companion animal infectious diseases. *Vet. Med. Intl.* 2011: 263768.

10

Cardiovascular Pharmacotherapeutics

Sunshine M. Lahmers

Department of Small Animal Clinical Sciences, Virginia-Maryland (VA-MD) College of Veterinary Medicine, Virginia Tech, Blacksburg, VA, USA

Key Points

- Degenerative valve disease, familial cardiomyopathies, and congenital heart disease affect veterinary patients and can result in congestive heart failure or arrhythmic sudden death in severely affected individuals.
- In contrast to human medicine, coronary artery disease is rare in veterinary medicine.
- Heartworm disease is the most common infectious cardiovascular disease in small animals, but the clinical disease, diagnosis, and treatment differ significantly between dogs and cats.
- Congestive heart failure is medically managed with diuretics, angiotensin-converting enzyme (ACE) inhibitors, aldosterone inhibitors, and the veterinary licensed inodilator pimobendan.

- Veterinary patients experience the same arrhythmias as people, with most tachyarrhythmias managed medically and most clinical significant bradyarrhythmias managed with pacemaker implantation.
- Systemic hypertension occurs in veterinary patients and is usually managed with the calcium-channel blocker amlodipine in cats.
- Thromboembolic consequences of cardiovascular disease occur most commonly in cats, and platelet inhibitors such as clopidogrel are used for thrombosis risk reduction.
- Because an MDR1 mutation exists in dogs and cats, MDR1 genotype should be considered when dispensing certain cardiovascular medications, including digoxin, dabigatran, and macrocyclic lactones.

10.1 Comparative Aspects of Cardiovascular Disease

Many of the congenital and acquired cardiovascular diseases that affect people also affect veterinary patients. The most notable exception is ischemic heart disease. Although ischemic heart disease is the leading cardiovascular disease of people, it rarely occurs in animals. Most non-infectious cardiac diseases are familial in veterinary species and therefore have strong breed associations. The most common infectious cardiovascular disease, heartworm disease, is rarely encountered in human medicine. A more detailed comparison of the common congenital and acquired cardiovascular diseases in veterinary patients will be discussed in the remainder of this section.

10.1.1 Congenital Heart Diseases

Congenital heart diseases occur in all species and are largely the same congenital heart diseases seen in children. The frequency of specific congenital heart diseases varies by species, with patent ductus arteriosus and subaortic stenosis being the most common congenital heart diseases in dogs and ventricular septal defect being the most common congenital heart disease in all other domesticated species. When possible, congenital heart diseases are treated with either surgical or interventional repair as the first line of therapy. Medical treatment of congenital heart disease in dogs and cats involves managing associated arrhythmias and congestive heart failure (CHF).

10.1.2 Degenerative Valve Disease

Degeneration of the mitral valve is the most common cardiac disease in companion animals. It is referred to as myxomatous mitral valve degeneration based on the pathologic changes that occur in the valve and is similar to mitral valve prolapse in people. Myxomatous mitral valve degeneration can affect most small-breed dogs over 10 years of age (Buchanan 1977; Borgarelli and Haggstrom 2010). Cavalier King Charles Spaniels are overrepresented and have an earlier onset of myxomatous mitral valve degeneration than other small-breed dogs (Beardow and Buchanan 1993; Pedersen and Haggstrom 2000). Myxomatous mitral valve degeneration occurs less commonly in large-breed dogs. Clinical signs attributable to myxomatous mitral valve degeneration are primarily the result of CHF, although syncope can also occur.

10.1.3 Cardiomyopathies

Dilated cardiomyopathy is primarily a hereditary disease of large- to giant-breed dogs, with Doberman Pinchers being overrepresented (Calvert et al. 1982). In contrast to human patients with dilated cardiomyopathy, veterinary patients almost never have ischemic cardiomyopathy. Dogs with dilated cardiomyopathy are primarily at risk for sudden death, the development of CHF, and/or atrial fibrillation. Treatment is largely focused on positive inotropic support and CHF management. Antiarrhythmic therapy is initiated when clinically necessary. Nutritional cardiomyopathies resulting in a dilated cardiomyopathy phenotype also occur but far less frequently. A taurine/carnitine responsive form of dilated cardiomyopathy has been identified in American Cocker Spaniels (Kittleson et al. 1997). This does not appear to be associated with a dietary insufficiency. Dilated cardiomyopathy due to a taurine-deficient diet can occur in cats (Pion et al. 1987, 1992c). Treatment for nutritionally responsive dilated cardiomyopathy is focused on nutrient supplementation.

Arrhythmogenic right ventricular cardiomyopathy occurs in veterinary patients. Similar to arrhythmogenic right ventricular cardiomyopathy in people, it is a familial disease in dogs and is primarily associated with increased risk of sudden death due to ventricular tachyarrhythmias. Arrhythmogenic right ventricular cardiomyopathy is a familial disease in Boxers and Bulldogs but has also been reported in cats (Fox et al. 2000; Basso et al. 2004; Santilli et al. 2009). In contrast to human patients, implantable cardioverter defibrillators have only rarely been implanted in veterinary patients, and medical management of ventricular arrhythmias is currently the mainstay of treatment (Nelson et al. 2006; Pariaut et al. 2011).

Among veterinary species, hypertrophic cardiomyopathy, is primarily a disease of cats. Familial forms have been reported in Maine Coons, Ragdoll, and Sphynx cats (Kittleson et al. 1999; Meurs et al. 2007; Silverman et al. 2012). There is overlap in the genetic mutations identified in people and in some breeds of cats with hypertrophic cardiomyopathy (Kittleson et al. 1999; Meurs et al. 2007; Silverman et al. 2012). Similar to hypertrophic cardiomyopathy in people, there is tremendous diversity in the manifestations of feline hypertrophic cardiomyopathy, with many cats remaining subclinical for life while others progress to heart failure or sudden death, or experience thromboembolic complications. Treatment for hypertrophic cardiomyopathy in cats primarily occurs in severely affected cats and focuses on CHF management or attempts to reduce risk of thromboembolism. Cats can also develop a hypertrophic cardiomyopathy phenotype secondary to systemic hypertension or hyperthyroidism.

10.1.4 Thyrotoxic Heart Disease

Similar to hyperthyroidism in people, cardiac changes can occur secondary to elevated thyroid hormone levels in domestic animals. This is referred to as thyrotoxic heart disease. In veterinary medicine, hyperthyroidism is almost exclusively a disease of cats. The clinical manifestation of thyrotoxic heart disease in cats can be similar to hypertrophic cardiomyopathy, but the cardiac changes largely resolve with successful treatment of hyperthyroidism (Bond et al. 1988).

10.1.5 Hypertensive Diseases

Systemic hypertension is usually a secondary disease in veterinary patients, with idiopathic/primary hypertension reported in only about 25% of cats (Huhtinen et al. 2015; Taylor et al. 2017). Underlying kidney disease is the most common systemic disease that increases the risk of systemic hypertension. Other underlying conditions associated with systemic hypertension include hyperthyroidism, diabetes mellitus, hyperadrenocorticism (common disease of dogs), primary hyperaldosteronism, and pheochromocytoma (Brown et al. 2007; Herring et al. 2014). Unlike in human patients, salt-sensitive systemic hypertension is not a significant entity in veterinary patients. Cats are more frequently affected by systemic hypertension, with evidence of target organ damage such as retinal detachment (Maggio et al. 2000). The American College of Veterinary Internal Medicine (ACVIM) Hypertension Consensus Panel defined the risk of target organ damage as severe with blood pressure (BP) >180/120 mmHg and as mild risk with BP <150/95 mmHg (Brown et al. 2007). Resting blood pressure in cats and dogs is similar to that in humans. The higher blood pressure cutoffs utilized in the veterinary consensus statement relative to human patients account for "white coat" influence on blood pressure, which is common in veterinary patients. Cardiac changes secondary to systemic hypertension largely resolve with normalization of systemic blood pressure.

Pulmonary arterial hypertension can be categorized into pre-capillary and post-capillary causes. Many of the causes of pulmonary arterial hypertension are similar between humans and animals, but some veterinary-specific causes exist as well. The most common pre-capillary causes in veterinary patients include heartworm disease, pulmonary thromboembolism, and reactive vasoconstriction due to hypoxic respiratory diseases. Myxomatous mitral valve degeneration is the most common cause of post-capillary pulmonary hypertension in dogs. In veterinary medicine, treatment is largely focused on addressing the underlying cause when possible.

10.1.6 Arrhythmic Diseases

10.1.6.1 Tachyarrhythmias

Atrial fibrillation is one of the most common arrhythmias encountered in veterinary medicine. It is usually the result of atrial enlargement secondary to congenital or acquired heart disease in small animal species, but it can occur spontaneously in giant-breed dogs and horses without heart disease and is similar to lone atrial fibrillation in people. Horses are particularly predisposed to lone atrial fibrillation due to their inherent large heart size and high vagal tone. Horses can also develop atrial fibrillation secondary to cardiac enlargement due to underlying heart disease. Cattle develop atrial fibrillation with increased vagal tone states, particularly when they have gastrointestinal disease. Therapy directed at correcting the gastrointestinal disease will usually resolve the atrial fibrillation. In all animals with underlying cardiac disease, medical management to achieve heart rate control is the treatment of choice. Electrical cardioversion is reserved for dogs or horses with lone atrial fibrillation.

Supraventricular tachyarrhythmias other than atrial fibrillation are associated either with underlying heart disease or with a congenital predisposition to ventricular pre-excitation and Wolff–Parkinson–White syndrome. Ventricular pre-excitation and associated reciprocating tachyarrhythmias have been reported in dogs and cats, with the Labrador Retriever being the most reported breed (Wright et al. 1996). Treatment by ablation is available at certain referral centers, but due to cost many dogs are managed pharmacologically.

Ventricular tachyarrhythmias and associated syncope or sudden death can occur in all mammalian species. In dogs, there are breed-associated ventricular tachyarrhythmias. Bulldogs and Boxers are predisposed to development of ventricular tachycardias associated with arrhythmogenic right ventricular cardiomyopathy, while Dobermans are at increased risk associated with dilated cardiomyopathy (Santilli et al. 2009; Meurs et al. 2014). Young German Shepherd dogs are predisposed to a heritable juvenile ventricular tachyarrhythmia (Moise et al. 1994). Ventricular arrhythmias can also be associated with certain noncardiac diseases in veterinary patients, including systemic inflammatory diseases, electrolyte abnormalities, gastric dilatation and volvulus, splenic disease, and drug side effects. Unlike people, drug-associated QT prolongation as a risk factor for ventricular tachyarrhythmias seems to be less common in veterinary patients. That said, sudden death associated with a specific gene mutation causing inherited QT interval prolongation occurs in English Springer Spaniels (Ware et al. 2015). Electrolyte abnormalities, particularly hypokalemia, can present a significant risk for ventricular tachyarrhythmias, especially in patients receiving digoxin. In contrast to people, only rarely are these ventricular tachyarrhythmias managed with implantation of an internal cardioverter defibrillator (Nelson et al. 2006; Pariaut et al. 2011). In veterinary patients, ventricular tachyarrhythmias are primarily managed pharmacologically (medically). Medical management has a demonstrated benefit of reducing collapse episodes, but whether or not medical management of ventricular tachyarrhythmias decreases the risk of sudden death in veterinary patients is unknown.

10.1.6.2 Bradyarrhythmias

Sick sinus syndrome occurs in dogs. Schnauzers and Cocker Spaniels are the breeds most commonly affected. The treatment of choice for symptomatic, non-atropine responsive sick sinus syndrome is pacemaker implantation (Ward et al. 2016). Medical management is pursued in many dogs in which a pacemaker is not an option or in dogs with atropine-responsive sick sinus syndrome.

Physiologic atrioventricular block (AV block) can occur in resting horses or in small animal species with increased vagal tone. In small animal species with increased vagal tone secondary to an underlying disease, management of the underlying disease is the treatment of choice, but medical management can be pursued when necessary. Non-atropine-responsive AV block that results in syncope is usually managed with pacemaker implantation (Schrope and Kelch 2006). Unlike sick sinus syndrome, pathologic AV block has a more significant risk of sudden death and is less likely to respond to medical management. However, given the cost of pacemaker implantation, medical therapy is attempted in many veterinary patients with pathologic AV block.

Atrial standstill is most commonly associated with hyperkalemia but can also occur with spontaneous atrial myocardial disease. Management of hyperkalemia is largely directed at correcting the underlying cause while normalizing serum potassium. Pacemaker implantation may be pursued for atrial standstill associated with myocardial disease (Cervenec et al. 2017).

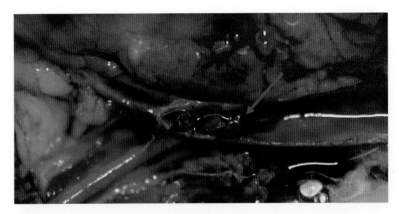

Figure 10.1 The terminal aorta in a cat with feline aortic thromboembolism (FATE). The thrombus can be seen at the bifurcation of the aorta (arrow). *Source:* Image provided courtesy of Dr. T. Cecere, Virginia Tech.

10.1.7 Thromboembolic Diseases

In dogs, protein-losing states, neoplastic conditions, and cortisol excess increase thromboembolic risk (Lake-Bakaar et al. 2012). Pulmonary thromboembolism and aortic thromboembolism are the most commonly identified sites of thromboembolism in dogs. In cats, cardiovascular disease resulting in left atrial enlargement is associated with significant risk of thromboembolic complications (Stokol et al. 2008). The forelimb and the terminal aorta (Figure 10.1) are the most commonly affected sites for thromboembolism in cats. In patients with increased thromboembolic risk, treatment focuses on management of underlying risk factors and shifting the hemostatic balance with antiplatelet or anticoagulant medications.

> **Dramatic difference**
>
> Dogs with cardiovascular disease, including those with atrial fibrillation, do not have increased risk of thromboembolic complications. This is in contrast to both humans and cats with cardiovascular disease, who do have an increased risk.

10.1.8 Infectious Cardiovascular Diseases

With the exception of heartworm disease, infectious cardiovascular disease is uncommon in veterinary patients. Infectious cardiovascular diseases reported in animals include heartworm disease, bacterial and fungal endocarditis and myocarditis, Chagas disease, Lyme disease, bartonella, leishmania, coccidioidomycosis, parvovirus, feline immunodeficiency virus, and herpes virus (Olson and Miller 1986; Levy and Duray 1988; Simpson et al. 2005; Church et al. 2007; Saunders et al. 2013; Costa et al. 2014; Rosa et al. 2014; Sime et al. 2015; Rolim et al. 2016; Santilli et al. 2017). Only heartworm disease has medical preventive measures. Treatment of infectious cardiovascular disease involves specific treatment directed at the infecting organism when possible.

10.1.8.1 Heartworm Disease

Heartworm disease is a mosquito-transmitted infection affecting dogs and cats in all parts of the USA with significant mosquito populations. Although the distribution of heartworm disease has not changed significantly, with the southern USA representing the most affected region, the incidence of disease is increasing despite readily available heartworm preventative medications. This increase appears to be primarily associated with failure of owners to administer preventative consistently (i.e. at monthly intervals) or at all.

Dirofilaria immitis is the parasite that causes heartworm disease. This parasite frequently harbors a Gram-negative, endosymbiotic bacteria, *Wolbachia* (Bazzocchi

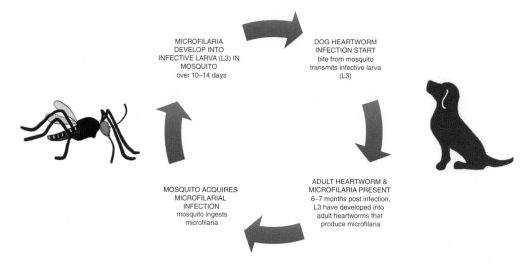

MICROFILARIA
DEVELOP INTO
INFECTIVE LARVA (L3) IN
MOSQUITO
over 10–14 days

DOG HEARTWORM
INFECTION START
bite from mosquito
transmits infective larva
(L3)

MOSQUITO ACQUIRES
MICROFILARIAL
INFECTION
mosquito ingests
microfilaria

ADULT HEARTWORM &
MICROFILARIA PRESENT
6–7 months post infection,
L3 have developed into
adult heartworms that
produce microfilaria

Figure 10.2 The lifecycle of *Dirofilaria immitis* in the dog. Heartworm prevention, testing, and treatment recommendations are based on the timeframes outlined in this lifecycle. Macrocyclic lactone heartworm preventatives block L3 and L4 development to adult worms. Heartworm antigen testing detects only adult, female heartworms and therefore can be used when adult worms are present, six months after inoculation with L3. Microfilaria testing with the modified Knott's test can detect infection once adult heartworms are present and producing microfilaria, six to seven months after inoculation with L3.

et al. 2008). Since *Wolbachia* is thought to contribute to both *D. immitis* survival and clinical heartworm disease, both *D. immitis* and *Wolbachia* must be treated in affected animals. Dogs are the normal definitive host for *D. immitis* (Henry and Dillon 1994). Although cats and ferrets are less suitable hosts, they can also be infected with *D. immitis*. Humans are rare incidental hosts (Jacob et al. 2016; Tumolskaya et al. 2016; Krstic et al. 2017; Mirahmadi et al. 2017). The heartworm cycle starts when an animal becomes infected with infective larvae (L3) when bitten by a mosquito carrying *D. immitis* (Figure 10.2). The larvae develop into adult heartworm about six to seven months after transmission in dogs. Adult heartworms reproduce in the pulmonary arteries, producing circulating microfilariae. The mosquito ingests the microfilariae with its blood meal, continuing the heartworm lifecycle.

The clinical manifestations of heartworm disease differ between dogs and cats (Knight et al. 2001; Nelson et al. 2005b; Venco et al. 2015). Dogs can have large numbers of *D. immitis* worms within their pulmonary arteries and sometimes right heart and vena cava (Figure 10.3). Clinical disease in dogs is a

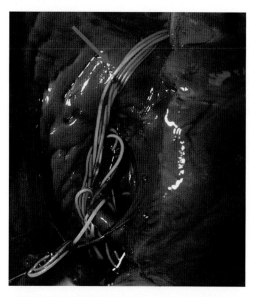

Figure 10.3 Heartworm infection in a dog. Numerous adult heartworms are present in the right ventricle (arrow). Adult heartworms primarily reside in the pulmonary arteries, with worms also present in the right heart with higher worm burdens. *Source:* Image provided courtesy of Dr. T. Cecere, Virginia Tech.

result of both the physical obstruction caused by the worms and the inflammatory response associated with *D. immitis* infection. In dogs, significant worm burden results in pulmonary hypertension, inflammatory pulmonary disease, and eventually secondary right heart disease/failure. Severity of heartworm disease in the dog is classified as class I (asymptomatic to mild disease), class II (moderate disease), class III (severe disease, including signs of right heart failure), and class IV (caval syndrome – obstruction due to worms). Secondary inflammatory pulmonary disease, immune-mediated anemia, and glomerular kidney disease can also occur in heartworm-positive dogs.

In contrast to dogs, cats usually have small worm burdens, and their disease is primarily related to the inflammatory response known as heartworm-associated respiratory disease. Infection with just a single adult heartworm can be fatal in a cat. In cats, the clinical manifestation occurs in two phases: (i) an early phase, three to four months after infection, due to an inflammatory response to the larvae; and (ii) a late phase, two to four years after infection, when adult worms die, resulting in pulmonary thromboemboli. The early (inflammatory) phase is characterized by asthma-like symptoms, including cough and wheeze, and is referred to as heartworm-associated respiratory disease. The late (thromboembolic) phase is characterized by acute respiratory distress. Interestingly, vomiting is also frequently reported in cats with heartworm disease, although the pathophysiology is not clear. Less common symptoms reported in the cat include neurologic symptoms and effusions.

The differences between heartworm disease in the dog and cat also extend to diagnosis and treatment. Commercially available antigen tests identify the adult female worm, while microfilaria tests (modified Knott's) identify circulating microfilaria. Antigen tests are the most sensitive and specific for identifying adult heartworm infection in dogs. In cats, because of the low worm burden and the possibility of infection with only male worms, both antigen and microfilarial testing are far less sensitive for detecting heartworm disease. Adulticide therapy, to kill the adult heartworm, is the treatment of choice in dogs. Due to the inflammatory nature of heartworm disease in cats, the benefit of adulticide therapy doesn't outweigh the risks, and it is therefore not currently recommended in cats.

10.1.8.2 Endocarditis

Infective endocarditis has been reported in many veterinary species. *Staphylococcus* spp., *Streptococcus* spp., *Escherichia coli*, and *Bartonella* spp. are the most commonly reported pathogens (Sykes et al. 2006; Chomel et al. 2009; Palerme et al. 2016). Clinical signs associated with infective endocarditis in veterinary patients include lethargy, inappetence, lameness, or signs of heart failure. Diagnosis for infective endocarditis in animals is similar to that for people (Topan et al. 2015).

10.2 Drug-Induced Cardiovascular Disease

Anthracycline-associated cardiomyopathy is the most commonly encountered drug-induced cardiovascular disease in veterinary patients. The cardiac effects are dose dependent in dogs, similar to in humans. However, dogs appear to develop doxorubicin-induced cardiomyopathy at much lower doses than people. The median cumulative dose at which cardiomyopathy occurs is $150\,mg\,M^{-2}$ (body surface area) in the dog (Mauldin et al. 1992; Chatterjee et al. 2010). Similar cardiac manifestations have also been reported with epirubicin at a total cumulative dose of $168\,mg\,M^{-2}$ (Lee et al. 2015). Clinical monitoring for evidence of cardiac dysfunction prior to each treatment and maintenance of a cumulative lifetime doxorubicin dose less than $150–180\,mg\,M^{-2}$ are recommended for dogs (Mauldin et al. 1992). Reducing the rate of doxorubicin administration is also recommended to avoid acute cardiac effects. Dexrazoxane can be used to decrease cardiotoxic effects of anthracyclines in dogs (Baldwin et al. 1992; Imondi et al. 1996; FitzPatrick et al. 2010).

Accidental ionophore intoxication of horses results in acute and long-term cardiomyopathy

(Bezerra et al. 1999; Hughes et al. 2009). This usually occurs when horses gain access to and consume cattle feed containing an ionophore such as monensin or lasolocid (Decloedt et al. 2012; Dorne et al. 2013). Ionophores are used in cattle feed to increase feed efficiency and body weight gain.

10.3 Cardiovascular Drug Pharmacogenomics

Similar to people, veterinary species have genetic alterations that influence their response to drugs. Genetic mutations/polymorphisms have been described that impact drugs used in the prevention and treatment of cardiovascular disease in dogs and cats.

A mutation in the MDR1 gene (also known as the ABCB1 gene) resulting in P-glycoprotein deficiency has been reported in dogs (Mealey et al. 2001). Less is known about the clinical impact of the nonsense MDR1 mutation in cats (Mealey and Burke 2015). The canine MDR1 mutation was first reported in Collies but has since been identified in multiple breeds (Mealey et al. 2001; Mealey and Meurs 2008). This mutation is of clinical importance in heartworm prevention because avermectin preventatives are P-glycoprotein-dependent drugs. Although standard preventative doses of ivermectin have been determined to be safe in all breeds, breeds with the MDR1 mutation receiving higher doses of ivermectin and/or dogs concurrently receiving a P-glycoprotein pump inhibitor are at increased risk of ivermectin toxicity (Mealey 2004, 2008, 2012; Mealey and Meurs 2008) The MDR1 mutation may also increase the risk of toxicity with other cardiovascular drugs that are transported by P-glycoprotein substrates, including digoxin, diltiazem, verapamil, losartan, propranolol, telmisartan, clopidogrel, warfarin, apixaban, and dabigatran (Henik et al. 2006; Stollberger and Finsterer 2015).

Polymorphisms have been identified in dogs and cats that could influence the response to other cardiovascular drugs. Polymorphisms in the beta-1 adrenergic receptor were identified in both dogs and cats (Maran et al. 2012, 2013; Meurs et al. 2015). An altered heart rate response was observed in dogs with this polymorphism (Meurs et al. 2015). Pharmacologic responsiveness in cats with this polymorphism has not been evaluated. An angiotensin-converting enzyme (ACE) polymorphism has also been identified in sled dogs, but the pharmacologic impact of this polymorphism is currently unknown (Huson et al. 2011). A polymorphism has been identified in the canine phosphodiesterase (PDE) 5A gene in healthy dogs. This polymorphism is associated with lower plasma cyclic guanosine monophosphate (cGMP) concentrations (Stern et al. 2014). Its role in pulmonary hypertension and impact on PDE inhibitors have not yet been investigated. Additional information about pharmacogenetics in companion animals can be found in Chapter 5.

10.4 Diagnostic Testing

The primary care veterinarian arrives at the preliminary diagnosis of canine and feline cardiovascular disease by utilizing readily available equipment and skills, including auscultation, blood biochemistry/biomarker evaluation, echocardiography, electrocardiogram (ECG), non-invasive blood pressure, and thoracic radiographs. Definitive diagnosis often requires echocardiography performed by a board-certified cardiologist. The following list includes available diagnostic testing modalities divided into their general availability.

Routinely available cardiovascular testing modalities (general veterinary practice):

- Auscultation
- Thoracic radiography
- Heartworm antibody/antigen testing
- Modified Knott's (microfilaria testing)
- Cardiac biomarkers (TnI and pro-BNP [brain natriuretic peptide])
- Taurine/carnitine plasma levels
- Blood pressure
- ECG.

Limited availability cardiovascular testing modalities (specialty veterinary practice):

- *Echocardiography:* 2D and 3D transthoracic and transesophageal
- Holter monitor, event monitor, or implantable loop recorder
- *Imaging:* Computed tomography (CT), magnetic resonance imaging (MRI; ECG-gated), and angiogram.

10.5 Pharmacological Treatment of Common Diseases

Medical therapy is the mainstay of treatment for acquired heart disease, arrhythmias, systemic hypertension, pulmonary hypertension, and thromboembolic and infectious cardiovascular diseases. In contrast, many congenital heart diseases are managed by interventional or surgical repair, with only a subset requiring ongoing medical management.

10.5.1 Heartworm Disease Prevention and Treatment

10.5.1.1 Prevention: Macrocyclic Lactones (MLs)

Heartworm preventative is a prescription medication requiring a valid client–patient relationship and documentation of a heartworm-negative status prior to initiating a preventative protocol. The American Heartworm Society recommends year-round heartworm preventative treatment to improve overall compliance and protection (Nelson et al. 2005b). Currently, the American Heartworm Society recommends both antigen and microfilaria tests for dogs prior to initiation of heartworm preventative. Testing for antigen is the most sensitive and specific test to identify heartworm infection in the dog. Testing for microfilaria is important to alert the veterinarian to the risk of an anaphylactoid reaction in microfilaremic dogs.

Guidelines for heartworm testing are based on the lifecycle of *D. immitis* (Figure 10.2). Because it takes a minimum of six months

from inoculation for adult worms to mature and produce microfilaria, dogs cannot test positive for heartworm disease prior to six months of age even if infected. Therefore, AHS does not recommend testing for puppies if preventative is initiated prior to eight weeks of age. Puppies started on preventative between two and six months of age should be tested six months after starting preventative. Puppies older than six months and adult dogs should be tested prior to initiation of preventative. Because of the low sensitivity of the antigen and microfilaria tests in cats, definitive determination of heartworm status prior to initiation of heartworm preventative is not currently possible. In addition, the safety of many of the preventatives is not known in heartworm-positive cats.

All heartworm preventative medications belong to the ML class of drugs, which includes both avermectins and milbemycins. MLs block the development of *D. immitis* larval stages (L3 and L4) (Figure 10.2). The most commonly used MLs for heartworm prevention in the USA include ivermectin (oral), milbemycin oxime (oral), selamectin (topical), and moxidectin (topical, long-acting injection). The oral (available in chewable and tablet formulations) and topical preventatives are administered monthly. The long-acting moxidectin-impregnated microsphere injection is administered every six months. Many heartworm preventative products are combined with other antiparasitics to combat internal and/or external parasites (e.g. fleas, ticks, roundworms, and tapeworms).

10.5.1.2 Treatment: Melarasamine and Doxycycline

Because the nature of *D. immitis* infection and the clinical disease it causes differ between cats and dogs, it is not surprising that the treatments differ as well. The disease in dogs is primarily influenced by the overall worm burden, so the treatment goal is to eliminate adult worms (adulticide treatment) and control secondary inflammation and thromboembolism associated with worm die-off. The current guidelines for treatment of heartworm disease in dogs include initial treatment with an antibiotic for *Wolbachia* (doxycycline) and a ML heartworm preventative, followed by an arsenical heartworm adulticide medication (melarsomine), anti-inflammatory doses of corticosteroids (prednisone), and strict cage rest to reduce thromboembolic complications (Figure 10.4). Dogs with "caval syndrome," obstruction of blood flow due to a very heavy worm burden, require urgent surgical removal of the worms. Although the combination of a ML, usually ivermectin at preventative doses, and doxycycline can be microfilaricidal and adulticidal over 2.5 years, the American Heartworm Society still recommends the treatment protocol described here because it results in earlier clearance of heartworm infection and avoids ongoing pathologic changes associated with the "slow kill" approach (Bazzocchi et al. 2008; Mavropoulou et al. 2014). The combination of 10% imidacloprid + 2.5% moxidectin (Advangate Multi®) and doxycycline is currently being evaluated as an alternative adulticide treatment protocol (Bendas et al. 2017).

Heartworm preventative MLs are administered to heartworm-positive dogs to both prevent new infections and eliminate heartworm larvae that are not susceptible to adulticide treatment. However, MLs can also have microfilaricidal activity, which can cause severe inflammatory responses if there is rapid microfilaria kill-off. By identifying the dog's microfilaria status prior to administration of a ML heartworm preventative, the veterinarian can pretreat the dog with diphenhydramine and prednisone to abrogate severe reactions and closely monitor the patient. For dogs that are still microfilaria-positive after adulticide treatment, topical 10% imidacloprid + 2.5% moxidectin (ADVANTAGE MULTI®) is FDA approved to treat circulating microfilaria in dogs (McCall et al. 2014). Although no adverse events were reported in the clinical trial, vomiting, diarrhea, dyspnea, and anaphylactoid reactions have been reported in post-approval experience (McCall et al. 2014).

Doxycycline has multiple benefits in the heartworm-infected dog. It reduces *Wolbachia*, decreasing the risk of *Wolbachia*-associated inflammatory disease; it is lethal to some heartworm larvae (L3 and L4); and it suppresses microfilaremia (Bazzocchi et al. 2008; McCall et al. 2014).

Melarsamine dihydrochloride (Immiticide®) is the recommended adulticide treatment in dogs. Melarsamine is administered by deep intramuscular injection in the lumbar muscles to reduce the incidence of injection site reactions. IMMITICIDE® has episodically been difficult to obtain over recent years due to manufacturing shortages, prompting veterinarians to pursue other treatment approaches or delay treatment. In the spring of 2017, Diroban™, an FDA-approved generic melarsamine dihydrochloride product labeled for use in dogs with Class I, II, or III heartworm disease, was released. Because of its recent release, there is very limited clinical experience with Diroban or its market availability.

In contrast to dogs, adulticide treatment is not recommended in heartworm-infected cats (Nelson et al. 2005a). This is largely because of a much higher incidence of life-threatening complications during adulticide treatment in cats. In addition, cats are more susceptible than dogs to melarsamine's adverse effects. In general, asymptomatic cats are not currently treated, and spontaneous clearance will occur in some of these cats. Symptomatic cats are treated with prednisolone to control respiratory signs, with the goal to taper down to the minimum effect dose. Symptomatic cats that are refractory to prednisolone have been treated with ivermectin. However, it is important to note that the impact on overall patient survival is unknown. The impact of doxycycline for management of *Wolbachia*-infected *D. immitis* in cats is also unknown.

> **Dramatic difference**
>
> Melarsamine dihydrochloride is the adulticide of choice for heartworm-positive dogs, but it is not recommended in heartworm-positive cats.

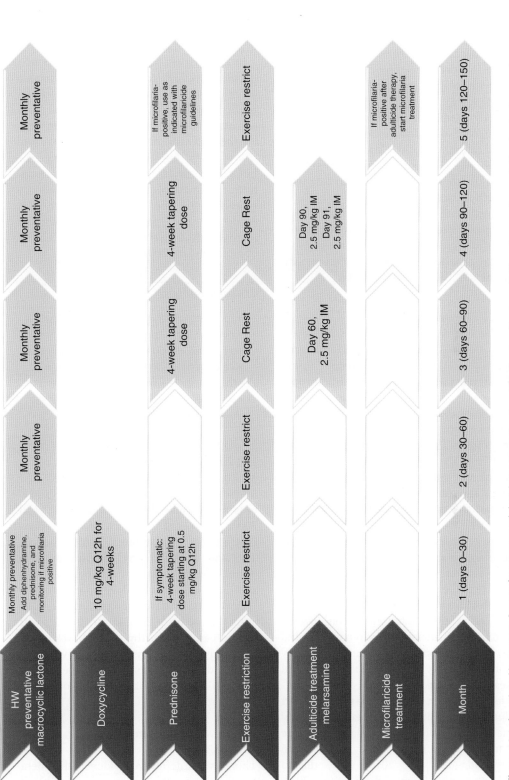

Figure 10.4 American Heartworm Society heartworm adulticide treatment protocol for the dog. Treatment of heartworm disease in the dog is a long and costly process that requires significant owner dedication to monitoring, exercise restriction, and frequent veterinary visits.

10.5.2 Delay Onset of Congestive Heart Failure

Despite decades of research to identify medications that delay the onset of heart failure in dogs with heart disease, only recently have studies identified drugs that demonstrate clinically significant benefits for dogs with myxomatous mitral valve degeneration and dilated cardiomyopathy. Unfortunately, studies have not yet identified medications that delay the onset of heart failure in cats with acquired heart disease.

Animals with secondary heart disease such as hyperthyroidism, systemic hypertension, or taurine-responsive dilated cardiomyopathy can experience disease resolution with treatment of the underlying cause.

10.5.2.1 Pimobendan

Pimobendan is an FDA-approved veterinary medication (Vetmedin®) indicated for treating dogs with CHF due to myxomatous mitral valve degeneration and dilated cardiomyopathy. It is a benzimidazole–pyridazinone derivative. Pimobendan is classified as an inodilator, providing both positive inotropic and vasodilatory effects. Pimobendan's inotropic effects result from its action as a PDE III inhibitor and calcium sensitizer. Inhibition of PDE III activity also causes vasodilation. It is available as a chewable tablet containing 1.25, 2.5, 5, or 10 mg of pimobendan. The chewable formulation is generally well accepted, and adverse effects are not commonly encountered. There is no generic formulation of pimobendan available in the USA at this time, and cost can be prohibitive in larger dogs.

Recently, pimobendan has been investigated in dogs with either myxomatous mitral valve degeneration or dilated cardiomyopathy prior to the onset of heart failure (preclinical disease). Multiple prospective, blinded studies identified both a delay in the onset of heart failure and an increased median survival time in dogs with cardiac enlargement due to myxomatous mitral valve degeneration (Boswood et al. 2016) or dilated cardiomyopathy (Summerfield et al. 2012; Vollmar and Fox 2016). Given these findings, pimobendan is regularly prescribed for preclinical dogs with myxomatous mitral valve degeneration or dilated cardiomyopathy.

In contrast to the veterinary experience, people with CHF treated with pimobendan experienced far more varied and riskier results. Despite improved exercise tolerance and quality of life noted in some human studies, the PICO trial demonstrated an increased risk of death (Lubsen et al. 1996). Later, the EPOCH study in Japan showed that long-term treatment with pimobendan reduced morbidity and improved physical activity in moderate heart failure patients without increased death in the treated group ("Effects of pimobendan" 2002).

Dramatic difference

Pimobendan delays the onset of CHF and is associated with improved survival times in dogs with CHF due to myxomatous mitral valve degeneration and dilated cardiomyopathy. An increased risk of death has not been identified in dogs treated with pimobendan, as it has in people.

10.5.2.2 ACE Inhibitors

Multiple clinical trials have evaluated ACE inhibitors in dogs with preclinical myxomatous mitral valve degeneration (Kvart et al. 2002; Atkins et al. 2007). These studies demonstrated at best minimal clinical benefit. Therefore, dogs with preclinical myxomatous mitral valve degeneration with heart enlargement should be managed with pimobendan.

Fewer studies have been performed evaluating the use of ACE inhibitors in dogs with dilated cardiomyopathy. A single retrospective study of Doberman Pinchers with preclinical dilated cardiomyopathy identified a delay to the onset of CHF in Dobermans receiving benazepril (O'Grady et al. 2009).

10.5.2.3 Beta-Adrenergic Receptor Antagonists

There is no definitive evidence that beta-adrenergic receptor antagonists (beta blockers) delay the onset of CHF in animals with cardiovascular disease. There have been only two published studies evaluating beta blockers in dogs with preclinical dilated cardiomyopathy or myxomatous mitral valve degeneration (Calvert et al. 1997; Oyama et al. 2007). Neither of these studies was designed to evaluate a delay in onset of heart failure.

Practiced but not proven
Although ACE inhibitors, beta blockers, or calcium-channel blockers have been prescribed in cats with preclinical hypertrophic cardiomyopathy, no study has documented a delay in onset of heart failure with any of these medications. In fact, no large, blinded, placebo-controlled studies have been performed in preclinical cats with hypertrophic cardiomyopathy.

Drugs commonly prescribed to delay the onset of CHF in dogs with dilated cardiomyopathy or myxomatous mitral valve degeneration:

Pimobendan: 0.25 mg/kg PO every 12 hours

*Enalapril:** 0.5 mg/kg PO every 12 hours.

*Enalapril may be used if pimobendan is cost prohibitive.

10.5.3 Congestive Heart Failure

Classification of heart failure severity in human patients uses the New York Heart Association (NYHA) system. In the veterinary literature, edema due to cardiac insufficiency is often referred to as one of the following: CHF, ACVIM stage C or D (Table 10.1), or ISACH (International Small Animal Cardiac Health Council) Class II or III A/B. Although included in some drug inserts, NYHA classification of heart failure is not routinely used, as it requires subjective evaluation that is challenging to assess in animals. Dogs with CHF are routinely treated with so-called triple therapy consisting of furosemide, pimobendan, and/or an ACE inhibitor. Cats with CHF are

Table 10.1 American College of Veterinary Internal Medicine (ACVIM) consensus classification system for heart disease.

ACVIM Stage	Description
A	Patient at high risk for developing heart disease due to breed predisposition but currently has no evidence of heart disease (no current heart disease)
B1	Patient with structural heart disease but no evidence of heart enlargement (asymptomatic heart disease)
B2	Patient with structural heart disease and evidence of heart enlargement but no evidence of congestive heart failure (advanced asymptomatic heart disease)
C	Patient with past or current congestive heart failure associated with heart disease (symptomatic heart disease)
D	Patient with refractory heart failure (end-stage heart disease)

routinely treated with furosemide and an ACE inhibitor to manage their CHF and antithrombotics to manage the increased thromboembolic risk.

10.5.3.1 Furosemide

Furosemide is the most commonly used diuretic in veterinary medicine. It is available under the trade name Salix®, labeled for the treatment of edema associated with cardiac insufficiency and acute non-inflammatory tissue edema in dogs, cats, and horses. Salix is available in 12.5 or 50 mg tablets, and 5.0% injectable solution. It is important to note that veterinary tablet strengths are not equivalent to human tablet strengths of furosemide (20 mg, 40 mg, and 80 mg tablets). Doses for all veterinary species are titrated to the minimum dose necessary to control signs associated with CHF. Other loop diuretics, including bumetanide, torsemide, and parenteral furosemide, are used in refractory heart failure cases.

Dramatic difference

Furosemide doses for human adults are much lower than canine doses, such that a 20 kg dog would receive a similar dose of furosemide as an adult human. Animal furosemide doses are more similar to pediatric doses.

10.5.3.2 Pimobendan

Pimobendan has been FDA approved for use in dogs with CHF since 2007. Since then, multiple clinical trials demonstrate that pimobendan treatment significantly improves survival time in dogs with CHF due to dilated cardiomyopathy or myxomatous mitral valve degeneration (Fuentes et al. 2002; Haggstrom et al. 2008). Accordingly, pimobendan is routinely used for treating CHF in dogs. When pimobendan is cost-prohibitive, canine CHF patients usually receive furosemide and an ACE inhibitor.

Extra-label use of pimobendan in cats with CHF has been reported in small, retrospective studies (Gordon et al. 2012; Reina-Doreste et al. 2014). Currently, it is primarily being used in cats with refractory heart failure. Pharmacokinetic studies in normal cats suggest that, compared with dogs, pimobendan is metabolized more slowly (Hanzlicek et al. 2012; Yata et al. 2016).

10.5.3.3 ACE Inhibitors

The ACE inhibitors benazepril and enalapril have been routinely used to manage clinical signs of CHF in dogs and cats. Multiple multicenter, placebo-controlled, blinded studies evaluating their use in dogs with CHF due to myxomatous mitral valve degeneration or dilated cardiomyopathy have demonstrated a morbidity and mortality benefit ("Acute and short-term" 1995; "Controlled clinical evaluation" 1995; Ettinger et al. 1998; "The effect of benazepril" 1999).

10.5.3.4 Spironolactone

The aldosterone antagonist spironolactone has been recently added to standard triple therapy (furosemide, pimobendan, and ACE inhibitor) as the consensus recommendation for treatment of CHF due to myxomatous mitral valve degeneration. Historically, this addition was often implemented with refractory heart failure. The reduced risk of death reported in human heart failure patients in the RALES trial, and the suggestion that spironolactone may improve survival in dogs with CHF, have led to this drug being added earlier in the course of CHF treatment (Juurlink et al. 2004; Bernay et al. 2010; Lefebvre et al. 2013).

Common Congestive Heart Failure Treatment Protocol: Dog

Drug	Class	Common starting dose (mg/kg dose)	Routine monitoring	Veterinary-labeled product
Furosemide	Loop diuretic	2 mg/kg Q12h	Renal function Electrolytes Blood pressure	Salix®
Enalapril	ACE inhibitor	0.5 mg/kg Q12h	Renal function Electrolytes Blood pressure	
Pimobendan	PDE III inhibitor/ calcium sensitizer (inodilator)	0.25 mg/kg Q12h		Vetmedin®
Spironolactone	Aldosterone inhibitor	1–2 mg/kg Q12h	Renal function Electrolytes Blood pressure	

ACE, Angiotensin-converting enzyme; PDE, phosphodiesterase; Q12h, every 12 hours.

Common Congestive Heart Failure/Thrombosis Risk Reduction Treatment Protocol: Cat

Drug	Class	Common starting dose (per cat dose[a])	Routine monitoring	Veterinary-labeled product
Furosemide	Loop diuretic	3.125–6.25 mg PER CAT TOTAL DOSE PO Q12 hours	Renal function Electrolytes Blood pressure	Salix®
Enalapril	ACE inhibitor	1.25–2.5 mg PER CAT TOTAL DOSE PO Q12 hours	Renal function Electrolytes Blood pressure	
Clopidogrel	Platelet inhibitor	18.75 mg PER CAT TOTAL DOSE PO Q24 hours	Evidence of bleeding	

ACE, Angiotensin-converting enzyme; PO, *per os* ("orally"); Q, every.
[a] Please note that since cat weights do not vary to the same degree as dogs, and since dosing is largely affected by tablet size, doses for cats are listed as a per-cat dose.

10.5.3.5 Angiotensin Receptor Blocker/Neprilysin Inhibitors

Although there are no published studies of the novel angiotensin receptor blocker/neprilysin inhibitor (valsartan/sacuitril; Entresto®) in dogs, a clinical trial for its use in dogs with CHF due to myxomatous mitral valve degeneration is currently enrolling patients.

10.5.3.6 Synthetic Canine Brain Natriuretic Peptide

A Phase I trial in healthy dogs and dogs with preclinical myxomatous mitral valve degeneration demonstrated that synthetic canine BNP was well tolerated and safe, but no studies of survival benefits have been published at this time (Oyama et al. 2017).

10.5.3.7 Beta-Adrenergic Receptor Antagonists

There is no definitive evidence that beta-adrenergic receptor antagonists (beta blockers) improve survival in animals with CHF. Beta blocker use can actually cause clinical decompensation in some animals with CHF. Small prospective studies of the use of beta blocker carvedilol in dogs with CHF due to dilated cardiomyopathy failed to demonstrate a mortality benefit (Oyama et al. 2007).

10.5.4 Systemic Hypertension

Since systemic hypertension is usually a secondary disease in veterinary patients, treatment is focused on management of underlying disease when possible and the use of vasodilators when needed. The dihydropyridine calcium-channel blockers such as amlodipine besylate and ACE inhibitors such as benazepril have been commonly used for the management of systemic hypertension in animals. The angiotensin receptor blocker Semintra® is the first FDA-approved drug for the management of systemic hypertension in cats (Snyder 1998; Brown et al. 2007). The goal of antihypertensive treatment in veterinary patients is gradual reduction in blood pressure to reduce the risk of systemic hypertension-induced organ damage. Since veterinary patients generally don't have sodium-responsive systemic hypertension, strict sodium restriction is not required, but avoidance of high-sodium diets is generally recommended.

> **Dramatic difference**
>
> Unlike human patients, diuretics are not used to treat systemic hypertension in animals.

10.5.4.1 Dihydropyridine Calcium-Channel Blockers

Amlodipine is the first-line therapy for cats with systemic hypertension (Taylor et al. 2017). A randomized, double-blinded, placebo-controlled study in cats demonstrated a clinically significant reduction in blood pressure with a chewable amlodipine tablet (Huhtinen et al. 2015). Similar results were reported in earlier studies with the human amlodipine tablet (Henik et al. 1997). A chewable formulation of amlodipine labeled for systemic hypertension in cats (Amodip® 1.25 mg) has recently been approved in the EU and UK. Due to insufficient evidence of efficacy, compounded transdermal formulations of amlodipine are not recommended.

10.5.4.2 ACE Inhibitors

ACE inhibitors are commonly used to treat systemic hypertension in dogs (Brown et al. 2007). ACE inhibitors tend to be less effective antihypertensives than amlodipine in veterinary patients; therefore, some canine patients with systemic hypertension will require the addition of a calcium-channel blocker. Because it is not highly dependent on renal excretion, benazepril is the recommended ACE inhibitor in patients with systemic hypertension associated with kidney disease.

10.5.4.3 Angiotensin Receptor Antagonists

There is limited information on the use of angiotensin type 1 receptor antagonists for treating systemic hypertension in animals as compared to people. Pharmacokinetics of the angiotensin receptor antagonists telmisartan, losartan, and valsartan were evaluated in normal dogs, with telmisartan having the longest systemic exposure (Baek et al. 2013). Anecdotal use of telmisartan in dogs with glomerular disease and in dogs with systemic hypertension has been reported (Bugbee et al. 2014). A liquid formulation of telmisartan, Semintra®, was recently FDA-approved for management of systemic hypertension in cats.

Common therapy for systemic hypertension in the cat:

Amlodipine: 0.625 mg PER CAT, TOTAL DOSE, PO every 24 hours.

Common systemic hypertension therapy options in the dog:

Benazepril: 0.5 mg/kg PO every 12–24 hours
Amlodipine: 0.1–0.25 mg/kg PO every 24 hours
Telmisartan: 1 mg/kg PO every 24 hours.

10.5.5 Pulmonary Hypertension

Treatment of pulmonary hypertension in dogs is primarily focused on management of the underlying disease when possible. Diseases associated with pulmonary hypertension in dogs include heartworm disease, other causes of pulmonary thromboembolism, some respiratory diseases, and left heart disease.

10.5.5.1 Pimobendan

Pimobendan has been shown to be beneficial for the management of post-capillary pulmonary hypertension secondary to left heart disease. In a small, blinded, placebo-controlled trial, pimobendan significantly reduced echocardiographically-assessed systolic pulmonary arterial pressure in dogs with moderate to severe pulmonary hypertension secondary to myxomatous mitral valve degeneration (Atkinson et al. 2009).

10.5.5.2 Sildenafil

The PDE-V inhibitor sildenafil has been minimally evaluated for the management of pulmonary hypertension in animals. Although some improvement has been reported in retrospective studies and small case series, no large, prospective, placebo-controlled clinical trials have been performed in dogs with pulmonary hypertension (Nakamura et al. 2011; Kellihan et al. 2015). A small, short-term, randomized, blinded, placebo-controlled study of sildenafil in dogs with pulmonary hypertension demonstrated increased quality-of-life scores (Brown et al. 2010). In this small study, estimates of pulmonary hypertension were reduced from baseline in sildenafil-treated dogs but were not significantly different from those in dogs receiving placebo.

Common treatment options for dogs with pulmonary hypertension:

Pimobendan (for post-capillary pulmonary hypertension):

Dog: 0.25 mg/kg every 12 hours.

Sildenafil (for pre-capillary pulmonary hypertension):

Dog: 0.5–1 mg/kg every 8–24 hours.

10.5.6 Thyrotoxic Heart Disease

Treatment of thyrotoxic heart disease of cats is primarily focused on normalization of thyroid levels. This can be achieved by radioactive iodine treatment, surgical removal of the thyroid glands, or medical control with methimazole (see Chapter 15). Resolution of heart disease is anticipated three to four months after normalization of thyroid levels.

10.5.7 Arrhythmias

No FDA-approved drugs are specifically indicated as antiarrhythmics for veterinary species. Drugs used to treat arrhythmias are often classified by mechanism of action using the Vaughn Williams classification. Table 10.2 summarizes the commonly used oral antiarrhythmics in veterinary medicine, their starting doses, their indications, and the species for which they are most commonly prescribed.

10.5.7.1 Atrial Fibrillation

Atrial fibrillation is one of the most common arrhythmias in veterinary medicine.

Table 10.2 Antiarrhythmic drugs, indications, and doses for dogs and cats.

Vaughn Williams classification	Drug	Dose	Antiarrhythmic indication	Species
1b (Na$^+$ channel blockers)	Mexiletine	5–8 mg/kg PO Q8 hours	VT	Dog
II (Beta-adrenergic receptor antagonists)	Atenolol	Dog: 0.1–1 mg/kg PO Q12–24 hours Cat: 6.25 mg PER CAT TOTAL DOSE PO Q 24 hours	SVT (A. Fib) VT	Dog and Cat
III (K$^+$ channel blockers)	Sotalol Amiodarone	1–3 mg/kg Q12 hours Loading dose: 8–10 mg/kg Q12 hours for 7–10 days Maintenance dose: 4–6 mg/kg Q24 hours	SVT (A. Fib) VT SVT (A. Fib) VT	Dog Dog
IV (Ca^{2+} channel blockers)	Diltiazem	Diltiazem: Dog: 0.5–1.5 mg/kg PO Q8 hours Cat: 7.5 mg PER CAT TOTAL DOSE PO Q8 hours Dilacor XR: Dog: 1–3 mg/kg Q12 hours Cat: 30 mg PER CAT TOTAL DOSE PO Q24 hours	SVT (A. Fib)	Dog and Cat

A. Fib, Atrial fibrillation; PO, per os (orally); Q, every; SVT, supraventricular tachycardia; VT, ventricular tachycardia.

The primary goal of therapy in patients with underlying cardiac disease is to control the heart rate. Many of these patients are concurrently receiving heart failure medications. The most common medications used for atrial fibrillation in dogs include digoxin, diltiazem, atenolol, and amiodarone (Table 10.4).

Medical therapy or electrical cardioversion can be considered in horses with atrial fibrillation in the absence of underlying heart disease (lone atrial fibrillation). In horses with lone atrial fibrillation, quinidine alone or in combination with digoxin can be used for conversion of atrial fibrillation to sinus rhythm. The duration of atrial fibrillation in horses is predictive of medical or electrical cardioversion outcome. Horses with shorter duration of atrial fibrillation have the best prognosis for successful conversion and maintenance of sinus rhythm. Medical cardioversion with quinidine in horses requires nasogastric tube drug administration and careful monitoring of quinidine plasma levels, ECG, and clinical status to avoid toxicity.

10.5.7.1.1 Digoxin

The cardiac glycoside digoxin is often the first-line therapy for atrial fibrillation in patients with dilated cardiomyopathy because it also has positive inotropic effects. The dosing considerations, side effect profile, and toxicity concerns are similar for human and veterinary patients. Digoxin is available in the veterinary formulation Cardoxin (Evsco). The elixir is generally not well tolerated in cats. Baseline lab work to evaluate renal function and electrolytes is important to determine the appropriate digoxin dose and to avoid arrhythmic complications associated with hypokalemia.

Many factors can influence serum digoxin levels and therefore digoxin dosing. Consideration of these factors is important to avoiding digoxin toxicity. Digoxin dosing is based on lean and dry body weight and reduced for patients with renal insufficiency or hypothyroidism. Owners should be aware that a digoxin dose may need to be reduced in the future if their pet loses weight or develops kidney disease or hypothyroidism. Digoxin is a substrate of P-glycoprotein, and therefore endogenous (MDR1 mutation) or exogenous (drugs that inhibit P-glycoprotein function) P-glycoprotein defects can affect digoxin levels. Digoxin can be involved

Table 10.3 Commonly used drugs (by class) that can INCREASE serum digoxin concentrations.

Drug class	Examples of commonly prescribed drugs (by class) that can increase digoxin concentrations
Antiarrhythmics	Amiodarone, Carvedilol, Diltiazem, Quinidine, Verapamil, Propafenone
Aldosterone inhibitor	Spironolactone
Antidepressants	Amitriptyline
Anticholinergics	Atropine, Cimetidine, Diphenhydramine, Cyproheptadine, Hydroxyzine, Hyoscyamine, Ranitidine, Scopolamine
Antihypertensive	Telmisartan
Anti-inflammatories (NSAIDS)	Rimadyl
Antimicrobials	Tetracycline, Erythromycin, Trimethoprim, Azithromycin
Antiulcer	Omeprazole
Anesthetic agents	Succinylcholine

Table 10.4 Common treatment options for atrial fibrillation.

Drug	Class	Monitoring	Drug-specific considerations
Digoxin	Cardiac glycoside Positive inotrope	Digoxin levels Renal values Electrolytes	First choice for dogs or cats with dilated cardiomyopathy Often used in combination with diltiazem if rate control insufficient alone Dose reduction with MDR1 mutation, some concurrent drugs, and reduced renal function Avoid use in hypokalemic patients.
Diltiazem	Calcium-channel blocker	GI side effects Blood pressure	Can be combined with digoxin in dogs Usually used alone in cats Do not use concurrently with atenolol.
Atenolol	Beta1 blocker	Blood pressure	Caution in cats and dogs with dilated cardiomyopathy or CHF Do not combine with diltiazem.
Amiodarone	Class III antiarrhythmic	CBC Serum chemistry T4	Primarily used in dogs Loading dose recommended Numerous adverse effects possible

CBC, Complete blood count; CHF, congestive heart failure; GI, gastrointestinal; T4, thyroid hormone.

in numerous drug–drug interactions, including other drugs used in the treatment of heart disease. Table 10.3 lists commonly used medications that increase serum digoxin levels. It is important that the owner understands the potential for drug interactions when their pet is receiving digoxin. Owners should notify the pharmacist and veterinarian when adding new medications or supplements, so that any necessary digoxin dose adjustments can be made to reduce the risk of toxicity.

Serum digoxin levels are measured seven days after initiation, six to eight hours post pill. Client education regarding signs of digoxin toxicity is essential. Clients should be instructed to discontinue digoxin and call the veterinarian if their pet develops new signs of inappetence, vomiting, diarrhea, syncope, seizures, or other neurologic symptoms. The pharmacist can play a key role in providing appropriate education to pet owners regarding monitoring for digoxin toxicity.

Digoxin dosages:

Dogs: 0.0025–0.003 mg/kg* PO every 12 hours. Target plasma concentration six to eight hours post pill of 0.8–1.3 nanograms/mL.

*Dry and lean body weight; dose reduction for patients with renal disease.

Cats: ¼ of a 0.125 mg tablet* PER CAT TOTAL DOSE PO every 48 hours.

*Dose reduction for patients with renal disease.

10.5.7.1.2 *Diltiazem*

The non-dihydropyridine calcium channel blocker diltiazem is commonly used for rate control in animals with atrial fibrillation. It can also be used in combination with digoxin when digoxin alone is insufficient to control heart rate (Gelzer et al. 2009). The oral bioavailability and plasma protein binding of diltiazem vary by formulation and between species (Piepho et al. 1982; Johnson et al. 1996). Standard diltiazem and the extended-release formulations Cardizem CD® and Dilacor XR® have been evaluated in cats and dogs (Johnson et al. 1996; Wall et al. 2005). It is important to note that the doses for the various diltiazem formulations are not the same, so switching between different diltiazem formulations is not advised without adjusting the dose accordingly. Additionally, administration of extended-release formulations of diltiazem to cats and smaller dogs may require opening the dispensed capsule to deliver a portion of the enclosed tablets. Therefore, care must be taken when dispensing diltiazem to ensure the appropriate formulation is dispensed. Counseling of owners may need to include instructions on more complicated administration requirements to manipulate human formulations to deliver the appropriate dose for a dog or cat.

10.5.7.1.3 Atenolol

Atenolol is a beta-1 selective adrenergic antagonist that can be used to control heart rate in patients with atrial fibrillation. Its use is generally limited to those animals not in CHF. Additionally, it is not used concurrently with diltiazem due to the combined negative inotropic effects.

10.5.7.1.4 Amiodarone

Amiodarone is a Class III antiarrhythmic with sodium, potassium, and calcium-channel-blocking effects that has been used for atrial fibrillation in dogs (Saunders et al. 2006). It is used in dogs undergoing cardioversion for atrial fibrillation or for rate control. Amiodarone has an extended plasma half-life in the dog (Latini et al. 1983; Brien et al. 1990). Dogs receiving chronic treatment with amiodarone should be monitored for the same adverse effects reported in people. CBC (complete blood count), liver enzyme values, and thyroid hormone concentrations are monitored in these patients. Serum amiodarone concentrations can also be evaluated in dogs (Pedro et al. 2012). Preservative-free injectable amiodarone is recommended when an injectable amiodarone formulation is necessary to minimize adverse effects (Levy et al. 2016).

10.5.7.2 Supraventricular Tachycardia

Supraventricular arrhythmias other than atrial fibrillation that can affect veterinary patients include atrial tachycardia and atrioventricular reciprocating tachycardia, resulting in a Wolf–Parkinson–White syndrome. Atrioventricular reciprocating tachycardia can be treated by catheter ablation, but due to cost and the limited number of veterinary facilities currently performing this procedure, medical management remains the primary therapy in veterinary patients. Common medical therapies for atrial tachycardia and atrioventricular reciprocating tachycardia include diltiazem, procainamide, and beta-adrenergic receptor antagonists (Atkins et al. 1995; Wright et al. 1996).

10.5.7.3 Ventricular Tachycardia

One should assume that all anti-arrhythmic drugs can have pro-arrhythmic effects. Examples of this include the variety of arrhythmias that can be caused by digoxin or the increased risk of mortality with medical arrhythmia suppression in the CAST trial in people (Echt et al. 1991). These challenges associated with antiarrhythmic therapy have contributed to the often-preferred use of cardioverter defibrillator implantation for managing significant ventricular arrhythmias in humans. Implantable cardioverter defibrillator placement has been performed in a few veterinary patients with ventricular tachycardia, but several factors limit this modality as a widespread approach for veterinary patients. Improvement of symptoms is a reasonable therapeutic goal of antiarrhythmic therapy in veterinary patients with ventricular tachycardia consisting of Vaughan-Williams Class Ib, Class II, and Class III antiarrhythmic drugs.

Practiced but not proven
Although antiarrhythmic drugs are commonly used to treat ventricular tachycardia in veterinary patients, their efficacy in preventing sudden death is unknown.

10.5.7.3.1 *Class Ib Antiarrhythmics*

Lidocaine is commonly used to treat acute ventricular tachycardia in dogs. It is generally well-tolerated and widely available in veterinary practices due to its use as a local anesthetic. Mexiletine alone or in combination with atenolol or sotalol can be used for patients with ventricular tachycardia (Meurs et al. 2002; Gelzer et al. 2010). When mexiletine is administered concurrently with sotalol, plasma mexiletine concentration can be expected to be higher (Gelzer et al. 2010). Unfortunately, practical limitations exist for mexiletine, which include its every-8-hour dosing schedule (difficult for many owners to comply with) and gastrointestinal side effects. The gastrointestinal effects in dogs can be decreased if the drug is administered with food, but they may still be significant enough in some dogs to discontinue the drug. Mexiletine is not used routinely in cats due to an apparent species-wide sensitivity to this class of drugs.

Dramatic difference

Class Ib antiarrhythmics, including mexiletine and lidocaine, can cause toxicity in cats.

10.5.7.3.2 *Class II Antiarrhythmics*

The beta-1 selective adrenergic antagonist atenolol can be used to treat dogs and cats with ventricular tachycardia. It should be avoided in patients with CHF, dilated cardiomyopathy, or asthma. It is a good choice for dogs with both supraventricular tachycardia and ventricular tachycardia as well as for cats (since Class Ib antiarrhythmics are not a good option). Atenolol is one of the few available antiarrhythmics that does not have to be compounded for use in cats because human formulations can be manipulated by owners to provide accurate doses. The ultra-short-acting beta-1 selective adrenergic antagonist esmolol may be used in acute situations requiring injectable formulation for management.

10.5.7.3.3 *Class III Antiarrhythmics*

Sotalol functions as both a beta-adrenergic antagonist and potassium-channel blocker. It is commonly used for long-term management of dogs with ventricular tachycardia, particularly in boxer dogs with arrhythmogenic right ventricular cardiomyopathy (Meurs et al. 2002). Sotalol must be used cautiously in patients with ventricular tachycardia associated with dilated cardiomyopathy because of its negative inotropic effect.

Amiodarone is becoming more widely used for ventricular arrhythmias in dogs despite its broad adverse effect profile. Among the most important benefits of amiodarone are its antifibrillatory effects, its ability to suppress concurrent supraventricular tachycardia and ventricular tachycardia, and its availability in both oral and injectable formulations.

10.5.8 Thrombosis Risk Reduction

As in humans, a prothrombotic state reflects an imbalance in procoagulant and anticoagulant factors. There are significant species differences in the underlying diseases that shift the balance to a procoagulant state, but the treatment approaches beyond addressing the underlying cause are similar. Antihemostatic agents include platelet inhibitors, anticoagulants, and fibrinolytics. In veterinary medicine, patients with increased risk of thromboembolism are primarily managed with platelet inhibitors and anticoagulants.

10.5.8.1 Platelet Inhibitors

Aspirin, a cyclooxygenase-1 (COX1) inhibitor, and clopidogrel, a platelet adenosine diphosphate (ADP) receptor antagonist, are the two most common platelet inhibitors used in veterinary medicine. The most common indication for their use is in cats with cardiac diseases that enhance the risk for thromboembolism (e.g. hypertrophic cardiomyopathy). Only one blinded, randomized study has compared aspirin and clopidogrel for secondary prevention of arterial thromboembolism in cats (Hogan et al. 2015).

Both drugs were well tolerated, but clopidogrel was significantly more likely to prevent recurrent aortic thromboembolism. Cats receiving clopidogrel had a longer median time to recurrence and reduced likelihood of aortic thromboembolism or death. Neither drug has been evaluated for efficacy in reducing the risk of a first thromboembolic event. Because of these limitations and simply the challenge of administering a daily medication to some cats, there is variability in treatment approaches. Ticlodipine is associated with a high incidence of gastrointestinal adverse effects in cats, limiting its clinical utility.

Dramatic difference

Aspirin has a very long elimination half-life in cats compared to dogs and humans, so it is administered once every two to three days.

Antiplatelet medication options most likely to be prescribed:
 Aspirin:

Dogs: 1 mg/kg PO every 24 hours
Cats: 20–81 mg PER CAT TOTAL DOSE PO every 48–72 hours.

 Clopidogrel:
Cats: 18.75 mg PER CAT TOTAL DOSE PO every 24 hours.

10.5.8.2 Antithrombotics (Heparins)

Antithrombotic medications, including unfractionated heparin and low-molecular-weight (fractionated) heparin, are used especially in the acute, critical care setting for veterinary patients with existing thrombosis or at increased thrombosis risk. There is significant individual variation in heparin pharmacokinetics in cats. The proposed benefit of low-molecular-weight heparin is greater bioavailability, longer half-life, and reduced bleeding and thrombocytopenia risk. Low-molecular-weight heparins have been evaluated in healthy cats and in

cats with heart disease (Smith et al. 2004; Alwood et al. 2007). An *in vivo* study in healthy cats demonstrated that cats may require higher doses and more frequent administration of low-molecular-weight heparin to meet the desired monitoring goal (anti-factor Xa activity) used in people. However, anti-factor Xa activity monitoring for cats is not well established. Dalteparin (one brand of low-molecular-weight heparin) administered to cats with heart disease was well tolerated (Smith et al. 2004). The impact of unfractionated heparin and low-molecular-weight heparin on clinical thrombosis and thrombosis risk reduction is still largely unknown. Monitoring clinical signs of bleeding and prothrombin time is recommended for cats receiving heparin therapy.

Antithrombotics most likely to be prescribed:

Heparin:
Mini-dose:
Dogs and cats: 75 Units/kg by subcutaneous injection every eight hours.
Standard dose (for existing thromboembolism):
Dogs: 150–250 Units/kg by subcutaneous injection every eight hours
Cats: 250–300 Units/kg by subcutaneous injection every eight hours.
Low-molecular-weight heparin:
Enoxaparin: Dogs and cats: 1 mg/kg by subcutaneous injection every 12 hours
Dalteparin: Dogs and cats: 100 IU/kg by subcutaneous injection every 12–24 hours.

10.5.8.3 Anticoagulants

Anticoagulant vitamin K antagonists such as warfarin have limited use in veterinary medicine. The risk of serious bleeding (it is difficult to limit the activity of veterinary patients relative to human patients), the cost of required monitoring, and the lack of definitive evidence of superior risk reduction are among the reasons that warfarin is not frequently used in veterinary patients. A study of warfarin in cats established a narrow therapeutic range and identified significant interindividual variation in pharmacokinetic and pharmacodynamic response (Smith et al. 2000a, 2000b). Because warfarin is highly protein bound, it has numerous drug interactions with other protein-bound drugs, increasing the risk of toxicity.

Mandatory monitoring

In patients receiving warfarin, prothrombin time, CBC, and monitoring for signs of bleeding – including occult blood in feces and urine – are recommended to reduce the risk of significant and potentially life-threatening hemorrhage.

10.5.8.4 Fibrinolytics

Fibrinolytic medications such as streptokinase and tissue plasminogen activator have been evaluated in clinical veterinary patients, particularly cats with thrombosis due to cardiac disease. Unfortunately, despite fibrinolytic efficacy, patients had an increased risk of death due to reperfusion injury when treated with these drugs (Welch et al. 2010).

10.5.9 Endocarditis and Myocarditis

Treatment for infective endocarditis is ideally based on bacterial culture and susceptibility results. Molecular diagnostic testing for *Bartonella* spp. is also recommended. When definitive identification of the causative agent is lacking, antibiotics with efficacy against *Staphylococcus* spp., *Streptococcus* spp., and *E. coli* are initiated. Patients with infective endocarditis should receive intravenous antibiotics for the first 72 hours, followed by a minimum of six weeks of oral antibiotic therapy. Patients that have CHF associated with infective endocarditis should also be treated for heart failure as outlined in this chapter. Whether or not antiplatelet medications reduce the risk of embolic complications in patients with infective endocarditis has not been established in veterinary medicine. Treatment for other causes of myocarditis is based on management of the underlying etiology when possible and supportive therapies.

10.6 Adverse Effects of Cardiovascular Drugs in Veterinary Species

Many of the adverse effects associated with cardiovascular medications in veterinary species are similar to those reported in people. This section will highlight both the commonly experienced and species-specific adverse effects.

10.6.1 Heartworm Preventatives

The ML heartworm preventatives are generally well tolerated. Rarely reported adverse effects include lethargy, anorexia, vomiting, diarrhea, and neurologic signs. According to the drug labels, hypersensitivity and anaphylactoid reactions have been reported in microfilaremic dogs receiving ML preventatives. Dermatologic adverse effects have been reported with the topical heartworm preventatives (selamectin and moxidectin), including alopecia, erythema, pruritus, and urticaria at the site of application. Dermatologic effects have also been reported in people administering the topical heartworm preventative. Pharmacists can play an important role in educating owners about safely administering topical drugs. Oral ingestion of topical heartworm preventatives can result in toxicity, so care should be taken to prevent the pet or other household pets from ingesting the medication after it has been applied. In cats, heartworm preventives may cause behavioral changes, hypersalivation, and coughing/gagging. The drug label for the injectable heartworm preventative moxidectin has a broader list of reported adverse events, including immune-mediated anaphylactoid reactions, anemia, thrombocytopenia, erythema multiforme, hepatopathy, and azotemia. The FDA temporarily restricted ProHeart-6® (injectable moxidectin) in

September 2004 due to reports of thousands of adverse reactions, including death (Kuehn 2004). In 2013, the FDA removed restrictions on ProHeart-6 following modifications in the drug's manufacturing process. Because the manufacturer requires veterinarians and veterinary staff to be certified to administer ProHeart-6, pharmacists should not dispense the drug directly to the public.

Ivermectin toxicity has been reported in dogs with the MDR1 mutation receiving concurrent P-glycoprotein pump inhibitors, with oral ingestion of topical heartworm preventatives, and with accidental ingestion and off-label administration of livestock ivermectin formulations (Hopkins et al. 1990). Signs of ivermectin toxicity include dilated pupils, ataxia, vomiting, drooling, disorientation, bradycardia, seizures, and coma (Hopper et al. 2002). The "lipid rescue" protocol has been used successfully for management of ivermectin toxicosis in dogs, but it is not successful in dogs with the MDR1 mutation.

10.6.2 Adulticide Heartworm Treatment

Melarsomine (Immiticide) is the only drug labeled to kill adult heartworms in dogs with heartworm disease. A recent retrospective study evaluated adverse effects during adulticide treatment following the American Heartworm Society–recommended treatment protocol (Maxwell et al. 2014). In this study, 52% of treated dogs experienced minor complications, including injection site reaction (pain, swelling, and reluctance to move), vomiting, diarrhea, inappetence, lethargy, and depression; 54% experienced respiratory signs, including coughing, dyspnea, and heart failure; and 14% died within the treatment period. Respiratory signs and death were attributed to thromboembolism, pulmonary inflammation associated with dying worms, and progression of heartworm disease during the treatment period. Activity level of the patient is a significant risk factor for post-adulticidal complications (Henry and Dillon 1994). From a practical standpoint,

strict exercise restriction/cage rest for five months can be one of the most challenging components of heartworm treatment. These findings illustrate the importance of appropriate client education prior to treatment and careful monitoring and cage rest during the treatment period.

10.6.3 Doxycycline

Doxycycline is used at standard antimicrobial doses to treat *Wolbachia* as a component of heartworm treatment. Adverse events associated with doxycycline administration during heartworm treatment are similar to what is reported in Chapter 9 and include inappetence, vomiting, diarrhea, and less commonly hepatotoxicity. To avoid esophageal irritation, a bolus of water or food should be given immediately after the doxycycline tablet or capsule to ensure it does not remain lodged in the esophagus.

10.6.4 Heart Failure Treatment

10.6.4.1 Loop Diuretics
Because loop diuretics can cause tremendous diuresis, the most common complaint of owners is managing their pet's increased need to urinate. Avoiding house soiling can be difficult, particularly because of a busy owner's work and sleep schedule. The pharmacist can play an important role in client education.

Other adverse effects of furosemide are similar in humans and animals (azotemia, hypokalemia, and hypotension). Hypokalemia is less frequent in patients that are concurrently treated with ACE inhibitors. Concurrent use of furosemide with other nephrotoxic drugs, such as aminoglycosides and nonsteroidal anti-inflammatory drugs (NSAIDs), enhances the risk of nephrotoxicity. Furosemide-induced ototoxicity can also occur in animals (Brown 1981), particularly at high doses. The risk of ototoxicity should be discussed with owners/handlers of service animals, because even subtle hearing loss may interfere with a service animal's performance.

Furosemide is occasionally administered subcutaneously by owners to their pets with refractory heart failure. Ulcerative dermatologic adverse effects have been sporadically reported in dogs after subcutaneous administration of furosemide. In a single case report, the lesions were only associated with a particular formulation of furosemide (Scruggs and Rishniw 2013). Although the cause of the ulcerative lesions was not determined, it was hypothesized that the more alkaline product was associated with tissue damage.

Other loop diuretics used in refractory heart failure cases, such as bumetanide and torsemide, have similar adverse effects to furosemide. The risk of hypokalemia and azotemia may be greater with these diuretics. Owners reporting their pet has developed inappetence, vomiting, or weakness after switching from furosemide to one of these diuretics should be alerted to the need to have their pet re-evaluated.

10.6.4.2 Pimobendan

Adverse effects are uncommonly reported with pimobendan in dogs and cats. In dogs with preclinical myxomatous mitral valve degeneration, adverse events reported were similar between the placebo and pimobendan groups and included vomiting, diarrhea, lethargy, and tachycardia (Boswood et al. 2016). Agitation, anorexia, hypotension, and constipation have also been reported in a small number of cats (Macgregor et al. 2011; Gordon et al. 2012; Reina-Doreste et al. 2014). In contrast to people, no increased risk of new arrhythmias has been identified, and blood pressure was unaffected at the label dose.

10.6.4.3 ACE Inhibitors

Similar to people, azotemia and electrolyte abnormalities (particularly hyperkalemia) can occur in animals treated with ACE inhibitors, although it is not common ("Controlled clinical evaluation" 1995; "The effect of benazepril" 1999). Still, evaluation of renal function, electrolytes, and blood pressure prior to initiation of ACE inhibitors is recommended. Patients with preexisting renal dysfunction are at increased risk of worsening azotemia.

Systemic hypotension is a concern for patients with CHF that are treated with both an ACE inhibitor and diuretic. In normal dogs, blood pressure reduction with an ACE inhibitor rarely exceeds 10 mmHg, but the risk of hypotension is greater when cardiac output is reduced due to either fluid loss associated with diuretic administration or poor output associated with underlying cardiac disease. Monitoring for hypotension is recommended for patients receiving furosemide and an ACE inhibitor.

10.6.4.4 Aldosterone Antagonists

Aldosterone antagonists are most frequently used in combination with other heart failure therapy, including pimobendan, loop diuretics, and ACE inhibitors. Concurrent treatment with an ACE inhibitor and spironolactone can increase the risk of electrolyte abnormalities, particularly hyperkalemia

(Juurlink et al. 2004). The concurrent use of a potassium-losing diuretic such as furosemide likely balances this risk. In a prospective, placebo-controlled study of dogs with CHF due to dilated cardiomyopathy or myxomatous mitral valve degeneration, no increase in adverse events, hyperkalemia, or azotemia was identified in dogs concurrently treated with receiving spironolactone, an ACE inhibitor, and furosemide (Lefebvre et al. 2013). Routine monitoring of electrolytes and renal function is still recommended for all CHF patients, including those receiving spironolactone.

Cats can experience a few unique adverse effects with spironolactone, including severe ulcerative facial dermatitis (Maine Coon Cats seem predisposed) and myelodysplasia (MacDonald et al. 2008). The skin lesions occur a few months after initiating treatment. The lesions usually resolve about a month after discontinuation of the medication.

Mandatory monitoring

Cats treated with spironolactone should be monitored for facial dermatitis.

10.6.5 Antiarrhythmics

10.6.5.1 Digoxin

Digoxin has a narrow margin of safety. Its dosing considerations, adverse effect profile, and toxicity concerns are similar to those observed in human patients. Cats tend to hypersalivate if given the elixir formulation of digoxin, so its use is not recommended. Any arrhythmia can occur with digoxin toxicity. AV block and life-threatening tachyarrhythmia are some of the most concerning. As in people, hypokalemia increases the risk of ventricular tachycardia. Most adverse effects reported are associated with toxic serum digoxin levels. Digoxin toxicity can be treated with discontinuation of the drug, supportive therapies, and administration of digoxin-specific antibodies (i.e. Digibind).

Mandatory monitoring

Because of digoxin's narrow margin of safety, client education regarding signs of toxicity is essential. Clients are instructed to discontinue digoxin and contact the veterinarian if their pet develops signs of inappetence, vomiting, diarrhea, syncope, seizures, or other neurologic symptoms. Serum digoxin levels are routinely monitored.

10.6.5.2 Class Ib Antiarrhythmics

Parenterally administered lidocaine is usually well tolerated in dogs. Cats are highly sensitive to lidocaine-induced neurological toxicity and should receive a reduced dose or an alternate antiarrhythmic.

In dogs, mexiletine can cause gastrointestinal symptoms, including anorexia and vomiting, especially when mexiletine is administered without food. In some patients, significant gastrointestinal symptoms persist, and a change in antiarrhythmic is required.

10.6.5.3 Class II Antiarrhythmics

Beta-adrenergic antagonists can cause lethargy, inappetence, syncope, or exacerbation of heart failure. Although a modest reduction of heart rate is often desired in patients receiving beta-adrenergic antagonists, excessive bradyarrhythmias can also occur. Nonselective beta-adrenergic antagonists (i.e. propranolol) are contraindicated in cats with asthma, but bronchoconstriction can even be caused by beta-1 selective adrenergic antagonists (i.e. atenolol) in some animals. Cats that develop asthma symptoms should discontinue drugs in this class and receive veterinary attention.

10.6.5.4 Class III Antiarrhythmics

The two most commonly used class III antiarrhythmics in veterinary medicine are amiodarone and sotalol. Their adverse effect profiles differ significantly, and therefore they will be discussed separately.

Generally, sotalol is well tolerated; however, some animals will experience new-onset syncope or worsening of syncope when sotalol is initiated. Owners should be made aware of this risk and the need to contact their veterinarian if this does occur.

Most adverse effects of amiodarone are similar to those observed in people and include: bradycardia, thyroid dysfunction, ocular abnormalities, neutropenia, anemia, gastrointestinal upset, and hepatopathies. Less is known about the potential for pulmonary fibrosis in veterinary patients. Monitoring liver enzyme values, CBC, and thyroid hormone levels is recommended. Serum amiodarone levels can also be monitored.

Preservative-free injectable amiodarone, such as Nexterone, is preferred if a parenteral formulation is required. Amiodarone prepared in solution with polysorbate 80 (Tween 80) and benzyl alcohol in 5% dextrose can cause life-threatening hypotension, anaphylaxis, other arrhythmias, acute hepatic necrosis, and death in people and dogs (Cober et al. 2009; Pedro et al. 2012).

10.6.5.5   Class IV Antiarrhythmics

Diltiazem is the most commonly used Class IV antiarrhythmic in veterinary medicine. Oral administration can cause gastrointestinal adverse effects, especially at higher doses. Owners should contact their veterinarian if significant gastrointestinal signs occur. Hypotension can occur, particularly in patients that are dehydrated, are receiving other vasodilators, or have poor cardiac output. If diltiazem is used in combination with digoxin, serum digoxin concentrations should be monitored because diltiazem can alter serum digoxin concentrations.

10.6.6   Antithrombotics

10.6.6.1   Platelet Inhibitors

Clopidogrel is generally well tolerated in cats (Hogan et al. 2004, 2015) and dogs (Mellett et al. 2011). Salivation or drug refusal due to the bitter taste are the most commonly reported problems associated with clopidogrel in cats. It can be administered in gelatin capsules to circumvent this problem. Rarely, cats may develop anorexia or vomiting when treated with clopidogrel, but this can be mitigated by administering with food. Although the risk of bleeding certainly should be considered, this has not been reported in small clinical trials in cats receiving clopidogrel (Hogan et al. 2015). If patients are receiving multiple platelet inhibitors, it is especially important to advise owners to seek veterinary care if their pet experiences bruising or bleeding.

Because "antiplatelet" doses of aspirin are much lower than anti-inflammatory doses, adverse effects are less frequent but may include inappetence, vomiting, and hematemesis (Smith et al. 2003). It is important to reiterate that the dosing interval of aspirin in cats is two to three days because of its extremely long elimination half-life.

10.6.6.2   Anticoagulants

Bleeding and thrombocytopenia can occur in dogs and cats treated with unfractionated heparin and low-molecular-weight heparin. Signs of epistaxis, melena, bruising, hematemesis, or other occult or overt bleeding in a patient receiving an anticoagulant indicate a need for medication adjustment, and the animal should receive veterinary care.

10.6.6.3   Antihypertensives

Adverse effects are uncommon with amlodipine, which is the most commonly used antihypertensive for systemic hypertension in veterinary medicine. There was no difference in adverse events in cats receiving chewable amlodipine compared to placebo (Huhtinen et al. 2015).

Sildenafil is the most commonly prescribed medication for management of severe precapillary pulmonary hypertension. Generally, it is well tolerated in dogs. Although systemic hypotension is a potential adverse effect, this has not been identified in small clinical studies of dogs with pulmonary hypertension receiving sildenafil (Brown et al. 2010). Cutaneous flushing in the inguinal region has been reported in dogs (Bach et al. 2006). Other side

Table 10.5 Summary of feline-specific considerations for the use of cardiovascular drugs.

Drug	Feline-specific adverse effect
Clopidogrel	Hypersalivation; can be administered in gelatin capsule
Aspirin	Inappetence, vomiting, and hematemesis even at antiplatelet doses
Digoxin elixir	Hypersalivation: use non-elixir formulation. Narrow therapeutic range, careful dosing, and drug interaction considerations
Class Ib antiarrhythmics (lidocaine, mexiletine)	Toxicity risk
Melarsomine	Toxicity risk and life-threatening adverse effects
Methimazole	Facial excoriations, hypersensitivity reactions, and hematologic and hepatic abnormalities
Spironolactone	Ulcerative facial dermatitis

Table 10.6 Summary of canine-specific considerations for the use of cardiovascular drugs.

Drug	Canine-specific adverse effect
Amiodarone (IV)[a]	Life-threatening adverse events with injectable amiodarone with preservative. Only use preservative-free injectable amiodarone.
Digoxin	Narrow therapeutic range, careful dosing, MDR1 mutation, and drug interaction considerations
Furosemide (subcutaneous)[a]	Ulcerative dermatitis. May be associated with certain furosemide formulations.

[a] The risk of these adverse effects in other veterinary species is unknown.

effects reported in people, including visual disturbances, dizziness, nasal congestion, and myalgia, are more difficult to assess in dogs.

Adverse effects of pimobendan (used for management of post-capillary pulmonary hypertension) are the same as those described in the "Congestive Heart Failure" section.

Species and breed-specific adverse effects are reported for many of the drugs used in the prevention and management of cardiovascular disease. Tables 10.5 and 10.6 summarize feline- and canine-specific considerations for the use of cardiovascular drugs.

10.7 Nutritional Supplements for Veterinary Cardiovascular Diseases

10.7.1 Omega-3 Fatty Acids

Because plasma omega-3 (n-3) concentration is decreased in some dogs with CHF, omega-3 supplements have been used in dogs with cardiac cachexia and Boxer dogs with arrhythmogenic right ventricular cardiomyopathy (Smith et al. 2007). Commercial fish oil supplements have variable eicosapentaenoic acid and docosahexaenoic acid content. A 1 g fish oil capsule that contains 180 mg of eicosapentaenoic acid and 120 mg of docosahexaenoic acid is recommended. Based on limited studies of omega-3 fatty acids in animals, cod liver oil and flax seed oil should not be used as sources of omega-3 fatty acids in dogs (Smith et al. 2007).

Studies evaluating serum fatty acid concentration in cats did not demonstrate decreased omega-3 concentration in cats with hypertrophic cardiomyopathy or CHF (Hall et al. 2014). Based on these results, omega-3 fatty acid supplementation is not routinely recommended in cats with heart disease.

10.7.2 CoEnzyme Q (Co-Q10)

No veterinary studies have evaluated the use of Co-Q10 in animal patients with cardiovascular disease.

10.7.3 Taurine

Dilated cardiomyopathy due to a taurine-deficient diet was first reported in cats in 1987 (Pion et al. 1987). Since this discovery, feline diets have been reformulated to include taurine (Pion et al. 1992b). Since then, dilated cardiomyopathy is uncommon in feline patients consuming a commercial cat food. Currently, when taurine-responsive dilated cardiomyopathy is diagnosed, it is usually identified in cats being fed dog food or homemade diets, or when improper production or storage conditions have occurred with commercial feline diets. Myocardial function can return to normal in cats with taurine-deficient myocardial failure following two to three months of taurine supplementation (Pion et al. 1992a). Therapy is continued until clinical resolution or establishment of normal plasma taurine levels. Some cats may require management for CHF prior to resolution of the taurine-deficient state.

Taurine dose in cats with taurine-deficient dilated cardiomyopathy:

Taurine: 250 mg TOTAL DOSE PO every 12 hours.

10.7.4 L-Carnitine

A diet-independent taurine-deficient and L-carnitine-responsive dilated cardiomyopathy has been reported in American Cocker Spaniels (Kittleson et al. 1997). All affected dogs had reduced plasma taurine concentrations and variable plasma carnitine levels. Improvement was noted in all dogs supplemented with taurine and L-carnitine. All dogs were able to be weaned off standard heart failure treatment.

Taurine and L-carnitine doses for American Cocker Spaniels with dilated cardiomyopathy:

Taurine: 500 mg TOTAL DOSE PO every 8–12 hours

L-Carnitine: 1 g TOTAL DOSE PO every 8–12 hours.

Myocardial function has also been reported to improve with L-carnitine supplementation in a subset of Boxer dogs affected with arrhythmogenic right ventricular cardiomyopathy with a dilated cardiomyopathy phenotype (Keene et al. 1991).

10.8 FDA-Approved Veterinary Drug Products with No Human Drug Equivalent

Brand name	Active ingredient(s)	Drug class	Rationale/notes
Salix® (Merck Animal Health)	Furosemide	Diuretic	Available as 12.5 mg or 50 mg tablets, or 5.0% injectable. Human formulations available in different tablet strengths.
HEARTGARD PLUS® (Merial)	Ivermectin + Pyrantel (oral)	Macrocyclic lactone heartworm preventative	Approved for use in dogs and cats as a monthly heartworm preventative. Also treats roundworms and hookworms.
IMMITICIDE® (Merial) DIROBAN™ (Zoetis)	Melarsamine dihydrochloride	Arsenical	Approved for use in heartworm-positive dogs as an adulticide heartworm treatment. Not recommended for use in cats.

(continued)

(continued)

Brand name	Active ingredient(s)	Drug class	Rationale/notes
INTERCEPTOR® (Elanco)	Milbemycin oxime (oral)	Macrocyclic lactone heartworm preventative	Approved for use in dogs and cats as a monthly heartworm preventative. Also treats whipworms, roundworms, and hookworms.
TRIFEXIS® (Elanco)	Milbemycin oxime + Spinosad (oral)	Macrocyclic lactone heartworm preventative	Approved for use in dogs as a monthly heartworm preventative. Also kills fleas and treats hookworms, roundworms, and whipworms.
ProHeart-6® (Zoetis)	Moxidectin (injection)	Macrocyclic lactone heartworm preventative	Approved for use in dogs as a twice-yearly injectable heartworm preventative. Restricted distribution program. Not to be administered in debilitated animals or animals with history of weight loss. It should not be administered concurrently with vaccination.
ADVANTAGE MULTI® (Bayer)	2.5% Moxidectin + 10% imidacloprid (topical)	Macrocyclic lactone heartworm preventative	Approved for use in dogs and cats as a monthly heartworm preventative. Approved as a microfilaricidal medication in dogs with heartworm infection. Also kills fleas and treats hookworms, roundworms, whipworms, and sarcoptic mange.
VETMEDIN® (Boehringer Ingelheim Vetmedica)	Pimobendan	Inodilator -PDE III inhibitor -Calcium sensitizer	Approved for use in dogs for CHF due to dilated cardiomyopathy or degenerative valve disease. Off-label use in cats with CHF and dogs with CHF due to other cardiac diseases.
REVOLUTION® (Zoetis)	Selamectin (topical)	Macrocyclic lactone heartworm preventative	Approved for use in dogs and cats as a monthly heartworm preventative. Also kills fleas, ear mites, and ticks and treats sarcoptic mange.

CHF, Congestive heart failure; PDE, phosphodiesterase.

Abbreviations

ACE	Angiotensin-converting enzyme	CAST	Cardiac arrhythmia suppression trial
ACVIM	American College of Veterinary Internal Medicine	CHF	Congestive heart failure
ADP	Adenosine diphosphate	COX	Cyclooxygenase
AHS	American Heartworm Society	EPOCH	Effects of pimobendan on chronic heart failure
AV	Atrioventricular		

FDA	Food and Drug Administration	NSAID	Nonsteroidal anti-inflammatory drug
cGMP	Cyclic guanosine monophosphate		
ISACHC	International Small Animal Cardiac Health Council	NYHA	New York Heart Association
		PO	Per os (orally)
L1,2,3, or 4	Heartworm larval stage 1, 2, 3, or 4	PDE	Phosphodiesterase
		RALES	Randomized aldactone evaluation study
MDR1	Multidrug resistance 1 gene (ABCB1 gene)		

References

Acute and short-term hemodynamic, echocardiographic, and clinical effects of enalapril maleate in dogs with naturally acquired heart failure: results of the Invasive Multicenter PROspective Veterinary Evaluation of Enalapril study: the IMPROVE Study Group. (1995) *J. Vet. Intern. Med.* 9: 234–242.

Alwood, A.J., Downend, A.B., Brooks, M.B. et al. (2007). Anticoagulant effects of low-molecular-weight heparins in healthy cats. *J. Vet. Intern. Med.* 21: 378–387.

Atkins, C.E., Kanter, R., Wright, K. et al. (1995). Orthodromic reciprocating tachycardia and heart failure in a dog with a concealed posteroseptal accessory pathway. *J. Vet. Intern. Med.* 9: 43–49.

Atkins, C.E., Keene, B.W., Brown, W.A. et al. (2007). Results of the veterinary enalapril trial to prove reduction in onset of heart failure in dogs chronically treated with enalapril alone for compensated, naturally occurring mitral valve insufficiency. *J. Am. Vet. Med. Assoc.* 231: 1061–1069.

Atkinson, K.J., Fine, D.M., Thombs, L.A. et al. (2009). Evaluation of pimobendan and N-terminal probrain natriuretic peptide in the treatment of pulmonary hypertension secondary to degenerative mitral valve disease in dogs. *J. Vet. Intern. Med.* 23: 1190–1196.

Bach, J.F., Rozanski, E.A., MacGregor, J. et al. (2006). Retrospective evaluation of sildenafil citrate as a therapy for pulmonary hypertension in dogs. *J. Vet. Intern. Med.* 20: 1132–1135.

Baek, I.H., Lee, B.Y., Lee, E.S. et al. (2013). Pharmacokinetics of angiotensin II receptor blockers in the dog following a single oral administration. *Drug Res. (Stuttg.)* 63: 357–361.

Baldwin, J.R., Phillips, B.A., Overmyer, S.K. et al. (1992). Influence of the cardioprotective agent dexrazoxane on doxorubicin pharmacokinetics in the dog. *Cancer Chemother. Pharmacol.* 30: 433–438.

Basso, C., Fox, P.R., Meurs, K.M. et al. (2004). Arrhythmogenic right ventricular cardiomyopathy causing sudden cardiac death in boxer dogs: a new animal model of human disease. *Circulation* 109: 1180–1185.

Bazzocchi, C., Mortarino, M., Grandi, G. et al. (2008). Combined ivermectin and doxycycline treatment has microfilaricidal and adulticidal activity against *Dirofilaria immitis* in experimentally infected dogs. *Int. J. Parasitol.* 38: 1401–1410.

Beardow, A.W. and Buchanan, J.W. (1993). Chronic mitral valve disease in cavalier King Charles Spaniels: 95 cases (1987–1991). *J. Am. Vet. Med. Assoc.* 203: 1023–1029.

Becker, T.J., Graves, T.K., Kruger, J.M. et al. (2000). Effects of methimazole on renal function in cats with hyperthyroidism. *J. Am. Anim. Hosp. Assoc.* 36: 215–223.

BENCH (BENazepril in Canine Heart disease) Study Group (1999). The effect of benazepril on survival times and clinical signs of dogs with congestive heart failure: Results of a multicenter, prospective, randomized, double-blinded, placebo-controlled, long-term clinical trial. *J. Vet. Cardiol.* 1: 7–18.

Bendas, A.J.R., Mendes-de-Almeida, F., Von Simson, C. et al. (2017). Heat pretreatment of canine samples to evaluate efficacy of imidacloprid + moxidectin and doxycycline in heartworm treatment. *Parasit. Vectors* 10: 246.

Bernay, F., Bland, J.M., Haggstrom, J. et al. (2010). Efficacy of spironolactone on survival in dogs with naturally occurring mitral regurgitation caused by myxomatous mitral valve disease. *J. Vet. Intern. Med.* 24: 331–341.

Bezerra, P.S., Driemeier, D., Loretti, A.P. et al. (1999). Monensin poisoning in Brazilian horses. *Vet. Hum. Toxicol.* 41: 383–385.

Bond, B.R., Fox, P.R., Peterson, M.E. et al. (1988). Echocardiographic findings in 103 cats with hyperthyroidism. *J. Am. Vet. Med. Assoc.* 192: 1546–1549.

Borgarelli, M. and Haggstrom, J. (2010). Canine degenerative myxomatous mitral valve disease: natural history, clinical presentation and therapy. *Vet. Clin. North Am. Small Anim. Pract.* 40: 651–663.

Boswood, A., Haggstrom, J., Gordon, S.G. et al. (2016). Effect of pimobendan in dogs with preclinical myxomatous mitral valve disease and cardiomegaly: the EPIC study – a randomized clinical trial. *J. Vet. Intern. Med.* 30: 1765–1779.

Brien, J.F., Jimmo, S., Brennan, F.J. et al. (1990). Disposition of amiodarone and its proximate metabolite, desethylamiodarone, in the dog for oral administration of single-dose and short-term drug regimens. *Drug Metab. Dispos.* 18: 846–851.

Brown, R.D. (1981). Comparative acute cochlear toxicity of intravenous bumetanide and furosemide in the purebred beagle. *J. Clin. Pharmacol.* 21: 620–627.

Brown, S., Atkins, C., Bagley, R. et al. (2007). Guidelines for the identification, evaluation, and management of systemic hypertension in dogs and cats. *J. Vet. Intern. Med.* 21: 542–558.

Brown, A.J., Davison, E., and Sleeper, M.M. (2010). Clinical efficacy of sildenafil in treatment of pulmonary arterial hypertension in dogs. *J. Vet. Intern. Med.* 24: 850–854.

Buchanan, J.W. (1977). Chronic valvular disease (endocardiosis) in dogs. *Adv. Vet. Sci. Comp. Med.* 21: 75–106.

Bugbee, A.C., Coleman, A.E., Wang, A. et al. (2014). Telmisartan treatment of refractory proteinuria in a dog. *J. Vet. Intern. Med.* 28: 1871–1874.

Calvert, C.A., Chapman, W.L. Jr., and Toal, R.L. (1982). Congestive cardiomyopathy in Doberman Pinscher dogs. *J. Am. Vet. Med. Assoc.* 181: 598–602.

Calvert, C.A., Pickus, C.W., Jacobs, G.J. et al. (1997). Signalment, survival, and prognostic factors in Doberman Pinschers with end-stage cardiomyopathy. *J. Vet. Intern. Med.* 11: 323–326.

Cervenec, R.M., Stauthammer, C.D., Fine, D.M. et al. (2017). Survival time with pacemaker implantation for dogs diagnosed with persistent atrial standstill. *J. Vet. Cardiol.* 19 (3): 240–246.

Chatterjee, K., Zhang, J., Honbo, N. et al. (2010). Doxorubicin cardiomyopathy. *Cardiology* 115: 155–162.

Chomel, B.B., Kasten, R.W., Williams, C. et al. (2009). *Bartonella* endocarditis: a pathology shared by animal reservoirs and patients. *Ann. NY Acad. Sci.* 1166: 120–126.

Church, W.M., Sisson, D.D., Oyama, M.A. et al. (2007). Third degree atrioventricular block and sudden death secondary to acute myocarditis in a dog. *J. Vet. Cardiol.* 9: 53–57.

Cober, R.E., Schober, K.E., Hildebrandt, N. et al. (2009). Adverse effects of intravenous amiodarone in 5 dogs. *J. Vet. Intern. Med.* 23: 657–661.

Controlled clinical evaluation of enalapril in dogs with heart failure: results of the Cooperative Veterinary Enalapril Study Group. The COVE Study Group (1995). *J. Vet. Intern. Med.* 9: 243–252.

Costa, A., Lahmers, S., Barry, S.L. et al. (2014). Fungal pericarditis and endocarditis secondary to porcupine quill migration in a dog. *J. Vet. Cardiol.* 16: 283–290.

Decloedt, A., Verheyen, T., De Clercq, D. et al. (2012). Acute and long-term cardiomyopathy and delayed neurotoxicity after accidental lasalocid poisoning in horses. *J. Vet. Intern. Med.* 26: 1005–1011.

DiBartola, S.P., Broome, M.R., Stein, B.S. et al. (1996). Effect of treatment of hyperthyroidism on renal function in cats. *J. Am. Vet. Med. Assoc.* 208: 875–878.

Dicpinigaitis, P.V. (2006). Angiotensin-converting enzyme inhibitor-induced cough: ACCP evidence-based clinical practice guidelines. *Chest* 129: 169s–173s.

Dorne, J.L., Fernandez-Cruz, M.L., Bertelsen, U. et al. (2013). Risk assessment of coccidostatics during feed cross-contamination: animal and human health aspects. *Toxicol. Appl. Pharmacol.* 270: 196–208.

Echt, D.S., Liebson, P.R., Mitchell, L.B. et al. (1991). Mortality and morbidity in patients receiving encainide, flecainide, or placebo: the cardiac arrhythmia suppression trial. *N. Engl. J. Med.* 324: 781–788.

Effects of Pimobendan on Chronic Heart Failure Study (EPOCH Study) (2002). Effects of pimobendan on adverse cardiac events and physical activities in patients with mild to moderate chronic heart failure: the effects of pimobendan on chronic heart failure study (EPOCH study). *Circ. J.* 66: 149–157.

Ettinger, S.J., Benitz, A.M., Ericsson, G.F. et al. (1998). Effects of enalapril maleate on survival of dogs with naturally acquired heart failure. The long-term investigation of veterinary enalapril (LIVE) study group. *J. Am. Vet. Med. Assoc.* 213: 1573–1575.

FitzPatrick, W.M., Dervisis, N.G., and Kitchell, B.E. (2010). Safety of concurrent administration of dexrazoxane and doxorubicin in the canine cancer patient. *Vet. Comp. Oncol.* 8: 273–282.

Fox, P.R., Maron, B.J., Basso, C. et al. (2000). Spontaneously occurring arrhythmogenic right ventricular cardiomyopathy in the domestic cat: a new animal model similar to the human disease. *Circulation* 102: 1863–1870.

Fuentes, V.L., Corcoran, B., French, A. et al. (2002). A double-blind, randomized, placebo-controlled study of pimobendan in dogs with dilated cardiomyopathy. *J. Vet. Intern. Med.* 16: 255–261.

Gelzer, A.R., Kraus, M.S., Rishniw, M. et al. (2009). Combination therapy with digoxin and diltiazem controls ventricular rate in chronic atrial fibrillation in dogs better than digoxin or diltiazem monotherapy: a randomized crossover study in 18 dogs. *J. Vet. Intern. Med.* 23: 499–508.

Gelzer, A.R., Kraus, M.S., Rishniw, M. et al. (2010). Combination therapy with mexiletine and sotalol suppresses inherited ventricular arrhythmias in German shepherd dogs better than mexiletine or sotalol monotherapy: a randomized cross-over study. *J. Vet. Cardiol.* 12: 93–106.

Gordon, S.G., Saunders, A.B., Roland, R.M. et al. (2012). Effect of oral administration of pimobendan in cats with heart failure. *J. Am. Vet. Med. Assoc.* 241: 89–94.

Haggstrom, J., Boswood, A., O'Grady, M. et al. (2008). Effect of pimobendan or benazepril hydrochloride on survival times in dogs with congestive heart failure caused by naturally occurring myxomatous mitral valve disease: the QUEST study. *J. Vet. Intern. Med.* 22: 1124–1135.

Hall, D.J., Freeman, L.M., Rush, J.E. et al. (2014). Comparison of serum fatty acid concentrations in cats with hypertrophic cardiomyopathy and healthy controls. *J. Feline Med. Surg.* 16: 631–636.

Hanzlicek, A.S., Gehring, R., Kukanich, B. et al. (2012). Pharmacokinetics of oral pimobendan in healthy cats. *J. Vet. Cardiol.* 14: 489–496.

Henik, R.A., Snyder, P.S., and Volk, L.M. (1997). Treatment of systemic hypertension in cats with amlodipine besylate. *J. Am. Anim. Hosp. Assoc.* 33: 226–234.

Henik, R.A., Kellum, H.B., Bentjen, S.A. et al. (2006). Digoxin and mexiletine sensitivity in a collie with the MDR1 mutation. *J. Vet. Intern. Med.* 20: 415–417.

Henry, C.J. and Dillon, R. (1994). Heartworm disease in dogs. *J. Am. Vet. Med. Assoc.* 204: 1148–1151.

Herring, I.P., Panciera, D.L., and Werre, S.R. (2014). Longitudinal prevalence of hypertension, proteinuria, and retinopathy in dogs with spontaneous diabetes mellitus. *J. Vet. Intern. Med.* 28: 488–495.

Hoffman, S.B., Yoder, A.R., and Trepanier, L.A. (2002). Bioavailability of transdermal methimazole in a pluronic lecithin organogel (PLO) in healthy cats. *J. Vet. Pharmacol. Ther.* 25: 189–193.

Hoffmann, G., Marks, S.L., Taboada, J. et al. (2003). Transdermal methimazole treatment in cats with hyperthyroidism. *J. Feline Med. Surg.* 5: 77–82.

Hogan, D.F., Andrews, D.A., Green, H.W. et al. (2004). Antiplatelet effects and pharmacodynamics of clopidogrel in cats. *J. Am. Vet. Med. Assoc.* 225: 1406–1411.

Hogan, D.F., Fox, P.R., Jacob, K. et al. (2015). Secondary prevention of cardiogenic arterial thromboembolism in the cat: the double-blind, randomized, positive-controlled feline arterial thromboembolism; clopidogrel vs. aspirin trial (FAT CAT). *J. Vet. Cardiol.* 17 (Suppl. 1): S306–S317.

Hopkins, K.D., Marcella, K.L., and Strecker, A.E. (1990). Ivermectin toxicosis in a dog. *J. Am. Vet. Med. Assoc.* 197: 93–94.

Hopper, K., Aldrich, J., and Haskins, S.C. (2002). Ivermectin toxicity in 17 collies. *J. Vet. Intern. Med.* 16: 89–94.

Hughes, K.J., Hoffmann, K.L., and Hodgson, D.R. (2009). Long-term assessment of horses and ponies post exposure to monensin sodium in commercial feed. *Equine Vet. J.* 41: 47–52.

Huhtinen, M., Derre, G., Renoldi, H.J. et al. (2015). Randomized placebo-controlled clinical trial of a chewable formulation of amlodipine for the treatment of hypertension in client-owned cats. *J. Vet. Intern. Med.* 29: 786–793.

Huson, H.J., Byers, A.M., Runstadler, J. et al. (2011). An SNP within the angiotensin-converting enzyme distinguishes between sprint and distance performing Alaskan sled dogs in a candidate gene analysis. *J. Hered.* 102 (Suppl. 1): S19–S27.

Imondi, A.R., Della Torre, P., Mazue, G. et al. (1996). Dose-response relationship of dexrazoxane for prevention of doxorubicin-induced cardiotoxicity in mice, rats, and dogs. *Cancer Res.* 56: 4200–4204.

Jacob, S., Parameswaran, A., Santosham, R. et al. (2016). Human pulmonary dirofilariasis masquerading as a mass. *Asian Cardiovasc. Thorac. Ann.* 24: 722–725.

Johnson, L.M., Atkins, C.E., Keene, B.W. et al. (1996). Pharmacokinetic and pharmacodynamic properties of conventional and CD-formulated diltiazem in cats. *J. Vet. Intern. Med.* 10: 316–320.

Juurlink, D.N., Mamdani, M.M., Lee, D.S. et al. (2004). Rates of hyperkalemia after publication of the randomized Aldactone evaluation study. *N. Engl. J. Med.* 351: 543–551.

Keene, B.W., Panciera, D.P., Atkins, C.E. et al. (1991). Myocardial L-carnitine deficiency in a family of dogs with dilated cardiomyopathy. *J. Am. Vet. Med. Assoc.* 198: 647–650.

Kellihan, H.B., Waller, K.R., Pinkos, A. et al. (2015). Acute resolution of pulmonary alveolar infiltrates in 10 dogs with pulmonary hypertension treated with sildenafil citrate: 2005–2014. *J. Vet. Cardiol.* 17: 182–191.

Kittleson, M.D., Keene, B., Pion, P.D. et al. (1997). Results of the multicenter spaniel trial (MUST): taurine- and carnitine-responsive dilated cardiomyopathy in American Cocker Spaniels with decreased plasma taurine concentration. *J. Vet. Intern. Med.* 11: 204–211.

Kittleson, M.D., Meurs, K.M., Munro, M.J. et al. (1999). Familial hypertrophic cardiomyopathy in Maine coon cats: an animal model of human disease. *Circulation* 99: 3172–3180.

Knight, D.H., Atkins, C.E., Atwell, R.B. et al. (2001). 1999 guidelines for the diagnosis, treatment, and prevention of heartworm (*Dirofilaria immitis*) infection in cats. *Vet. Ther.* 2: 78–87.

Krstic, M., Gabrielli, S., Ignjatovic, M. et al. (2017). An appraisal of canine and human cases reveals an endemic status of dirofilariosis in parts of Serbia. *Mol. Cell. Probes* 31: 37–41.

Kuehn, B.M. (2004). Fort Dodge recalls ProHeart 6, citing FDA safety concerns. Advisory committee to review FDA findings. *J. Am. Vet. Med. Assoc.* 225: 1157–1158.

Kvart, C., Haggstrom, J., Pedersen, H.D. et al. (2002). Efficacy of enalapril for prevention of congestive heart failure in dogs with myxomatous valve disease and asymptomatic mitral regurgitation. *J. Vet. Intern. Med.* 16: 80–88.

Lake-Bakaar, G.A., Johnson, E.G., and Griffiths, L.G. (2012). Aortic thrombosis in dogs: 31 cases (2000–2010). *J. Am. Vet. Med. Assoc.* 241: 910–915.

Latini, R., Connolly, S.J., and Kates, R.E. (1983). Myocardial disposition of amiodarone in the dog. *J. Pharmacol. Exp. Ther.* 224: 603–608.

Lee, Y.R., Kang, M.H., and Park, H.M. (2015). Anthracycline-induced cardiomyopathy in a dog treated with epirubicin. *Can. Vet. J.* 56: 571–574.

Lefebvre, H.P., Ollivier, E., Atkins, C.E. et al. (2013). Safety of spironolactone in dogs with chronic heart failure because of degenerative valvular disease: a population-based, longitudinal study. *J. Vet. Intern. Med.* 27: 1083–1091.

Levy, S.A. and Duray, P.H. (1988). Complete heart block in a dog seropositive for *Borrelia burgdorferi*. Similarity to human Lyme carditis. *J. Vet. Intern. Med.* 2: 138–144.

Levy, N.A., Koenigshof, A.M., and Sanders, R.A. (2016). Retrospective evaluation of intravenous premixed amiodarone use and adverse effects in dogs (17 cases: 2011–2014). *J. Vet. Cardiol.* 18: 10–14.

Lubsen, J., Just, H., Hjalmarsson, A.C. et al. (1996). Effect of pimobendan on exercise capacity in patients with heart failure: main results from the pimobendan in congestive heart failure (PICO) trial. *Heart* 76: 223–231.

MacDonald, K.A., Kittleson, M.D., Kass, P.H. et al. (2008). Effect of spironolactone on diastolic function and left ventricular mass in Maine Coon Cats with familial hypertrophic cardiomyopathy. *J. Vet. Intern. Med.* 22: 335–341.

Macgregor, J.M., Rush, J.E., Laste, N.J. et al. (2011). Use of pimobendan in 170 cats (2006–2010). *J. Vet. Cardiol.* 13: 251–260.

Maggio, F., DeFrancesco, T.C., Atkins, C.E. et al. (2000). Ocular lesions associated with systemic hypertension in cats: 69 cases (1985–1998). *J. Am. Vet. Med. Assoc.* 217: 695–702.

Maran, B.A., Meurs, K.M., Lahmers, S.M. et al. (2012). Identification of beta-1 adrenergic receptor polymorphisms in cats. *Res. Vet. Sci.* 93: 210–212.

Maran, B.A., Mealey, K.L., Lahmers, S.M. et al. (2013). Identification of DNA variants in the canine beta-1 adrenergic receptor gene. *Res. Vet. Sci.* 95: 238–240.

Mauldin, G.E., Fox, P.R., Patnaik, A.K. et al. (1992). Doxorubicin-induced cardiotoxicosis. Clinical features in 32 dogs. *J. Vet. Intern. Med.* 6: 82–88.

Mavropoulou, A., Gnudi, G., Grandi, G. et al. (2014). Clinical assessment of post-adulticide complications in Dirofilaria immitis-naturally infected dogs treated with doxycycline and ivermectin. *Vet. Parasitol.* 205: 211–215.

Maxwell, E., Ryan, K., Reynolds, C. et al. (2014). Outcome of a heartworm treatment protocol in dogs presenting to Louisiana State University from 2008 to 2011: 50 cases. *Vet. Parasitol.* 206: 71–77.

McCall, J.W., Arther, R., Davis, W. et al. (2014). Safety and efficacy of 10% imidacloprid+2.5% moxidectin for the treatment of Dirofilaria immitis circulating microfilariae in experimentally infected dogs. *Vet. Parasitol.* 206: 86–92.

Mealey, K.L. (2004). Therapeutic implications of the MDR-1 gene. *J. Vet. Pharmacol. Ther.* 27: 257–264.

Mealey, K.L. (2008). Canine ABCB1 and macrocyclic lactones: heartworm prevention and pharmacogenetics. *Vet. Parasitol.* 158: 215–222.

Mealey, K.L. (2012). ABCG2 transporter: therapeutic and physiologic implications in veterinary species. *J. Vet. Pharmacol. Ther.* 35: 105–112.

Mealey, K.L. and Burke, N.S. (2015). Identification of a nonsense mutation in feline ABCB1. *J. Vet. Pharmacol. Ther.* 38: 429–433.

Mealey, K.L. and Fidel, J. (2015). P-glycoprotein mediated drug interactions in animals and humans with cancer. *J. Vet. Intern. Med.* 29: 1–6.

Mealey, K.L. and Meurs, K.M. (2008). Breed distribution of the ABCB1-1Delta (multidrug sensitivity) polymorphism among dogs undergoing ABCB1 genotyping. *J. Am. Vet. Med. Assoc.* 233: 921–924.

Mealey, K.L., Bentjen, S.A., Gay, J.M. et al. (2001). Ivermectin sensitivity in collies is associated with a deletion mutation of the mdr1 gene. *Pharmacogenetics* 11: 727–733.

Mellett, A.M., Nakamura, R.K., and Bianco, D. (2011). A prospective study of clopidogrel therapy in dogs with primary immune-mediated hemolytic anemia. *J. Vet. Intern. Med.* 25: 71–75.

Meurs, K.M., Spier, A.W., Wright, N.A. et al. (2002). Comparison of the effects of four antiarrhythmic treatments for familial ventricular arrhythmias in boxers. *J. Am. Vet. Med. Assoc.* 221: 522–527.

Meurs, K.M., Norgard, M.M., Ederer, M.M. et al. (2007). A substitution mutation in the myosin binding protein C gene in ragdoll hypertrophic cardiomyopathy. *Genomics* 90: 261–264.

Meurs, K.M., Stern, J.A., Reina-Doreste, Y. et al. (2014). Natural history of arrhythmogenic right ventricular cardiomyopathy in the boxer dog: a prospective study. *J. Vet. Intern. Med.* 28: 1214–1220.

Meurs, K.M., Stern, J.A., Reina-Doreste, Y. et al. (2015). Impact of the canine double-deletion beta1 adrenoreceptor polymorphisms on protein structure and heart rate response to atenolol, a beta1-selective beta-blocker. *Pharmacogenet. Genomics* 25: 427–431.

Mirahmadi, H., Maleki, A., Hasanzadeh, R. et al. (2017). Ocular dirofilariasis by Dirofilaria immitis in a child in Iran: a case report and review of the literature. *Parasitol. Int.* 66: 978–981.

Moise, N.S., Meyers-Wallen, V., Flahive, W.J. et al. (1994). Inherited ventricular arrhythmias and sudden death in German Shepherd dogs. *J. Am. Coll. Cardiol.* 24: 233–243.

Nakamura, K., Yamasaki, M., Ohta, H. et al. (2011). Effects of sildenafil citrate on five dogs with Eisenmenger's syndrome. *J. Small Anim. Pract.* 52: 595–598.

Nelson, C.T., McCall, J.W., Rubin, S.B. et al. (2005a). 2005 guidelines for the diagnosis, prevention and management of heartworm (*Dirofilaria immitis*) infection in cats. *Vet. Parasitol.* 133: 267–275.

Nelson, C.T., McCall, J.W., Rubin, S.B. et al. (2005b). 2005 guidelines for the diagnosis, prevention and management of heartworm (*Dirofilaria immitis*) infection in dogs. *Vet. Parasitol.* 133: 255–266.

Nelson, O.L., Lahmers, S., Schneider, T. et al. (2006). The use of an implantable cardioverter defibrillator in a boxer dog to control clinical signs of arrhythmogenic right ventricular cardiomyopathy. *J. Vet. Intern. Med.* 20: 1232–1237.

O'Grady, M.R., O'Sullivan, M.L., Minors, S.L. et al. (2009). Efficacy of benazepril hydrochloride to delay the progression of occult dilated cardiomyopathy in Doberman Pinschers. *J. Vet. Intern. Med.* 23: 977–983.

Olson, G.R. and Miller, L.D. (1986). Studies on the pathogenesis of heart lesions in dogs infected with pseudorabies virus. *Can. J. Vet. Res.* 50: 245–250.

Oyama, M.A., Sisson, D.D., Prosek, R. et al. (2007). Carvedilol in dogs with dilated cardiomyopathy. *J. Vet. Intern. Med.* 21: 1272–1279.

Oyama, M.A., Solter, P.F., Thorn, C.L. et al. (2017). Feasibility, safety, and tolerance of subcutaneous synthetic canine B-type natriuretic peptide (syncBNP) in healthy dogs and dogs with stage B1 mitral valve disease. *J. Vet. Cardiol.* 19 (3): 211–217.

Palerme, J.S., Jones, A.E., Ward, J.L. et al. (2016). Infective endocarditis in 13 cats. *J. Vet. Cardiol.* 18: 213–225.

Pariaut, R., Saelinger, C., Queiroz-Williams, P. et al. (2011). Implantable cardioverter-defibrillator in a German shepherd dog with ventricular arrhythmias. *J. Vet. Cardiol.* 13: 203–210.

Pedersen, H.D. and Haggstrom, J. (2000). Mitral valve prolapse in the dog: a model of mitral valve prolapse in man. *Cardiovasc. Res.* 47: 234–243.

Pedro, B., Lopez-Alvarez, J., Fonfara, S. et al. (2012). Retrospective evaluation of the use of amiodarone in dogs with arrhythmias (from 2003 to 2010). *J. Small Anim. Pract.* 53: 19–26.

Peterson, M.E., Kintzer, P.P., and Hurvitz, A.I. (1988). Methimazole treatment of 262 cats with hyperthyroidism. *J. Vet. Intern. Med.* 2: 150–157.

Piepho, R.W., Bloedow, D.C., Lacz, J.P. et al. (1982). Pharmacokinetics of diltiazem in selected animal species and human beings. *Am. J. Cardiol.* 49: 525–528.

Pion, P.D., Kittleson, M.D., Rogers, Q.R. et al. (1987). Myocardial failure in cats associated with low plasma taurine: a reversible cardiomyopathy. *Science* 237: 764–768.

Pion, P.D., Kittleson, M.D., Thomas, W.P. et al. (1992a). Response of cats with dilated cardiomyopathy to taurine supplementation. *J. Am. Vet. Med. Assoc.* 201: 275–284.

Pion, P.D., Kittleson, M.D., Skiles, M.L. et al. (1992b). Dilated cardiomyopathy associated with taurine deficiency in the domestic cat: relationship to diet and myocardial taurine content. *Adv. Exp. Med. Biol.* 315: 63–73.

Pion, P.D., Kittleson, M.D., Thomas, W.P. et al. (1992c). Clinical findings in cats with dilated cardiomyopathy and relationship of findings to taurine deficiency. *J. Am. Vet. Med. Assoc.* 201: 267–274.

Reina-Doreste, Y., Stern, J.A., Keene, B.W. et al. (2014). Case-control study of the effects of pimobendan on survival time in cats with hypertrophic cardiomyopathy and congestive heart failure. *J. Am. Vet. Med. Assoc.* 245: 534–539.

Rolim, V.M., Casagrande, R.A., Wouters, A.T. et al. (2016). Myocarditis caused by feline immunodeficiency virus in five cats with hypertrophic cardiomyopathy. *J. Comp. Pathol.* 154: 3–8.

Rosa, F.A., Leite, J.H., Braga, E.T. et al. (2014). Cardiac lesions in 30 dogs naturally infected with Leishmania infantum chagasi. *Vet. Pathol.* 51: 603–606.

Santilli, R.A., Bontempi, L.V., Perego, M. et al. (2009). Outflow tract segmental arrhythmogenic right ventricular cardiomyopathy in an English Bulldog. *J. Vet. Cardiol.* 11: 47–51.

Santilli, R.A., Battaia, S., Perego, M. et al. (2017). *Bartonella*-associated inflammatory cardiomyopathy in a dog. *J. Vet. Cardiol.* 19: 74–81.

Saunders, A.B., Miller, M.W., Gordon, S.G. et al. (2006). Oral amiodarone therapy in dogs with atrial fibrillation. *J. Vet. Intern. Med.* 20: 921–926.

Saunders, A.B., Gordon, S.G., Rector, M.H. et al. (2013). Bradyarrhythmias and pacemaker therapy in dogs with Chagas disease. *J. Vet. Intern. Med.* 27: 890–894.

Schrope, D.P. and Kelch, W.J. (2006). Signalment, clinical signs, and prognostic indicators associated with high-grade second- or third-degree atrioventricular block in dogs: 124 cases (January 1, 1997–December 31, 1997). *J. Am. Vet. Med. Assoc.* 228: 1710–1717.

Scruggs, S.M. and Rishniw, M. (2013). Dermatologic adverse effect of subcutaneous furosemide administration in a dog. *J. Vet. Intern. Med.* 27: 1248–1250.

Silverman, S.J., Stern, J.A., and Meurs, K.M. (2012). Hypertrophic cardiomyopathy in the sphynx cat: a retrospective evaluation of clinical presentation and heritable etiology. *J. Feline Med. Surg.* 14: 246–249.

Sime, T.A., Powell, L.L., Schildt, J.C. et al. (2015). Parvoviral myocarditis in a 5-week-old dachshund. *J. Vet. Emerg. Crit. Care (San Antonio)* 25: 765–769.

Simpson, K.E., Devine, B.C., and Gunn-Moore, D. (2005). Suspected toxoplasma-associated myocarditis in a cat. *J. Feline Med. Surg.* 7: 203–208.

Smith, S.A., Kraft, S.L., Lewis, D.C. et al. (2000a). Pharmacodynamics of warfarin in cats. *J. Vet. Pharmacol. Ther.* 23: 339–344.

Smith, S.A., Kraft, S.L., Lewis, D.C. et al. (2000b). Plasma pharmacokinetics of warfarin enantiomers in cats. *J. Vet. Pharmacol. Ther.* 23: 329–337.

Smith, S.A., Tobias, A.H., Jacob, K.A. et al. (2003). Arterial thromboembolism in cats: acute crisis in 127 cases (1992–2001) and long-term management with low-dose aspirin in 24 cases. *J. Vet. Intern. Med.* 17: 73–83.

Smith, C.E., Rozanski, E.A., Freeman, L.M. et al. (2003). Use of low molecular weight heparin in cats: 57 cases (1999–2003). *J. Am. Vet. Med. Assoc.* 225: 1237–1241.

Smith, C.E., Freeman, L.M., Rush, J.E. et al. (2007). Omega-3 fatty acids in boxer dogs with arrhythmogenic right ventricular cardiomyopathy. *J. Vet. Intern. Med.* 21: 265–273.

Snyder, P.S. (1998). Comparison of some pharmacokinetic parameters of 5 angiotensin-converting enzyme inhibitors in normal beagles. *J. Vet. Intern. Med.* 12: 478.

Stern, J.A., Reina-Doreste, Y., Chdid, L. et al. (2014). Identification of PDE5A:E90K: a polymorphism in the canine phosphodiesterase 5A gene affecting basal cGMP concentrations of healthy dogs. *J. Vet. Intern. Med.* 28: 78–83.

Stokol, T., Brooks, M., Rush, J.E. et al. (2008). Hypercoagulability in cats with cardiomyopathy. *J. Vet. Intern. Med.* 22: 546–552.

Stollberger, C. and Finsterer, J. (2015). Relevance of P-glycoprotein in stroke prevention with dabigatran, rivaroxaban, and apixaban. *Herz* 40 (Suppl. 2): 140–145.

Summerfield, N.J., Boswood, A., O'Grady, M.R. et al. (2012). Efficacy of pimobendan in the prevention of congestive heart failure or sudden death in Doberman Pinschers with preclinical dilated cardiomyopathy (the PROTECT study). *J. Vet. Intern. Med.* 26: 1337–1349.

Sykes, J.E., Kittleson, M.D., Pesavento, P.A. et al. (2006). Evaluation of the relationship between causative organisms and clinical characteristics of infective endocarditis in dogs: 71 cases (1992–2005). *J. Am. Vet. Med. Assoc.* 228: 1723–1734.

Taylor, S.S., Sparkes, A.H., Briscoe, K. et al. (2017). ISFM consensus guidelines on the diagnosis and management of hypertension in cats. *J. Feline Med. Surg.* 19: 288–303.

Topan, A., Carstina, D., Slavcovici, A. et al. (2015). Assessment of the Duke criteria for the diagnosis of infective endocarditis after twenty-years: an analysis of 241 cases. *Clujul Med.* 88: 321–326.

Tumolskaya, N.I., Pozio, E., Rakova, V.M. et al. (2016). *Dirofilaria immitis* in a child from the Russian Federation. *Parasite* 23: 37.

Venco, L., Marchesotti, F., and Manzocchi, S. (2015). Feline heartworm disease: A 'Rubik's-cube-like' diagnostic and therapeutic challenge. *J. Vet. Cardiol.* 17 (Suppl. 1): S190–S201.

Vollmar, A.C. and Fox, P.R. (2016). Long-term outcome of Irish Wolfhound dogs with preclinical cardiomyopathy, atrial fibrillation, or both treated with pimobendan, benazepril hydrochloride, or methyldigoxin monotherapy. *J. Vet. Intern. Med.* 30: 553–559.

Wall, M., Calvert, C.A., Sanderson, S.L. et al. (2005). Evaluation of extended-release diltiazem once daily for cats with hypertrophic cardiomyopathy. *J. Am. Anim. Hosp. Assoc.* 41: 98–103.

Ward, J.L., DeFrancesco, T.C., Tou, S.P. et al. (2016). Outcome and survival in canine sick sinus syndrome and sinus node dysfunction: 93 cases (2002–2014). *J. Vet. Cardiol.* 18: 199–212.

Ware, W.A., Reina-Doreste, Y., Stern, J.A. et al. (2015). Sudden death associated with QT interval prolongation and KCNQ1 gene mutation in a family of English springer spaniels. *J. Vet. Intern. Med.* 29: 561–568.

Welch, K.M., Rozanski, E.A., Freeman, L.M. et al. (2010). Prospective evaluation of tissue plasminogen activator in 11 cats with arterial thromboembolism. *J. Feline Med. Surg.* 12: 122–128.

Wright, K.N., Atkins, C.E., and Kanter, R. (1996). Supraventricular tachycardia in four young dogs. *J. Am. Vet. Med. Assoc.* 208: 75–80.

Yata, M., McLachlan, A.J., Foster, D.J. et al. (2016). Single-dose pharmacokinetics and cardiovascular effects of oral pimobendan in healthy cats. *J. Vet. Cardiol.* 18: 310–325.

Yusuf, S., Pitt, B., Davis, C.E. et al. (1991). Effect of enalapril on survival in patients with reduced left ventricular ejection fractions and congestive heart failure. *N. Engl. J. Med.* 325: 293–302.

11

Respiratory Pharmacotherapeutics

Katrina L. Mealey

College of Veterinary Medicine, Washington State University, Pullman, WA, USA

Key Points

- Both infectious and non-infectious (asthma-like) inflammatory diseases of the airways are common in veterinary species.
- Corticosteroids are the mainstay of treatment of non-infectious inflammatory airway disease, but there are important species differences in oral bioavailability of corticosteroid formulations and in susceptibility to corticosteroid-induced adverse reactions.
- Most over-the-counter cough and cold preparations formulated for people are not used in dogs or cats because they are either ineffective or toxic in commercially available formulations.

11.1 Comparative Aspects of Respiratory Disease

Many diseases of the respiratory system that afflict people can also afflict veterinary species – pneumonia (viral, bacterial, fungal, and protozoal), non-infectious inflammatory disorders of the trachea and/or bronchi (asthma or asthma-like diseases), and pulmonary hypertension. Other respiratory diseases that occur with some frequency in people, chronic obstructive pulmonary disease (COPD; characterized by both chronic bronchitis and emphysema) and cystic fibrosis, are rare or nonexistent in dogs and cats (Williams and Roman 2016). This may be related to behavior and/or genetic differences between people and their pets. For example, the fact that chronic smoking is the primary cause of COPD in people explains why the disease is not seen in dogs and cats (dogs and cats don't smoke). But what about exposure of pets to secondhand smoke? While there is some documentation that secondhand smoke may cause respiratory pathology in dogs and cats, the relatively short lifespan of these species (roughly 10 and 20 years, respectively) likely precludes development of emphysema, which is not typically diagnosed in people until their sixth or seventh decade. Another relatively common pulmonary disease that afflicts both humans and dogs is pulmonary arterial hypertension. In both species, the disease can be primary (idiopathic, heritable, or drug-induced) but most often occurs secondary to other diseases of the lungs or heart (e.g. left-sided valvular diseases).

Pharmacotherapeutics for Veterinary Dispensing, First Edition. Edited by Katrina L. Mealey.
© 2019 John Wiley & Sons, Inc. Published 2019 by John Wiley & Sons, Inc.

Causes of pulmonary hypertension unique to people include HIV infection and sleep disorders (Duggan et al. 2017), while heartworm (*Dirofiliaria immitis*) is unique to dogs (Venco et al. 2014). With respect to cystic fibrosis, which afflicts humans, the functional genetic defects in the cystic fibrosis transmembrane conductance regulator that cause the disease in people have not been identified in dogs or cats (Sosnay et al. 2017).

Cats and dogs are predisposed to some respiratory diseases that are distinct from those in people because of differences in their behaviors, environments, and genetic makeup. For example, fungal (*Aspergillus* and *Penicillium*) and even parasitic (the nasal mite *Pneumonyssoides*) infections are relatively common causes of nasal disease in dogs and cats (Cohn 2014) but certainly not in people. These infectious diseases are likely more common in pets than in people because they use their noses more extensively and for different purposes than people do. This is truer of dogs than cats, as anyone who has observed a dog sniffing around at a dog park

can attest. Genetics also plays a role in predisposition to some canine and feline respiratory diseases. Some dogs and cats have been bred for particular physical characteristics such that, over time, these animals have accumulated a constellation of anatomical abnormalities affecting the upper respiratory tract, including the nares, soft palate, trachea, and nasopharyngeal turbinates (Meola 2013). These abnormalities are collectively referred to as brachycephalic airway syndrome ("brachy" meaning short and "cephalic" meaning head) and occur in certain breeds of dogs (Pugs, Boxers, Pekingese, etc.) or cats (Himalayan, Persian, etc.) with "smushed" faces. On the opposite end of the spectrum are the dolichocephalic dog breeds ("dolicho" meaning long), which include Collies, Greyhounds, Borzoi, and others. Dolichocephalic breeds are thought to be at greater risk for nasal cavity tumors than brachycephalic breeds. The tremendous anatomic differences between the nasal cavities of different dog breeds can be seen in Figure 11.1. Because of these tremendous anatomic differences, it

(a) (b)

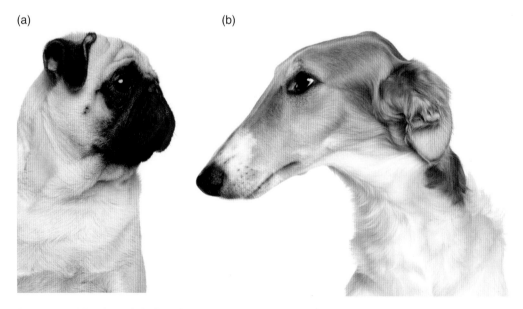

Figure 11.1 A brachycephalic breed represented by a Pug (a), and a dolichocephalic breed represented by a Borzoi (b). Breed susceptibilities to certain types of respiratory disease are not surprising considering the anatomic differences in the nares, nasal cavity, nasal sinuses, and nasopharynx between brachycephalic and dolichocephalic breeds. *Source:* CanStock Photo.

should not be surprising that there is such a strong association between breed and certain upper respiratory diseases in dogs.

Another genetically linked condition that occurs in dogs, but not cats or humans, is tracheal collapse. Tracheal collapse is a condition commonly seen in small dog breeds (Pomeranian, Yorkshire Terrier, etc.). The functional integrity of tracheal cartilage is compromised, resulting in dynamic collapse and severe narrowing of the tracheal lumen, particularly during inspiration (Tappin 2016). The normally O-shaped lumen of the trachea flattens into an oval (Figure 11.2), and in severe cases, the "roof" of the trachea can actually touch the "floor" of the trachea, essentially obliterating the lumen. While the definitive treatment requires surgical implantation of prosthetics, symptomatic treatment is common and may include antitussives, corticosteroids, and bronchodilators.

Despite genetic, anatomic, and functional variations between the respiratory tract of humans, dogs, and cats, pathophysiologic responses to similar insults are comparable. Allergen-specific activation of immune cells in airways stimulates inflammation and bronchoconstriction that can result in cough,

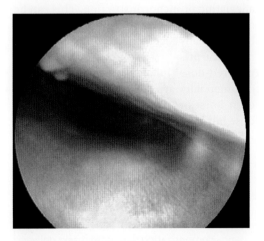

Figure 11.2 Bronchoscopic image of trachea at the thoracic inlet at peak expiration. The tracheal diameter is narrowed by the dorsal membrane (grade III/IV tracheal collapse), and a small amount of mucus is present. *Source:* Courtesy of Simon Tappin, Dick White Referrals, UK.

wheezing, and, in severe instances, respiratory distress in each of these species. Consequently, asthma in humans and the respective reactive airway diseases in cats and dogs are often treated similarly. Corticosteroids are used to combat airway inflammation, and bronchodilators are used as needed for episodes of bronchoconstriction (Reinero and Nafe 2011).

11.1.1 Drug-Induced Pulmonary Disease

In all species, drug therapy carries a risk of adverse events or collateral damage. The lungs are sometimes the victim of that collateral damage (Taylor et al. 2016). Some drugs that induce pulmonary disease in people can induce the same disease in dogs. Cats, however, are an entirely different animal with respect to drug-induced pulmonary disease. Cisplatin (Knapp et al. 1987), a chemotherapy drug, and potassium bromide (Boothe et al. 2002), a drug used to treat canine epilepsy and previously used to treat epilepsy in people (Ryan and Baumann 1999), can cause fatal pulmonary disease in cats, but apparently cause no pathology to the respiratory tract of dogs or people. Over 300 drugs have been implicated in causing lung disease in people; however, many of these are drugs of abuse or other agents not used frequently in dogs or cats. Table 11.1 shows some known similarities and differences of drug-induced pulmonary disease in dogs, cats, and people.

11.2 Diagnostic Testing

Definitive diagnosis of canine and feline respiratory diseases may be sufficiently limited by owner finances, such that treatment based on the most likely cause may be initiated without the veterinarian ever having established a true diagnosis. Ideally, however, diagnostic testing might include the following procedures, some of which are unique to veterinary species. For example, because

Table 11.1 Species similarities and differences in drug-induced pulmonary disease.

	Tyrosine kinase inhibitors	Bleomycin	Opioids	Cisplatin	Potassium bromide[a]
Human	Interstitial lung disease	Pneumonitis and fibrosis	Respiratory depression	None reported	Not used
Dog	Tachypnea reported	Pneumonitis and fibrosis	Respiratory depression	None reported	None reported
Cat	None reported	Unknown	Respiratory depression	Acute, fulminant pulmonary edema	Severe asthma-like reaction

[a] Used to treat canine epilepsy and previously used to treat epilepsy in people.

parasites (heartworm, lungworm, and nasal mites) cause respiratory disease much more frequently in veterinary patients than in human patients in the USA, diagnostic testing for parasites is routine in dogs and cats.

- Auscultation
- Radiography
- Complete blood count (helpful for infectious and parasitic diseases)
- Fecal analysis (helpful for some parasitic diseases)
- Heartworm antibody/antigen testing
- Cytological analysis of respiratory fluid (transtracheal wash or bronchoalveolar lavage)
- Allergy testing (serum or intradermal)
- Advanced imaging, such as computerized tomography (CT) and magnetic resonance imaging (MRI)
- Endoscopic visualization (bronchoscopy and nasal endoscopy)
- Pulmonary function testing (rarely used in dogs and cats because of limited availability).

11.3 Pharmacological Treatment of Common Diseases

Pharmacotherapy of non-infectious, inflammatory airway disease of the cat (feline asthma) and dog (canine allergic bronchitis); pulmonary hypertension and symptomatic treatment of cough (antitussives) in dogs; and rhinitis (nasal decongestants)

in cats will be presented in this chapter. Pharmacotherapy of the most common bacterial, fungal, protozoal, and parasitic pathogens involved in respiratory diseases of dogs and cats is presented in Chapters 7 and 9. A number of pharmacotherapeutic principles are shared between species with respect to treating respiratory diseases. Nonpharmacological management includes avoiding known allergens, minimizing environmental pollutants such as smoke or noxious fumes, and dietary measures to treat or prevent obesity, which limits lung function. Key principles of asthma pharmacotherapy include decreasing airway inflammation and alleviating bronchoconstriction. This can be accomplished systemically (oral or injectable) or locally (aerosolized drug delivery). It may surprise some pharmacists that metered-dose inhaler spacer devices are commercially available for cats, dogs, and even horses for use with human metered-dose inhaler formulations (Chapter 25).

> **Practiced but not proven**
>
> Aerosol chambers are commercially available for dogs, cats, or horses and are intended for use with metered-dose inhalers formulated for human patients. I am not aware of evidence demonstrating that these masks deliver appropriately sized droplets to the appropriate anatomic location within the airways, but clinical experience suggests their use improves clinical outcome in veterinary patients.

Symptomatic treatment of cough and rhinitis in people with over-the-counter "cough and cold" products is a billion-dollar industry. Most over-the-counter products are not effective for the corresponding condition in dogs and cats, and some of these widely available human products are actually deadly for dogs and cats. Products containing acetaminophen or aspirin must not be used in cats, while products containing the sweetener xylitol must not be used in dogs because of species-dependent susceptibility to toxicosis. Ingestion of even small amounts can be fatal. See Chapter 6 for additional information regarding over-the-counter drug products that can be toxic to pets. Dextromethorphan, the active ingredient in over-the-counter cough suppressant products labeled for people, is ineffective as a cough suppressant in dogs or cats (Papich 2009). Likewise, guaifenesin has not been shown to be an effective expectorant in dogs or cats (Papich 2009). Decongestants such as pseudoephedrine have a narrow therapeutic index in dogs and cats. Doses of pseudoephedrine available in human products are excessive for use in cats and many dogs. For example, a pseudoephedrine tablet intended for human patients (30 mg is the lowest strength available) would be excessive for dogs weighing less than 44 pounds (Plumb 2015). Topical decongestants such as pediatric phenylephrine nasal drops are sometimes used in cats with viral or idiopathic rhinitis. Antihistamines in human formulations such as diphenhydramine, loratadine, and others, while generally not considered effective for treating canine or feline respiratory disease, are used for treating atopic dermatitis (pruritic allergic skin disease) in dogs and cats. See Chapter 18 for information on the use of antihistamines in dermatologic pharmacotherapy. However, a US Food and Drug Administration (FDA)-approved combination product containing the antihistamine trimeprazine and prednisolone (Temaril-P®) has a label indication as an antitussive as well as for treatment of pruritic allergic skin disease in dogs.

11.3.1 Feline Asthma

The community pharmacist is not likely to be involved in emergency management of an acute crisis such as status asthmaticus, so this discussion will be limited to chronic pharmacotherapy of feline asthma.

11.3.1.1 Controlling Airway Inflammation

Corticosteroids, inhaled or systemic, are the mainstay for combatting the inflammatory component of feline asthma despite the plethora of adverse effects they can cause (Olah 2015). Although many corticosteroid-associated adverse effects seen in cats are similar to those that occur in human patients, some adverse effects that occur in humans are rare or do not occur in cats. In particular, osteoporosis has not been identified in cats receiving systemic corticosteroid therapy, even after long-term treatment. Corticosteroid-associated adverse effects that are somewhat unique to cats include the development of diabetes mellitus and thin, fragile skin, particularly with prolonged treatment. Inhaled corticosteroid formulations for human asthma sufferers are used preferentially over systemic corticosteroids because adverse effects are minimal in human patients. Inhaled corticosteroids are delivered with a feline-specific spacer concurrently with human metered-dose inhalers (Figure 11.3). The same may not be true for cats where some systemic absorption may occur. This is probably because the dose of drug delivered by a metered-dose inhaler is the same for a feline patient (roughly 3–5 kg) and a human patient (roughly 30–70 kg), resulting in a relative dose that is 10-fold higher in the cat than the person. Because inhaled corticosteroids are extremely potent (1000-fold greater than cortisol), even minute quantities absorbed by a very small patient (i.e. a cat) may induce systemic corticosteroid effects. For this reason, cat owners should be warned of the potential for systemic corticosteroid effects in cats treated with inhaled corticosteroids. Additionally, cats have developed bacterial infections and mite infestations of

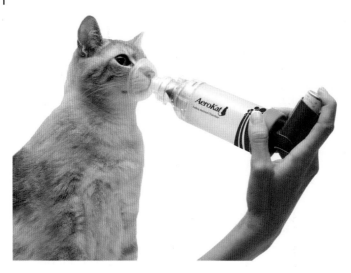

Figure 11.3 Demonstration of the use of a human drug formulation (a corticosteroid metered-dose inhaler) in combination with a feline-specific "spacer" to deliver inhalation therapy to a cat with asthma. *Source:* Photo courtesy of Trudell Medical International.

the skin underneath the masks used for delivering inhaled corticosteroids (Bizikova 2014). This is presumed to result from localized immunosuppression caused by nebulized corticosteroid droplets that come in contact with the skin. Currently, there are no other options for addressing airway inflammation in asthmatic cats. Alternative anti-inflammatory agents, sometimes used for treating asthma in people, are not currently used in cats. Leukotriene modifiers have not demonstrated efficacy in feline asthma (Reinero et al. 2005), and the human recombinant anti-immunoglobulin E (IgE) antibody omalizumab is currently too expensive for most cat owners.

Dramatic difference

Because prednisone has low oral bioavailability in cats and horses, prednisolone or methylprednisolone should be used instead.

11.3.1.2 Systemic Corticosteroids
Most Likely to Be Prescribed
Prednisolone: 1–2 mg/kg PO (orally) every 24 hours (once daily or divided). The goal is to gradually wean the patient off the medication, if possible, or use the lowest effective dose.

Methylprednisolone: 0.8–2.2 mg/kg PO every 24 hours (once daily or divided). The goal is to gradually wean the patient off medication, if possible, or use the lowest effective dose.

Dexamethasone: 0.1–0.2 mg/kg PO every 24 hours. The goal is to gradually wean the patient off the medication, if possible, or use the lowest effective dose. Use of dexamethasone is less desirable than prednisolone or methylprednisolone because it is more likely to cause diabetes mellitus (Lowe et al. 2009).

11.3.1.3 Aerosolized Corticosteroids
Most Likely to Be Prescribed
Note: Inhaled corticosteroids are not recommended for acute management of asthma-induced respiratory distress because their effects are delayed.

Fluticasone propionate: Metered-dose inhaler: 110 micrograms every 12–36 hours as needed.

The drug delivery technique for metered-dose inhalers is found in Chapter 25.

Bronchodilators: Acute bronchoconstriction resulting in respiratory distress can be a feature of feline asthma. The primary use of bronchodilators on an outpatient basis is as an early intervention in an acute asthmatic crisis. This is typically accomplished with administration as a parenteral injection (owners can be trained to administer terbutaline subcutaneously; see Chapter 25) or aerosolized inhalant. Use of orally administered bronchodilators on a chronic basis has fallen out of favor for long-term management of feline asthma. Beta adrenergic receptor agonists (preferably β_2-selective ones) are preferred as bronchodilators relative to methylxanthines (i.e. theophylline and aminophylline) for a number of reasons: lack of convenient dosing forms (sustained-release preparations formulated for human patients do not provide predictable plasma drug concentrations in cats), narrow therapeutic index necessitating therapeutic drug monitoring, and their potential involvement in numerous drug interactions.

11.3.1.4 Bronchodilators Most Likely to Be Prescribed

Terbutaline:

Parenteral injection: 0.01 mg/kg subcutaneously (SC)

Oral tablets: 0.1–0.2 mg/kg PO every 8–12 hours.

Albuterol: Metered-dose inhaler: 90 micrograms every 30 minutes as needed for up to eight treatments. The drug delivery technique for metered-dose inhalers is described in Chapter 25.

11.3.2 Canine Chronic Bronchitis

Canine sterile or noninfectious bronchitis is characterized by a chronic cough for which a specific cause (e.g. infection, congestive heart failure, heartworm disease, or neoplasia) is not identified. Coughing is often triggered by environmental irritants and allergens, as with feline asthma, but severe bronchoconstriction resulting in respiratory distress is not typically associated with the disease. The cough, while not life-threatening, is presumed to decrease the dog's quality of life and is certainly distressful to owners (particularly at bedtime if the dog sleeps in the owners' bedroom). Pharmacotherapeutic goals are to suppress airway inflammation and decrease the frequency and severity of coughing for the benefit of both the dog and the owner. Antitussives are presented in Section 11.3.2.1.1. Corticosteroids, administered systemically (oral) or by inhalation (metered-dose inhaler), are used to decrease airway inflammation.

11.3.2.1 Drugs Most Commonly Prescribed to Decrease Airway Inflammation

Prednisone or prednisolone: 0.5 mg/kg PO every 12 hours as needed. The goal is to gradually wean the patient off the medication, if possible, or use the lowest effective dose.

Fluticasone: Metered-dose inhaler: 110–220 micrograms every 8–12 hours.

The drug delivery technique for metered-dose inhalers is found in Chapter 25.

11.3.2.1.1 Antitussives

Antitussives are indicated relatively frequently for dogs but less so in cats. Coughing in cats tends to be a sign of a disease that requires more definitive treatment (e.g. asthma, cardiac disease, or pneumonia). Cough suppression in dogs is indicated for a variety of diseases, including sterile bronchitis, viral and mild bacterial bronchitis ("kennel cough"), tracheal collapse, and even some cardiac diseases (while concurrently treating the underlying cardiac disorder). Antitussives should be used cautiously in dogs with a productive cough, since this could indicate an underlying infection that could be exacerbated if the cough reflex is suppressed. Opioids are the only class of drugs that are effective for suppressing cough in dogs. Butorphanol is available in a FDA-approved veterinary formulation with a label indication for treating chronic cough in dogs. It is a US Drug Enforcement Agency (DEA) Schedule IV controlled substance.

The most commonly prescribed antitussives are:

Butorphanol tablets: 0.05–0.12 mg/kg PO every 8–12 hours (dogs)

Hydrocodone: 0.22 mg/kg PO every 6–12 hours (dogs).

11.3.3 Tracheal Collapse

Tracheal collapse is a disease involving progressive degeneration of cartilage composing the tracheal rings. It results in flattening and collapse of the trachea, which can severely narrow the tracheal lumen. It is most often seen in small dog breeds, with clinical signs varying depending on the severity of the disease. Dogs may experience mild airway inflammation, which progresses to a "goosehonk" cough and, potentially, respiratory distress and dyspnea. In severe cases, definitive treatment involves tracheal ring prostheses or intratracheal stenting. Medical management involves weight loss, use of harnesses rather than collars, judicious use of corticosteroids, bronchodilators, and antitussives (Tappin 2016). Specific agents and doses are as listed for canine chronic bronchitis (Section 11.3.2.1).

11.3.4 Rhinitis

Nasal decongestants: Nasal decongestants are rarely indicated in veterinary species (in contrast to people), owing to the fact that rhinitis is usually caused by something that requires more definitive treatment (bacterial, parasitic, or neoplastic causes). Systemic decongestants should not be administered to dogs or cats because of the narrow therapeutic index in these species. Topical (pediatric nasal drops) decongestants such as phenylephrine are sometimes used to treat viral or idiopathic rhinitis in cats once other causes of nasal discharge have been ruled out.

11.3.5 Pulmonary Hypertension

Sildenafil: Treatment of underlying disorders, if possible, should be the focus for appropriate management of secondary pulmonary hypertension. For primary hypertension, and when other treatments fail to adequately control secondary pulmonary hypertension, sildenafil (a phosphodiesterase-5 inhibitor) has been used in dogs (Stern et al. 2014). This drug is not FDA approved for use in dogs, nor is there evidence based on randomized, controlled clinical trials that it is effective for treating pulmonary hypertension in dogs. However, there are no other therapeutic options.

11.4 Adverse Drug Effects in Veterinary Species

11.4.1 Corticosteroids

As is the case with human patients, the likelihood of detrimental effects of corticosteroids in veterinary patients increases as the dose and duration of treatment increase. Ideal treatment consists of balancing the benefits of corticosteroid therapy with potential adverse effects. Ideally, systemic corticosteroids are administered as pulse therapy (an anti-inflammatory dose for one to two weeks) to augment inhaled corticosteroid therapy, because adverse effects are less likely, although still possible, with inhaled corticosteroids. In particular, suppression of the hypothalamic–pituitary–adrenal axis has been documented with inhaled corticosteroids in dogs and cats (Galler et al. 2013; Melamies et al. 2012).

Potential adverse effects of corticosteroids in dogs and cats are, for the most part, similar to those in humans with some notable differences. Adverse effects common to all species include immunosuppression, delayed wound healing, hypertension, and metabolic effects. Specific metabolic adverse effects include protein catabolism and gluconeogenesis (observed in the patient as muscle wasting and abdominal redistribution of fat). Osteoporosis, which is a common sequela of chronic corticosteroid use in people, does not seem to be a problem in dogs or cats. Adverse effects that are somewhat canine-specific include polyuria and polydipsia, which lead to house soiling so owners should be forewarned; panting; and a higher risk for gastrointestinal (GI) ulceration, particularly with dexamethasone (Sorjonen et al. 1983). Dogs receiving corticosteroids should not concurrently be given nonsteroidal anti-inflammatory drugs (NSAIDs), as this greatly enhances the risk of severe GI ulceration. Cats are very susceptible to the diabetogenic effects of corticosteroids, particularly dexamethasone, so owners should be counseled to monitor for signs of diabetes (polyuria/polydipsia, weight loss despite good appetite, and lethargy) and seek veterinary care should they occur (Lowe et al. 2009). Cats may also experience dramatic thinning of the skin, resulting in skin fragility such that it may actually tear with routine handling.

11.4.2 Bronchodilators

The most common adverse effects of terbutaline and albuterol, despite the fact that they are selective β_2 adrenergic receptor agonists, involve the heart (β_1 adrenergic stimulation). Tachycardia should be expected with systemic administration of terbutaline and may also occur when albuterol is administered via inhalation. Consequently, patients with hyperthyroidism (a very common endocrinopathy in cats), hypertension, or preexisting cardiac disease (various cardiomyopathies can be common among certain cat breeds) should undergo vigilant monitoring if treated with β_2 adrenergic receptor agonists. Use of long-acting inhaled β_2 adrenergic receptor agonists is not routine in veterinary medicine, so it is unknown whether or not the FDA black box warning against the use of this drug class as sole therapy is applicable to veterinary patients.

Use of methylxanthines such as theophylline for feline asthma, canine bronchitis, or tracheal collapse in dogs has declined (Rozanski 2014) for the reasons described in this chapter, but they are still prescribed by some veterinarians. Adverse effects are similar to those in human patients (tremors, tachycardia, inappetence, tachyarrhythmias, and seizures), but dogs and cats seem to be at greater risk for experiencing toxicity. Pharmacists may provide an important service to the pet, owner, and veterinarian by suggesting use of a β_2 adrenergic receptor agonist as an alternative bronchodilator.

11.4.3 Antitussives

Lack of efficacy is an adverse drug event; therefore, dextromethorphan should be mentioned here because it exerts no cough-suppressive effects in veterinary patients. The only drug class that has shown efficacy in suppressing cough in veterinary patients is the opioids, butorphanol in particular. In fact, there is an FDA-approved product for dogs with a label indication for the relief of coughing. It is more effective than codeine (Cavanagh et al. 1976) and safer than most other opioid agents because, as a partial rather than full opioid agonist, it does not depress the respiratory center and does not cause histamine release. It may, however, cause central nervous system (CNS) depression in dogs. Butorphanol is labeled as an analgesic, not antitussive, in cats. Physical dependence in veterinary patients is not perceived to be likely. However, pharmacists should be wary of owners who request refills at shorter intervals than expected based on the prescribed dosing regimen in order to prevent diversion.

> **Dramatic difference**
>
> Interestingly, butorphanol and other opioids can cause CNS excitation and dysphoria in cats (and horses), rather than CNS depression as they do in other species such as dogs and people. In cats, opioids are typically administered concurrently with a tranquilizer or sedative.

11.4.4 Decongestants

Pseudoephedrine has a narrow therapeutic index, so it is not recommended for use as a systemic decongestant in veterinary patients. Systemic dosing of phenylephrine should be avoided also. Adverse effects include agitation, hypertension, tachycardia, seizures, hyperthermia, and cardiac arrhythmias (Plumb 2015). Phenylephrine in topical (nasal drops) human pediatric formulations may be used cautiously in cats with viral or idiopathic rhinitis, but owners should be cautioned against redosing even if they

Table 11.2 Drugs that are FDA approved for respiratory disease in a veterinary species but are not available in a human formulation.

Brand name	Active ingredient(s)	Drug class	Rationale/ notes
Ventpulmin	Clenbuterol	β_2 adrenergic agonist	Not approved for human use in the USA. Clenbuterol may be abused by athletes for its repartitioning effects. Its use in humans has been associated with severe cardiovascular and neurological adverse effects. Approved for use in horses.
Temaril-P*	Trimeprazine, prednisolone	Antihistamine/ phenothiazine and corticosteroid	Trimeprazine-containing products labeled for human use may be available outside the USA. Approved for use in dogs.

believe most of the drop was not delivered into the nares. Absorption can occur from the nasal mucosa with sufficient bioavailability to cause systemic signs.

11.5 Nutritional Supplements for Veterinary Respiratory Diseases

Vitamin D insufficiency has been associated with more poorly controlled asthma in children (Hollenbach and Cloutier 2015). Omega-3 fatty acids, or fish oils, are occasionally recommended as adjunct therapy in feline asthma, as they are purported to nonspecifically blunt inflammatory responses. I am not aware of any studies investigating the use of vitamin D, omega-3 fatty acids, or any other nutritional supplements for asthma or other respiratory diseases in veterinary patients.

11.6 FDA-Approved Veterinary Drug Products with No Human Drug Equivalent

See Table 11.2.

Abbreviations

CNS   Central nervous system
COPD   Chronic obstructive pulmonary disease

DEA   Drug Enforcement Agency
FDA   Food and Drug Administration
PO   per os ("by mouth," or orally)

References

Bizikova, P. (2014). Localized demodecosis due to Demodex cati on the muzzle of two cats treated with inhalant glucocorticoids. *Vet. Dermatol.* 25 (3): 222–225.

Boothe, D.M., George, K.L., and Cough, P. (2002). Disposition and clinical use of bromide in cats. *J. Am. Vet. Med. Assoc.* 221 (8): 1131–1135.

Cavanagh, R.L., Gylys, J.A., and Bierwagen, M.E. (1976). Antitussive properties of butorphanol. *Arch. Int. Pharmacodyn. Ther.* 220 (2): 258–268.

Cohn, L.A. (2014). Canine nasal disease. *Vet. Clin. North Am. Small Anim. Pract.* 44 (1): 75–89.

Duggan, S.T., Kearn, S.J., and Burness, C.B. (2017). Selexipag: a review in pulmonary hypertension. *Am. J. Cardiovasc. Drugs* 17 (1): 73–80.

Galler, A., Shibly, S., Bilek, A. et al. (2013). Inhaled budesonide therapy in cats with naturally occurring chronic bronchial disease (feline asthma and bronchitis). *J. Small Anim. Pract.* 54 (10): 531–536.

Hollenbach, J.P. and Cloutier, M.M. (2015). Childhood asthma management and environmental triggers. *Pediatr. Clin. N. Am.* 62 (5): 1199–1214.

Knapp, D.W., Richardson, R.C., DeNicola, D.B. et al. (1987). Cisplatin toxicity in cats. *J. Vet. Intern. Med.* 1 (1): 29–35.

Lowe, A.D., Graves, T.K., Campbell, K.L. et al. (2009). A pilot study comparing the diabetogenic effects of dexamethasone and prednisolone in cats. *J. Am. Anim. Hosp. Assoc.* 45 (5): 215–224.

Melamies, M., Vainio, O., Spillman, T. et al. (2012). Endocrine effects of inhaled budesonide compared with inhaled fluticasone propionate and oral prednisolone in healthy beagle dogs. *Vet. J.* 194 (3): 349–353.

Meola, S.D. (2013). Brachycephalic airway syndrome. *Top. Companion Anim. Med.* 39 (3): 91.

Olah GA. (2015). Which drugs are used to treat feline asthma? Plumb's Therapeutics Brief, May 18–30.

Papich, M.G. (2009). Drugs that affect the respiratory system. In: *Veterinary Pharmacology and Therapeutics*, 9e (ed. J.E. Riviere and M.G. Papich), 1295–1311. Ames, IA: Wiley-Blackwell.

Plumb, D.C. (ed.) (2015). *Plumb's Veterinary Drug Handbook*, 8e. Ames, IA: Wiley-Blackwell.

Reinero, C. and Nafe, L. (2011). Asthma, cat. In: *Clinical Veterinary Advisor*, 2e (ed. E. Côté). St, Louis, MO: Elsevier.

Reinero, C.R., Decile, K.C., Byerly, J.R. et al. (2005). Effects of drug treatment on inflammation and hyperreactivity of airways and on immune variables in cats with experimentally induced asthma. *Am. J. Vet. Res.* 66 (7): 1121–1127.

Rozanski, E. (2014). Canine chronic bronchitis. *Vet. Clin. N. Am. Small Anim. Pract.* 44 (1): 107–116.

Ryan, M. and Baumann, R.J. (1999). Use and monitoring of bromides in epilepsy treatment. *Pediatr. Neurol.* 21 (2): 523–528.

Sorjonen, D.C., Dillon, A.R., Powers, R.D. et al. (1983). Effects of dexamethasone and surgical hypotension on the stomach of dogs: clinical, endoscopic and pathologic evaluations. *Am. J. Vet. Res.* 44 (7): 1233–1237.

Sosnay, P.R., Salinas, D.B., White, T.B. et al. (2017). Applying cystic fibrosis transmembrane conductance regulator genetics and CFTR2 data to facilitate diagnoses. *J. Pediatr.* 181: S27–S32. doi: 10.1016/jpeds.09.063.

Stern, J.A., Reina-Doreste, Y., Chdid, L. et al. (2014). Identification of PDE5A:E90K: a polymorphism in the canine phosphodiesterase 5A gene affecting basal cGMP concentrations of healthy dogs. *J. Vet. Intern. Med.* 28 (1): 78–83.

Tappin, S.W. (2016). Canine tracheal collapse. *J. Small Anim. Pract.* 57 (1): 9–17.

Taylor, A.C., Verma, N., Slater, R. et al. (2016). Bad for breathing: a pictorial of drug-induced pulmonary disease. *Curr. Probl. Diagn. Radiol.* 45 (6): 429–432.

Venco, L., Mihaylova, L., and Boon, J.A. (2014). Right pulmonary artery distensibility index (RPAD) index. A field study of an echocardiographic method to detect early development of pulmonary hypertension and its severity even in the absence of regurgitant jets for doppler evaluation in heartworm-infected dogs. *Vet. Parasitol.* 206 (1–2): 60–66.

Williams, K. and Roman, J. (2016). Studying human respiratory disease in animals-role of induced and naturally occurring models. *J. Pathol.* 238 (2): 220–232.

12

Gastrointestinal, Hepatic, and Pancreatic Pharmacotherapeutics

Michael D. Willard

Department of Small Animal Clinical Sciences, College of Veterinary Medicine & Biomedical Sciences, Texas A&M University, College Station, TX, USA

Key Points

- Proton pump inhibitors are the most effective drugs for decreasing gastric acid secretion and hence are the best drugs for treating erosive esophagitis and for treating or preventing gastric ulceration/erosion. However, they are frequently prescribed inappropriately.
- Maropitant is the most effective antiemetic approved for use in dogs and cats; whenever possible, it should be used instead of other antiemetics.

- Antidiarrheal opiates are seldom needed or indicated in small animal patients.
- Tylosin and metronidazole are useful in chronic small-bowel antibiotic-responsive enteropathy (also called antibiotic-responsive diarrhea and dysbiosis), but they are seldom indicated in acute diarrhea.
- Therapeutic trials for exocrine pancreatic insufficiency with pancreatic enzymes are not recommended.

12.1 Comparative Aspects of Gastrointestinal Disease

Like their human counterparts, cats and dogs experience diseases of the gastrointestinal (GI) tract, liver, and pancreas that result from inflammatory, infectious, neoplastic, and other etiologies. However, diseases that are defined based on clinical symptoms (i.e. description of what the patient is experiencing) are obviously more difficult to document in veterinary patients. For example, gastroesophageal reflux disease (GERD) in people is often defined, classified, and treated based on how troublesome the symptoms are perceived to be by the patient. This approach is not reasonable in dogs or cats. Similarly, disease conditions of the GI tract, liver, pancreas, or gall bladder that cause symptoms of abdominal pain or nausea but no obvious clinical signs (i.e. vomiting, diarrhea, and hyporexia) are likely to go undetected in dogs or cats unless the pain becomes severe enough that the owners can detect it or the disease progresses to include clinical signs (e.g. hyporexia).

Acute gastroenteropathies causing diarrhea and/or vomiting in dogs and cats are relatively poorly defined compared to people. With the exception of parvoviral enteritis (a very severe, highly contagious viral infection), most causes of acute diarrhea

---

Pharmacotherapeutics for Veterinary Dispensing, First Edition. Edited by Katrina L. Mealey.
© 2019 John Wiley & Sons, Inc. Published 2019 by John Wiley & Sons, Inc.

that are not due to parasites are seldom definitively diagnosed, even when there is obvious contagion. More importantly, finding a "pathogen" in diarrheic feces does not necessarily allow confidence in establishing cause and effect. Bacteria recognized as pathogens causing gastroenteritis in people (e.g. *Salmonella* spp. and *Campylobacter* spp.) are commonly found in normal feces from clinically normal dogs and cats. Even when specific bacteria are strongly tied to an acute diarrheal syndrome (e.g. acute hemorrhagic diarrhea syndrome [AHDS], previously called hemorrhagic gastroenteritis, an acute GI disease in adult, small-breed dogs), antibacterial therapy is not necessarily beneficial. Therefore, finding a recognized "pathogen" in the feces of a diarrheic patient does not necessarily justify antibiotic therapy. As is the case in people, many acute gastroenteropathies causing diarrhea and/or vomiting in dogs and cats are self-limiting and do not require pharmacological management.

Acute colitis or exacerbation of chronic ulcerative colitis in people is sometimes treated with products containing 5-aminosalicylic acid (i.e. sulfasalazine, mesalamine, and olsalazine). Use of this drug is relatively sporadic in veterinary medicine compared to human medicine, where it is more commonly used. Toxic megacolon can be a complication of ulcerative colitis in people but is not described as a complication of so-called inflammatory bowel diseases in dogs or cats. Cats do develop megacolon; however, it tends to be associated with mechanical obstruction such as a pelvic fracture compressing the colon or from primary neurological disorders. The latter is thought to be the case in tailless breeds such as Manx cats.

The biggest differences between people and small animals in the treatment of GI disorders are seen in the chronic gastroenteropathies. While the names of the chronic GI diseases that commonly affect people may sound similar to the nomenclature used for dogs and cats (e.g. inflammatory bowel disease [IBD], irritable bowel syndrome [IBS], and gastric ulceration/erosion [GUE]), the actual diseases

and their causes are often quite different. Great care must be taken when extrapolating from human medicine to veterinary medicine. For example, in human medicine, IBD primarily refers to Crohn's disease and ulcerative colitis, two diseases for which there are no good counterparts in veterinary medicine. In dogs, so-called IBD (now often better referred to as chronic enteropathy) is usually considered to be dietary-responsive and/or antibiotic-responsive. IBS in people is a multifaceted problem, while so-called IBS in dogs is usually a fiber-responsive, large-bowel diarrhea. GUE in people is primarily caused by use of nonsteroidal anti-inflammatory drugs (NSAIDs) or infection with *Helicobacter pylori*. Dogs are renowned for GUE caused by NSAID exposure, but *Helicobacter* spp. are almost never a cause of GUE in dogs or cats. Therefore, antibiotics are not a component of pharmacological management of GUE in dogs or cats.

Breed predilections abound for certain GI diseases. Notable examples include lymphangiectasia in Yorkshire Terriers and Norwegian Lundehunds, histiocytic ulcerative colitis in Boxer dogs and French Bulldogs, protein-losing enteropathy in Soft Coated Wheaton Terriers and Yorkshire Terriers, IBD in Shar Peis, and immunoproliferative enteropathy in Basenjis. However, the statistically significant association of a particular disease with a particular breed does not allow one to confidently treat without first obtaining a definitive diagnosis.

The major hepatic diseases of dogs and cats tend to be very different than the major hepatic diseases found in people. Viral causes of chronic hepatic disease are exceedingly important in human beings but are almost never diagnosed (or at least almost never recognized) in dogs or cats. Alcoholic steatohepatitis is a very important hepatic disease of people, but dogs and cats obviously do not develop alcohol-related hepatic disease. There are well-documented cases of breed-associated hepatic diseases (e.g. copper intoxication in Bedlington Terriers, West Highland White Terriers, Labrador Retrievers, and

Dalmatians; early-onset cirrhosis in Cocker Spaniels; congenital portovascular anomalies in Yorkshire Terriers; and vacuolar hepatopathy and hepatocellular carcinoma in Scottish Terriers). More recently, a breed predilection for gallbladder disease, gallbladder mucocele formation, has been recognized in Shetland Sheepdogs and Schnauzers.

12.2 Specific GI Diseases of Importance in Small-Animal Veterinary Medicine

"Megaesophagus" is a relatively common problem in dogs but very uncommon in cats. Most cases of megaesophagus in the dog are idiopathic. This is in distinction to people with esophageal retention, who are typically afflicted with achalasia of the lower esophageal sphincter (LES) (or "high-pressure zone"). Achalasia is best treated with therapies designed to "loosen" the LES (e.g. balloon dilation or injection with medicinal botulinum toxin). Once thought to be rare, achalasia is being diagnosed more frequently over the last 3 years; idiopathic megaesophagus seen in dogs typically produces chalasia, rather than achalasia, of the LES. Therefore, dogs infrequently respond to therapies used in people. Prokinetic drugs such as cisapride do not enhance canine esophageal motility, but they do "tighten up" the LES. Therefore, a subset of dogs with idiopathic megaesophagus that apparently have concurrent gastroesophageal reflux (GER) seemingly benefit from cisapride therapy. Some dogs develop acquired megaesophagus because of a localized myasthenia gravis, which only affects the esophagus or pharynx; this is less common in people.

Spontaneous GER is a common human malady. Dogs and cats are seldom recognized to have spontaneous GER that is causing discernible symptoms. In contrast, dogs and cats sporadically experience severe acid reflux during anesthetic procedures, which can produce severe esophagitis that in turn causes cicatrix-induced benign strictures in the esophagus, nasopharynx, and/or nasal choana. Regardless of the cause, therapy in people and dogs/cats for benign strictures is somewhat similar. Because gastric acid is a major factor in causing esophagitis and strictures, therapy is aimed at eliminating acid secretion (i.e. chemical clearance) and preventing reflux of other gastric secretions back into the esophagus (i.e. volume clearance). Proton pump inhibitors (PPIs) are the mainstay of prophylaxis as well as therapy for chemical clearance of acid in patients with esophagitis. PPIs are recognized to be clearly superior to H-2 receptor antagonists (H2RAs). Volume clearance is accomplished by prokinetics. Cisapride, which is only available in compounded formulations, is the preferred gastric prokinetic. Cisapride was sold as a US Food and Drug Administration (FDA)-approved drug for treating gastroparesis in people under the name Propulsid™ but was withdrawn for its association with long-QT syndrome and fatal arrhythmias. There have been no reports of cardiac arrhythmias associated with the use of cisapride in dogs or cats.

GUE is a relatively common problem in dogs (Figure 12.1) but a much less frequent problem in cats. NSAIDs are important

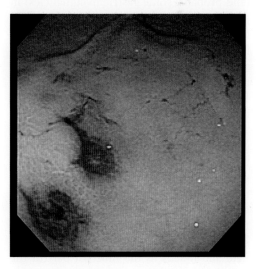

Figure 12.1 An endoscopic view of a cat's gastric mucosa with obvious ulceration of unknown origin.

causes of GUE in both dogs and people. Dogs are very sensitive to NSAIDs (even the so-called Cox-2 selective NSAIDs), and GUE is a common side effect; hence, dogs to be treated with NSAIDs for prolonged times or that are known to have demonstrated previous sensitivity to NSAIDs commonly receive prophylactic therapy. PPIs are generally considered the prophylactic drugs of choice in both people and dogs. Despite the fact that misoprostol is FDA approved for reducing the risk of NSAID-induced gastric ulcers in people, it is infrequently used in veterinary patients because it is more expensive and has more side effects. Some corticosteroids (especially dexamethasone) are notorious for causing GUE in dogs. Relatively little work has been done to determine how to prevent corticosteroid-induced GUE, and what has been published to date has not shown any drug to be an effective preventative. However, it is possible that raising the gastric pH may help stabilize blood clots and help decrease gastric bleeding when GUE develops.

Human beings and dogs/cats are very different regarding *Helicobacter*-induced gastric diseases. People are primarily infected with *H. pylori*, while dogs and cats have non–*H. pylori* helicobacter (NHPH) in their stomachs. *H. pylori* is a major cause of GUE (and probably some gastric malignancies) in people. Current thought is that NHPH can cause gastritis with subsequent vomiting/hyporexia in some dogs and cats, but it almost never causes GUE. Furthermore, unlike the treatment of *H. pylori* in people, PPIs do not augment the treatment of NHPH in dogs or cats.

Horses are also commonly treated for gastric ulcers. The equine stomach is particularly prone to ulcers because part of their gastric lining is composed of squamous epithelial cells rather than the gastric mucosal epithelial lining of other species. Ulceration tends to involve the squamous portion of the stomach, which is not protected by bicarbonate and mucus as the mucosal part of the stomach is. GI ulceration is so common in performance horses (i.e. racing or other strenuous competitive events) during training that there are FDA-approved products labeled specifically for horses. One product is indicated for preventing gastric ulcers in horses and is available over-the-counter (OTC), while the other is indicated for treatment of gastric ulcers in horses and requires a veterinary prescription. Omeprazole is the active ingredient in both products, which are formulated as pastes rather than tablets or capsules for ease of administration to horses. The only difference in the two products is the recommended dose and duration of treatment.

Compared to the syndrome in people, IBD can be confusing in veterinary medicine. First, there is not a universally agreed-upon definition of IBD in the dog or the cat. Most diagnoses have been based upon histology of the intestines, which is unfortunate because seemingly almost every dog and cat that has had its intestines biopsied has been diagnosed with a lymphocytic-plasmacytic inflammation to a greater or lesser extent. Because the intestinal tract is the largest lymphoid organ in the body, a lymphocytic-plasmacytic infiltrate is the expected response of the intestines to almost every chronic insult or irritation. Most chronic enteropathies are ultimately found to be dietary-responsive and/or antibiotic-responsive, and the vast majority of dogs with so-called IBD can be controlled with carefully designed therapeutic trials of exclusion diets (including but not limited to hydrolyzed or limited/novel antigen diets) and/or antibacterial drugs (especially but not exclusively tylosin). Some patients' clinical signs cannot be controlled with such therapy, either because the inflammation is extremely severe or because the owners cannot strictly comply with dietary recommendations or cannot administer the medications (especially to cats). In such patients, anti-inflammatory drugs, usually glucocorticoids but sometimes other immunosuppressive drugs, are administered. Some clinicians have opted to use progressively stronger and stronger anti-inflammatory or immunosuppressive drugs instead of work with clients to ensure good dietary/antibacterial therapeutic trials. This tendency has caused some severe iatrogenic illness, especially from the catabolic effects of glucocorticoids. The importance of dietary and antibacterial therapy cannot be overstated for most of these patients. The pharmacist can play an important role in educating pet owners about the importance of eliminating extraneous treats and even flavored/chewable drug products from the controlled diets of dogs or cats being treated for IBD. Introduction of even a seemingly trivial quantity of beef or chicken protein, for example, can exacerbate signs of IBD.

Protein-losing enteropathies (PLEs) due to primary GI disease are generally uncommon in human beings, but they are reasonably common in dogs. Lymphangiectasia (Figure 12.2) in particular is well documented in dogs. There are nuances in distinguishing primary from secondary lymphangiectasia that are potentially important from a therapeutic standpoint. Some dog breeds have an obvious predilection for primary lymphangiectasia (e.g. Yorkshire Terrier). Ultra-low-fat diets are the cornerstone of therapy for primary lymphangiectasia, but formation of lipogranulomas in the intestinal wall typically necessitates the use of anti-inflammatory and/or immunosuppressive drug therapy.

Exocrine pancreatic insufficiency (EPI) in dogs is either breed associated (e.g. pancreatic acinar atrophy in German Shepherds) or secondary to chronic pancreatitis. Approximately 15% of affected dogs never respond well to pancreatic enzyme supplementation. This makes it important to have a definitive diagnosis instead of attempting a therapeutic trial. A readily available assay for species-specific trypsin-like immunoreactivity is often diagnostic for EPI. Many dogs that have EPI but do not respond to a therapeutic trial end up undergoing a variety of costly and sometimes invasive diagnostic procedures, including exploratory laparotomy. Complicating the matter is the fact that not all pancreatic enzyme supplements are of equal efficacy. Powders tend to have better efficacy than tablets or capsules. Although a specially formulated diet is not required, a high-quality (premium) diet is likely to be more easily digested than low-cost, store-brand-type foods. Cats are affected less frequently than dogs.

Lymphoma of the GI tract, while important in dogs, is extremely important in cats. Large-cell lymphoma (i.e. lymphoblastic or prolymphocytic lymphoma) is relatively easy to diagnose but hard to effectively treat in both dogs and cats. Several chemotherapy protocols have been proposed, but none are consistently effective in achieving long-term remissions in either species. In contrast, feline small-cell lymphoma of the GI tract is currently a source of confusion and controversy. Diagnosis of feline small-cell lymphoma is not straightforward and often requires advanced techniques such as polymerase chain reaction (PCR) testing of clonality (PCR of antigen receptor rearrangement [PARR]). Anecdotally, current therapy for feline small-cell lymphoma, rightly or wrongly, is usually very similar to that prescribed for severe lymphocytic and plasmacytic enteritis (e.g. prednisolone and

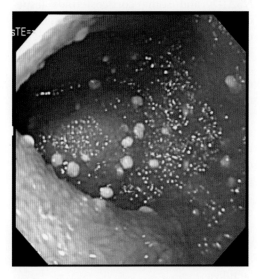

Figure 12.2 An endoscopic view of the duodenal mucosa of a French Bulldog with obvious lymphangiectasia (i.e. the large white "bumps" are dilated lacteals filled with chyle).

chlorambucil). However, this may change as more data are accumulated.

Histiocytic ulcerative colitis is somewhat similar to Whipple's disease in people. In dogs, it is most commonly found in Boxer dogs and French Bulldogs, with other breeds being rarely affected. A few years ago, it was reliably cured with a prolonged course of enrofloxacin; however, the adherent-invasive *Escherichia coli* responsible for histiocytic colitis has become increasingly more resistant to the fluoroquinolones, to the point that it is now a requirement to culture colonic mucosa (not feces) to find an antibiotic to which the bacteria are sensitive.

Chronic hepatitis of dogs is typically idiopathic but may also be due to copper intoxication and sometimes from iatrogenic drug administration. Chronic hepatitis in people is primarily due to viral hepatitis or alcohol. It is important to look for a cause before pronouncing a patient to have idiopathic disease and then treating with anti-inflammatory/immunosuppressive therapy, considering the fact that these drugs can cause serious adverse reactions, including liver insults. Copper-associated chronic hepatitis is particularly important to recognize because it may be resolved by copper chelation therapy such as d-penicillamine. Various hepatosupportive therapies are available. While therapy solely with hepatosupportive drugs seldom resolves primary hepatic diseases of dogs and cats, these drugs can be very beneficial when combined with therapy directed against the primary disease. Ursodeoxycholic acid (i.e. ursodiol) is a hydrophilic bile acid that helps patients through several mechanisms, including helping to displace hydrophobic bile acids (e.g. lithocholic acid) from the hepatocyte membrane. S-adenosyl-L-methionine (SAMe) is a cysteine donor that enhances intracellular glutathione production, thus acting as an antioxidant. Silybin is another antioxidant that helps to protect the hepatocyte membrane.

Gall bladder diseases of dogs have become increasingly recognized over the last 10–15 years and can be a major cause of morbidity and mortality. Gall bladder mucoceles in people are primarily due to biliary outflow obstruction (usually associated with a gallstone). In dogs, the cause is probably multifactorial, but outflow obstruction is not considered an important cause. In dogs, there are definite associations with select breeds (i.e. Shetland Sheepdogs and Schnauzers) and endocrinopathies (i.e. hyperadrenocorticism and hypothyroidism). Diagnosis of early, incipient mucoceles often allows medical resolution (ursodiol with or without the nutritional supplement SAMe), while mature mucoceles require surgery.

12.2.1 Drug-Induced GI, Hepatic, and Pancreatic Disease

Drug-induced esophagitis with subsequent cicatrix causing a benign stricture is well recognized in cats receiving doxycycline therapy. Cats in particular are renowned for retaining tablets or capsules in the esophagus unless their administration is followed by a syringeful of water, broth, or food. As mentioned in this chapter, dogs are particularly sensitive to the ulcerogenic potential of NSAIDs and some corticosteroids (especially dexamethasone). Co-administration of corticosteroids with NSAIDs is a recipe for severe GI ulceration in dogs and is generally contraindicated. Antibiotic-associated diarrhea occurs in dogs and cats, but it tends to be of minimal severity. It is probably due to disruption of the GI microbiome, but some drugs (e.g. erythromycin) have prokinetic effects that can cause vomiting and diarrhea. *Clostridium difficile*–associated pseudomembranous colitis is closely associated with clindamycin therapy in people and horses, but the disease is essentially undescribed in dogs and cats. Constipation may occur from drugs like sucralfate, and diarrhea may result from excessive use of lactulose.

While some drugs have been suspected to cause pancreatitis, azathioprine is definitely recognized as a potential cause.

Several drugs are well recognized for their marked hepatotoxic potential (i.e. phenobarbital, sulfa drugs, Cox-2 selective NSAIDs, lomustine, and acetaminophen), and many others are recognized for their occasional involvement with hepatic damage (e.g. diazepam in cats, doxycycline, clindamycin, itraconazole, amiodarone, azathioprine, rifampin, and others). However, almost all drugs have been reported to cause hepatotoxicity, even if it is only very, very rarely.

12.3 Diagnostic Testing

Definitive diagnosis of canine and feline GI diseases may be sufficiently limited by owner finances, such that treatment based on the most likely cause may be initiated without the veterinarian ever having established a true diagnosis. Ideally, however, diagnostic testing might include some of the following procedures:

- Abdominal palpation/digital rectal examination
- Thoracic and/or abdominal radiography (plain and/or contrast-enhanced)
- Thoracic and/or abdominal fluoroscopy
- Abdominal ultrasound
- Complete blood count (helpful for some acute disorders)
- Serum biochemical profile (especially looking for evidence of PLE [hypoalbuminemia and hypocholesterolemia] or increased alanine aminotransferase [ALT])
- Serum bile acids (looking for otherwise occult hepatic disease)
- Serum cortisol (hypoadrenocorticism may closely mimic primary GI disease)
- Fecal flotation/direct smear (important because parasites may be the primary disease or may be contributing to signs from other diseases)
- Serum trypsin-like immunoreactivity (TLI)
- Fecal parvovirus enzyme-linked immunosorbent assay (ELISA)
- Fecal ELISA for giardia

- Serum cobalamin and folate concentrations
- Endoscopic visualization/biopsy of upper and lower GI tract
- Laparoscopic hepatic biopsy
- Capsule endoscopy of the GI

12.4 Pharmacological Treatment of Common Diseases

Pharmacotherapy of patients with esophageal disorders that are regurgitating consists primarily of treating either (i) dogs with megaesophagus caused by localized myasthenia gravis, or (ii) dogs or cats with erosive esophagitis. Treatment of localized myasthenia causing megaesophagus is aimed at symptomatically strengthening esophageal smooth muscle with cholinergic drugs (specifically, pyridostigmine) and occasionally co-administering immunosuppressives to decrease antibody titers to the acetylcholine receptor (but not glucocorticoids). Treatment of esophagitis primarily consists of suppressing gastric acid secretion (PPIs) and increasing gastric emptying to minimize GER (prokinetics). Esophageal pain relief is effected with sucralfate suspensions and/or oral, viscous lidocaine, which is available as an OTC preparation.

12.4.1 Cholinergic Drugs Most Likely to Be Prescribed

Pyridostigmine: 0.5–3 mg/kg PO (orally) every 8–12 hours. There is some danger of overdosage causing a cholinergic crisis; therefore, start at the low end of the dose, and gradually increase it. Do not use neostigmine or physostigmine because there is greater risk of cholinergic crisis with these drugs.

12.4.2 Acid Suppression Drugs Most Likely to Be Prescribed

Omeprazole: 1 mg/kg PO every 12 hours; twice-daily administration is important. Co-administration of H2RA is not helpful and may decrease omeprazole's efficacy. While it requires two to five days for omeprazole to achieve maximum efficacy, the acid suppression occurring on the first day of therapy is generally superior to that achieved with high-dose H2RA. There is minimal evidence of the reported drug-related adverse effects noted in people occurring in dogs and cats.

Pantoprazole: 1 mg/kg intravenously (IV) every 12–24 hours. Generally administered when a near-immediate effect is needed and/or when oral administration of omeprazole is inappropriate.

Famotidine: 0.2–0.5 mg/kg PO every 12 hours. Clearly inferior to PPIs for acid suppression and should not be used for treating esophagitis. Tachyphylaxis occurs.

12.4.3 Prokinetic Drugs Most Likely to Be Prescribed

Cisapride: 0.1–0.5 mg/kg PO every 8–12 hours. The drug must be obtained from a veterinary compounding pharmacy. It is currently the most effective prokinetic in veterinary medicine for enhancing gastric, small-intestinal, and large-intestinal motility. However, cisapride does not stimulate motility in the canine esophagus. There is minimal evidence of adverse drug effects on the canine heart, in contrast to people.

Metoclopramide: 0.25–0.5 mg/kg IV every 6–8 hours or 1 mg/kg/hour as constant rate infusion (CRI). This drug primarily enhances gastric emptying of liquids.

Erythromycin: 0.5–1.0 mg/kg PO or IV every 8–12 hours. Primarily effective in the stomach and upper duodenum, this is probably a more effective prokinetic in dogs than metoclopramide.

Ranitidine: 2 mg/kg PO or IV every 8 hours. Prokinetic effects are inconsistent between patients, but some patients respond very well. Nizatidine also has some prokinetic activity, but the other H2RAs do not.

12.4.4 Antiemetics Most Likely to Be Prescribed

Pharmacotherapy of acutely vomiting patients primarily consists of parenteral administration of fluids, if needed. If the vomiting is causing excessive loss of fluids/electrolytes or is causing severe nausea (or if the owners just want it stopped now), then antiemetic drugs are indicated. Maropitant, which is approved for use in dogs and cats, is a very effective antiemetic. Ondansetron, a drug approved for use in people, is typically the second choice. If these are ineffective, using metoclopramide as an add-on is usually effective. PPIs are not anti-emetics. They may have some anti-dyspeptic effects, but maropitant is probably superior to a PPI in this regard.

Chronically vomiting patients by definition are not generally going to resolve their disease with symptomatic antiemetic drugs. They need to be diagnosed and the underlying disease resolved.

Maropitant: 1 mg/kg subcutaneously (SC) every 24 hours; 2 mg/kg PO every 24 hours. Parenteral administration is more effective than PO but is painful. The drug is so effective that it will often stop vomiting even if caused by foreign body obstruction, which can result in GI perforation; therefore, it is important to eliminate such problems before starting therapy. It also has visceral analgesic effects.

Ondansetron: 0.25–0.5 mg/kg IV every 8–12 hours. Because there is first-pass metabolism, parenteral administration is superior to oral administration. In most patients, it is not as effective as maropitant. The drug has been noted to cause sedation in dogs with the MDR1 mutation.

Metoclopramide: 0.25–0.5 mg/kg IV every 6–8 hours or 1 mg/kg/hour as CRI. This is a relatively weak antiemetic and is especially ineffective in cats. Metoclopramide is best used as an "add-on" to maropitant or ondansetron when they are ineffective by themselves. Administering metoclopramide as a CRI is typically more effective than administering it as an intermittent bolus. Excessive administration of metoclopramide may cause extrapyramidal signs (i.e. the dog will act like it has an overdose of methamphetamine).

12.4.5 Gastroprotectant Drugs Most Likely to Be Prescribed

GUE is best treated by eliminating the underlying cause, whenever that is possible. Most patients with GUE will heal within two to four days once the cause is removed, unless the ulcer is so deep or necrotic that the gastric mucosal epithelium can no longer establish itself over the ulcer base. If the cause cannot be eliminated or if it is important to resolve the ulceration as quickly as possible, then pharmacotherapy is indicated.

Omeprazole: 1 mg/kg PO every 12 hours; twice-daily administration is important. While it requires two to five days for omeprazole to achieve maximum efficacy, the acid suppression occurring on the first day of therapy is generally superior to that achieved with high-dose H2RA. Co-administration of H2RA is not helpful and may decrease omeprazole's efficacy. Co-administration with other gastroprotectants is not recommended except perhaps in the case of an acute overdose of an NSAID (in which case misoprostol might be a reasonable add-on).

Pantoprazole: 1 mg/kg IV every 12–24 hours. Generally administered when a near-immediate effect is needed and/or when oral administration of omeprazole is inappropriate.

Sucralfate: 0.5–1 g PO every 8–24 hours. The suspension tends to be more effective than the tablet. Co-administration with other drugs may delay their absorption. Sucralfate tends to cause constipation, especially if the patient is dehydrated.

Famotidine: 0.2–0.5 mg/kg PO every 12 hours. This is the most potent of the H2RAs, but it is clearly inferior to all PPIs in suppressing gastric acid secretion. Tachyphylaxis is documented to occur in dogs within 5–15 days.

Misoprostol: 2–5 microgram/kg PO every 12 hours. A prostaglandin E analogue, it was specifically developed as a prophylaxis for NSAID-induced ulceration; however, it can be used to treat GUE. Multiple side effects lessen its desirability as a therapeutic modality. PPIs tend to be as effective as misoprostol in preventing NSAID-induced GUE.

12.4.6 Antiparasite Drugs Most Likely to Be Prescribed (See Also Chapter 7)

Pyrantel pamoate: 5 mg/kg PO, once. Pyrantel pamoate is an effective and exceedingly safe anthelmintic for roundworms and hookworms, even in lactating and very young animals.

Fenbendazole: 50 mg/kg PO every 24 hours for three to five days. Fenbendazole is a very effective and safe anthelmintic for hookworms, roundworms, and whipworms, even in young dogs. It is used off-label in cats and is effective for treating giardia.

Praziquantel: 5 mg/kg PO once for dogs >6.8 kg; 7.5 mg/kg PO once for dogs <6.8 kg. Praziquantel is very effective against all cestodes as well as *Schistosoma* spp. It is a relatively safe drug (even in pregnant animals), but avoid using in kittens and puppies younger than six weeks or four weeks of age, respectively.

Sulfadimethoxine: 55 mg/kg PO once (loading dose), followed by 27.5 mg/kg PO every 12 hours. Sulfa drugs have a plethora of side effects; therefore, the patient should be monitored during therapy. Sulfadimethoxine is a long-acting sulfonamide that is excreted unchanged in the urine, making it somewhat safer than most other sulfonamides. There are preparations of sulfadimethoxine combined with ormetoprim that are usually more effective than the sulfa drug administered by itself.

Metronidazole: 15 mg/kg PO every 12 hours for 8 days. Metronidazole is used off-label in dogs and cats. Must watch for drug toxicity manifested by central vestibular signs. No evidence of carcinogenesis in dogs or cats. Tablets are very distasteful to cats; therefore, reformulating as a flavored suspension is often tried.

Ronidazole: 30 mg/kg PO every 24 hours for 2 weeks (cats). Ronidazole is the best treatment for feline *Tritrichomonas* spp., and it is effective against giardia. It is not available for therapeutic use; it must be obtained from a veterinary compounding pharmacy.

12.4.7 Antidiarrheal Drugs Most Likely to Be Prescribed

Acute diarrhea is typically best treated with a multimodal approach of eliminating any parasites (even if they are not causing the diarrhea outright, their presence may contribute to the decompensation of the GI tract), feeding an easily digested diet, and stopping vomiting if it is excessive. Antidiarrheal drugs such as loperamide are seldom needed or administered. Despite their frequent use, antibiotics are almost never needed unless the patient has parvoviral enteritis and is at risk for septicemia. Probiotics have been shown to shorten the duration of acute diarrheas in puppies and kittens.

Loperamide: 0.12 mg/kg PO every 12 hours in dogs. Available OTC, it can cause constipation. Dogs lacking P-glycoprotein due to MDR mutation are at increased risk for toxicity.

Bismuth subsalicylate: 1–3 ml/kg every 24 hours (divided into two to three doses/day). Available OTC, bismuth subsalicylate is a very effective antidiarrheal drug. Most dogs and essentially all cats detest the taste and end up putting as much on the carpet as they swallow. The NSAID moiety is absorbed and can result in toxicity (cats) or adverse drug interactions (dogs).

Chronic diarrheas in dogs and cats are most commonly due to parasites, diet, and/or bacteria.

12.4.8 Pancreatic Enzyme Supplements Most Likely to Be Prescribed

Viokase: 1–2 tsp./meal, PO. There are numerous products with various potencies. Some experimentation may be needed to find an effective product. Viokase tends to be as effective as, or more effective than, other products. There is no good evidence that preincubation of the enzymes with food makes a major difference in efficacy. Excessive administration may produce a reversible stomatitis. Administration of pancreatic enzyme supplements does not alter TLI test results. Some dogs with chronic small-bowel diarrhea that is not due to EPI have some degree of response to pancreatic enzyme replacement.

12.4.9 Antibacterial Drugs Most Likely to Be Prescribed

Tylosin: 10–20 mg/kg PO daily. Tylosin is FDA approved for use in turkeys and pigs and is used off-label in dogs and cats. There have been multiple publications documenting this drug's effectiveness in canine chronic or recurrent diarrheas. It is typically sprinkled on the food, but it tends to have a bitter taste; therefore, some animals will only accept it if it is compounded into capsules and administered by hand.

Metronidazole: 15 mg/kg PO daily. Metronidazole is particularly unpalatable to cats, but compounding it into a flavored suspension usually makes it possible for owners to administer the drug. Care must be taken to avoid overdosing this drug, as it has severe adverse central nervous system (CNS) effects (i.e. central vestibular effects).

12.4.10 Anti-Inflammatory/Immunosuppressive Drugs Most Likely to Be Prescribed

Prednisolone: 1.1–2.2 mg/kg PO daily. Be sure to use prednisolone and not prednisone (the latter has much lower bioavailability than prednisolone). Cats tend to have fewer adverse effects than dogs.

Budesonide: 0.125 mg/kg PO every 8–24 hours. Primarily metabolized by first-pass metabolism in the liver, the main indication for this drug is that the patient is known to respond to prednisolone but cannot tolerate its systemic side effects (e.g. a male diabetic cat that has IBD but cannot tolerate the insulin resistance occurring due to the glucocorticoid).

Chlorambucil: 4–6 m/M^2 PO every 24 hours for first 7–21 days, then slowly decrease. This drug is gradually replacing azathioprine for use in canine chronic enteropathies; it appears to be more effective with fewer side effects.

Azathioprine: 2 mg/kg PO every 24 hours for 5–7 days, then every 48 hours. This drug should not be used in cats. It can cause severe hepatitis, bone marrow suppression, and pancreatitis.

Cyclosporine: 2–6 mg/kg PO every 12 hours. A very effective drug for some chronic canine enteropathies. Expense often limits its usefulness. There is a marked variation in the bioavailability of different brands and different formulations of cyclosporine.

Sulfasalazine: 10–30 mg/kg PO every 8–12 hours. The sulfa drug portion may be absorbed and cause side effects. Do not use with azathioprine.

Mesalamine: 5–10 mg/kg PO every 8–12 hours. Not approved for use in dogs, it is sometimes used off-label in an effort to avoid side effects due to the sulfa drug portion of sulfasalazine.

12.4.11 Osmotic Laxative Drugs Most Likely to Be Prescribed

Constipation, especially in dogs, is often due to issues that can be resolved (e.g. diet, prostatomegaly, and rectal/anal pain). In contrast to dogs, cats sometimes develop idiopathic megacolon, which requires chronic therapy. The typical laxatives used by people (e.g. phenophathelines and bisacodyl) are not useful in this disorder. Rather, osmotic laxatives (e.g. lactulose) and colonic prokinetics are the mainstay of managing megacolon that cannot be managed with diet alone.

Dramatic difference

Commercially available enemas formulated for people (even human infants) can be deadly in cats and small dogs. Fleet™ and other brands that contain electrolytes such as sodium and phosphorous (often in the form of phosphate) can create severe electrolyte imbalances, dehydration, and hypotension.

Lactulose: 1 ml/4.5 kg PO every 8 hours or 15 ml/cat/day. Care must be taken to not overdose dogs lest a severe osmotic catharsis causes hypernatremic dehydration. Cats are hard to overdose, and relatively large doses are often needed to soften feline feces. Most cats detest the taste of lactulose.

12.4.12 Hepatoprotective Drugs Most Likely to Be Prescribed

Ursodeoxycholic acid: 15 mg/kg PO daily. A hydrophilic bile acid with numerous beneficial effects, it is used in almost all canine and feline hepatic diseases. It is very safe and has also been used to try to dissolve incipient gall bladder mucoceles.

12.5 Adverse Drug Effects in Veterinary Species

12.5.1 Pyridostigmine

Overdoses can lead to a cholinergic crisis with GI signs, weakness, bradycardia, and bronchoconstriction.

12.5.2 Metronidazole

Metronidazole can cause severe, dose-dependent central vestibular signs in dogs and cats. If the drug is withdrawn quickly after the onset of adverse signs, the signs typically abate. Metronidazole is a potential carcinogen in people, but dogs and cats do not live long enough to see such effects. There is no evidence of metronidazole-induced malignancy in dogs or cats.

12.5.3 Metoclopramide

Metoclopramide can cause behavioral changes/excitation when large doses are administered IV or if the patient is unable to excrete the drug through the kidneys.

12.5.4 Loperamide

Relatively safe, except in dogs with the MDR1 mutation and diminished P-glycoprotein. In such animals, loperamide may cause severe sedation.

12.5.5 Sulfasalazine, Mesalamine, and Olsalazine

Sulfasalazine has a sulfa drug moiety and can cause any of the numerous side effects attributed to sulfa drugs. All of these drugs have been anecdotally connected to keratoconjunctivitis sicca in dogs.

12.5.6 Misoprostol

Misoprostol is a prostaglandin E analogue. Its most important side effect is causing abortions in pregnant females (animals and people). It can also cause vomiting, diarrhea, and/or abdominal discomfort.

12.5.7 Azathioprine

Some animals do not have the enzymes necessary to metabolize azathioprine. These are at increased risk for myelosuppression, hepatitis/hepatic failure, and pancreatitis. Cats are especially susceptible; azathioprine should not be used in this species.

12.5.8 Cyclosporine

It is hard to anticipate the blood levels after oral administration of cyclosporine. Therefore, it is possible that the blood levels will be higher than anticipated. The most common side effect is severe hyporexia. However, very high blood levels can produce immunosuppression, and opportunistic infections (especially fungal) are reported in dogs. Hepatic and renal toxicity common in people are very uncommon in dogs and cats. Gingival hyperplasia is reported. The drug should not be administered to pregnant females. There are numerous important drug interactions, and one should always check before administering cyclosporine to a patient already receiving other drugs.

12.5.9 Bismuth Subsalicylate

The salicylate moiety is absorbed; therefore, all the side effects of aspirin are possible.

12.5.10 Corticosteroids

Adverse effects that are somewhat canine-specific include polyuria and polydipsia, which lead to house soiling so owners should be forewarned; panting; and a higher risk for GI ulceration, particularly with dexamethasone. Dogs receiving corticosteroids should not concurrently be given NSAIDs, as this greatly enhances the risk of severe GI ulceration. Cats are very susceptible to the diabetogenic effects of corticosteroids, particularly dexamethasone, so owners should be counseled to monitor for signs of diabetes (e.g. polyuria, polydipsia, weight loss despite good appetite, and lethargy) and seek veterinary care should they occur.

12.6 Nutritional Supplements for Veterinary Gastrointestinal Diseases

Probiotics include a very large number of commercially available products that range from almost useless to those of excellent quality. When comparing different probiotic formulations, an important factor is the amount of bacteria to be administered. Large numbers of live bacteria should be administered with each dose (e.g. approximately 1 000 000 000/treatment). Generally, the clinician should seek to administer several different species of bacteria and preferably different strains of the same bacteria. Probiotics have been demonstrated to shorten the duration of acute diarrheas in dogs and cats.

Several nutritional supplements are touted as "hepatoprotectants," including SAMe and silymarin. Both compounds are antioxidants. SAMe is a methyl donor and is administered to increase intracellular glutathione levels. Whether or not this actually results in hepatoprotection has not been consistently demonstrated. For example, SAMe treatment was no different than placebo in blunting liver enzyme elevation in dogs treated with prednisolone (Center et al. 2005). However, it has minor, generally unimportant side effects. It is important to note that it has extremely low oral bioavailability and must be administered to a

Table 12.1 Drugs that are FDA approved for gastrointestinal disease in a veterinary species but are not available in a human formulation.

Brand name	Active ingredient(s)	Drug class	Rationale/notes
Cerenia (Zoetis)	Maropitant	Neurokinin-1 receptor antagonist (antiemetic)	FDA approved for dogs and cats
Many	Tylosin	Macrolide antibiotic	FDA approved for use in chickens, turkeys, swine, and honeybees
Gastrogard and Ulcergard (Merial)	Omeprazole	Proton pump inhibitor	Formulated as a buffered paste for administration to horses

fasting animal in order to achieve even low systemic concentrations. Many veterinarians fail to counsel pet owners on appropriate dosing of this compound, so it is likely that many veterinary patients do not benefit whatsoever from SAMe products.

Silymarin is considered an antioxidant and free-radical scavenger that is administered to help protect the hepatocyte membrane. Silymarin is also known as milk thistle. Similar to SAMe, there are no peer-reviewed, placebo-controlled clinical trials to support these claims, but silymarin is very unlikely to cause harm. A product that combines SAMe and silymarin, however, has been demonstrated to have some benefit in decreasing the severity of lomustine-induced hepatotoxicity in tumor-bearing dogs based on liver enzyme activity (Skorupski et al. 2011).

Practiced but not proven
Nutritional supplements that are touted as "hepatoprotectants" are widely used in veterinary medicine. Essentially, any dog or cat that may have liver disease of any kind is often given SAMe and/or silymarin. Although these products are not likely to cause harm, it is reasonable to fully disclose to the pet owner that the efficacy of these products for all liver diseases has not yet been demonstrated. The philosophy tends to be "It might help and it won't hurt."

12.7 FDA-Approved Veterinary Drug Products with No Human Drug Equivalent

See Table 12.1.

Abbreviations

AHDS	Acute hemorrhagic diarrheal syndrome
CRI	Constant rate infusion
GI	Gastrointestinal
GUE	Gastric ulceration/erosion
H2RA	Histamine-2 receptor antagonist
IBD	Inflammatory bowel disease
IBS	Irritable bowel syndrome
LES	Lower esophageal sphincter
NHPH	Non–*Helicobacter pylori* helicobacter
NSAID	Nonsteroidal anti-inflammatory drug
OTC	Over-the-counter
PARR	PCR of antigen receptor rearrangement
PLE	Protein-losing enteropathy
PPI	Proton pump inhibitor
PO	Per os ("by mouth," or orally)
TLI	Trypsin-like immunoreactivity

Bibliography

Center, S.A., Warner, K.L., McCabe, J. et al. (2005). Evaluation of the influence of S-adenosylmethionine on systemic and hepatic effects of prednisolone in dogs. *Am. J. Vet. Res.* 66 (2): 330–341.

Craven, M., Mansfield, C.S., and Simpson, K.W. (2011). Granulomatous colitis of boxer dogs. *Vet. Clin. North Am.* 41: 433–445.

Dandrieux, J.R.S., Noble, P.J.M., Scase, T.J. et al. (2013). Comparison of a chlorambucil-prednisolone combination with an azathioprine-prednisolone combination for treatment of chronic enteropathy with concurrent protein-losing enteropathy in dogs: 27 cases (2007–2010). *J. Am. Vet. Med. Assoc.* 242: 1705–1714.

Dye, T.L., Diehl, K.J., Wheeler, S.L. et al. (2013). Randomized, controlled trial of budesonide and prednisone for the treatment of idiopathic inflammatory bowel disease in dogs. *J. Vet. Intern. Med.* 27: 1385–1391.

Favarato, E.S., Souza, M.V., Costa, P.R.S. et al. (2012). Evaluation of metoclopramide and ranitidine on the prevention of gastroesophageal reflux episodes in anesthetized dogs. *Res. Vet. Sci.* 93: 466–467.

Fiechter, R., Deplazes, P., and Schnyder, M. (2012). Control of Giardia infections with ronidazole and intensive hygiene management in a dog kennel. *Vet. Parasitol.* 187: 93–98.

Foy, D.S., Trepanier, L.A., and Shelton, G.D. (2011). Cholinergic crisis after neostigmine administration in a dog with acquired focal myasthenia gravis. *J. Vet. Emerg. Crit. Care* 21: 547–551.

Jenkins, E.K., Lee-Fowler, T.M., Angle, T.C. et al. (2016). Effects of oral administration of metronidazole and doxycycline on olfactory capabilities of explosives detection dogs. *Am. J. Vet. Res.* 77: 906–912.

Kempf, J., Lewis, F., Reusch, C.E. et al. (2014). High-resolution manometric evaluation of the effects of cisapride and metoclopramide hydrochloride administered orally on lower esophageal sphincter pressure in awake dogs. *Am. J. Vet. Res.* 75: 361–366.

Kilpinen, S., Spillmann, T., and Westermarck, E. (2014). Efficacy of two low-dose oral tylosin regimens in controlling the relapse of diarrhea in dogs with tylosin-responsive diarrhea: a prospective, single-blinded, two-arm parallel, clinical field trial. *Acta Vet. Scand.* 56: 43. doi:10.1186/s13028-014-0043-5.

Kilpinen, S., Spillmann, T., Syrja, P. et al. (2011). Effect of tylosin on dogs with suspected tylosin-responsive diarrhea: a placebo-controlled, randomized, double-blinded, prospective clinical trial. *Acta Vet. Scand.* 53: 26. doi:10.1186/1751-0147-53-26.

KuKanich, K. and KuKanich, B. (2015). The effect of sucralfate tablets vs. suspension on oral doxycycline absorption in dogs. *J. Vet. Pharmacol. Ther.* 38: 169–173.

Leonard, E.K., Pearl, D.L., Finley, R.L. et al. (2011). Evaluation of pet-related management factors and the risk of *Salmonella* spp. carriage in pet dogs from volunteer households in Ontario (2005–2006). *Zoonoses Public Health* 58: 140–149.

Parkinson, S., Tolbert, K., Messenger, K. et al. (2015). Evaluation of the effect of orally administered acid suppressants on intragastric pH in cats. *J. Vet. Intern. Med.* 29: 104–112.

Procter, T.D., Pearl, D.L., Finley, R.L. et al. (2014). A cross-sectional study examining *Campylobacter* and other zoonotic enteric pathogens in dogs that frequent dog parks in three cities in South-Western Ontario and risk factors for shedding *Campylobacter* spp. *Zoonosis Public Health* 61: 208–218.

Rossi, G., Pengo, G., Caldin, M. et al. (2014). Comparison of microbiological, histological, and Immunomodulatory parameters in response to treatment with either combination therapy with prednisone and metronidazole or probiotic VSL#3 strains in dogs with idiopathic inflammatory bowel disease. *PLoS One* 9 (4): e94699.

Sedlacek, H.S., Ramsey, D.S., Boucher, J.F. et al. (2008). Comparative efficacy of maropitant and selected drugs in preventing emesis induced by centrally or peripherally acting emetogens in dogs. *J. Vet. Pharmacol. Ther.* 31: 533–537.

Sekis, I., Ramstead, K., Rishniw, M. et al. (2009). Single-dose pharmacokinetics and genotoxicity of metronidazole in cats. *J. Feline Med. Surg.* 11: 60–68.

Skorupski, K.A., Hammond, G.M., Irish, A.M. et al. (2011). Prospective randomized clinical trial assessing the efficacy of denamarin for prevention of CCNU-induced hepatopathy in tumor-bearing dogs. *J. Vet. Intern. Med.* 25: 838–835.

Tolbert, M.K., Odunayo, A., Howell, R.S. et al. (2015). Efficacy of intravenous administration of combined acid suppressants in healthy dogs. *J. Vet. Intern. Med.* 29: 556–560.

Tolbert, M.K., Graham, A., Odunayo, A. et al. (2017). Repeated famotidine administration results in a diminished effect on intragastric pH in dogs. *J. Vet. Intern. Med.* 31: 117–123.

Tolbert, K., Bissett, S., King, A. et al. (2011). Efficacy of oral famotidine and 2 omeprazole formulations for the control of intragastric pH in dogs. *J. Vet. Intern. Med.* 25: 47–54.

Ullal, T.V., Kass, P.H., Conklin, J.L. et al. (2016). High-resolution manometric evaluation of the effects of cisapride on the esophagus during administration of solid and liquid boluses in awake healthy dogs. *Am. J. Vet. Res.* 77: 817–826.

Wallisch, K. and Trepanier, L.A. (2015). Incidence, timing, and risk factors of azathioprine hepatotoxicosis in dogs. *J. Vet. Intern. Med.* 29: 513–518.

13

Pharmacotherapy of Renal and Lower Urinary Tract Disease

Joe Bartges

Department of Small Animal Medicine and Surgery, College of Veterinary Medicine, University of Georgia, Athens, GA, USA

Key Points

- Renal disease occurs commonly in dogs and cats, and the etiology, pathophysiology, and treatment share some similarities with human renal disease.
- Renal replacement therapy (i.e. dialysis, hemofiltration, etc.) is often performed in human patients with acute kidney injury (AKI) for removal of potential nephrotoxins and to provide time for renal recovery;

- unfortunately, this is not widely available for veterinary patients.
- Nonsteroidal anti-inflammatory drugs (NSAIDs) are important causes of drug-induced renal injury in both human and veterinary patients, but cyclosporine is an important cause of drug-induced renal injury only for human patients.

Part I Renal Disease

13.1 Comparative Aspects of Renal Disease

Dogs and cats are affected with renal disease, of which many, but not all, are analogous to those in human beings. There are several pathophysiological processes that result in renal disease and, using the DAMNIT scheme, these are: degenerative (e.g. chronic tubulointerstitial disease), anatomic (e.g. unilateral renal agenesis), metabolic (e.g. hepatorenal syndrome), neoplastic (e.g. lymphoma), infectious (e.g. bacterial pyelonephritis)/inflammatory (e.g. non-immune-mediated nephritis)/immune-mediated (e.g. immune-mediated glomerulonephritis), and toxic

(e.g. ethylene glycol)/traumatic (e.g. renal fracture due to trauma). Some of these occur more commonly in dogs than in cats, and vice versa (e.g. renal lymphoma occurs more commonly in cats than in dogs, and immune-medicated glomerulonephritis occurs more commonly in dogs than in cats). Some have an age predilection (e.g. cancer occurs more commonly in older dogs and cats) (Polzin 2011; Bartges 2012; Brown et al. 2016). Lastly, some result in acute decompensation of renal function (acute kidney injury [AKI]), while others are associated with chronic kidney disease (CKD). Occasionally, an owner may not notice subtle signs of renal disease, and by the time the animal is examined by a veterinarian, the disease has progressed to the chronic stage. This "acute-on-chronic" situation may

Pharmacotherapeutics for Veterinary Dispensing, First Edition. Edited by Katrina L. Mealey.
© 2019 John Wiley & Sons, Inc. Published 2019 by John Wiley & Sons, Inc.

make the pet owner feel frustrated, perhaps even guilty, for not identifying the problem earlier. CKD is considered the most common renal disease occurring in dogs and cats. Usually, the cause(s) is/are not known. Diabetic nephropathy, a common cause of CKD in human beings, does not seem to occur in diabetic dogs or cats. Glomerulonephropathy occurs in dogs but is rare in cats. Approximately 50% of canine cases are immune-mediated in nature, either primary or secondary to another condition, and 50% are non-immune-mediated in nature (Table 13.1). Nephroureterolithiasis ("kidney stones") occurs in dogs and cats; however, it is not a common cause of renal disease, as approximately 98% of uroliths in dogs and cats occur in the lower urinary tract.

Table 13.1 Causes of glomerulonephropathy in dogs.

Familial

Doberman Pinscher, Samoyeds (X-linked dominant), Bull Terrier (autosomal dominant), Soft-Coated Wheaton Terrier, Greyhound, Burmese Mountain Dog, Rottweiler, English Cocker Spaniel (autosomal dominant), Norwegian Elkhound, Brittany Spaniel (autosomal dominant): Deficiency of C3 results in recurrent bacterial urinary tract infections and membranoproliferative glomerulonephritis

Neoplastic

Lymphosarcoma, mastocytosis, hemangiosarcoma, adenocarcinoma

Infectious

Bacterial endocarditis, infectious canine hepatitis, brucellosis, dirofilariasis, ehrlichiosis, systemic fungal or bacterial infection, feline infectious peritonitis, feline leukemia virus

Inflammatory

Systemic lupus erythematosus, chronic pancreatitis, chronic pyoderma, chronic otitis externa, polyarthritis

Miscellaneous

Hyperadrenocorticism, chronic glucocorticoid treatment, systemic arterial hypertension, idiopathic

---

13.2 Drug-Induced Renal Disease

The kidneys are susceptible to hypoxia and necrosis from hypoperfusion/hypovolemia due to the fact that approximately 20% of cardiac output circulates through the kidneys. Therefore, drugs that cause hypotension or modulate renal blood flow can be indirectly nephrotoxic. The kidneys are also susceptible to direct drug-induced toxicity because of a high renal metabolic rate. Some medications are inherently nephrotoxic; however, others induce nephrotoxicity associated only with high dosage or concurrent dehydration. There are numerous drugs that have the potential to cause nephrotoxicity in human beings, dogs, and cats (Table 13.2). Some of the well-documented drugs that cause nephrotoxicity in veterinary patients will be discussed further here.

Aminoglycoside antimicrobials may induce AKI, especially when other risk factors such as dehydration, age, and preexisting renal disease are present (Riviere et al. 1981). They demonstrate a hierarchal nephrotoxicity according to the number of cationic groups and ability to be internalized by renal epithelial cells. Neomycin is most nephrotoxic, followed by gentamicin, tobramycin, amikacin, netilimicin, and streptomycin. Concurrent administration of a diuretic increases risk of nephrotoxicity.

Nonsteroidal anti-inflammatory drugs (NSAIDs) are frequently prescribed for dogs, cats, and horses. NSAID-induced AKI can occur in each of these species, but it is more commonly reported in cats and horses than dogs. Dehydration, hypotension, and concurrent administration of other potentially nephrotoxic drugs increase the risk of AKI. Meloxicam, which is US Food and Drug Administration (FDA) approved for use in cats, has a boxed warning on the product's label stating, "Repeated use of meloxicam in cats has been associated with acute renal failure and death. Do not administer additional doses of injectable or oral meloxicam to cats."

Table 13.2 Potential nephrotoxins and mechanisms of nephrotoxicity.

Class of agent	Examples
Antimicrobials	Aminoglycosides (ATN, AIN), aztreonam (AIN), bacitracin (ATN), carbapenems (AIN), cephalosporins (AIN), colistin (ATN), penicillins (AIN), polymixin (ATN), quinolones (AIN), rifampin (AIN), sulfonamides (AIN, Cry), tetracyclines (AIN, Fanconi), vancomycin (AIN, ATN)
Antiprotozoals	Dapsone (AIN), pentamidine (ATN), sulfadiazine (AIN, Cry), thiacetarsamide, trimethoprim–sulfamethoxazole (AIN, Cry)
Antifungals	Amphotericin B (ATN, HD)
Antivirals	Acyclovir (Cry, ATN), foscarnet (Cry, ATN), indivir (Cry), cidofovir (ATN), tenovir (ATN)
Chemotherapeutics	Azathioprine (AIN), cis- or carboplatin (ATN), cytosine arabinoside (AIN), doxorubicin, gemcitabine (Vasc), ifosfamide (ATN), methotrexate (Cry), mitomycin (Vasc), oxaliplatin (ATN), pentostatin (ATN), antivascular endothelial growth factor (bevacizumab and others)
Immunosuppressives	Cyclosporine (HD, ATN, CIN, Vasc), interleukin-2, rapamycin (Vasc), tacrolimus (HD, ATN, CIN, Vasc)
Nonsteroidal anti-inflammatory drugs	All (HD, AIN, GN)
Angiotensin-converting enzyme inhibitors and angiotensin receptor antagonists	All (HD, GN), captopril (AIN)
Diuretics	All (HD), furosemide (AIN), thiazides (AIN), triamterene (Cry), acetazolamide (AIN)
Diagnostic agents	Radiocontract agents (ATN, HD, Osm), gadolinium (high dose), oral sodium phosphate solution
Miscellaneous therapeutics	Acetaminophen (AIN), allopurinol (nephrolithiasis, AIN), carbamazepine (AIN, ATN), cimetidine (AIN), clopidogrel (Vasc), deferoxamine, dextran (Osm), diltiazem (HD), dopamine (HD), ε-aminocaproic acid, epinephrine (HD), hydralazine (GN), hydroxyethyl starch (Osm), IVIg (Osm), lipid-lowering agents (AIN), lithium, mannitol (Osm, HD), methoxyflurane, methyldopa (AIN), pamidronated (GN), penicillamine (GN), phenobarbitol (AIN), phenytoin (AIN), phosphorus-containing urinary acidifiers, propanolol (HD), propylthiouracil (GN), proton pump inhibitors (AIN), ranitidine (AIN), streptokinase (AIN), ticlopidine (Vasc), topiramate (nephrolithiasis), quinine/quinidine (Vasc), vitamin D_3 analogs (psoriasis medications), warfarin (AIN), zoledronate
Heavy metals	Antimony, arsenic (ATN), bismuth salts, cadmium, chromium, copper, gold (GN), lead, mercury (HD), nickel, silver, thallium, uranium
Organic compounds	Carbon tetrachloride and other chlorinated hydrocarbons, chloroform, ethylene glycol (ATN), herbicides, pesticides, solvents
Miscellaneous toxins	Bee venom (ATN), disphosphonates, gallium nitrate, lilies, germanium, grapes and raisins, vitamin C, melamine cyanurate (Cry), mushrooms (Gyomitra), silicon, snake venom (HD), sodium fluoride, superphosphate fertilizer, vitamin D_3–containing rodenticides (HD)
Endogenous toxins	Hemoglobin, myoglobin

(Continued)

Table 13.2 (Continued)

Class of agent	Examples
Illicit drugs	Amphetamines*, cocaine* (HD), heroin*, barbiturates*, phencyclidine* *AKI from rhabdomyolysis
Herbal/natural products	Herbal: *Akebia* sp., Aristolchic acid (fibrosis), *Ephedra* sp. (ma huang), Cape aloes, *Uno degatta*, *Glycyrrhiza* sp., *Datura* sp., Chinese yew (*Taxus celbica*) extract, impila (*Callilepis laureola*), morning cypress (*Cupressus funebris Endl*), St. John's wort (*Hypericum perforatum*), thundergod vine (*Tripterygium wilfordii hook F*), tribulus (*Tribulus terrestris*), wormwood (*Artemisia herba-alba*), and *Solanum nigrum.* Adulterants: mefenamic acid, dichromate, cadmium, phenylbutazone

ATN, Acute tubular necrosis; AIN, acute interstitial nephritis; CIN, chronic interstitial nephritis; Cry, obstructive nephropathy (crystal formation); GN, glomerular; HD, hemodynamic; ON, osmotic nephrosis; Vas, vascular.
Source: Modified from Cowgill and Langston (2011).

Pharmacists should know that there are no data to suggest that other NSAIDs are less nephrotoxic than meloxicam. In fact, meloxicam is probably safer than most NSAIDs for cats because it relies on oxidative metabolism, rather than glucuronidation, for elimination. Since cats are deficient in most glucuronidation enzymes, the elimination half-life of NSAIDs tends to be prolonged in cats relative to other species. It is truly unfortunate that veterinarians have to choose between using meloxicam, which carries a label warning against repeated use but has been used safely for long-term administration in many cats, and other NSAIDs that are more likely to be toxic to cats but that do not carry a warning simply because they are not FDA approved for use in cats.

Drugs that are well-known nephrotoxins in human patients include amphotericin B, cyclosporine, and cisplatin. Each has a unique perspective with regard to veterinary use that pharmacists should be made aware of. Liposomal formulations of amphotericin B are less likely to cause nephrotoxicity than standard (aqueous) amphotericin B. However, the expense of liposomal formulations severely limits their use in veterinary patients. In human patients, renal impairment is the primary limitation to long-term use of cyclosporine (Colombo et al. 2017), whereas in dogs and cats, nephrotoxicity is extremely rare. Cisplatin carries such a high risk of nephrotoxicity that, for both humans and dogs, hydration protocols are used to prevent cisplatin-induced nephrotoxicity. Whether or not cats are susceptible to cisplatin-induced nephrotoxicity is actually unknown because cats succumb to fulminant pulmonary edema before renal toxicity develops (see Chapter 20 for more information about cisplatin pulmonary toxicity in cats).

13.3 Diagnostic Testing

Evaluation of veterinary patients with renal disease is directed at determining the cause and metabolic derangements that occur in association with renal disease. Identifying the cause may be critical for determining the most appropriate treatment. For example, leptospirosis is a treatable cause of AKI in dogs but is an uncommon cause of AKI in human beings. Diagnostic testing for leptospirosis involves polymerase chain reaction (PCR) on urine and microscopic agglutination antibody testing, and these are routine components of the diagnostic approach for AKI in dogs, but would not be for human beings. Another factor that differs between dogs and humans is the fact that dogs are often vaccinated against three to five leptospiral serovars; therefore, interpretation of MAT results may be skewed by vaccinal antibodies. Conversely, determination of glomerular filtration rate (GFR) from serum creatinine concentration is not performed in dogs and cats, as it is in human beings, due to lack of correlation with actual measured GFR. A new biomarker, symmetric dimethylarginine, may reflect GFR better than creatinine concentration (Yerramilli et al. 2016). Diagnostically, testing of dogs and cats with renal disease may include some or all of the following:

- Complete blood cell counts
- Serum or plasma biochemical analysis
- Plasma symmetric dimethylarginine concentration
- Ionized calcium concentration, parathyroid hormone concentration, and vitamin D concentration
- Urinalysis
- Urine protein-to-creatinine (UPC) ratio
- Aerobic bacteriological culture
- Blood pressure
- Abdominal imaging, such as radiography, ultrasonography, computed tomography (CT), or contrast studies
- Infectious disease testing: tick-borne diseases (Rocky Mountain spotted fever, Lyme disease, and ehrlichiosis) and leptospirosis
- Ethylene glycol
- Renal biopsy.

Abnormalities associated with renal disease may include some or all of the following:

- Physical examination:
  - Normal to decreased body condition
  - Abnormal renal palpation
  - Signs of chronic disease (e.g. unkempt haircoat or sarcopenia)
  - Dehydration
  - Uremic stomatitis or glossitis
- Serum biochemistry values:
  - Azotemia
  - Hyperphosphatemia
  - Hypokalemia or hyperkalemia
  - Hypocalcemia or hypercalcemia
  - Metabolic acidosis
  - Anemia (normocytic or normochromic) or polycythemia
  - Hyperglobulinemia

- Hypoalbuminemia
- Proteinuria
- Normal or increased parathyroid hormone concentration
- Imaging:
  - Small, normal, or enlarged kidney(s)
  - Mineralization of soft tissue
  - Nephroureterolithiasis
- Systemic arterial hypertension.

13.4 Pharmacological Treatment of Common Renal Diseases

The etiology and progression of renal disease in dogs and cats share many similarities with those occurring in human beings; however, there are differences. Thus, medical management of renal disease in veterinary patients can differ from that of human patients. Pharmacotherapy of common canine and feline renal diseases will be discussed. Pharmacotherapy of the most common bacterial, fungal, protozoal, and parasitic pathogens involved in renal diseases of dogs and cats are presented in the infectious disease and parasitic disease chapters (Chapters 7 and 9, respectively). Pharmacotherapy of neoplastic renal diseases of dogs and cats is presented in Chapter 20.

13.4.1 Acute Kidney Injury

Acute kidney injury (AKI) is defined as a severe and sudden decline in GFR, usually with signs of uremia. AKI may be due to pre-renal, renal, and post-renal causes (Ross 2011). Pre-renal AKI is a result of hypovolemia and decreased renal perfusion, which is usually reversible but can lead to irreversible renal failure. Intrinsic AKI is a primary insult to or a failure of nephrons caused by toxins, ischemia, infectious agents, or "acute-on-chronic" failure. Post-renal AKI is a result of bilateral ureteral obstruction or urethral obstruction, which is also usually reversible but can lead to irreversible renal failure.

Table 13.3 Veterinary International Renal Interest Society (IRIS) AKI grading criteria.

AKI grade	Blood creatinine	Clinical description
Grade I	<1.6 mg/dL (<140 micromoles/L)	Non-azotemic AKI: a) Documented AKI (historical, clinical, laboratory, or imaging evidence of AKI, clinical oliguria/anuria, volume responsiveness[a]) and/or b) Progressive nonazotemic increase in blood creatinine: ≥0.3 mg/dL (≥26.4 micromoles/L) within 48 hours c) Measured oliguria (<1 mL/kg/h)[b] or anuria over 6 hours
Grade II	1.7–2.5 mg/dL (141–220 micromoles/L)	Mild AKI: a) Documented AKI and static or progressive azotemia b) Progressive azotemic: increase in blood creatinine; ≥0.3 mg/dL ≥ 26.4 micromoles/L) within 48 hours), or volume responsiveness[a] c) Measured oliguria (<1 mL/kg/h) or anuria over 6 hours
Grade III	2.6–5.0 mg/dL (221–439 micromoles/L)	Moderate to severe AKI: a) Documented AKI and increasing severities of azotemia and functional renal failure
Grade IV	5.1–10.0 mg/dL (440–880 micromoles/L)	
Grade V	>10.0 mg/dL (>880 micromoles/L)	

[a] Volume responsive is an increase in urine production to >1 mL/kg/h over 6 hours; and/or decrease in serum creatinine to baseline over 48 hours.

[b] Each grade of AKI is further subgraded as:
1) Non-oliguric (NO) or oligo-anuric (O)
2) Requiring renal replacement therapy (RRT).

AKI may be staged using a system that is modified from human medicine and promoted by the veterinary International Renal Interest Society, or IRIS (Table 13.3; http://www.iris-kidney.com).

The abrupt decline in renal function occurs because of several mechanisms, including afferent arteriolar vasoconstriction in response to decreased circulating volume, damaged glomerular surface area and filtration properties, vasodilation of efferent arterioles, tubular back leak of luminal substances, and tubular obstruction due to cell swelling, crystals, casts, and/or cellular debris. If the tubular epithelial cell basement membrane is intact, then recovery may occur with re-epithelialization and return to function (partial or complete). The most common causes of AKI result from hypovolemia and/or hypotension, ischemia, nephrotoxins, infections, outflow obstruction, and acute-on-chronic.

Renal replacement therapy (e.g. dialysis or hemofiltration) is often performed in human patients with AKI for removal of potential nephrotoxins and to provide time for renal recovery; this is not widely available in veterinary medicine. Many nephrotoxins have no specific therapy other than supportive care, so without renal replacement therapy as an option, many dogs and cats with AKI are euthanized or simply die from complications of renal failure.

Ethylene glycol (antifreeze) induces AKI by crystal-induced tubular obstruction and cellular damage due to metabolism of the ethylene glycol (Hewlett et al. 1989). Dogs and cats can ingest ethylene glycol in garages or in puddles on the road or driveways, where leakage or spills have occurred. Ethylene glycol intoxication is a medical emergency – even if the dog or cat has not ingested a large volume. Initially, dogs and cats exposed to ethylene glycol experience

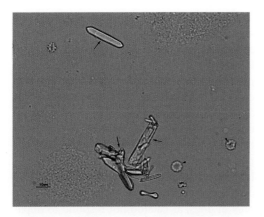

Figure 13.1 Urine from a dog with ethylene glycol toxicity demonstrating characteristic calcium oxalate monohydrate crystal (arrow); red blood cell (arrowhead) indicated for size comparison (400×).

vomiting, anorexia, and central nervous system signs. If not treated aggressively, metabolites of ethylene glycol induce AKI and seizures. Patients present with a high anion gap metabolic acidosis and often have calcium oxalate or hippuric acid crystalluria (Figure 13.1). Pharmacotherapy may be beneficial if instituted within the first 12 hours after ingestion. The strategy of pharmacotherapy is to prevent metabolism of ethylene glycol to its nephrotoxic metabolites, glycolic acid and oxalate. Ethanol or 4-methylpyrazole (Dial et al. 1994; Connally et al. 1996) is used to inhibit the enzyme alcohol dehydrogenase, which is the rate-limiting step in the metabolism of ethylene glycol. Pharmacists may be asked to compound 4-methylpyrazole to have "on hand" in case of emergency ethylene glycol exposures. "Formulations" of ethanol can be either reagent grade 95% or 190 proof liquor, depending on which is more readily available.

95% Ethanol:

- *Dogs:* 5.5 mL/kg intravenous (IV) of a 20% solution every 4 hours (q4h) for 5 treatments, then q6h for 4 additional treatments as CRI over 1 hour. *Alternatively:* 8.6 mL/kg of a 7% ethanol solution, slowly IV followed by a CRI of 1.43 mL/kg/h for at 36–48 hours.
- *Cats:* 5 mL/kg IV of a 20% solution q6h for 5 treatments, then q8h for 4 additional

treatments as CRI over 1 hour. *Alternatively:* Administer a 7% ethanol solution as described for dogs.

4-methylpyrazole (4-MP; Fomepizole):

- *Dogs:* Initially 20 mg/kg IV; at 12 hours post initial dose, give 15 mg/kg IV; at 24 hours post initial dose, give another 15 mg/kg IV; and, at 36 hours after initial dose, give 5 mg/kg. May give additional 5 mg/kg doses as necessary.
- *Cats:* Initially, 125 mg/kg slow IV; at 12, 24, 36 hours, give 31.25 mg/kg IV. In addition, treat supportively with supplemental fluids. Cats must be treated within three hours of ingestion. Cats whose treatment began four hours post ethylene glycol had 100% mortality with either fomepizole or ethanol therapy.

Infectious AKI is often bacterial in origin. *Escherichia coli* is the most common cause of bacterial pyelonephritis associated with AKI in dogs and cats (Pressler and Bartges 2010). Bacterial pyelonephritis may cause AKI or be associated with CKD, and it may be caused by other organisms. Aerobic bacteriologic culture with antimicrobial susceptibility testing should be performed on patients suspected of having pyelonephritis. Choice of antimicrobial therapy is based on susceptibility testing. Empiric therapy most commonly involves a veterinary fluoroquinolone, such as enrofloxacin or marbofloxacin, for its spectrum of activity and ability to achieve therapeutic concentrations in tissue and urine.

Dramatic difference
Diuretics are often administered to human beings with pyelonephritis; however, most dogs and cats with acute pyelonephritis have dilute urine and renal azotemia, so diuretics are not recommended.

Another infectious cause of AKI that is relatively common in dogs is leptospirosis (Sykes et al. 2011). Leptospirosis is a worldwide zoonotic disease that affects many organ systems in infected dogs, including the kidneys. Treatment involves supportive care and antimicrobial administration (Adin and Cowgill 2000). Penicillin (e.g. ampicillin or penicillin G) is administered during the acute phase for two weeks, and doxycycline is administered after two weeks for two additional weeks to treat the carrier phase. Alternatively, doxycycline may be administered as a single agent to treat the acute and carrier phases, although IV doxycycline is associated with adverse events. Pharmacists should be aware that leptospirosis is a zoonotic disease, and pet owners may be infected simply by sharing the same environment as their pet or from exposure to their pet's urine. Pharmacists can provide important client education and counseling to prevent exposure and alert owners to potential symptoms they may experience if infected. Clinical signs of human disease are often mild and flu-like; however, leptospirosis may cause more serious clinical signs.

When possible, treatment of AKI should be directed at addressing and/or eliminating the specific cause. Supportive treatment regardless of the cause also includes management of AKI-induced derangements in homeostasis, and conversion of oligo-anuria to non-oligo-anuria. After collection of diagnostic samples, a four-step process of AKI management is undertaken, and confounding factors are addressed. Intensive therapy is usually required. The four-step process involves (i) rehydration, (ii) differentiating AKI from end-stage CKD and oligo-anuria from non-oligo-anuria, (iii) inducing diuresis, and (iv) managing established oligo-anuric AKI. Pharmacological therapy is heavily involved in step (iii) and will be discussed in more detail. Pharmacotherapeutic attempts to induce diuresis begin with FDA-approved human formulations of mannitol, an osmotic diuretic. Mannitol expands vascular volume by osmotically inducing fluid movement from the interstitial space into the vascular space. It improves renal blood flow and GFR as well as tubular flow. It is filtered at the glomerulus and has an osmotic effect throughout the entire nephron. Furosemide is a loop diuretic that increases

sodium excretion and diuresis at the thick ascending loop of Henle. Furosemide is FDA approved for dogs, cats, and horses, but human formulations are also used in veterinary patients. Furosemide's effect is enhanced with concurrent administration of a vasodilatory agent such as dopamine. Renal blood flow and therefore GFR may be increased by administration of a vasodilatory agent. At low infusion rates, dopamine selectively dilates renal vasculature, increasing sodium excretion and urine output, but has minimal effect on GFR. Use only in dogs, as cats do not respond to dopamine constant rate infusion (CRI).

Dramatic difference

Cats have a putative dopamine receptor D1 (DRD1) that differs from those of dogs and human beings; as a result, they do not respond to dopamine administration (Flournoy et al. 2003).

Fenoldopam is a synthetic benzodiazepine derivative approved for human use that acts as a selective DRD1 agonist. It is an antihypertensive agent that can be used in an extra-label manner to induce renal artery vasodilation in cats and dogs (Nielsen et al. 2015; O'Neill et al. 2016). Calcium channel blockers selectively dilate the afferent arteriole, increasing renal blood flow to glomerular capillaries. Since there are no calcium channel blockers that are FDA approved for use in veterinary patients, their use is considered extra-label.

Practiced but not proven

Aggressive therapy with vasodilators and diuretics has not been shown to improve outcome for patients with AKI.

Mannitol: Should be used only after correcting fluid, electrolyte, and acid–base balance. 0.25–0.5 g/kg as a slow IV bolus over 10–20 minutes. If substantial diuresis occurs, can be administered as a CRI at 60–120 mg/kg/hour IV or administered as intermittent repeated boluses (0.25–0.5 g/kg) every 4–6 hours.

Furosemide:

- *Dogs:* Initial IV bolus of 1–2 mg/kg (up to 4 mg/kg in dogs if no response observed within 30–60 minutes), followed by a CRI of 0.1–2 mg/kg/hour, depending on patient's response.
- *Cats:* Bolus of 1–2 mg/kg IV, and, if effective, start a CRI at 0.25–1 mg/kg/hour, depending on patient's response.

Dopamine: Dogs: 1–5 micrograms/kg/min CRI IV

Fenoldopam:

- *Dogs:* 0.8 micrograms/kg/min CRI IV
- *Cats:* 0.1–1 micrograms/kg/min CRI IV

Calcium channel blocker:

- *Diltiazem:*
  - *Dogs:* 1–4 mg/kg PO ("per os," or orally) every 8 hours of prompt-release diltiazem. A common starting dose is 2 mg/kg every 8 hours.
  - *Cats:* 7.5–15 mg PER CAT PO every 8 hours of prompt-release diltiazem
- *Amlodipine:*
  - *Dogs:* 0.1–0.5 mg/kg PO every 12–24 hours. Maximum dose: 1 mg/kg/day
  - *Cats:* 0.625–1.25 mg PER CAT PO every 12–24 hours.

Hyperkalemia is a potential complication of oligo-anuria and can cause serious cardiac arrhythmias. Pharmacological treatment of hyperkalemia involves inducing a transcellular shift of potassium from the vascular system into cells using glucose, glucose and regular insulin, or bicarbonate. If hyperkalemic arrhythmias occur, treatment involves establishing normal sinus rhythm by counteracting the effect of hyperkalemia at the sinoatrial node using calcium gluconate. Each of these drugs is FDA approved for human use only; their use in veterinary patients constitutes extra-label drug use.

Dextrose: 0.5–1 g/kg body weight IV with or without regular insulin

Insulin and glucose: 0.06–0.5 Units/kg IV, with 50% dextrose (4 mL dextrose per unit insulin)

Bicarbonate: 1–2 milliequivalents/kg IV infused over 15–20 minutes

Calcium gluconate: 0.5–1 mL/kg of the 10% solution (this corresponds to 50–100 mg/kg of calcium gluconate) IV infused over 10–20 minutes; monitor electrocardiograph (ECG).

Systemic arterial hypertension has been reported to occur in over 50% of veterinary patients with AKI (Cole et al. 2017). It is important for pharmacists to understand that normal blood pressure values in humans do not apply to most veterinary patients. Antihypertensive therapy is indicated if systolic blood pressure is greater than 170–180 mmHg (Bartges et al. 1996). Renin–angiotensin–aldosterone system (RAAS) antagonists may be used; they decrease systolic blood pressure by an average of 10 mmHg, while calcium channel blockers decrease systolic blood pressure by an average of 50 mmHg in dogs and cats (Stepien 2011). The only antihypertensive that is FDA approved for veterinary use is enalapril.

Angiotensin-converting enzyme (ACE) inhibitors (dogs and cats unless otherwise indicated):

- *Enalapril:* 0.25–1.0 mg/kg PO every 12–24 hours
- *Benazapril:* 0.25–1.0 mg/kg PO every 12–24 hours
- *Remipril:* 0.125–0.25 mg/kg PO every 24 hours
- *Captopril:* 0.5–1.5 mg/kg PO every 8–24 hours
- *Lisinopril:* 0.5 mg/kg PO every 12–24 hours
- *Imidapril: Dogs only:* 0.25 mg/kg PO every 24 hours

Angiotensin II receptor antagonists (dogs and cats):

- *Telmisartan:* 1 mg/kg PO every 12–24 hours
- *Irbesartan:* 5 mg/kg PO every 12–24 hours
- *Losartan:* 0.125–1 mg/kg PO every 12–24 hours
- *Candesartan:* 1 mg/kg PO every 24 hours

Calcium channel blockers:

- *Amlodipine:*
  - *Dogs:* 0.1–0.5 mg/kg PO every 12–24 hours. Maximum dose 1 mg/kg/day
  - *Cats:* 0.625–1.25 mg PER CAT PO every 12–24 hours.

13.4.2 Chronic Kidney Disease

CKD implies irreversible renal failure that remains stable for a period of time but ultimately progresses. Although there are many potential causes of CKD, by the time CKD is diagnosed, the cause(s) is/are no longer present or treatable. CKD can occur as a result of congenital or acquired renal diseases or a combination thereof. Because the kidneys are intimately involved with homeostasis, CKD affects the animal's overall well-being. Clinical signs of CKD involve primarily alteration in water balance (polyuria and polydipsia) and gastrointestinal signs (hyporexia, anorexia, vomiting, and/or halitosis); general signs of chronic disease may also be present (weight loss, sarcopenia, loss of body condition, and/or an unkempt appearance). Laboratory evaluation often reveals azotemia, dilute urine, hyperphosphatemia, metabolic acidosis, hypokalemia, non-regenerative anemia, hypo- or hyper-calcemia, and proteinuria. Systemic hypertension may also occur.

The cause(s) of progression of CKD is/are not completely known. A likely scenario is that CKD results from repeated insults over time that result in sequential loss of nephrons. The compensatory response is an increase in single-nephron GFR by remaining nephrons, which results in maintenance of total GFR despite loss of functional renal tissue and reserve. Afferent arteriolar dilation occurs, increasing intraglomerular pressure and resulting in increased renal blood flow and GFR. There are trade-offs to this compensation. Increased intraglomerular pressure increases the likelihood of proteinuria with production of growth factors that promote tubulointerstitial fibrosis and glomerulosclerosis. These adaptations result in further loss of nephrons and eventual progression to end-stage CKD.

IRIS (http://www.IRIS-kidney.com) has developed a staging system for animals with CKD and treatment based on staging. CKD is staged by magnitude of renal dysfunction and further modified (substaged) by the presence or absence of proteinuria and/or hypertension (Table 13.4).

The goals of CKD management are to minimize electrolyte and metabolic byproduct excesses and deficits induced by CKD in order to improve quality and quantity of the patient's life. Veterinary therapeutic kidney diets are a mainstay of CKD management in dogs and cats. In comparison to regular pet foods, they are formulated to be replete in potassium and water-soluble vitamins; be more calorically dense; contain omega-3 fatty acids and fiber; have lower protein, phosphorous, and sodium content; and have alkalinizing effects.

Pharmacologic therapy of CKD in dogs and cats is multifactorial and symptomatic. Uremic gastroenteritis may be associated with hyporexia to complete anorexia and/or vomiting. Gastric acid secretion inhibitors are often administered, including histamine-2 receptor antagonists and proton pump inhibitors. Sucralfate may be used if gastric ulceration is suspected. Although gastric hyperacidity is thought to occur with CKD, data are inconsistent as to whether this is actually the case in veterinary patients. If the patient is vomiting, antiemetics may be warranted. The antiemetic maropitant citrate is a neurokinin receptor antagonist that is FDA approved for dogs and cats. Appetite stimulants may also be prescribed to support CKD patients. The two drugs most likely to be prescribed are mirtazapine, a human drug, and capromorelin, a ghrelin receptor agonist that is FDA approved for dogs, but has also been used in an extra-label manner in cats.

Dramatic difference

Diabetes mellitus is not a cause of chronic kidney disease in dogs and cats, as it can be in human beings.

Practiced but not proven

Despite the fact that they are frequently prescribed, the efficacy of gastric acid secretion inhibitors for decreasing gastric hyperacidity in dogs and cats with CKD is unproven.

Table 13.4 International Renal Insufficiency Society (IRIS) CKD grading criteria.

Stage	Plasma creatinine mg/dL		Comments
	Dogs	Cats	
1	<1.4	<1.6	Non-azotemic. Some other renal abnormality present, e.g. inadequate concentrating ability without identifiable non-renal cause; abnormal renal palpation and/or abnormal renal imaging findings; proteinuria of renal origin; abnormal renal biopsy results.
2	1.4–2.0	1.6–2.8	Mild renal azotemia [lower end of the range lies within the reference range for many labs, but the insensitivity of creatinine as a screening test means that animals with creatinine values close to the upper limit of normality often have excretory failure]. Clinical signs usually mild or absent.
3	2.1–5.0	2.9–5.0	Moderate renal azotemia. Many systemic clinical signs may be present.
4	>5.0	>5.0	Severe renal azotemia. Many extra-renal clinical signs present.

UPC value		Substage
Dogs	Cats	
<0.2	<0.2	Non-proteinuric (NP)
0.2–0.5	0.2–0.4	Borderline proteinuric (BP)
>0.5	>0.4	Proteinuric (P)

Systolic BP mmHg	Diastolic BP mmHg	Adaptation when breed-specific reference range is available *	Substage
<150	<95	<10 mmHg above reference range	AP0: Minimal risk (N)
150–159	95–99	10–20 mmHg above reference range	AP1: Low risk (L)
160–179	100–119	20–40 mmHg above reference range	AP2: Moderate risk (M)
=180	=120	=40 mmHg above reference range	AP3: High risk (H)
No evidence of end organ damage/complications			No complications (nc)
Evidence of end organ damage/complications			Complications (c)
Blood pressure not measured			Risk not determined (RND)

Histamine 2 receptor antagonists (dogs and cats):

Famotidine: 1 mg/kg PO every 12–24 hours

Ranitidine: 1–3.5 mg/kg PO every 8–12 hours

Proton pump inhibitors (dogs and cats):

Omeprazole: 0.5–1 mg/kg PO every 24 hours

Esomeprazole: 0.5–1.5 mg/kg PO every 24 hours

Sucralfate: 0.5–2 g PER dog or cat PO every 6–8 hours

Maropitant: 1 mg/kg injected subcutaneously (SC) every 24 hours; 2–4 mg/kg PO every 24 hours

Mirtazapine:

Dogs: 0.17–1.33 mg/kg PO every 24 hours, not to exceed 30 mg PER DOG per day

Capromerelin:

Dogs: 3 mg/kg PO every 24 hours.

Hypokalemia may occur in CKD patients, especially cats, due to anorexia, increased renal and fecal losses, chronic metabolic acidosis, and activation of RAAS. Pharmacists may receive prescriptions for oral potassium supplements or even injectable potassium chloride that is added to parenteral fluids that owners can administer to their pet SC at home. See Chapter 25 for additional information about SC fluid administration to dogs and cats. *Potassium citrate:* 75 mg/kg PO every 12 hours initially; adjust to urine pH of approximately 7.5

Potassium gluconate: 0.5–1 mg/kg PO every 12 hours mixed with food.

Metabolic acidosis occurs with CKD due to retention of organic acids, decreased renal ability to regenerate and reclaim bicarbonate, and decreased ammoniagenesis. Treatment is not usually necessary unless blood pH is less than 7.2. Potassium citrate may be prescribed to serve both as a source of potassium and as an alkalizer.

Proteinuria occurs commonly with CKD. Treatment is indicated if the UPC ratio is >0.5 in dogs or >0.4 in cats. Inhibitors of RAAS (angiotensin-converting enzyme inhibitors or angiotensin II receptor antagonists) are typically prescribed to decrease the severity of proteinuria, since they dilate glomerular efferent arterioles, resulting in decreased intraglomerular pressure (see Section 13.4.1).

Mineral imbalance (hyperphosphatemia and hypocalcemia) occurs with CKD from phosphorous retention and decreased vitamin D metabolism, respectively. As in human patients, the kidneys convert vitamin D pro-hormone to calcitriol, the active form of vitamin D that is necessary for calcium homeostasis and prevention of renal secondary hyperparathyroidism.

Hyperphosphatemia is associated with progression of CKD. The goal of treatment is to decrease the serum/plasma phosphorous concentration to normal ranges through dietary phosphorous restriction and oral administration of phosphate binders. Conventionally, aluminum hydroxide is prescribed as a phosphate binder, as aluminum toxicity is a rare occurrence in dogs and cats. Use of calcium-containing phosphate binders is effective; however, hypercalcemia may occur. Noncalcium and non-aluminum phosphate binders such as the human drug products lanthanum carbonate and sevelamer hydrochloride are used in dogs and cats with CKD. Evidence supporting the benefit of addressing vitamin D deficiency in veterinary patients is contradictory. Calcitriol has been shown to improve survival in dogs in IRIS stage 3 or 4 CKD, but not in cats with any stage of CKD. When dispensing calcitriol to patients with CKD, it is important for pharmacists to work with veterinarians to ensure that serum/plasma phosphorous concentrations are within the normal range. Additionally, pharmacists should counsel pet owners to monitor for clinical signs of hypercalcemia, which may be difficult for the owner to discern from clinical signs of CKD (polyuria, polydipsia, weakness, lethargy, and inappetence). Vitamin D analogs that are sometimes used in human patients with CKD have not been evaluated in veterinary patients.

Dramatic difference

Aluminum toxicity is a rare occurrence in dogs and cats treated with aluminum hydroxide, and aluminum can be used safely.

13.4.2.1 Phosphate Binders

Aluminum hydroxide: 10–35 mg/kg PO administered with meals (typically every 8–12 hours) for a daily cumulative dose of 30–100 mg/kg

Calcium acetate: 20–30 mg/kg PO administered with meals (typically every 12 hours) for a daily cumulative dose of 60–90 mg/kg

Chitosan and calcium carbonate: 150–200 mg/kg PO administered with meals (typically every 12 hours) for a daily cumulative dose of 400 mg/kg

Lanthanum carbonate: 4–30 mg/kg PO administered with meals (typically every 12 hours) for a daily cumulative dose of 12.5–95 mg/kg

Sevelamer hydrochloride: 10–25 mg/kg administered with meals (typically every 12 hours) for a daily cumulative dose of 30–80 mg/kg.

13.4.2.2 Vitamin D Supplementation

Calcitriol: 2.5–3.5 nanograms per kg PO every 24 hours (fasting); alternatively, 9 nanograms per kg PO every 3–5 days.

As is the case in human CKD, normocytic, normochromic, non-regenerative anemia often occurs in dogs and cats as CKD progresses. It may also induce progression of CKD due to decreased blood flow, stagnation of blood, oxidative stress, decreased oxygen diffusion, and induction of fibrosis. Anemia occurs due to decreased erythropoietin production, nutritional imbalances from hyporexia or anorexia, and blood loss due to uremic gastroenteritis. Treatment involves decreasing gastrointestinal blood loss, improving nutritional status, and stimulating red blood cell production. Anabolic steroids are relatively ineffective in stimulating red blood cell production and may be hepatotoxic, so they are no longer recommended. Erythropoietic-stimulating agents such as recombinant human erythropoietin or darbepoetin are effective in dogs and cats with CKD. Iron should be prescribed for dogs and cats treated with erythropoietic-stimulating agents.

Dramatic difference

Because recombinant human erythropoietin is recognized by the immune system as a foreign protein in dogs and cats, its use is associated with anti-erythropoietin antibody production in approximately 20% of cats and 40% of dogs, resulting in potentially severe, refractory anemia. Antibody production is rare with darbepoetin.

Pharmacists should counsel owners of dogs or cats treated with recombinant human erythropoietin to monitor for refractory anemia (lethargy, weakness, tachypnea, pale mucous membranes, and/or tachycardia). See Appendix C for normal respiratory and heart rates of dogs and cats based on body size and weight. The reader may wonder why recombinant human erythropoietin would be prescribed for veterinary patients instead of darbepoetin. The reason is that most pet owners do not have insurance or other third-party payment options, so darbepoetin may not be an affordable option.

13.4.2.3 Anemia

Recombinant human erythropoietin: 100 International Units per kg injected SC three times per week until target hematocrit achieved, then 75–100 IU/kg SC two times per week as maintenance

Darbepoetin: 1–1.5 micrograms per kg SC every 7 days until target hematocrit achieved, then decrease frequency until the longest interval is reached that maintains desired hematocrit.

Iron dextran:

Dogs: 100–300 mg/dog injected intramuscularly (IM) every 2–4 weeks
Cats: 50–100 mg/cat injected IM every 2–4 weeks.

13.4.2.4 Systemic arterial hypertension

Systemic arterial hypertension is reported to occur in 65–75% of dogs and cats with CKD. It occurs due to activation of RAAS, activation of the sympathetic nervous system, and increased antidiuretic hormone secretion due to hypovolemia. Risk of hypertensive-associated complications increases as systolic hypertension worsens. These complications include ophthalmic damage (retinal vessel tortuosity, intraocular hemorrhage, and retinal detachment), renal damage (proteinuria and progression of CKD), left ventricular hypertrophy and possible left-sided congestive heart failure, and ischemic encephalopathy (seizures and death). The goal of treatment is to decrease systolic blood pressure to less than 150 mmHg using calcium channel blockers and RAAS inhibitors; calcium channel blockers may be more effective (see Section 13.4.1). Other drugs, such as alpha- and beta-adrenergic antagonists, direct arteriolar vasodilators, and diuretics, are not as effective as first-line treatment, but may be used in combination to control systemic arterial hypertension. Diuretics are not used typically in veterinary patients with CKD due to the risk of inducing dehydration, which can exacerbate CKD.

Propranolol:

Dogs: 0.5–2 mg/kg PO every 8–12 hours
Cats: 0.2–1 mg/kg PO every 8–12 hours

Atenolol:

Dogs: 0.25–1 mg/kg PO every 12 hours
Cats: 6.25–12.5 mg PER CAT PO every 12 hours

Hydralazine:

Dogs: 0.5–3 mg/kg PO every 12 hours
Cats: 2.5–10 mg PER CAT PO every 12 hours.

Other treatments for CKD in dogs and cats that are used occasionally or are being evaluated include chronic hemodialysis, renal transplantation, and stem cell therapy.

13.4.3 Protein-Losing Glomerulonephropathy

The presence of protein in urine is an abnormal finding. The protein pad on urine dipsticks detects protein, primarily albumin, in the range of 30–3000 mg/dL. Micro-albuminuria refers to albuminuria of less than 30 mg/dL, that is, below the limit of detection by routine urine dipstick analysis. Microalbuminuria is an indication of developing renal disease associated with poorly controlled diabetes mellitus and primary systemic arterial hypertension in human beings; however, these do not occur in dogs or cats. Quantitation of urine protein may be done by determining 24-hour excretion, but this is difficult to perform in dogs and cats because they are usually not cooperative in supplying urine samples. In veterinary medicine, the UPC is used, with normal being less than 0.2 and borderline being 0.2–0.4 in cats and 0.2–0.5 in dogs. A UPC greater than these is abnormal. Proteinuria may occur because of several different processes. Pre-renal proteinuria may be physiologic (e.g. exercise, stress, fever, etc.) or overload (e.g. hyperproteinemia, myoglobinemia, hemoglobinemia, etc.) in nature. Post-renal proteinuria is the most common reason for proteinuria in veterinary patients and is associated with inflammation, infection, or hemorrhage (e.g. bacterial urinary tract infection [UTI], urolithiasis, neoplasia, etc.). Renal proteinuria may be glomerular, tubular, or interstitial in origin. To assess proteinuria, it is important to exclude post-renal causes first. If the proteinuria is localized to the kidneys, then determination of the underlying cause directs treatment. Proteinuria has prognostic implications whether azotemia is present or not. Renal biopsy is often performed in human patients with proteinuria, and while it is being performed more in dogs and cats, it is not performed commonly.

Proteinuria is a hallmark finding with glomerular disease. Clinical signs associated with glomerular disease are variable. Azotemia may or may not be present. With moderate proteinuria (serum/plasma albumin concentration greater than 1.5 g/dL but less than 2.5 mg/dL), clinical signs often include weight loss, sarcopenia, lethargy, and polyuria. With more severe proteinuria (serum/plasma albumin concentration less than 1.5 g/dL), clinical signs and laboratory abnormalities are more severe and may include edema/ascites, sarcopenia, weight loss, anorexia, hypercholesterolemia, and hyperlipidemia.

Treatment of glomerular disease in veterinary medicine is often frustrating because of the unpredictable response to therapy and the variable biologic course. The goals of therapy are similar to those for CKD, with an additional goal of increasing serum albumin concentration and minimizing likelihood of nephrotic syndrome. When possible, identifying and treating the primary cause are important (see Table 13.1). Even with treatment of the primary process, glomerular proteinuria may not resolve or may worsen. For example, Lyme nephritis in dogs, which is a cause of glomerular proteinuria, does not often respond to therapy with doxycycline and immune suppression. Renal biopsy is beneficial in identifying the underlying renal pathology (immune-mediated versus non-immune-mediated versus amyloid); however, as mentioned, this is often not performed due to expense and complications in dogs and cats. Approximately 50% of glomerulonephropathy in dogs is immune-mediated in origin, while the other 50% is non-immune-mediated in origin. Amyloidosis occurs rarely in dogs and cats; however, certain breeds have a predisposition, including Shar Pei dogs and Abyssinian cats. Although diabetes mellitus is an important cause of glomerular injury in humans, diabetic dogs and cats do not appear to be at increased risk of glomerular injury.

Nutritionally, feeding a therapeutic kidney diet (see Section 13.6) is beneficial. Pharmacotherapeutically, RAAS inhibitors reduce the degree of proteinuria, increase plasma/serum albumin concentration, and improve quality and quantity of life (see Section 13.4.1). Antithrombotic therapy is often prescribed to combat the increased risk of thromboembolism due to urinary loss of antithrombin III. Conventionally, a low dose of aspirin is used; however, the human approved drug clopidogrel, an inhibitor of the P2Y$_{12}$ subtype of the adenosine diphosphate (ADP) receptor involved in platelet activation, may be prescribed.

Practiced but not proven

Administration of low-dose aspirin or clopidogel has not been shown to decrease risk of thromboembolic disease in veterinary patients with glomerular proteinuria.

Given the fact that approximately 50% of canine glomerulonephropathies are immune-mediated in nature, immunosuppressive therapy may be warranted. There are no studies documenting the best immunosuppressive drug for glomerulonephropathy in dogs. In most patients, glucocorticoid administration worsens proteinuria; however, in acute cases of severe glomerulonephropathy, immunosuppressive dosages of a glucocorticoid are suggested. For long-term management, mycophenolate is often prescribed; however, other immunosuppressives may be used, such as azathioprine or cyclosporine. Cyclosporine was not shown to be effective in a randomized controlled clinical trial of dogs with glomerular proteinuria, however. Chapter 14 provides more detailed information regarding immunosuppressant therapy. With ascites or pleural effusion,

diuretic therapy may be used to control fluid retention, although the mechanism for fluid retention with glomerular proteinuria is decreased plasma oncotic pressure due to hypoalbuminemia and not increased hydrostatic pressure. Often a combination of furosemide, a loop diuretic (see Section 13.4.1), with spironolactone, an aldosterone receptor antagonist, is prescribed. The goal of managing a patient with protein-losing glomerulonephropathy is to ideally reduce the UPC to less than 0.5; however, a more realistic goal is to decrease the UPC by at least 50%.

13.4.3.1 Platelet Aggregation Inhibitors

Acetylsalicylic acid (aspirin):

Dogs: 0.25–0.5 mg/kg PO every 12–24 hours
Cats: 40–81 mg PER CAT PO every 3 days (the long dose interval is due to prolonged elimination half-life in cats)

Clopridogrel:

Dogs: 1–2 mg/kg PO every 24 hours
Cats: 18–75 mg PER CAT PO every 24 hours.

13.4.3.2 Immunosuppressants

(See Chapter 14 for additional information.)

Prednisone and prednisolone: 2 mg/kg PO every 24 hours or divided in equal doses every 12 hours (prednisolone, not prednisone, must be used in cats because prednisone is not orally bioavailable).

Dexamethasone: 0.2 mg/kg injected SC every 24 hours; *or*
Mycophenolate mofetil:

Dogs: 10–20 mg/kg PO every 12 hours
Cats: 10 mg/kg PO every 12 hours

Cyclosporine:

Dogs: 5 mg/kg PO every 24 hours initially. Dose may be reduced to every other day or twice weekly, depending on response; some dogs will require daily treatment.
Cats: 1–4 mg/kg PO every 12 hours. Measure whole blood trough concentration, and adjust dose to therapeutic level of

300–500 nanograms/mL; maintain this dose, then taper to approximately 250 nanograms/mL for maintenance.

Azathioprine: Dogs only: 2 mg/kg PO every 24 hours; 50 mg/m^2 PO every 24–48 hours (see Appendix H for a body surface area conversion table for dogs).

Chlorambucil:

Dogs: 2–6 mg/m^2 PO every 24–48 hours, then taper dose (see Appendix H for a body surface area conversion table for dogs)

Cats: 2 mg/m^2 PO every 24–48 hours, then taper dose; 20 mg/m^2 PO q14–21d (see Appendix H for a body surface area conversion table for cats).

13.4.3.3 Diuretics

Spironolactone: 2 mg/kg PO every 12–24 hours.

13.4.4 Renal Tubular Disorders

The renal tubules, composed of the proximal convoluted tubule, loop of Henle, distal convoluted tubule, and collecting ducts, modify the glomerular filtrate. While renal function is often thought of in terms of azotemia, a reflection of glomerular function, tubular function is responsible for the final composition of urine through reabsorption and secretion of various molecules (e.g. electrolytes, glucose, and water). Renal tubules are also involved in metabolism of hormones (e.g. erythropoietin and renin) and in maintaining systemic acid–base balance. Tubulopathies can be classified as either isolated or complex defects, and as congenital or acquired. They may involve alteration in carbohydrate, nitrogen, electrolyte, mineral, fluid, and acid-based metabolism. There are several underlying principles of tubulopathies: (i) Tubular disorders involve an abnormality of transport function; (ii) clinical and biochemical abnormalities reflect the site of tubular function; (iii) inherited tubular disorders involve loss of function of a transport protein or an error of metabolism; (iv) diseases that perturb energy production or structural integrity of tubular cells result in

complex disorders; (v) therapeutic principles are simple and involve replacement of the substance lost in urine or avoidance of the toxic substance; and (vi) dose requirements for replacement therapy are directly proportional to the function of the defective tubular site. If the defective site is responsible for bulk reabsorption, larger replacement doses will be required than at a site with less reclamation of a lost molecule. Those tubulopathies that require pharmacotherapeutic management will be discussed here.

13.4.4.1 Hypercarnitinuria

Carnitine is a nonessential sulfur-containing amino acid. Although carnitine is reabsorbed in the proximal renal tubule, similar to other amino acids, it is reabsorbed at a rate less than that for other mammals (approximately 75% reabsorption in dogs compared with >90% in other mammals). Dilated cardiomyopathy has been associated with systemic carnitine deficiency in dogs. Hypercarnitinuria likely represents a proximal renal tubular transport defect. Treatment for carnitine deficiency includes feeding a diet with adequate or increased carnitine content, or supplementation with L-carnitine.

L-Carnitine: 50–100 mg/kg PO every 8 hours.

13.4.4.2 Hyperaldosteronism

Increased aldosterone production and secretion stimulate tubular reabsorption of Na$^+$ and excretion of K$^+$ and H$^+$, resulting in hypokalemia and metabolic alkalosis. Hyperaldosteronism may occur as a result of an adrenal tumor or hyperplasia (primary aldosteronism and Conn's syndrome), hyperreninism due to a tumor of the juxtaglomerular apparatus, or renovascular hypertension from Bartter's syndrome (characterized by hyperreninemia, metabolic acidosis, increased secretion of vasodilatory prostaglandins, and normal systemic arterial blood pressure) or from exogenous mineralocorticoid administration. Treatment involves removal of the tumor if possible, K$^+$ supplementation, and administration of spironolactone (see Section 13.4.2).

13.4.4.3 Methylmalonic Aciduria Secondary to Vitamin B$_{12}$ Deficiency

Methylmalonic aciduria has been observed in Giant Schnauzers with intestinal malabsorption of vitamin B$_{12}$ (cobalamin). Vitamin B$_{12}$ deficiency occurs due to the lack of intrinsic factor–B$_{12}$ receptors in the ileum. The trait appears to be autosomal recessive in nature. Affected puppies exhibit inappetence and failure to thrive between 6 and 12 weeks of age. Megaloblastic anemia occurs. Treatment involves administration of vitamin B$_{12}$, which is a cofactor necessary for normal methylmalonic acid intermediate metabolism.

Vitamin B$_{12}$ (cobalamin):

Dogs: 25–250 micrograms/kg PO every 24 hours; 500 micrograms PER DOG injected SC every 7 days for dogs ≤15 kg and 1000 micrograms PER DOG SC every 7 days for dogs >15 kg

Cats: 250 micrograms PER CAT SC every 7 days.

13.4.5 Disorders of Water Metabolism

Nephrogenic diabetes insipidus (nDI) is a term used to describe any disorder in which there is a structural or functional defect in the ability of the kidneys to respond to antidiuretic hormone (ADH). These animals produce large volumes of dilute urine (polyurina). Numerous drugs (e.g. furosemide, glucocorticoids, and methoxyflurane), toxins (e.g. *E. coli* endotoxin), and conditions (e.g. hypokalemia, hypercalcemia, medullary cystic disease, interstitial nephritis, and bacterial pyelonephritis) can result in nDI. Congenital nDI describes a condition where patients have structurally defective or absent ADH receptors. Animals with nDI are unable to respond to exogenous ADH, which would normally result in concentrated urine. Treatment consists of unlimited access to water, dietary Na$^+$ restriction, and, paradoxically, use of thiazide diuretics. Thiazide diuretics induce a mild dehydration, enhanced proximal renal tubular reabsorption of Na$^+$, decreased delivery of tubular fluid to the distal nephron, and reduced urine output. Reduction of dietary Na$^+$ and protein may reduce the amount of solute that must be excreted in urine, and may further reduce obligatory water loss and polyuria.

Central diabetes insipidus (cDI) describes insufficient ADH secretion. Like patients with nDI, these animals are polyuric, However, patients with cDI respond to exogenous ADH therapy and are able to produce concentrated urine. Since ADH is a peptide hormone, oral bioavailability is less than 1% in dogs. Bioavailability of ADH after sublingual administration is 10–20%. Onset of action in dogs occurs within one hour of administration, with peak effects at two to six hours, and duration of action 10–27 hours. Despite poor absorption of oral ADH, some dogs will respond to orally administered ADH.

Thiazide diuretics:

Chlorothiazide: 4.5–9 mg/kg PO every 12 hours

Hydrochlorothiazide: 0.5–1 mg/kg PO every 12 hours

Exogenous ADH (desmopressin acetate, DDAVP):

Nasal drops: 5–20 micrograms (2–4 drops PER DOG per day) intranasally or into subconjunctival sac – this dose is generally divided and administered every 12 hours (Chapter 25 describes drug administration into the subconjunctival sac).

Tablets: 0.1 mg PER DOG PO every 8 hours initially. May require increasing dose up to 0.2 mg. Some dogs will require 0.1–0.2 mg PER DOG PO every 8–12 hours for long-term management.

13.4.5.1 Fanconi Syndrome

Urinary hyperexcretion of amino acids, phosphate, glucose, bicarbonate, calcium, potassium, and other ions, and proteins of molecular weights under 50 000 Da, in conjunction with renal tubular acidosis (RTA) and ADH-resistant polyuria, define the complex tubulopathy termed Fanconi syndrome. There are inherited and acquired forms of Fanconi syndrome. The pathogenesis of the syndrome regardless of its cause involves one of two basic mechanisms. The first is that renal tubular membranes become leaky, allowing less efficient reabsorption of solutes. The second hypothesis suggests that the intracellular metabolism of renal tubule cells fails to produce sufficient energy to support transport. Any substance that could be "toxic" and alter renal tubular metabolism, such as heavy metals (e.g. lead, copper, mercury, organomercurials, Lysol, and maleic acid) and drugs (e.g. gentamicin, cephalosporins, outdated tetracycline, cisplatin, and salicylate), could impair transport processes. Fanconi syndrome may also occur with malignancies (e.g. multiple myeloma), monoclonal gammopathies, hyperparathyroidism, potassium depletion, amyloidosis, nephrotic syndrome, vitamin D deficiency, or interstitial nephritis associated with antitubular basement membrane antibodies, or as a complication of renal transplantation.

Dramatic difference

Inherited Fanconi syndrome occurs in up to 30% of the Basenji dog breed, but it is rare in humans, cats, and other dog breeds.

Dogs with Fanconi syndrome have deficient fractional reabsorption of many solutes, including glucose, phosphate, and amino acids. Aminoaciduria is generalized in most dogs, but occasionally is limited to cystinuria with minor defects in reabsorption of methionine, glycine, and some dibasic amino acids. Many dogs also have variably severe reabsorptive defects for bicarbonate, sodium, potassium, and uric acid. Defective urinary concentrating ability in dogs with Fanconi syndrome represents a form of nDI. This defect may precede development of glucosuria. Glomerular filtration rate is normal in some affected dogs and reduced in others. Progression of the disease in affected dogs is variable. Some dogs develop chronic renal failure within a few months of diagnosis, and others remain stable for several years. Rapid progression and death may result from acute

renal failure and papillary necrosis or acute pyelonephritis. Treatment of dogs with Fanconi syndrome is limited to control of metabolic acidosis, appropriate antibiotic therapy for UTIs, and conservative medical management of CKD. It may be difficult to control acidosis, even with high doses of alkali therapy. This is a consequence of the marked bicarbonaturia (bicarbonate wasting) that occurs when bicarbonate supplementation normalizes plasma bicarbonate concentrations. Potassium citrate therapy provides both alkalinization and K^+ supplementation.

13.4.5.2 Alkali Replacement

Bicarbonate: Dosages in excess of 11 mEq/kg/day may be required to correct plasma bicarbonate concentration in patients with proximal RTA (pRTA). Lower doses are required for distal RTA (dRTA): 1–5 mEq/kg/day.

Mandatory monitoring

Severe hypokalemia can develop as a result of bicarbonaturia that is exacerbated by bicarbonate supplementation.

Potassium citrate: 75 mg/kg PO every 12 hours initially. One 540 mg tablet provides 5 mEq of potassium and 1.7 mEq of citrate, and its metabolism yields 5 mEq of bicarbonate.

13.4.6 Nephroureterolithiasis

Unlike in human beings, the majority of uroliths occur in the lower urinary tract of dogs and cats; however, dogs and cats do develop nephroureteroliths (Figure 13.2). As in human beings, the most common mineral found in nephroureteroliths is calcium oxalate, although other minerals such as struvite, urate, cystine, and compound or mixed uroliths do occur. Discussion of medical management of urolithiasis will be covered in Part II of this chapter, which covers lower urinary tract diseases; however, there are several pharmacotherapeutic agents that are prescribed for nephroureterolithiasis in dogs

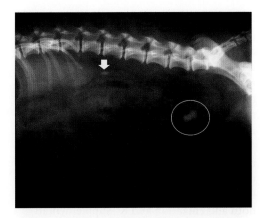

Figure 13.2 Calcium oxalate urocystoliths (bladder stone; circled) and ureterolith (arrow) in an older Miniature Schnauzer. *Source:* Image courtesy of Dr. Joe Bartges, University of Georgia.

and cats, and these will be discussed here. A 50-fold increase in nephroureteroliths reported in dogs and cats occurred between 1980 and 2000. While the presence of nephroliths is not associated with higher mortality or progression of CKD in cats, the presence of ureteroliths is. For ureteroliths that are obstructing urine flow, surgical removal or interventional radiologic techniques such as placement of a ureteral stent or subcutaneous bypass device are indicated. Pharmacotherapeutics are aimed at addressing excesses and deficiencies associated with decreased renal function, as described in Sections 13.4.1 and 13.4.2 on AKI and CKD, respectively. Additionally, medical expulsion therapy of ureteroliths can be attempted. This is less successful than in human beings due to the internal diameters of canine and feline ureters. Cat ureters are normally less than 0.1 mm in diameter, and dog ureters are normally less than 1.4 mm in diameter and correlate with the overall size of the patient. Supportive treatment for ureteral obstruction involves fluid therapy, analgesia, and managing potential concurrent conditions such as hyperkalemia, vomiting, systemic arterial hypertension, and UTIs. Many cats with ureteral obstruction also have underlying CKD that must also be managed long term.

Medical expulsion therapy is attempted by administering IV fluids, diuretics, ureteral smooth muscle relaxants, and anti-inflammatories. The diuretic mannitol is often administered (see Section 13.4.1). For ureteral smooth muscle relaxation, alpha-adrenergic antagonists (usually prazosin) and amitriptyline may be prescribed, but none have been shown to be effective in dogs and cats with ureteral obstruction. Amitriptyline has been shown to relax urethral smooth muscle and is assumed to decrease ureteral smooth muscle tone as well. Glucagon has been evaluated in cats with ureteroliths but was not shown to be effective despite its ability to increase ureteral smooth muscle contraction. Anti-inflammatories may decrease inflammation of the ureteral wall where the ureterolith is wedged; however, there are risks. Glucocorticoids are catabolic and increase risk of bacterial infection, while nonsteroidal anti-inflammatory drugs may exacerbate azotemia in patients with preexisting renal disease by decreasing renal blood flow. A new FDA-approved veterinary-specific analgesic, grapiprant, is a selective prostaglandin E EP4 receptor antagonist that could be used in patients with renal disease because it may not affect renal blood flow.

Prazosin: 1 mg per 15 kg (33 lbs.) body weight PO every 8–24 hours

Amitriptyline:

Dogs: 1–2 mg/kg PO every 12–24 hours
Cats: 0.5–1 mg/kg PO every 12–24 hours

Dexamethasone: 0.05–0.1 mg/kg IV every 24 hours

Meloxicam: 0.05–0.1 mg/kg injected SC or IV every 24 hours

Grapiprant: Dogs only: 2 mg/kg PO every 24 hours.

13.4.7 Neoplasia

The most common neoplastic renal diseases include lymphoma and carcinoma (adenocarcinoma and transitional cell carcinoma). Rarely, nephroblastoma and other neoplasms may occur. If the cancer is unilateral, then unilateral nephrectomy is performed. If both kidneys are involved or if unilateral nephrectomy is not an option, chemotherapy is administered based on type of neoplasm (Chapter 20). Transitional cell carcinoma is relatively common in dogs but rare in cats. Scottish terriers have up to a 20-fold greater risk than other breeds for developing transitional cell carcinoma. Intravehicular therapy with bacillus Calmette–Guérin (BCG), which is often used in human patients, is not effective in dogs. The NSAID piroxicam, either alone or in combination with other chemotherapy agents, has been the most effective treatment for canine transitional cell carcinoma.

13.5 Adverse Drug Effects in Veterinary Species

RAAS inhibitors: In general, RAAS inhibitors are associated with gastrointestinal upset and hyperkalemia as potential adverse effects.

Diuretics: Diuretics may be associated with dehydration, azotemia, and electrolyte imbalances, primarily hypokalemia and hyponatremia. Thiazide diuretics may also be associated with hypercalcemia due to increased calcium absorption in the distal convoluted tubule.

Spironolactone has been associated with an unusual idiosyncratic reaction. In one study, approximately 25% of Maine Coon cats developed severely pruritic facial ulcerative dermatitis requiring drug discontinuation (MacDonald et al. 2008). Other cat breeds do not seem to be affected.

Vasodilators: Hydralazine may induce vomiting in up to 30% of dogs. It may also cause reflex stimulation of RAAS with associated sodium and water retention.

Calcium channel blockers: Hypotension is a potential complication but is difficult to induce when administering antihypertensive agents because of systemic hypertension. Amlodipine, a calcium channel blocker, is associated with inducing reversible (when the drug is discontinued) gingival hyperplasia in some dogs.

Erythropoeitin-stimulating agents: Erythropoeitin-stimulating agents may induce polycythemia and systemic arterial hypertension if the erythrocyte count/hematocrit is not monitored closely. Pain and irritation may occur at the injection site. Human recombinant erythropoietin may induce anti-erythropoietin in approximately 20% of cats and 40% of dogs. These antibodies also cross-react with native erythropoietin and may result in severe anemia. Darbepoetin has not been associated with antibody production in dogs and cats.

Immunosuppressants: In general, immunosuppressants increase risk of infections. Chlorambucil is usually well tolerated by dogs and cats, but it may be associated with adverse effects, including bone marrow suppression (e.g. leukopenia, neutropenia, lymphopenia, and thrombocytopenia), neurologic signs (seizures, tremors, and muscle twitching), dermatologic signs (pyoderma, otitis externa, and rashes), gastrointestinal signs (anorexia, vomiting, and diarrhea), respiratory signs (pulmonary fibrosis, pneumonia, and pulmonary edema), urinary signs (Fanconi syndrome in cats, sterile cystitis, hematuria, polyuria, and polydipsia), hypersensitivity, hepatotoxicity, bradycardia, and fever. Cyclosporine has potential for side effects, most commonly infections; however, other potential side effects include gastrointestinal signs (vomiting, diarrhea, and anorexia), lethargy, urticaria, anaphylaxis, hyperactivity and restlessness, seizures, hepatopathy, lameness and myositis, diabetes mellitus (West Highland White Terriers are the most common breed), weight loss, azotemia, and proteinuria in dogs. In cats, adverse effects of cyclosporine include vomiting, diarrhea, weight loss, hepatopathy, hemolytic-uremia syndrome, and lameness. Mycophenolate has been associated with gastrointestinal signs (hemorrhagic diarrhea, anorexia, and weight loss) and myelosuppression. More detailed information about immunosuppressive agents can be found in Chapter 14.

Practiced but not proven

There are no controlled studies demonstrating the effectiveness of immunosuppressants in dogs with glomerular proteinuria.

13.6 Nutritional Supplements for Veterinary Renal Disease

Nutritional therapy is a mainstay of managing dogs and cats with renal disease. So-called "therapeutic kidney diets" are formulated to manage the excesses and deficiencies that occur with chronic kidney disease, to ameliorate clinical signs, and to slow down progression. In general, therapeutic kidney diets contain decreased quantities of protein, phosphorous, sodium, fiber, and calcium, and increased quantities of B vitamins, potassium, alkalinization, omega-3 fatty acids, and energy density. These diets contain a more balanced amino acid composition, resulting in a higher bioavailability and decreased dietary content of dietary protein.

Many causes of renal disease are associated with inflammation and intraglomerular hypertension. Omega-3 fatty acids may be beneficial in decreasing inflammation and intraglomerular hypertension and increasing GFR. An omega-6 to omega-3 fatty acid ratio of 1:1–5:1 is beneficial. The dose can be increased but can result in diarrhea and flatulence, which adversely impact pet owners' enthusiasm for these "natural" anti-inflammatory therapies.

Omega-3 fatty acids: 300 mg of the sum of eicosapentaenoic acid and docosahexaenoic acid per 4.5 kg body weight per day (300 mg per each 10 lbs. of body weight per day).

Probiotics with or without prebiotics have been purported to be beneficial for animals with CKD, including claims that they improve azotemia. Studies to date have not proven this claim.

L-Carnitine is used to treat renal tubular defects associated with hypercarnitinuria, while vitamin B_{12} is used to treat methylmalonic aciduria secondary to vitamin B_{12} deficiency.

13.7 FDA-Approved Veterinary Drug Products with No Human Drug Equivalent

Brand name	Active ingredient(s)	Drug class	Rationale/ notes
Cerenia	Maropitant	Neurokinin-1 inhibitor	Acts at emetic center; was initially approved for emesis associated with motion sickness
Entyce	Capro-merelin	Ghrelin receptor agonist	Appetite stimulant; also stimulates growth hormone secretion
Galliprant	Grapaprant	Prostaglandin E EP4 receptor antagonist	Selective analgesic that does not affect gastrointestinal tract or renal blood flow

Part II Pharmacotherapeutics of Lower Urinary Tract Disease

Key Points

- The majority of uroliths occurring in dogs and cats occur in the lower urinary tract, while the majority of uroliths occurring in human beings occur in the upper urinary tract.
- Similar to human beings, *E. coli* is the most common bacterial organism causing urinary tract infections in dogs and cats.

- Cats have an idiopathic cystitis that is similar but not identical to interstitial cystitis in human beings.
- Urinary incontinence in human and veterinary patients can have similar causes and share many of the same pharmacological treatment options. However, many pet owners are unable or unwilling to tolerate urinary incontinence in an indoor cat or dog because of the damage the urine does to furniture, flooring, or other household items.
- Benign prostatic hypertrophy in intact male dogs is similar to that in human beings; however, prostatic cancer tends to be malignant in dogs.

13.8 Comparative Aspects of Lower Urinary Tract Disease

Lower urinary tract diseases occur commonly in dogs and cats, and many mirror what occurs in human beings (Bartges 2000). Bacterial cystitis, prostate disease (in dogs), urinary incontinence, and idiopathic cystitis (so-called interstitial cystitis in human beings) are similar; however, other diseases are different. Urolithiasis primarily occurs in the lower urinary tract in dogs and cats, as opposed to involving the kidneys in human beings. Neoplastic lower urinary tract disease is often benign in nature in human beings; however, it tends to be malignant and aggressive in dogs and rare in cats. An aspect of lower urinary tract disease that most pharmacists have not considered is the fact that urinary incontinence (which may occur secondary to all lower urinary tract diseases) may carry the "death penalty" in dogs and cats. Dealing with the consequences of urinary incontinence in a pet (e.g. urine-stained carpet or furniture, and urine soiling of the pet's fur) may not be consistent with many pet owners' lifestyles. Thus, urinary incontinence can be considered a life-threatening condition for many pets, since owners may choose to euthanize the pet rather than attempt treatment.

13.9 Drug-Induced Lower Urinary Tract Disease

There are not many drug-induced lower urinary tract diseases in dogs and cats. Immunosuppressive drugs and diuretics increase the risk of bacterial UTIs. Cyclophosphamide is associated with sterile hemorrhagic cystitis (Crow et al. 1977) and is discussed in more detail in Chapter 20.

13.10 Diagnostic Testing

Clinical signs of lower urinary tract diseases in dogs and cats are similar regardless of cause and include difficulty urinating, straining to urinate, inappropriate urination, urgency, hematuria, and possibly urinary obstruction. For dogs, "inappropriate" urination would be urinating in the house instead of outside (presumably due to urgency). For cats, inappropriate urination would be urinating outside the litterbox (presumably due to the cat associating the current litterbox with a painful experience). It is also important to note that for cats and female dogs, many owners attribute their animal's squatting posture to indicate constipation rather than dysuria. Pharmacists can help educate clients on clinical signs to monitor when dispensing drugs for lower urinary tract disease.

Some lower urinary tract diseases are associated with upper urinary tract diseases. For example, patients with nephroureteroliths often have urocystoliths, and dogs and cats with CKD may have concurrent bacterial cystitis. Veterinarians should include rectal palpation as part of the physical examination in dogs to evaluate the prostate (male dogs) and intrapelvic urethra (males and females). It is not possible to perform rectal palpation in a non-anesthetized cat.

Diagnostically, testing of dogs and cats with lower urinary tract disease may include some or all of the following:

- Complete blood cell counts
- Serum or plasma biochemical analysis

- Plasma symmetric dimethylarginine concentration (SDMA)
- Ionized calcium concentration, parathyroid hormone concentration, and vitamin D concentration
- Urinalysis
- Aerobic bacteriological culture
- If uroliths are retrieved, quantitative urolith analysis
- Blood pressure
- Abdominal imaging, such as radiography, ultrasonography, CT, or contrast studies
- Cystoscopy with biopsy or lithotripsy
- Ejaculate, prostatic wash, prostatic aspirate, or biopsy.

Abnormalities associated with renal disease may include some or all of the following:
- Physical examination:
  - Normal to decreased body condition
  - Abnormal renal palpation
  - Signs of chronic disease (e.g. unkempt haircoat and sarcopenia)
  - Dehydration
  - Large urinary bladder
  - Enlarged prostate (male dogs) and/or distended and firm pelvic urethra on rectal palpation
- Laboratory values:
  - Azotemia
  - Hyperphosphatemia
  - Hypokalemia or hyperkalemia
  - Hypocalcemia or hypercalcemia
  - Metabolic acidosis
  - Anemia (normocytic, normochromic) or polycythemia
  - Hyperglobulinemia
  - Hypoalbuminemia
  - Proteinuria
  - Increased SDMA
  - Hematuria
  - Crystalluria
  - Bacteriuria
  - Positive aerobic bacteriologic culture
- Imaging:
  - Small, normal, or enlarged kidney(s)
  - Nephroureterolithiasis and/or urocystolithiasis and/or urethroliths (see Figure 13.3)
  - Prostatomegaly (male dogs)
  - Bladder and/or urethral mass
  - Cystoscopy may reveal uroliths, masses, bladder mucosal hemorrhages (glomerulations), or strictures
- Systemic arterial pressure.

13.11 Pharmacological Treatment of Common Diseases

Pharmacological treatment of lower urinary tract diseases in dogs and cats is dependent on the underlying disease process. For example, some types of uroliths may be

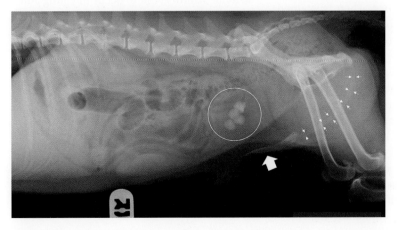

Figure 13.3 Calcium oxalate urocystoliths (bladder stones; circle) in a male dog. Note that male dogs have a bone in their penis called the os-penis (large arrow) and that there is a urinary catheter present (small arrows).

medically dissolved and managed long term using a combination of diet and drug therapy. As in human beings, potassium citrate and thiazide diuretics may be used to manage patients with calcium oxalate uroliths. Pharmacotherapy of the most common bacterial, fungal, protozoal, and parasitic pathogens of dogs and cats are presented in Chapters 7 and 9, respectively. A number of newer drug therapies are available for treating urinary incontinence in human patients, but they are not routinely used in veterinary patients because of the expense (most dogs and cats are not covered by insurance, and no other third-party payment systems are available).

13.11.1 Urolithiasis

Urolithiasis is common in dogs and cats, and approximately 98% of cases occur within the lower urinary tract, although sometimes patients will have upper and lower urinary tract uroliths (Figure 13.2) (Bartges and Callens 2015). Unlike upper urinary tract uroliths and human urolithiasis, where over 80% are composed of calcium oxalate, over 80% of lower urinary tract uroliths in dogs and cats are struvite (magnesium ammonium phosphate hexahydrate) or calcium oxalate; urate accounts for 5–8%, cystine for 0.2–2%, and other minerals make up the remaining. As is the case in human beings, urolith formation occurs when sustained alterations in urine composition promote supersaturation of one or more urinary substances, resulting in precipitation and subsequent organization and growth into uroliths. While urine oversaturation is necessary for urolith formation, there are other factors involved, including decreased inhibitors or increased promoters of lithogenesis (Bartges 2011). Factors involved with urolith formation include the state of saturation of the lithogenic minerals, the urine's pH, inhibitors and promoters of urolith formation, complexors, and macrocrystalline matrixes. Urolithiasis may occur in association with metabolic disease. Hypercalcemia and hyperadrenocorticism are associated with calcium oxalate formation. Diseases associated with bacterial UTIs may be associated with struvite formation. Urate uroliths may occur in patients with liver disease, especially congenital liver diseases such as portovascular anomaly (Lulich et al. 2011).

Dramatic difference

Approximately 98% of uroliths occur in the lower urinary tract in dogs and cats, while the majority of uroliths occur in the upper urinary tract in human beings.

13.11.1.1 Struvite Uroliths

There are two types of struvite uroliths – infection-induced and sterile (Palma et al. 2009, 2013). Human beings form infection-induced struvite (also called "infection stones"). Dogs tend to form infection-induced struvite, while cats tend to form sterile struvite (Bartges et al. 1992). Infection-induced struvite uroliths occur as a consequence of a bacterial UTI with a urease-producing organism. Urease metabolizes urea to ammonia, with subsequent generation of ammonium ion, alkaluria, and a shift in ionization state of phosphorous promoting magnesium ammonium phosphate hexahydrate precipitation and urolith formation (Figure 13.4) (Osborne et al. 1985). Infection-induced struvite uroliths tend to occur in young adult female dogs, but any dog at risk for developing bacterial UTIs may form them. The most common urease-producing organisms

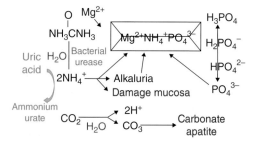

Figure 13.4 Mechanism of infection–induced struvite urolith formation.

in dogs and cats are *Staphylococcus* spp.; *Proteus* spp., which is the main organism associated with infection stones in human beings, may be involved as well. Cats tend to form sterile struvite uroliths. They tend to form in young adult cats and are associated with an alkaline and highly concentrated urine, with abnormally high amounts of magnesium, ammonium, and phosphorous. Unlike human beings, where urine specific gravity is often 1.010–1.030, dogs typically have a urine specific gravity greater than 1.030 and cats greater than 1.035.

Dramatic difference

Dogs tend to form infection-induced struvite uroliths, while cats tend to form sterile (non-infection-associated) struvite uroliths.

Struvite uroliths may be managed by surgery or by minimally invasive techniques, such as cystoscopy with laser lithotripsy (Adams et al. 2008) or percutaneous cystolithotomy (Bartges et al. 2014); however, they are also amenable to medical dissolution. Infection-induced struvite urocystoliths dissolve in an average of eight weeks by feeding a diet that induces urine undersaturation with magnesium, ammonium, and phosphorous, and induces an acidic dilute urine (Osborne et al. 1999a). Administration of an appropriate antimicrobial agent is necessary, as causative bacteria are trapped within the matrix of the stone and are released as the stones dissolve. Uroliths dissolve in a manner similar to ice cubes dissolving in water, that is, from the outer layers to the inner layers. Typically, amoxicillin–clavulanic acid is an appropriate antimicrobial agent for initial treatment, but results of aerobic bacteriologic culture with antimicrobial susceptibility should be used to guide therapy. An alternative dissolution protocol evaluated in a small clinical study used a urinary acidifier, d,l-methionine, with amoxicillin–clavulanic acid without changing diet in dogs with infection-induced struvite (Bartges and Moyers 2010).

Sterile struvite uroliths typically dissolve in one to four weeks by feeding a struvite dissolution diet, many of which are commercially available. In contrast to management of infection-induced struvite uroliths, additional pharmacologic treatment is not usually necessary unless pharmacological manipulation of bladder or urethral muscle tone is required (see Section 13.11.4 on micturition disorders). A struvite dissolution diet is formulated to result in urine that is undersaturated with magnesium, ammonia, and phosphorous, thereby promoting struvite urolith dissolution; it is not effective against other types of uroliths.

d,l-Methionine: 100 mg/kg PO every 24 hours (dogs).

13.11.1.2 Urate Uroliths

Urate comprises 5–8% of uroliths retrieved from dogs and cats (Bartges et al. 1999b). In human beings, uric acid is the primary mineral found in urate stones; however, in dogs and cats, ammonium urate is the primary salt.

Dramatic difference

In nonprimate mammals, allantoin is the end product of purine metabolism, while in primates uric acid is the end product. This likely explains why urate is the predominant urolith formed in human beings, but not in dogs and cats.

Purines are a class of nitrogen-containing compounds widely occurring in nature. For example, the nucleotide bases, adenine and guanine, are purines. Sources of purines include diet, cell turnover, and de novo synthesis from nonpurine precursors. Related compounds are methylxanthines (bronchodilators), caffeine, and theobromine. As shown in Figure 13.5, purines are metabolized to hypoxanthine. Hypoxanthine is converted to xanthine and xanthine to uric acid by xanthine oxidase. Uric acid is converted to allantoin by hepatic uricase, which is absent in primates (Figure 13.5). Allantoin

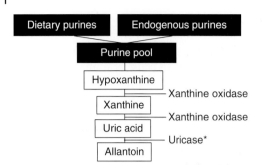

Figure 13.5 Schematic representation of purine metabolism. Note that metabolism of uric acid to allantoin does not occur in primates because they lack hepatic uricase (asterisk).

is a highly water-soluble compound that is renally excreted.

Urate urolith formation in dogs and cats is dependent, in part, on urinary oversaturation with ammonia and uric acid, which can occur due to genetic predisposition or liver disease. Patients with liver disease, especially congenital portosystemic shunts, are predisposed to urate urolith formation, since hepatic uricase is necessary for conversion of relatively insoluble urate to soluble allantoin. Some dogs have a genetic predisposition to form urate uroliths despite having normal liver function. Dalmatians, English bulldogs, and Black Russian Terriers have a mutation in the SLC2A9 gene that encodes a uric acid transporter. Defective function of this uric acid transporter, which is normally expressed in both the kidney and liver, is associated with increased risk of urate uroliths (Bannasch et al. 2008). In other dog breeds and in cats with liver disease that have urate uroliths, the underlying defect is not known. In patients with liver disease, medical dissolution is not successful, and uroliths must be removed if they are causing medical problems for the patient (Bartges et al. 1999a). In patients without liver disease, treatment combining dietary modification (low purine, alkalinizing) and allopurinol results in successful dissolution of urate uroliths in approximately 40% of patients. Allopurinol, a xanthine oxidase inhibitor approved for human use, decreases conversion of xanthine to uric acid, thus reduc-

ing plasma and urine uric acid levels, but leads to a buildup of xanthine (Figure 13.5). Thus, there is a risk that allopurinol may induce xanthine urolith formation, especially if a low-purine diet is not fed concurrently. Ammonium urate is more soluble in alkaline pH, and an alkalinizing agent, such as potassium citrate (see Section 13.4.4 on renal tubular disorders), may be administered to achieve a urine pH greater than 7. The safety and efficacy of allopurinol have not been evaluated in cats, and it should not be administered.

Allopurinol: Dogs only:

Dissolution: 15 mg/kg PO every 12 hours
Prevention: 5–7 mg/kg PO every 12 hours.

13.11.1.3 Cystine Uroliths

Cystine accounts for less than 0.1% of uroliths in cats and approximately 2% of uroliths in dogs (Osborne et al. 1999b). Cystine is an amino acid, and cystinuria represents a proximal renal tubular defective reabsorption of cystine. In dogs, there are four types of cystinuria based on the underlying genetic defect (Brons et al. 2013).

Cystine uroliths can be dissolved medically using a low-protein, alkalinizing diet and administering a thiol-containing drug. Typically, 2-mercaptopropionylglycine (2-MPG) is administered (Hoppe and Denneberg 2001). Alternatively, D-penicillamine can be used. These drugs break the disulfide bond of cystine and bind the sulfhydryl groups of the resultant cysteine monomers to form a soluble compound, resulting in decreased urinary excretion and saturation. 2-MPG should not be administered to cats, as it has been associated with a Heinz body anemia. D-penicillamine is another chelator used for not only cystine but also copper and other metals. Prevention of cystine urolith formation involves castration (if androgen dependent) or feeding a low-protein, alkalinizing diet with or without chelation therapy. Cystine solubility increases exponentially above a urine pH of 7.2; therefore, administering potassium citrate, a urinary alkalinizing agent (see Section 13.4.4), may be beneficial.

2-mercaptopropionyl glycine: Dogs only:

Dissolution: 40 mg/kg PO every 12 hours
Prevention: 20–30 mg/kg PO every 12 hours

D-penicillamine:

Dogs: 15 mg/kg PO every 12 hours
Cats: 10–15 mg/kg PO every 12 hours.

13.11.1.4 Calcium Oxalate Uroliths

Calcium oxalate accounts for 40–45% of uroliths and greater than 80% of nephrouret-eroliths (Bartges et al. 2004). Risk factors include increased urinary calcium excretion, increased oxalate excretion, and/or decreased inhibitors of calcium oxalate formation (Smith 1990). Calcium oxalate urolith formation tends to occur in middle-aged or older dogs and cats, especially small-breed dogs and long-haired cat breeds. Hypercalcemia occurs in approximately 5% of dogs and 20–35% of cats. In dogs, primary hyperparathyroidism and hyperadrenocorticism are the most common causes of hypercalcemia with calcium oxalate uroliths; in cats, idiopathic hypercalcemia is the most common associated cause. There are no medical dissolution protocols for calcium oxalate. If calcium oxalate uroliths are causing clinical problems, then they must be removed physically (by surgery or other methods).

Approximately 30% of patients will have a recurrence of calcium oxalate uroliths within a one year, and approximately 60% will have a recurrence by five years. Preventative measures are dictated by the presence or absence of hypercalcemia as well as the underlying cause of hypercalcemia. In dogs with calcium oxalate uroliths and hypercalcemia, the two most common causes are primary hyperparathyroidism and hyperadrenocorticism. Management of these endocrine disorders is discussed in Chapter 15. In cats with idiopathic hypercalcemia, no single treatment has been shown to be uniformly effective. Feeding a high-fiber, mineral-restricted diet may help. Administering potassium citrate, an inhibitor of calcium oxalate formation and a urinary alkalinizing agent, may help. Some cats appear to respond to alendronate, a bis-phosphonate. Alendronate is not FDA approved for cats and may have serious adverse effects (see Section 13.12).

> **Practiced but not proven**
>
> Alendronate, a bis-phosphonate that is FDA approved for human use, has been recommended for managing idiopathic hypercalcemia in cats, but safety and efficacy data are lacking.

Alendronate:

Dogs: 0.5–1 mg/kg PO every 24 hours on an empty stomach

Cats: 5–20 mg PER CAT PO every 7 days. Administer after a 12-hour fast; following administration, give 6 mL water PO and dab a small amount of butter on cat's lips to promote transit of tablet to stomach; do not feed for two hours following administration. Cats are susceptible to esophageal stricture.

In dogs and cats with calcium oxalate uroliths but normocalcemia, dietary management is recommended. Commercial diets formulated specifically for calcium oxalate prevention are available. Uroliths may recur despite appropriate dietary management. As in human beings, pharmacotherapeutic agents may be prescribed. Potassium citrate is a urinary alkalinizing agent, and citrate is an inhibitor of calcium oxalate formation (Bartges et al. 2013). The goal of treatment is to achieve a urine pH of 7.5. Thiazide diuretics may be prescribed to manage calcium oxalate uroliths, as in human beings. Thiazide diuretics are distal tubule diuretics with weak diuretic effects; however, they promote tubular calcium reabsorption, thereby decreasing urinary calcium excretion. Thiazide diuretics are not FDA approved for dogs or cats, so their safety and efficacy have not been evaluated extensively in these species (Lulich et al. 2001; Hezel et al. 2007). Pyridoxine (vitamin B_6) is involved in normal oxalate metabolism. However, while there are no data that dogs or cats with calcium oxalate uroliths have pyridoxine deficiency, it is sometimes pre-scribed by veterinarians for patients with calcium oxalate uroliths.

Practiced but not proven

There are no dietary or pharmacological therapies that have been shown to decrease recurrence rates of calcium oxalate uroliths in dogs and cats. However, potassium citrate, thiazide diuretics, and/or pyridoxine are often prescribed for this purpose.

Potassium citrate: 75 mg/kg PO every 12 hours initially; titrate dose to achieve a urine pH of approximately 7.5.

Thiazide diuretics:

Chlorothiazide: 4.5–9 mg/kg PO every 12 hours

Hydrochlorothiazide: 0.5–1 mg/kg PO every 12 hours

Pyridoxine (vitamin B_6):

Dogs: 25–50 mg PO every 24 hours.

13.11.2 Infectious Cystitis

UTIs are typically bacterial in nature; how-ever, occasionally parasitic, viral, and fungal infections do occur. The urinary tract is in contact with the external environment, and bacteria normally reside in the distal urogen-ital tract. Development of a UTI depends on a balance between the infectious agent and host resistance. As is the case with human patients, a UTI can be simple or uncomplicated in nature or complicated. Additionally, asymptomatic bacteriuria occurs.

13.11.2.1 Bacterial UTI

Bacterial UTI has been estimated to occur in 2–3% of dogs, with female dogs more likely to be affected than male dogs (Pressler and Bartges 2010). The incidence of bacterial UTI in cats is not known; however, in cats younger than 10 years of age, only 1–4% of cats with lower urinary tract signs have a bacterial UTI, while in cats older than 10 years of age, bacterial UTI occurs in 40–45% of cats with lower urinary tract

signs. Bacterial UTI may be diagnosed on routine urinalysis, but aerobic microbiologi-cal culture with susceptibility testing is the gold standard. As with human beings, *E. coli* is the most common isolate from dogs and cats with bacterial UTI, accounting for approximately 40–60% of isolates. Gram-positive cocci, e.g. *Staphylococcus* spp. and *Enterococcus* spp., are next most common, accounting for 25–35% of isolates; other organisms account for the remaining (e.g. *Proteus* spp. and *Klebsiella* spp.). Treatment of symptomatic bacterial UTI depends on identifying and correcting the break(s) in host defenses and appropriate antimicrobial therapy (drug, dose, duration, etc.) based on whether the bacterial UTI is simple or com-plicated in nature (Weese et al. 2011, 2015).

Dramatic difference

There is one major difference in the classifi-cation of UTIs as complicated or uncompli-cated in veterinary patients compared to human patients. Bacterial UTIs are consid-ered complicated if they occur in reproduc-tively intact dogs (especially males, where prostatic infection may be present).

Additionally, bacterial UTI in cats is con-sidered complicated, as cats are innately resistant to bacterial UTI. Other factors in the classification scheme are similar between species, such as identifiable defects in sys-temic or local host defenses, or recurrent bacterial UTI.

Conventionally, a simple bacterial UTI is treated for 10–14 days with an antimicrobial agent based on an empiric choice or on results of aerobic microbiological culture and susceptibility results. Empirically, amox-icillin or trimethoprim–sulfamethoxazole may be administered based on the fact that *E. coli* is the most common isolate. There is evidence that a three-day course of enroflox-acin, a veterinary-specific fluoroquinolone, is no less effective than a 14-day course of amoxicillin–clavulanic acid (Westropp et al. 2012). Treatment of a complicated bacterial

Table 13.5 Antimicrobial agents commonly used to treat urinary tract infections in dogs and cats, and the dose, route, and mean urine concentration achieved.

Agent	Dose	Mean (SD) urine concentration (micrograms/mL)
Amoxicillin	15 mg/kg PO every 8 hours	202 (93)
Ampicillin	25 mg/kg PO every 8 hours	309 (55)
Cephalexin	18 mg/kg PO every 8 hours	500
Chloramphenicol	*Dog:* 40 mg/kg PO every 8 hours *Cat:* 33 mg/kg PO every 8 hours	124 (40)
Enrofloxacin	*Dog:* 5 mg/kg PO every 12–24 hours *Cat:* 2.5–5 mg/kg every 25 hours	40
Nitrofurantoin	4 mg/kg PO every 8 hours	100
Tetracycline	15 mg/kg PO every 8 hours	138 (35)
Trimethoprim + (sulfamethoxazole or sulfadiazine)	15 mg/kg PO every 12 hours	246

PO, "Per os" (orally); SD, standard deviation.

UTI should be based on results of aerobic microbiological culture and susceptibility testing. Identifying a break in systemic or local host defenses and correcting or controlling it are beneficial and should be pursued. Examples of breaks in systemic host defenses include diabetes mellitus, hyperadrenocorticism, and chronic kidney disease; examples of breaks in local host defenses include urolithiasis, urinary bladder cancer, and vaginal disease. Conventionally, complicated bacterial UTI is treated for three to six weeks and sometimes longer, depending on the patient. There is evidence that for UTIs not causing clinical signs, withholding treatment may be warranted since, in some studies, more than 80% of asymptomatic bacteriuria will resolve without treatment. The incidence of asymptomatic bacteriuria is 10–15% in older cats and up to 25% in morbidly obese dogs. Antimicrobial treatment failure may be due to: (i) inappropriate drug, dose, or duration of therapy; (ii) failure of antimicrobial agent to reach sufficient concentration at site of infection; (iii) presence of nidus of infection that is capable of recolonizing the urinary tract once antimicrobial therapy is withdrawn; (iv) presence of anatomical or functional abnormalities of the urinary tract that lower resistance to bacterial colonization; and/or (v) misdiagnosis of bacterial UTI (Table 13.5).

Practiced but not proven

There are no controlled studies evaluating the outcomes of treatment or no treatment of asymptomatic bacteriuria in dogs and cats.

Dramatic difference

Conventionally, a 10–14-day course of antimicrobial agent is administered to dogs and cats with uncomplicated bacterial UTI on the belief that the infection may be deep-seated when compared with more conventional three-day courses of antimicrobial agents in human beings with uncomplicated UTI.

Prevention of bacterial UTI encompasses several elements, starting with avoiding or minimizing conditions that impair host defenses. Some veterinarians prescribe prophylactic antimicrobial therapy that involves either a therapeutic dosage of an antimicrobial agent for one out of every four weeks or administering a subtherapeutic dosage of an antimicrobial agent (typically one-third to one-half of the therapeutic dosage) at night after the pet has urinated. There are no data to support the efficacy of either approach, and there is a risk of inducing antimicrobial resistance. Other drugs sometimes prescribed for preventing UTI include methenamine or nitrofurantoin. Methenamine, which is not FDA approved for veterinary use, is a cyclic hydrocarbon that is hydrolyzed to formaldehyde at a urine pH less than 6.5. It is formulated in combination with an acidifier (either hippurate or mendelate). It is effective against many organisms except urease-producing organisms, as they induce alkaluria, which interferes with drug activation. Methenamine may induce metabolic acidosis and should not be used in patients who have or are at risk of metabolic acidosis. Nitrofurantoin is not used often in veterinary medicine, primarily due to the risk of adverse effects (see Section 13.12), but many organisms are susceptible. Attempts to improve host defenses in female dogs may involve hormone replacement therapy with estrogen in order to address recurrent vagocystitis. Estrogens may increase uroepithelial turnover, thereby decreasing bacterial counts in the distal urogenital tract as well as increase urethral tone. There are no data documenting the effectiveness of estrogens in preventing recurrent UTI. Urinary acifidiers are often recommended for prevention of bacterial UTI in both human and veterinary patients; however, bacteria can survive in pH values of 4.0–9.0, and dogs and cats cannot acidify urine to less than 5.5. One mechanism of bacterial antimicrobial resistance is production of biofilm by the bacteria. Clarithromycin is a macrolide antimicrobial agent that has been shown to degrade biofilm, thereby exposing the bacterial community to antimicrobial agents in urine. It often causes emesis in dogs and cats and should be administered with an antiemetic.

Methenamine:

Hippurate:
Dog: 500 mg PO every 12 hours
Cat: 250 mg PO every 12 hours
Mendelate: 10–20 mg/kg PO every 6–12 hours

Nitrofurantoin: 3–4 mg/kg PO every 24 hours
Estrogen:
Estriol: Dogs only: 1 mg PER DOG PO every 24 hours for 7 days. If incontinence is not resolved, increase to 2 mg PER DOG every 24 hours for 7 days. Do not exceed 2 mg in a 24-hour period. If initial 1 mg dose is successful, reduce to 0.5 mg PER DOG every 24 hours for 7 days. Once effective daily dose is established, decreasing dose frequency to every 48 hours or 72 hours may be attempted. If no response to 2 mg PER DOG every 24 hours, the diagnosis should be reconsidered.

Diethylstilbesterol:
Dogs: Initially, 0.1–1 mg PER DOG PO every 24 hours for 5 days, then decrease to once every 4–14 days.
Cats: 0.5 mg PO every 24 hours for 5 days, then decrease to once every 4–14 days.
Conjugated estrogens (e.g. Premarin): Dogs only:
Small breeds (1–40 lbs.): One 0.9 mg tablet PER DOG PO every 24 hours for 7 days, then 1 tablet PO every 7–14 days
Large breeds (greater than 40 lbs.): One 1.25 mg tablet PER DOG PO every 24 hours for 7 days, then 1 table PO every 7–14 days.

Bacteria are the most common cause of cystitis in dogs and cats; however, occasionally, viral, fungal, and parasitic cystitis occurs. There are no known treatments for viral cystitis; therefore, they will not be discussed further here. Treatment of fungal infections is discussed in Chapter 9.

13.11.2.2 Parasitic UTI

While extremely rare in human medicine in North America, filarial parasitic infections do occur in veterinary patients. There are several parasites associated with lower urinary tract signs in dogs and cats. *Capillaria pica* and *Capillaria felis-cati* are small thread-like

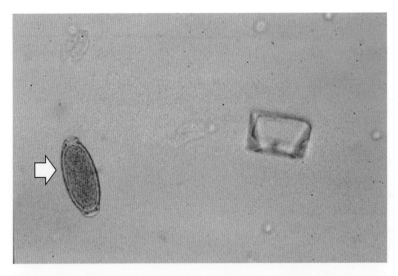

Figure 13.6 Capillaria egg (arrow) in urine sediment from a cat.

yellowish parasites that live within the lumen of the urinary bladder (Figure 13.6). Most dogs and cats with urinary capillariasis are asymptomatic but may develop lower urinary tract signs. Treatment of urinary capillariasis is unwarranted if asymptomatic. A single dose of ivermectin has been effective in some dogs. Prolonged treatment with albendazole was effective in 85% of dogs.

Ivermectin: Dogs: 0.2 mg/kg injected subcutaneously one time. Do not administer this dose to dogs or cats with MDR1 polymorphisms (see Chapters 5 and 7).

Albendazole: 50 mg/kg PO every 12 hours for 30 days (cats may experience neurological adverse effects with albendazole).

13.11.3 Idiopathic Cystitis

Some cats have an idiopathic inflammatory cystitis analogous to interstitial cystitis in human beings. It tends to occur in young adult cats (Forrester and Towell 2015). There are two current hypotheses concerning the etiopathogenesis of feline idiopathic cystitis: a cell-associated viral UTI (Kruger and Osborne 1990) or centrally mediated neurogenic inflammation (Westropp and Tony Buffington 2004). Clinical signs of feline idiopathic cystitis are similar to those caused by

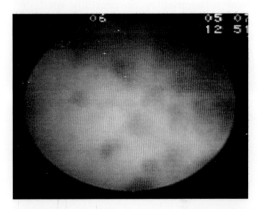

Figure 13.7 Glomerulations (pinpoint hemorrhages) visualized by cystoscopy in the bladder of a cat with feline idiopathic cystitis.

other lower urinary tract diseases. Diagnostic testing reveals hematuria, inflammation in the urinary bladder wall, occasionally urinary bladder mucosal ulcers (called Hunner's ulcers in human interstitial cystitis), and pinpoint hemorrhages (called glomerulations) of the urinary bladder mucosa visualized by cystoscopy (Figure 13.7). It is considered idiopathic because a specific cause for the lesions or clinical signs has not been identified in affected patients. The diagnosis of feline idiopathic cystitis is made by exclusion of other causes (e.g. uroliths, bacterial UTI, or cancer). Feline idiopathic cystitis exists in two forms. The acute self-limiting form accounts for approximately 90% of cases. Clinical signs are acute in onset and resolve within seven days regardless of treatment. The chronic form, characterized by highly recurrent episodes or persistent clinical signs, accounts for approximately 10% of cases (Figure 13.7).

Many treatments have been proposed; however, very few have been evaluated in randomized controlled clinical trials. Because the disease is often acute and self-limiting, resolving within seven days regardless of treatment, response to proposed treatments in uncontrolled studies is difficult to accurately determine. Drugs used to treat feline idiopathic cystitis are aimed at addressing either local inflammation or centrally mediated inflammation (stress/anxiety). The most commonly prescribed drugs used to treat feline idiopathic cystitis will be briefly discussed here. Most are drugs that are FDA approved for human patients and used in an extra-label manner in cats. Although antimicrobial agents are often prescribed, UTIs are uncommon because young adult cats are innately resistant to bacterial UTIs – and if a bacterial UTI were present, then the diagnosis of feline idiopathic cystitis would be excluded. Urinary antiseptics and analgesics (such as methenamine and phenazopyridine) should not be dispensed to cats due to adverse events, including vomiting, diarrhea, anorexia, and hemolytic anemia. Antispasmodics such as propantheline or alpha-adrenergic sympatholytic agents such as phenoxybenzamine or prazosin are often prescribed for cats with acute feline idiopathic cystitis, even though there are no data to support their efficacy. Propantheline is an anticholinergic agent that decreases bladder contraction, while phenoxybenzamine and prazosin decrease spasm of the smooth muscle of the proximal urethra (Barsanti et al. 1982). Skeletal muscle relaxants, such as diazepam and dantrolene, may be prescribed to decrease spasm of the skeletal muscle of the mid to distal urethra; however, only dantrolene has been documented to decrease skeletal muscle urethral tone (Straeter-Knowlen et al. 1995). In addition to sedation, diazepam may induce hepatic necrosis in cats (see Section 13.12).

Anti-inflammatory agents may be prescribed to cats with feline idiopathic cystitis despite lack of evidence of efficacy. Prednisolone did not decrease duration of clinical signs or time to resolution of hematuria in cats with feline idiopathic cystitis in a placebo-controlled randomized clinical trial. There are no studies evaluating NSAIDs for treatment of feline idiopathic cystitis. Amitriptyline, a tricyclic antidepressant that may stabilize mast cells, decrease inflammation, and have analgesic properties, is used in women with idiopathic cystitis. One uncontrolled study in cats with chronic feline idiopathic cystitis showed improvement in clinical signs in 9 of 15 cats, while another study of cats with acute feline idiopathic cystitis showed an improvement in clinical signs but an increase in recurrence rates in cats treated with amitriptyline compared with placebo-treated cats (Chew et al. 1998; Kruger et al. 2003).

Glycosaminoglycans are beneficial for approximately 35% of women with idiopathic cystitis versus 9% receiving placebo. There are two placebo-controlled randomized clinical trials evaluating glycosaminoglycans in cats with feline idiopathic cystitis. One study evaluated pentosan polysulfate, a polysulfated glycosaminoglycan, which was not found to be more efficacious than placebo (Gunn-Moore and Shenoy 2004; Chew et al. 2009). Another study evaluated glucosamine and yielded similar results. Anecdotally, however, there are some cats with chronic feline idiopathic cystitis that appear to benefit from pentosan administration.

Behavior-modifying drugs (Chapter 16) such as fluoxetine and clomipramine are used to treat cats with inappropriate urination (i.e. cats that urinate outside the litterbox or on furniture, carpet, clothing, etc.), although these drugs have not been evaluated in cats with feline idiopathic cystitis. Feline facial pheromones in the form of sprays and diffusers are also used for behavior modification in cats. One study evaluated facial pheromones for cats with feline idiopathic cystitis, but a benefit was not detected (Gunn-Moore and Cameron 2004). Because of the association of acute episodes of feline idiopathic cystitis with stress, environmental modification to decrease stressors (Chapter 16) may be beneficial in some cats.

Practiced but not proven

Most recommended treatments for feline idiopathic cystitis have not been evaluated in placebo-controlled clinical trials, and those that have been evaluated have not been shown to be more effective than placebo.

Amitriptyline: 0.5–1 mg/kg PO every 24 hours

Clomipramine: 0.25–0.5 mg/kg PO every 24 hours

Dantrolene: 0.5–2 mg/kg PO every 8–12 hours

Diazepam: 1–5 mg PO every 8–12 hours

Fluoxetine: 0.5–1 mg/kg PO every 24 hours

Glucosamine: 125 mg PO every 24 hours

Pentosan polysulfate: Approximately 8 mg/kg PO every 12 hours

Phenoxybenzamine: 2.5–7.5 mg PER CAT PO every 8 hours

Prazosin: 0.25–1 mg/kg PO every 8–24 hours

Propantheline: 0.25–0.5 mg/kg PO every 8–12 hours.

13.11.4 Micturition Disorders

The function of the lower urinary tract involves urine retention and urine expulsion; micturition is the consciously controlled reflex of urine expulsion. Disorders of micturition may involve either abnormal urine retention or urine leakage (Fischer and Lane 2011). General principles of lower urinary tract function are: (i) the urinary bladder and urethra normally function opposite to each other, that is, when the urinary bladder is relaxed, the urethra is contracted, and vice versa; (ii) micturition is a reflex involving autonomic nervous system control of smooth muscle; (iii) smooth muscle

of the urinary bladder is predominantly under parasympathetic control, while urethral smooth muscle (internal urethral sphincter) is predominantly under sympathetic control; (iv) micturition is consciously controlled with the mid to distal urethra, composed of skeletal muscle under somatic nervous system control; and (v) in general terms, parasympathetic tone promotes peeing, while sympathetic tone promotes storage.

13.11.4.1 Urine Retention

Inappropriate retention of urine occurs with either decreased bladder function (detrusor atony) or increased urethral tone (functional or mechanical) (Lane 2000). Bladder atony may be due to neurogenic and/or myogenic causes. Overdistension of the urinary bladder disrupts tight junctions between myocytes, resulting in bladder atony. Neurogenic bladder atony can be caused by central neurologic lesions (e.g. due to trauma or neoplasia) above the proximal lumbar spinal cord. Treatment of an atonic urinary bladder involves keeping the urinary bladder empty with urinary catheterization and stimulating bladder contraction using a parasympathomimetic drug, bethanechol. When bethanechol is used, a urethral relaxant, such as phenoxybenzamine or prazosin, should be administered to promote urine expulsion.

Urethral outflow obstruction resulting in urine retention may be either functional or mechanical in nature. Functional urethral obstruction is often due to a spinal cord lesion above the proximal lumbar region. Alpha-adrenergic receptor antagonists and sometimes skeletal muscle relaxants are prescribed to relax the urethra. Tamsulosin, approved for use in human medicine as an alpha-adrenergic antagonist, is being used with increased frequency in veterinary patients with urinary retention. Acepromazine, a veterinary-approved drug, is a phenothiazine tranquilizer that also has alpha-adrenergic antagonistic effects and can be used to relax urethral smooth muscle. Baclofen is approved for use in human medicine as a skeletal muscle relaxant. While it can be prescribed for dogs with urinary retention, it should not be used in cats. Reflex dyssynergia refers to a syndrome whereby a patient begins urination with a normal stream, but during urination the stream decreases to drops or stops completely, implying premature closure of the urethral sphincter before the urinary bladder is emptied. Treatment involves relaxing the urethra with alpha-adrenergic receptor antagonists and possibly skeletal muscle relaxants. Some dogs with this condition develop partial or complete detrusor atony due to chronic urine retention, so bethanechol may be prescribed concurrently.

Mechanical urethral obstruction may occur with urethroliths, strictures, or neoplasia. Neoplastic disease occurs more commonly in dogs than in cats (Cannon and Allstadt 2015). In dogs, transitional cell carcinoma often occurs in female dogs, while prostatic carcinoma occurs in male dogs (Henry 2003). There are several chemotherapeutic protocols that may be tried for these patients (see Chapter 20). Most patients with transitional cell carcinoma will be treated with an NSAID because urinary carcinomas often express cyclooxygenase-2. Piroxicam is most commonly prescribed (Knapp et al. 1994); however, others may be used as well. In addition to pharmacotherapy, placement of a cystostomy tube or a urethral stent may be employed.

13.11.4.2 Urine Leakage

Inability to retain urine may be caused by decreased bladder capacity, decreased urethral tone, or a congenital anomaly (Byron 2015). Congenital anomalies include ectopic ureter and urethral hypoplasia, among others. Congenital anatomic abnormalities are managed using an appropriate intervention, whether surgical or a minimally invasive approach such as laser ablation of an ectopic ureter.

Bladder hyperexcitability results in an involuntary inability to adequately store urine (e.g. cystitis and urocystolithiasis). The treatment approach is to relax bladder smooth muscle using parasympatholyic or antispasmodic agents, such as propantheline, oxybutynin, or flavoxate. Each of these drugs is approved for

use in human medicine but used in an extra-label manner in veterinary patients. Tricyclic antidepressants may improve urinary bladder storage through several mechanisms, including anticholinergic, alpha-adrenergic, and beta-adrenergic effects. Amitriptyline has been prescribed most commonly in veterinary medicine, but other tricyclic antidepressants may also be used.

Urine leakage may also occur due to urethral sphincter mechanism incompetency. Incontinence in women is most often stress incontinence, while in men it is most often due to prostatic disease. It occurs rarely in cats. In female dogs, urinary incontinence is most often due to a decrease in internal urethral sphincter tone and pressure. This is a disease of spayed female dogs and is thought to result from alteration in hormonal influences after ovariohysterectomy. Pharmacotherapeutically, estrogens and sympathomimetics are prescribed. Phenylpropanolamine, which has been withdrawn from the market for human use, is FDA approved for use in spayed female dogs with urinary incontinence. It may be associated with behavior changes and systemic arterial hypertension. Estrogens increase receptors for norepinephrine, increase sensitivity of adrenergic receptors to norepinephrine, and increase secretions and folding of the urethra to increase urethral tone. Estrogens can have severe adverse effects if not dosed appropriately (see Section 13.12 on adverse effects). Gonadotropin-releasing hormone analogs may be efficacious in spayed female dogs as well. If medical therapy is ineffective or loses effectiveness, alternative treatments include cystoscopic urethral bulking and surgical implantation of a hydraulic urethral occluder.

Acepromazine: 0.01–0.05 mg/kg IV, IM, or SC or 0.5–2 mg/kg PO as needed

Amitriptyline:

Dogs: 1–2 mg/kg PO every 12–24 hours
Cats: 0.5–1 mg/kg PO every 24 hours

Baclofen: Dogs: 1–2 mg/kg PO every 8 hours or 5–10 mg PER DOG every 8 hours

Bethanechol:

Dogs: 5–15 mg PO every 8 hours
Cats: 1.25–7.5 mg PO every 8 hours

Clomipramine:

Dogs: 1–2 mg/kg PO every 12 hours for 2 weeks, then 3 mg/kg PO every 24 hours if needed
Cats: 0.25–0.5 mg/kg PO every 24 hours

Dantrolene:

Dogs: 1–5 mg/kg PO every 8 hours
Cats: 0.5–2 mg/kg PO every 8–12 hours

Diazepam:

Dogs: 2–10 mg PO every 8 hours
Cats: 1–5 mg PO every 8–12 hours

Estrogens:
Estriol: Dogs only: 1 mg PER DOG PO every 24 hours for 7 days. If unsuccessful, increase to 2 mg PER DOG every 24 hours for 7 days. Do not exceed 2 mg PER DOG in a 24-hour time period. If initial 1 mg dose is successful, reduce to 0.5 mg PER DOG every 24 hours for 7 days. Once effective daily dose is established, dose interval should be extended to every 48 or 72 hours if possible. Minimum dose should not be less than 0.5 mg PER DOG. If no response to 2 mg per dog every 24 hours, the diagnosis should be reconsidered (e.g. it could be a neurological disorder or bladder neoplasia).
Diethylstilbesterol:
Dogs: Initially, 0.1–1 mg PER DOG PO every 24 hours for 5 days, then decrease to every 4–14 days (longest interval that adequately controls signs)
Cats: 0.5 mg PER CAT PO every 24 hours for 5 days, then decrease to every 4–14 days (longest interval that adequately controls signs)
Conjugated estrogens: Dogs only:
Small breeds (1–40 lbs.): 1 tablet (0.9 mg/tablet) PO q24h for 7 days, then 1 tablet PO q7–14d
Large breeds (greater than 40 lbs.): 1 tablet (1.25 mg/tablet) PO q24h for 7 days, then 1 tablet PO q7–14d

Flavoxate: Dogs: 100–200 mg PER DOG PO every 6–8 hours
Fluoxetine:

Dogs: 1–2 mg/kg PO every 24 hours
Cats: 0.5–1 mg/kg PO every 24 hours

Imipramine:

Dogs: 5–20 mg PER DOG PO every 12 hours
Cats: 2.5–5 mg PER CAT PO every 12 hours

Oxybutinin: 0.1–0.2 mg/kg PO every 8–12 hours
Pentosan polysulfate: Approximately 8 mg/kg PO every 12 hours
Phenylpropanolamine: Dogs only: 1–2.2 mg/kg PO every 8–24 hours
Prazosin:

Dogs: 0.07 mg/kg PO every 8–24 hours
Cats: 0.25–1 mg PER CAT PO every 8–24 hours

Propantheline: Dogs and cats: 0.25–0.5 mg/kg PO every 8–24 hours
Phenoxybenzamine:

Dogs: 5–15 mg PER DOG PO every 8 hours
Cats: 2.5–7.5 mg PER CAT PO every 8 hours

Piroxicam:

Dogs: 0.3 mg/kg PO every 24 hours
Cats: 0.3 mg/kg PO every 48–72 hours

Tamsulosin:

Dogs: 0.1 mg per 10 kg body weight PO every 12–24 hours or 0.4–0.8 mg PER DOG PO every 12–24 hours
Cats: 0.004–0.006 mg/kg (4–6 micrograms per kg) PO every 12–24 hours.

13.11.5 Prostate Disease

Prostatic disease is uncommon in veterinary medicine because many dogs, at least in the USA, are castrated (Johnston et al. 2000). Cats have prostatic tissue but rarely have disease. Intact male dogs are prone to bacterial prostatitis and benign prostatic hypertrophy. When castrated male dogs are affected by prostatic disease, it is usually prostatic cancer rather than infection or benign prostatic hyperplasia (BPH).

BPH is an increase in epithelial cell number and size in intact male dogs. It begins in dogs as young as 2.5 years of age. Scottish terriers have a prostate that is four times larger than that of other dogs of similar body weight. Approximately 30% of dogs with BPH have hematuria, and if the prostate enlarges to a sufficient size, urethral obstruction and tenesmus may occur. Castration is curative, and there is a 50% reduction in prostate size within three weeks, with complete atrophy by four to six months. If castration is not feasible, the human drug finasteride, a 5 alpha-reductase inhibitor, which is the final enzyme in the synthetic pathway for dihydrotestosterone, results in reduction of prostate size and resolution of clinical signs within two to four weeks, with no apparent side effects and no effect on sperm quantity or quality (Sirinarumitr et al. 2001). The human drug flutamide, an anti-androgen, may also be effective but has been used infrequently in veterinary medicine (Frank et al. 2004). Progestins, such as megesterol acetate, have been used but are not advised due to a high incidence of complications, such as feminization and diabetes mellitus.

Finasteride: 0.5–1 mg/kg PO every 24 hours
Flutamide: 5 mg/kg PO every 24 hours.

Acute and chronic prostatitis are inflammatory diseases of the prostate gland that are usually caused by bacterial infection (Smith 2008). Bacterial prostatitis is most commonly caused by *E. coli*. Other potential causative organisms include *Staphylococcus* spp., *Klebsiella* spp., and *Proteus* spp. *Brucella canis* is associated with prostatitis in dogs and is a zoonotic organism. Male dogs with acute prostatitis usually act sick and are febrile with an enlarged and painful prostate. Male dogs with chronic prostatitis typically have a history of recurrent hematuria and cystitis but are not typically systemically ill. Prostatic infection may develop into a prostatic abscess at any time and may cause sepsis. Treatment of acute prostatitis includes supportive care and appropriate antimicrobial therapy based on culture and susceptibility. Empiric treatment should consist of an antimicrobial drug effective against *E. coli*. Adequate penetration of the antimicrobial into the prostate may be limited by the blood–prostate barrier; however, with acute prostatitis, the barrier is disrupted, and most antimicrobials are able to penetrate adequately. Chronic bacterial prostatitis is more difficult to treat because the barrier is intact. Antimicrobials that are lipid soluble, are not highly protein bound, and ionize at the pH of prostate tissue will penetrate and be retained within the prostate. Most antimicrobial agents do not penetrate abscesses well, so abscesses must be surgically drained in order to treat them effectively. Because *E. coli* is the most common inciting organism, fluoroquinolones are the first line of therapy, followed by potentiated sulfonamides.

Prostatic neoplasia is usually epithelial in origin (i.e. a carcinoma), although other cell types occur (Argyle 2009). Prostatic adenocarcinoma is malignant, and the presence of metastasis is often detected by the time a diagnosis is made. Prostatectomy is not an option, typically due to resultant urinary incontinence (Basinger et al. 1987). Radiation therapy, especially stereotactic or intensity-modulated, is the treatment of choice. Chemotherapy may be attempted, as with other urothelial neoplasias (Chapter 20). Dogs with prostate cancer may require treatment with an alpha-adrenergic receptor antagonist to improve urethral urine flow. If urethral obstruction occurs, urethral stenting can be performed.

13.12 Adverse Effects in Veterinary Species

Most of the potential adverse events associated with use of the pharmacotherapeutic agents mentioned in this chapter are the same as those that can occur in human patients. This section will primarily focus on adverse effects that either are unique to or may be more severe in veterinary patients. Additionally, since veterinary patients cannot verbally convey symptoms of adverse drug reactions, this section will discuss clinical signs to watch for, so that pharmacists can counsel and help pet owners to monitor for adverse effects. For example, parasympathomimetics such as bethanechol may cause gastrointestinal symptoms such as cramping/pain and clinical signs such as diarrhea. Abdominal pain in dogs and cats may manifest as a decrease in the pet's level of activity, decreased appetite, abdominal splinting, or aggression. Sympathomimetics may be associated with systemic arterial hypertension, while sympatholytics may be associated with hypotension.

Bisphosphonates: Aledronate, like other bisphosphonates, has been associated with esophagitis and bone necrosis in human patients. The FDA has set forth strict dosing and administration guidelines for these drugs in human patients that involve measures to ensure that the drug passes through the esophagus to the stomach (i.e. drinking 6–8 ounces of water with the tablet, and avoiding lying down for 60 minutes for gravitational assistance). Because they are not FDA approved for use in dogs and cats, there are no administration guidelines for bisphosphonates in these species. Canine and feline anatomy increases the risk of retaining the drug in the esophagus, since it is oriented horizontally rather than vertically as in humans. The pharmacist can play a key role in preventing serious esophageal complications in dogs and cats by educating their owners on the importance of ensuring the animal drinks a sufficient volume of water after drug administration.

Diazepam: Although uncommon, oral administration of diazepam to some cats can cause fulminant hepatic necrosis. Clinical signs (inappetence, vomiting, and jaundice) were noted within the first two weeks of treatment (Center et al. 1996).

Estrogens: Estrogens are generally well tolerated in dogs and cats; however, high doses in dogs can results in life-threatening myelotoxicity or pyometra. Clinical signs of myelosuppression can be vague (e.g. inappetence and depression) or more explicitly related to anemia (pale mucous membranes), thrombocytopenia (petechial hemorrhages,

epistaxis, and vaginal bleeding), or neutropenia (fever and sepsis). Refer to Appendix C for additional information on monitoring parameters for veterinary species. Pyometra (literal translation is "pus in the uterus") can be fatal if not addressed rapidly. Intact female dogs (and occasionally spayed female dogs with residual uterine tissue) are susceptible; they should be monitored for inappetence, fever, and depression, and they often have a purulent to hemorrhagic vaginal discharge. Pharmacists should urge pet owners to seek immediate veterinary care if either of these complications from estrogen treatment is suspected.

Nitrofurantoin: At therapeutic dosages, adverse events occur commonly and include gastrointestinal upset, hepatopathy, blood dyscrasias, and peripheral neuropathy that resolve with drug discontinuance.

Potassium citrate: Potassium citrate may be associated with gastrointestinal signs (hyporexia, anorexia, vomiting, and/or diarrhea). This appears to be associated with the form of potassium citrate administered rather than the dose. If adverse effects occur with potassium citrate, switching to a different formulation often helps.

Thiazide diuretics: Potential adverse events associated with thiazide diuretics include dehydration and electrolyte imbalances, the most likely of which is hypercalcemia. Therefore, serum/plasma calcium concentration should be monitored. An important difference for pharmacists to keep in mind for veterinary versus human patients is that veterinary patients cannot communicate early symptoms of hypercalcemia. Pharmacist should educate owners to monitor for inappetence, weakness, and lethargy.

Urinary antiseptics and analgesics: Methenamine can cause severe gastrointestinal signs in cats, so it should not be used in that species. Phenazopyridine can cause severe oxidative damage to feline erythrocytes, resulting in methemoglobinemia and hemolysis. Hepatic toxicity is also a potential risk in cats. Phenazopyridine should never be administered to cats.

13.13 Nutritional Supplements for Veterinary Lower Urinary Tract Disease

A number of nutritional supplements are promoted for use in veterinary renal and lower urinary tract disease. Some of these compounds and products are briefly described in this section.

13.13.1 Urinary Tract Infection

Cranberry extract that contains proanthocyanidins may prevent adhesion of bacteria to uroepithelium by binding to the PapG pilli of bacteria that is present in 25–50% of canine *E. coli*. Since not all bacteria express this urovirulence factor, proanthocyanidins may be of no benefit in the majority of canine UTIs. Proanthocyanidins from cranberry are often used for management of bacterial UTIs, although there are minimal data to support their use in dogs or cats.

D-mannose is a sugar that binds to glycosaminoglycans of *E. coli*. By doing so, the bacteria are purported to lack the ability to adhere to the urinary tract and bladder. D-mannose has shown some benefit in rodent models of bacterial UTI and in some human patients, but it has not been sufficiently evaluated in veterinary patients.

Cranberry extract: Approximately 1 mg/kg of proanthocyanidin per kg body weight PO every 24 hours

D-mannose: Approximately 15 mg/kg PO every 12 hours.

13.13.2 Feline Idiopathic Cystitis

The only treatment shown to have efficacy in cats with feline idiopathic cystitis is dietary modification (enhanced omega-3 fatty acids and antioxidants) in conjunction with alpha-casozepine. This protocol decreased recurrence rates by approximately 90% (Lulich et al. 2013). Alpha-casozepine is an extract from casein and has been shown to have a calming effect in cats, potentially decreasing centrally mediated bladder inflammation and pain.

Alpha-casozepine: Cats: 75 mg PO every 24 hours.

Glycosaminoglycans are often recommended for management of cats with idiopathic cystitis; however, there are no data to support their use.

Glucosamine: 125 mg PO every 24 hours.

13.13.3 Benign Prostatic Hyperplasia

Phytotherapies such as saw palmetto, which is highly touted for BPH in men, is not effective in male dogs (Barsanti et al. 2000).

13.13.4 Miscellaneous

Ecotherapeutics include probiotics, prebiotics, and symbiotics (a combination of probiotics and prebiotics). They change the gastrointestinal microbiota, which induces changes in whole-body metabolism and immune function. Although they are not associated with adverse events, there are no data to support their efficacy for renal or lower urinary tract disease in dogs and cats. There are dog- and cat-specific probiotics; however, there are no data that a species-specific probiotic is necessary, and many veterinarians use human probiotics due to the increased number of organisms and strains present in human probiotic products.

13.14 FDA-Approved Veterinary Drug Products with No Human Drug Equivalent

Brand name	Active ingredient(s)	Drug class	Rationale/ notes
Proin	Phenylpropanolamine	Sympathomimetic	Used for urinary incontinence. May induce systemic arterial hypertension
Incurin	Estriol	Reproductive hormone	Only FDA-approved estrogen for use in spayed female dogs with urinary incontinence

References

Adams, L.G., Berent, A.C., Moore, G.E. et al. (2008). Use of laser lithotripsy for fragmentation of uroliths in dogs: 73 cases (2005–2006). *J. Am. Vet. Med. Assoc.* 232 (11): 1680–1687.

Adin, C.A. and Cowgill, L.D. (2000). Treatment and outcome of dogs with leptospirosis: 36 cases (1990–1998). *J. Am. Vet. Med. Assoc.* 216 (3): 371–375.

Argyle, D.J. (2009). Prostate cancer in dogs and men: a unique opportunity to study the disease. *Vet. J.* 180 (2): 137–138.

Bannasch, D., Safra, N., Young, A. et al. (2008). Mutations in the SLC2A9 gene cause hyperuricosuria and hyperuricemia in the dog. *PLoS Genet.* 4 (11): e1000246.

Barsanti, J.A., Finco, D.R., Shotts, E.B. et al. (1982). Feline urolgoic syndrome: further investigations into therapy. *J. Am. Anim. Hosp. Assoc.* 18: 387–390.

Barsanti, J.A., Finco, D.R., Mahaffey, M.M. et al. (2000). Effects of an extract of *Serenoa repens* on dogs with hyperplasia of the prostate gland. *Am. J. Vet. Res.* 61 (8): 880–885.

Bartges, J.W. (2000). Diseases of the urinary bladder. In: *Saunders Manual of Small Animal Practice* (ed. S.J. Birchard and R.G. Sherding), 943–957. Philadelphia: WB Saunders.

Bartges, J.W. (2011). Urinary saturation testing. In: *Nephrology and Urology of Small Animals* (ed. J. Bartges and D.J. Polzin), 75–85. Ames, IA: Wiley-Blackwell.

Bartges, J.W. (2012). Chronic kidney disease in dogs and cats. *Vet. Clin. North Am. Small Anim. Pract.* 42 (4): 669–692, vi.

Bartges, J.W. and Callens, A.J. (2015). Urolithiasis. *Vet. Clin. North Am. Small Anim. Pract.* 45 (4): 747–768.

Bartges J, Moyers T. (2010). Evaluation of d,l-methionine and antimicrobial agents for dissolution of spontaneously-occurring infection-induced struvite urocystoliths in dogs. Paper presented at the ACVIM Forum, Anaheim, CA.

Bartges, J.W., Osborne, C.A., and Pozin, D.J. (1992). Recurrent sterile struvite urocystolithiasis in three related Cocker Spaniels. *J. Am. Anim. Hosp. Assoc.* 28: 459–469.

Bartges, J.W., Willis, A.M., and Pozin, D.J. (1996). Hypertension and renal disease. *Vet. Clin. North Am. Small Anim. Pract.* 26 (6): 1331–1345.

Bartges JW, Cornelius LM, Osborne CA (eds). (1999a). Ammonium urate uroliths in dogs with portosystemic shunts. In *Current Veterinary Therapy XIII*, Bartges JW, Cornelius LM, Osborne CA (eds). WB Saunders, Philadelphia.

Bartges, J.W., Osborne, C.A., Lulich, J.P. et al. (1999b). Canine urate urolithiasis. Etiopathogenesis, diagnosis, and management. *Vet. Clin. North Am. Small Anim. Pract.* 29 (1): 161–191, xii–xiii.

Bartges, J.W., Kirk, C., and Lane, I.F. (2004). Update: management of calcium oxalate uroliths in dogs and cats. *Vet. Clin. North Am. Small Anim. Pract.* 34 (4): 969–987, vii.

Bartges, J.W., Kirk, C.A., Cox, S.K. et al. (2013). Influence of acidifying or alkalinizing diets on bone mineral density and urine relative supersaturation with calcium oxalate and struvite in healthy cats. *Am. J. Vet. Res.* 74 (10): 1347–1352.

Bartges, J.W., Sura, P.S., and Callens, A. (2014). Minilaparotomy-assisted cystotomy. In: *Current Veterinary Therapy XV* (ed. J.D. Bonagura and E.C. Feldman), 905–909. St. Louis, MO: Saunders-Elsevier.

Basinger, R.R., Rawlings, C.A., Barsanti, J.A. et al. (1987). Urodynamic alterations after prostatectomy in dogs without clinical prostatic disease. *Vet. Surg.* 16 (6): 405–410.

Brons, A.K., Henthorn, P.S., Raj, K. et al. (2013). SLC3A1 and SLC7A9 mutations in autosomal recessive or dominant canine cystinuria: a new classification system. *J. Vet. Intern. Med.* 27 (6): 1400–1408.

Brown, C.A., Elliott, J., Schmiedt, C.W. et al. (2016). Chronic kidney disease in aged cats: clinical features, morphology, and proposed pathogenesis. *Vet. Pathol.* 53 (2): 309–326.

Byron, J.K. (2015). Micturition disorders. *Vet. Clin. North Am. Small Anim. Pract.* 45 (4): 769–782.

Cannon, C.M. and Allstadt, S.D. (2015). Lower urinary tract cancer. *Vet. Clin. North Am. Small Anim. Pract.* 45 (4): 807–824.

Center, S.A., Elston, T.H., Rowland, P.H. et al. (1996). Fulminant hepatic failure associated with oral administration of diezepam in 11 cats. *J. Am. Vet. Med. Assoc.* 209 (3): 618–625.

Chew, D.J., Buffington, C.A., Kendall, M.S. et al. (1998). Amitriptyline treatment for severe recurrent idiopathic cystitis in cats. *J. Am. Vet. Med. Assoc.* 213 (9): 1282–1286.

Chew, D.J., Bartges, J.W., Adams, L.G. et al. (2009). Randomized placebo-controlled clinical trial of pentosan polysulfate sodium for treatment of feline interstitial (idiopathic) cystitis. *J. Vet. Intern. Med.* 23: 690.

Cole, L., Jepson, R., and Humm, K. (2017). Systemic hypertension in cats with acute kidney injury. *J. Small Anim. Pract.* 58 (10): 577–581.

Colombo, D., Banfi, G., Cassano, N. et al. (2017). The GENDER ATTENTION Observational Study: gender and hormonal status differences in the incidence of adverse events during cyclosporine treatment in psoriatic patients. *Adv. Ther.* 34 (6): 1349–1363.

Connally, H.E., Thrall, M.A., Forney, S.D. et al. (1996). Safety and efficacy of 4-methylpyrazole for treatment of suspected or confirmed ethylene glycol intoxication in dogs: 107 cases (1983–1995). *J. Am. Vet. Med. Assoc.* 209 (11): 1880–1883.

Cowgill, L.D. and Langston, C. (2011). Acute kidney insufficiency. In: *Nephrology and Urology of Small Animals* (ed. J.W. Bartges and D.J. Polzin), 472. Ames, IA: Wiley-Blackwell.

Crow, S.E., Theilen, G.H., Madewell, B.R. et al. (1977). Cyclophosphamide-induced cystitis in the dog and cat. *J. Am. Vet. Med. Assoc.* 171 (3): 259–262.

Dial, S.M., Thrall, M.A., and Hamar, D.W. (1994). Efficacy of 4-methylpyrazole for treatment of ethylene glycol intoxication in dogs. *Am. J. Vet. Res.* 55 (12): 1762–1770.

Fischer, J. and Lane, I.F. (2011). Micturition disorders. In: *Nephrology and Urology of Small Animals* (ed. J.W. Bartges and D.J. Polzin), 755–777. Ames, IA: Wiley-Blackwell.

Flournoy, W.S., Wohl, J.S., Albrecht-Schmitt, T.J. et al. (2003). Pharmacologic identification of putative D1 dopamine receptors in feline kidneys. *J. Vet. Pharmacol. Ther.* 26 (4): 283–290.

Forrester, S.D. and Towell, T.L. (2015). Feline idiopathic cystitis. *Vet. Clin. North Am. Small Anim. Pract.* 45 (4): 783–806.

Frank, D., Sharpe, N., Scott, M.C. et al. (2004). Chronic effects of flutamide in male beagle dogs. *Toxicol. Pathol.* 32 (2): 243–249.

Gunn-Moore, D.A. and Cameron, M.E. (2004). A pilot study using synthetic feline facial pheromone for the management of feline idiopathic cystitis. *J. Feline Med. Surg.* 6 (3): 133–138.

Gunn-Moore, D.A. and Shenoy, C.M. (2004). Oral glucosamine and the management of feline idiopathic cystitis. *J. Feline Med. Surg.* 6 (4): 219–225.

Henry, C.J. (2003). Management of transitional cell carcinoma. *Vet. Clin. North Am. Small Anim. Pract.* 33 (3): 597–613.

Hewlett, T.P., Jacobsen, D., Collins, T.D. et al. (1989). Ethylene glycol and glycolate kinetics in rats and dogs. *Vet. Hum. Toxicol.* 31 (2): 116–120.

Hezel, A., Bartges, J.W., Kirk, C.A. et al. (2007). Influence of hydrochlorothiazide on urinary calcium oxalate relative supersaturation in healthy young adult female domestic shorthaired cats. *Vet. Ther.* 8 (4): 247–254.

Hoppe, A. and Denneberg, T. (2001). Cystinuria in the dog: clinical studies during 14 years of medical treatment. *J. Vet. Intern. Med.* 15 (4): 361–367.

Johnston, S.D., Kamolpatana, K., Root-Kustritz, M.V. et al. (2000). Prostatic disorders in the dog. *Anim. Reprod. Sci.* 60–61: 405–415.

Knapp, D.W., Richardson, R.C., Chan, T.C. et al. (1994). Piroxicam therapy in 34 dogs with transitional cell carcinoma of the urinary bladder. *J. Vet. Intern. Med.* 8 (4): 273–278.

Kruger, J.M. and Osborne, C.A. (1990). The role of viruses in feline lower urinary tract disease. *J. Vet. Intern. Med.* 4 (2): 71–78.

Kruger, J.M., Conway, T.S., Kaneene, J.B. et al. (2003). Randomized controlled trial of the efficacy of short-term amitriptyline administration for treatment of acute, nonobstructive, idiopathic lower urinary tract disease in cats. *J. Am. Vet. Med. Assoc.* 222 (6): 749–758.

Lane, I.F. (2000). Diagnosis and management of urinary retention. *Vet. Clin. North Am. Small Anim. Pract.* 30 (1): 25–57, v.

Lulich, J.P., Osborne, C.A., Lekcharoensuk, C. et al. (2001). Effects of hydrochlorothiazide and diet in dogs with calcium oxalate urolithiasis. *J. Am. Vet. Med. Assoc.* 218 (10): 1583–1586.

Lulich, J.P., Osborne, C.A., and Albasan, H. (2011). Canine and feline urolithiasis: diagnosis, treatment, and prevention. In: *Nephrology and Urology of Small Animals* (ed. J. Bartges and D.J. Polzin), 687–706. West Sussex, UK: Wiley-Blackwell.

Lulich, J.P., Kruger, J.M., Macleay, J.M. et al. (2013). Efficacy of two commercially available, low-magnesium, urine-acidifying dry foods for the dissolution of struvite uroliths in cats. *J. Am. Vet. Med. Assoc.* 243 (8): 1147–1153.

MacDonald, K.A., Kittelson, M.D., Kass, P.H. et al. (2008). Effect of spironolactone on diastolic function and left ventricular mass in Maine Coon cats with familial hypertrophic cardiomyopathy. *J. Vet. Intern. Med.* 22 (2): 335–341.

Nielsen, L.K., Bracker, K., and Price, L.L. (2015). Administration of fenoldopam in critically ill small animal patients with acute kidney injury: 28 dogs and 34 cats (2008–2012). *J. Vet. Emerg. Crit. Care (San Antonio)* 25 (3): 396–404.

O'Neill, K.E., Labato, M.A., and Court, M.H. (2016). The pharmacokinetics of intravenous fenoldopam in healthy, awake cats. *J. Vet. Pharmacol. Ther.* 39 (2): 202–204.

Osborne, C.A., Polzin, D.J., Abdullahi, S.U. et al. (1985). Struvite urolithiasis in animals and man: formation, detection, and dissolution. *Adv. Vet. Sci. Comp. Med.* 29: 1–101.

Osborne, C.A., Lulich, J.P., Polzin, D.J. et al. (1999a). Medical dissolution and prevention

of canine struvite urolithiasis. Twenty years of experience. *Vet. Clin. North Am. Small Anim. Pract.* 29 (1): 73–111, xi.

Osborne, C.A., Sanderson, S.L., Lulich, J.P. et al. (1999b). Canine cystine urolithiasis. Cause, detection, treatment, and prevention. *Vet. Clin. North Am. Small Anim. Pract.* 29 (1): 193–211, xiii.

Palma, D., Langston, C., Gisselman, K. et al. (2009). Feline struvite urolithiasis. *Compend Contin. Educ. Vet.* 31 (12): 542–552.

Palma, D., Langston, C., Gisselman, K. et al. (2013). Canine struvite urolithiasis. *Compend Contin. Educ. Vet.* 35 (8): E1.

Polzin, D.J. (2011). Chronic kidney disease. In: *Nephrology and Urology of Small Animals* (ed. J. Bartges and D.J. Polzin), 433–471. Ames, IA: Wiley-Blackwell.

Pressler, B. and Bartges, J.W. (2010). Urinary tract infection. In: *Textbook of Small Animal Internal Medicine* (ed. S.J. Ettinger and E.C. Feldman), 2036–2047. St. Louis, MO: Elsevier-Saunders.

Riviere, J.E., Hinsman, E.J., Coppoc, G.L. et al. (1981). Single dose gentamicin nephrotoxicity in the dog: early functional and ultrastructural changes. *Res. Commun. Chem. Pathol. Pharmacol.* 33 (3): 403–418.

Ross, L. (2011). Acute kidney injury in dogs and cats. *Vet. Clin. North Am. Small Anim. Pract.* 41 (1): 1–14.

Sirinarumitr, K., Johnston, S.D., Kustritz, M.V. et al. (2001). Effects of finasteride on size of the prostate gland and semen quality in dogs with benign prostatic hypertrophy. *J. Am. Vet. Med. Assoc.* 218 (8): 1275–1280.

Smith, L.H. (1990). The pathophysiology and medical treatment of urolithiasis. *Semin. Nephrol.* 10 (1): 31–52.

Smith, J. (2008). Canine prostatic disease: a review of anatomy, pathology, diagnosis, and treatment. *Theriogenology* 70 (3): 375–383.

Stepien, R.L. (2011). Feline systemic hypertension: diagnosis and management. *J. Feline Med. Surg.* 13 (1): 35–43.

Straeter-Knowlen, I.M., Marks, S.L., Rishniw, M. et al. (1995). Urethral pressure response to smooth and skeletal muscle relaxants in anesthetized, adult male cats with naturally acquired urethral obstruction. *Am. J. Vet. Res.* 56 (7): 919–923.

Sykes, J.E., Hartmann, K., Lunn, K.F. et al. (2011). 2010 ACVIM small animal consensus statement on leptospirosis: diagnosis, epidemiology, treatment, and prevention. *J. Vet. Intern. Med.* 25 (1): 1–13.

Weese, S.J., Blondeau, J.M., Boothe, D. et al. (2011). Antimicrobial use guidelines for treatment of urinary tract disease in dogs and cats: antimicrobial guidelines working group of the International Society for companion animal infectious diseases. *Vet. Med. Int.* 2011: 263768.

Weese, J.S., Giguere, S., Guardabassi, L. et al. (2015). ACVIM consensus statement on therapeutic antimicrobial use in animals and antimicrobial resistance. *J. Vet. Intern. Med.* 29 (2): 487–498.

Westropp, J.L. and Tony Buffington, C.A. (2004). Feline idiopathic cystitis: current understanding of pathophysiology and management. *Vet. Clin. North Am. Small Anim. Pract.* 34 (4): 1043–1055.

Westropp, J.L., Sykes, J.E., Irom, S. et al. (2012). Evaluation of the efficacy and safety of high dose short duration enrofloxacin treatment regimen for uncomplicated urinary tract infections in dogs. *J. Vet. Intern. Med.* 26 (3): 506–512.

Yerramilli, M., Farace, G., Quinn, J. et al. (2016). Kidney disease and the nexus of chronic kidney disease and acute kidney injury: the role of novel biomarkers as early and accurate diagnostics. *Vet. Clin. N. Am. Small Anim. Pract.* 46 (6): 961–993.

14

Pharmacotherapeutics of Immune-Mediated Disease

Katrina R. Viviano

Department of Medical Sciences, School of Veterinary Medicine, University of Wisconsin, Madison, WI, USA

Key Points

- Dogs and cats can be afflicted with the same or similar immune-mediated diseases that affect people, including immune-mediated cytopenias, immune-mediated polyarthritis, inflammatory bowel disease, and others.
- Corticosteroids are considered the initial treatment of choice for most immune-mediated/inflammatory diseases of dogs

and cats; however, adverse effects are common and can be species-dependent.
- Although multiple biological therapeutic agents are available for people with immune-mediated diseases, only one FDA-approved veterinary biologic agent is available, and that one is specific for canine atopy (see Chapter 18).

14.1 Comparative Aspects of Immune-Mediated Disease

Systemic immune-mediated diseases are a heterogeneous and diverse group of diseases that affect dogs, cats, and people (McCullough 2003; Cerquetella et al. 2010; Cooper 2017). Immune-mediated diseases in all species result when the body's immune system, in response to self or foreign antigens, damages solitary cell types (i.e. erythrocytes), tissues, or organs. In some cases (e.g. systemic lupus erythematosus), multiple tissues and organs can be targeted by the abnormal immune response. The pathophysiology of immune-mediated diseases in veterinary patients is thought to be similar to that in people and

may involve genetic predisposition, environmental exposures, exposure to certain drugs or immunizations, hormones, and epigenetic changes that influence cytokine expression (Gershwin 2007; Huang et al. 2012; Day 2013). The inappropriate immune response can involve either humoral and/or cellular arms of the immune system, directed toward specific target cells, organs, or tissues, or can be caused by deposition of antigen–antibody complexes within certain tissues or organs (Whitley and Day 2011). These complexes activate the complement cascade, leading to further tissue damage. Infections, inflammation, or neoplasia can serve as trigger to stimulate an inappropriate immune response. Proposed mechanisms have included exposure

Pharmacotherapeutics for Veterinary Dispensing, First Edition. Edited by Katrina L. Mealey.

to sequestered self-antigens, altered self-antigens, cross-reactivity to self-antigens (molecular mimicry), and/or altered antigen processing (Gershwin 2007; Huang et al. 2012; Day 2013). Comparatively, there are some similarities in the types and frequency of immune-mediated disease between species, but there are also important differences. Some of the more common immune-mediated diseases affecting dogs versus cats, and where applicable the corresponding condition recognized in people, are briefly described in the remainder of this section.

14.1.1 Immune-Mediated Cytopenias

Immune-mediated anemias and thrombocytopenia occur in dog, cats, and people, but patient characteristics and disease frequency differ between species. In dogs, for example, immune-mediated anemias are more commonly diagnosed in middle-aged or older animals and include idiopathic hemolytic anemia (IMHA) or precursor-directed anemia. In cats, pure red cell aplasia (PRCA) occurs more commonly (Weiss 2002; McCullough 2003; Viviano and Webb 2011; Lucidi et al. 2017) and tends to occur in young cats. However, in people, both types of immune-mediated anemias occur (Means 2016a, 2016b; Go et al. 2017; Liebman and Weitz 2017), with autoimmune hemolytic anemia sharing similarities with IMHA in dogs (Figure 14.1), while PRCA may be congenital (i.e. Diamond–Blackfan anemia) or acquired. Aplastic anemia (Weiss 2003; Boddu and Kadia 2017), immune-mediated thrombocytopenia (IMT) (Jordan et al. 1993; Kohn et al. 2000; Putsche and Kohn 2008; Cines et al. 2009; Cooper 2017), and immune-mediated neutropenia (Brown and Rogers 2001; Waugh et al. 2014; Dale and Bolyard 2017; Devine et al. 2017) can occur in many species. Therapeutic goals are similar between species. In severe cases, supplemental oxygen (Figure 14.2) and transfusions (Figure 14.3) may be necessary. It may surprise pharmacists to know that transfusion medicine (blood typing, blood banking,

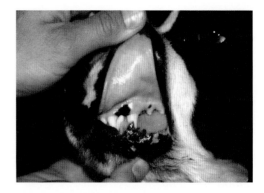

Figure 14.1 Springer Spaniel with immune-mediated hemolytic anemia. Increased breakdown of hemoglobin in destroyed red blood cells causes increased bilirubin levels and icteric (jaundiced) mucous membranes. *Source:* Photo courtesy of Dr. Katrina Mealey, Washington State University College of Veterinary Medicine.

cross-matching, and screening blood donors for hematogenous infectious disease) is available for dogs and cats at many veterinary hospitals.

14.1.2 Immune-Mediated Arthritides

Immune-mediated polyarthritis is relatively common in dogs (Stull et al. 2008; Colopy et al. 2010) and rare in cats (Oohashi et al. 2010). Neither occurs as frequently as the corresponding immune-based polyarthritic disease that occurs in people (rheumatoid arthritis) (Scott et al. 2010). In both dogs and people, chronic inflammation resulting from immune-mediated polyarthritis affects the synovial lining of the joint capsule initially then progresses to involve cartilage and underlying bone. The pattern of joint involvement is similar, with distal joints being most commonly affected, including the wrist, ankle, and digits of the hand and feet in people or the carpus, hock, and digits of the paws in dogs (Wahl and Schuna 2014). The relatively recent introduction of biological agents for treating rheumatoid arthritis in people (etanercept, infliximab, adalimumab, and other agents) has improved therapeutic outcomes in affected patients. Canine-specific biologics for

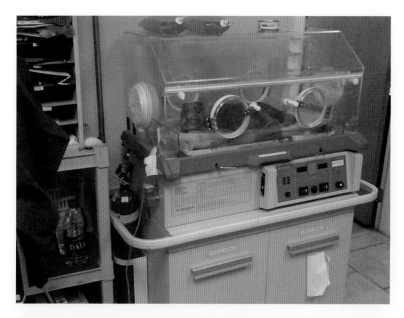

Figure 14.2 Severely anemic cat (hematocrit, 13%; reference range, 24–45%) in an incubator to provide supplemental oxygen. *Source:* Photo courtesy of Dr. Dave Luttinen, Wheaton Way Veterinary Hospital.

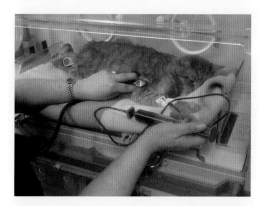

Figure 14.3 The same cat in Figure 14.2 receiving a whole blood transfusion after being cross-matched with the donor cat. The cat's post-transfusion hematocrit was 23%. *Source:* Photo courtesy of Dr. Dave Luttinen, Wheaton Way Veterinary Hospital.

immune-mediated polyarthritis are not available for dogs.

14.1.3 Inflammatory Bowel Disease

Inflammatory bowel disease (IBD) in people includes two separate forms of disease: ulcerative colitis (affects rectum and colon) and Crohn's disease (can affect the gastrointestinal [GI] tract from the mouth to the anus). The chronic inflammatory GI diseases of dogs and cats have similarities but also significant differences compared to Crohn's disease and ulcerative colitis (Cerquetella et al. 2010; Jergens 2012; Jergens and Simpson 2012). Segments of the GI tract most commonly affected by IBD in dogs include the small intestine, colon, and perianal area (fistulas) (Ellison 1995; Patricelli et al. 2002; Dalal and Schwartz 2016), but the stomach can also be affected. In cats, the small intestine and colon are the segments most commonly involved. As is the case with other immune-mediated diseases that affect animals and people, the etiology is believed to involve a combination of environmental (infectious agents and dietary antigens), genetic, and immunologic factors. Some subtypes of IBD occur almost exclusively in one particular dog breed (e.g. histiocytic colitis in Boxers), suggesting that genetics likely plays a large role in the pathophysiology of that particular subtype. IBD is considered a common disease in dogs. In cats, IBD can occur in combination with cholangiohepatitis and pancreatitis, resulting in the nickname "triaditis." Clinical signs of IBD in veterinary patients typically reflect the GI segment involved and can be mild or severe, ranging from periodic inappetence to severe vomiting, diarrhea, and dramatic weight loss. Management of IBD involves a combination of dietary modifications and pharmacological therapy.

14.1.4 Systemic Lupus Erythematosus

Systemic lupus erythematosus (SLE) in people occurs most frequently in young women. SLE is extremely rare in cats, and the disease in dogs occurs with equal frequency in both males and females. Whether this is due to the fact that most dogs in the USA are neutered at an early age (blunting hormonal influences) is not known. SLE in both species can involve multiple tissues and organs, including skin, erythrocytes, leukocytes, kidneys, joints, heart, nervous system, and others. In people and dogs, patients with renal, cardiac, and nervous system involvement tend to have a poorer prognosis. Unfortunately, SLE is not considered a "curable" disease in either species. Therapeutic goals are to prevent disease flare-ups, minimize organ damage, and try to maintain remission status.

The approach to treatment of immune-mediated disease is first to identify and address any identified underlying triggers resulting in secondary immune dysfunction. In veterinary patients, this includes insidious infections (e.g. tickborne diseases – *Anaplasma* spp. and *Ehrlichia* spp.), neoplasia (e.g. lymphosarcoma), or drugs (e.g. sulfonamides [dogs], methimazole [cats], or vaccines). Primary or idiopathic immune-mediated disease is common in veterinary patients, meaning no underlying trigger is identified. In these cases, treatment is focused on the suppression of the body's immune response, which may include a variety of immunosuppressive drugs (discussed further in the "Pharmacological Treatment of Common Immune-Mediated Diseases" section).

14.1.5 Drug-Induced Immune-Mediated Disease

Numerous drugs from a variety of drug classes can precipitate immune-mediated diseases in people and veterinary patients. These are generally considered idiosyncratic reactions and are often caused by a reactive metabolite formed in a susceptible individual (likely due to pharmacogenetics). In dogs and cats, drug-induced immune-mediated diseases often target the skin, liver, bone marrow (hematopoietic stem cells), and kidney. The most commonly prescribed drugs that are associated with immune-mediated disease in dogs and cats include sulfonamides, nonsteroidal anti-inflammatory drugs (NSAIDs), anticonvulsants, and methimazole. Adverse reactions involving methimazole, and recommendations for monitoring, are discussed in Chapter 15.

Sulfonamides can cause hepatopathy, fever, blood dyscrasias, skin eruptions, uveitis, polyarthropathy, glomerulonephritis, and uveitis. Because Doberman Pinschers appear to be particularly susceptible, it is reasonable for the pharmacist to ask the veterinarian if he or she wants to consider a different drug if presented with a prescription for a sulfonamide for that breed. At minimum, the pharmacist should counsel the owner to be vigilant for clinical signs that might indicate an idiosyncratic adverse reaction so that the sulfonamide can be immediately discontinued.

NSAIDs, many of which are exclusively labeled for use in animals, have been associated with idiosyncratic toxicity in dogs or cats. Phenylbutazone (labeled for horses) can cause aplastic anemia in dogs and is not recommended for use in either cats or dogs. Meloxicam, labeled for dogs, cats, and people, has been reported to cause severe skin eruptions in dogs (rare). Hepatotoxicity, including acute hepatic necrosis, in dogs has been associated with many veterinary NSAIDs (carprofen, deracoxib, firocoxib, meloxicam, and robenacoxib). Most dogs are affected within the first few weeks of treatment.

The pharmacist can play a key role in adverse event monitoring by suggesting liver enzyme (alanine aminotransferase [ALT] and alkaline phosphatase [ALP]) monitoring one to two weeks after these drugs are initiated.

Hepatotoxicity has also been associated with anticonvulsants in dogs and/or cats, including zonisamide (dogs), diazepam (cats), and phenobarbital (dogs and cats). Phenobarbital can also cause skin eruptions and blood dyscrasias.

It is important to note that virtually any drug can cause an immune-mediated adverse event. Pharmacists can encourage pet owners to monitor for the development of fever, skin eruptions, blisters or ulcers of mucocutaneous areas, and signs of liver or kidney disease.

14.2 Diagnostic Testing

Definitive diagnosis of some immune-mediated diseases in veterinary patients is elusive. In some situations, a presumptive diagnosis is made by ruling out infectious diseases and/or neoplasia. A complete diagnostic work-up is recommended to include:

- Thorough history and physical examination
- Complete blood count (reticulocyte count if anemia is present)
- Biochemical profile
- Urinalysis
- Serology to rule out infectious diseases
- Imaging if indicated (radiograph joints if polyarthritis is present; chest radiographs and advanced imaging such as ultrasonography, computed tomography [CT], or magnetic resonance imaging [MRI] if suspicious of neoplasia)
- Cytologic and/or histopathology of identified lesions (skin, mucous membranes, GI tract, bone marrow, or arthrocentesis).

Serologic testing for autoantibodies is generally not sufficiently sensitive or specific in veterinary patients. Diagnostics performed and considered gold standard in each case may vary depending on the organ system(s)

impacted. For IBDs, histopathologic diagnosis is the gold standard, with biopsies collected using celiotomy, laparoscopy, or endoscopy.

14.3 Pharmacological Treatment of Common Immune-Mediated Diseases

Biological therapeutics or immunotherapy agents that selectively target specific molecules of the inflammatory pathway or immune system have proven beneficial for treating many immune-mediated diseases in people. Novel biological therapies or immunotherapies are on the horizon for the treatment of immune-mediated diseases in dogs (Swann and Garden 2015; Mizuno 2016; Baker and Isaacs 2017). For example, there is only one FDA-approved biologic agent for canine immune-mediated disease, and that one is specific for atopy (see Chapter 18). At the time of this writing, no FDA-approved biologic therapeutics or immunotherapies are available or appear to be under development for feline immune-mediated diseases. Therefore, immune-mediated diseases in veterinary patients are treated with drugs that nonspecifically inhibit the immune system. With the exception of corticosteroids, this entails extra-label use of FDA-approved drugs for people.

Glucocorticoids are considered the first-line therapy in dogs and cats with immune-mediated disease, with additional second-line (i.e. cyclosporine, azathioprine, and chlorambucil) or third-line (i.e. mycophenolate mofetil and leflunomide) agents used in cases that are severe, or not sufficiently responsive to glucocorticoids, or in patients that experience significant glucocorticoid-induced adverse effects.

Practiced but not proven
The choice of second- or third-line immunosuppressive agents is largely clinician

dependent, as there is no definitive evidence or consensus as to which drug is most effective in the treatment of a particular immune-mediated disease in dogs and cats. Available clinical prospective studies that objectively evaluate the safety or efficacy of these immunosuppressive drugs in dogs and cats are limited. Treatment recommendations are often extrapolated from human medicine or anecdotal clinical experience. Appropriately trained pharmacists could be instrumental in organizing clinical trials to assess the efficacy of immunosuppressive agents in dogs and cats.

There are exceptions; for example, the recommended treatment for perianal fistulas in dogs is cyclosporine, and there is evidence-based data on the use of leflunomide in the treatment of IMPA in dogs. This section will describe the most commonly prescribed immunosuppressive drugs used for chronic management of immune-mediated/inflammatory diseases in dogs and cats. Table 14.1 summarizes the dosages typically used in dogs and cats. As disease remission is achieved, drug doses are slowly tapered to the lowest dose that sufficiently controls disease. In some cases, it is possible to taper off drug therapy completely.

Table 14.1 Recommended dosage for the common immunosuppressive drugs used in dogs and cats.

Drug	Dosage(s)
Prednisone[a]/prednisolone	*Dogs and cats:* *Immunosuppressive dose:* 2 mg/kg/day (total daily dose usually administered at 1 mg/kg PO every 12 hours. Maximum daily dose of 60 mg/day for large to giant breed dogs) *Anti-inflammatory dose:* 0.5–1 mg/kg/day PO *Physiologic replacement dose:* 0.1–0.2 mg/kg/day PO
Methylprednisolone (oral tablets)	*Dogs and cats:* Dose as prednisone/prednisolone above. Methylprednisolone acetate (depo injection) is not recommended.
Dexamethasone	*Dogs and cats:* Calculated prednisone/prednisolone dose divided by 7
Budesonide	Empirical PO dosing based on estimated body size. *Dogs:* *Toy/small breeds:* 1 mg PER DOG/day (compounded) *Medium breeds:* 2 mg PER DOG/day (compounded) *Large/giant breeds:* 3 mg PER DOG/day *Cats:* 0.5–1 mg PER CAT/day (compounded)
Cyclosporine A, modified[b]	*Dogs and cats:* 4 mg/kg PO every 12 hours In dogs with perianal fistula, cyclosporine (2.5 mg/kg PO every 12 hours) is often combined with ketoconazole (8 mg/kg PO every 24 hours) (Patricelli et al. 2002).
Azathioprine	*Dogs:* 2 mg/kg PO every 24 hours for 5–7 days, then 1 mg/kg PO every other day *Cats:* Do not use azathioprine in cats.
Chlorambucil	*Cats:* 2 mg/cat PO every 48–72 hours or 20 mg/m² PO every 14 days (Stein et al. 2010)
Mycophenolate mofetil	*Dogs:* 10 mg/kg PO every 12 hours
Leflunomide	*Dogs:* 1–2 mg/kg PO every 24 hours (Sato et al. 2017)

As disease remission is achieved, drug doses are slowly tapered to the lowest dose to control disease, and in some cases tapering-off therapy may be possible.
[a] Prednisone has low oral bioavailability in cats (Center et al. 2013); prednisolone should be used instead.
[b] Cyclosporine oral bioavailability varies based on formulation (i.e. cyclosporine modified versus cyclosporine in oil) (Whalen et al. 1999; Palmeiro 2013). The oral absorption of cyclosporine modified is more predictable and is therefore the recommended formulation for dogs and cats.

14.3.1 Corticosteroids

Corticosteroids are considered first-line therapy for immune-mediated or autoimmune diseases (e.g. immune-mediated anemias, IMT, and IMPA) in dogs and cats. Advantages of corticosteroids are their systemic impact on both innate and acquired immunity and their relatively rapid onset of action, thereby affirming their role in the acute management of inflammatory and immune-mediated diseases. Corticosteroid dosing strategies used in dogs and cats are variable depending on the particular disease being treated. It is important for the pharmacist to understand the three general classifications of corticosteroid dosing in dogs and cats based on the desired pharmacological goal: physiologic replacement, anti-inflammatory, and immunosuppressive. The dosages of individual corticosteroids required to achieve the pharmacological goal in veterinary patients depend on the relative potency of those agents as well as their oral bioavailability, which can vary between species (Table 14.2).

Corticosteroid products vary in their potency, relative glucocorticoid-to-mineralocorticoid activity, route of administration, and duration of action (Plumb 2011). For treating immune-mediated diseases, intermediate-acting oral corticosteroids are typically used in dogs and cats. The most common oral, intermediate-acting systemic corticosteroids used in veterinary medicine include prednisone and prednisolone. Alternatively, oral methylprednisolone or dexamethasone have less mineralocorticoid activity than prednisone or prednisolone, so it may be preferred for treating patients with underlying cardiovascular disease or diseases associated with fluid retention (e.g. hypoalbuminemia and portal hypertension). In cats, oral bioavailability of prednisolone is four to five times greater compared to the pro-drug oral prednisone (Graham-Mize and Rosser 2004). A similar phenomenon is observed in horses. Therefore, prednisolone is recommended in cats or horses.

In patients suspected to have severe malabsorption, or in patients with life-threatening immune-mediated disease, dexamethasone sodium phosphate may be administered by injection. However, because of its potency (dexamethasone is 4–10 times more potent than prednisone or prednisolone; Ballard et al. 1975; Cantrill et al. 1975) and duration of action (up to 48 hours), there is a risk of overdosing dogs and cats. Therefore, pharmacists should question prescriptions for dexamethasone for dogs or cats that implicate chronic administration. Prednisone/prednisolone or methylprednisolone may be a better option.

Budesonide, a prescription drug labeled for people, is an oral, locally active, high-potency glucocorticoid absorbed at the level of the enterocyte. In people, budesonide is metabolized by the liver, resulting in limited systemic absorption. However, dogs treated with budesonide (3 mg per meter^2) for 30 days experienced suppression of the hypothalamic-pituitary-adrenal axis, indicating systemic corticosteroid exposure (Tumulty et al. 2004; Stroup et al. 2006). When used in cats or dogs, therefore, tapering of the drug may be necessary prior to discontinuation. Budesonide is used to manage Crohn's disease and ulcerative colitis in people (De Cassan et al. 2012), and inflammatory bowel disease in dogs (Pietra et al. 2013) and cats (Trepanier 2009). Although there is some evidence of efficacy, budesonide is more expensive than prednisone/prednisolone and other corticosteroids, so it may not be a viable option for some pet owners. Dosing of budesonide for dogs and cats is listed in Tables 14.1 and 14.2. On a case-by-case basis, corticosteroids may be used in combination with other immunosuppressive agents for treating immune-mediated/autoimmune diseases in dogs and cats, especially in patients that do not respond sufficiently to corticosteroids alone or those with severe life-threatening disease (Viviano and Webb 2011; Swann and Skelly 2012). In these cases, the veterinarian must balance the benefit of added drug therapy to control the disease

Table 14.2 Most commonly used oral glucocorticoids in dogs, cats, and horses, and doses used to achieve various pharmacological effects.

	Physiologic replacement	Anti-inflammatory	Immunosuppressive
Prednisone	*Dogs*: 0.1–0.25 mg/kg/day *Cats*: Inconsistent oral bioavailability *Horses*: Inconsistent oral bioavailability	*Dogs*: 0.5–1 mg/kg/day *Cats*: Inconsistent oral bioavailability *Horses*: Inconsistent oral bioavailability	*Dogs*: 2 mg/kg/day. Maximum daily dose of 60 mg/day *Cats*: Inconsistent oral bioavailability *Horses*: Inconsistent oral bioavailability
Prednisolone	*Dogs*: 0.1–0.25 mg/kg/day *Cats*: Rarely indicated *Horses*: Rarely indicated	*Dogs*: 0.5–1 mg/kg/day *Cats*: 1–2 mg/kg/day *Horses*: 0.25–1 mg/kg/day	*Dogs*: 2 mg/kg/day. Maximum daily dose of 60 mg/day *Cats*: 2 mg/kg/day *Horses*: Rarely indicated
Methylprednisolone	*Dogs*: 0.1–0.2 mg/kg/day *Cats*: Rarely indicated *Horses*: Oral formulations not used	*Dogs*: 0.5–1 mg/kg/day *Cats*: 0.8–1.6 mg/kg/day *Horses*: Oral formulations not used	*Dogs*: 1.6–2 mg/kg/day *Cats*: 1.6–2 mg/kg/day *Horses*: Oral formulations not used
Dexamethasone[a]	N/A	*Dogs*: Not recommended *Cats*: Not recommended *Horses*: 0.05–0.1 mg/kg/day	*Dogs*: Not recommended *Cats*: Not recommended *Horses*: 0.1–0.2 mg/kg/day
Budesonide[b] (Use limited to inflammatory bowel disease)	N/A	*Dogs*: *Toy or small breeds*: 1 mg PER DOG once daily *Medium breeds*: 2 mg PER DOG once daily *Large or giant breeds*: 3 mg PER DOG once daily *Cats*: 1 mg PER CAT once daily	N/A

N/A, Not applicable.

[a] Dexamethasone may be administered acutely (a single dose) but is typically not used chronically in dogs and cats because of perceived increased risks of adverse events compared to other oral glucocorticoids.

[b] Systemic absorption of budesonide occurs in dogs and cats to a greater degree than in humans.

with the potential risk for serious adverse effects. Adverse effects of corticosteroids and other immunosuppressive drugs are described in the "Adverse Drug Effects" section later in this chapter. In particular, adverse effects that are not typically observed in people will be emphasized.

14.3.2 Cyclosporine A, Modified

Cyclosporine A, modified (Atopica®) is FDA approved as an oral capsule for treating dogs with atopic dermatitis. The comparable FDA-approved cyclosporine formulation for people is Neoral® or Gengraf®, a modified formulation from cyclosporine in oil (Sandimmune®). This modified formulation is a microemulsion with more predictable oral absorption and improved stability. Modified cyclosporine A is used off-label as a second-line agent in the treatment of immune-mediated diseases such as IMHA (Grundy and Barton 2001), PRCA (Viviano and Webb 2011), IMT (Nakamura et al. 2012), and IBD (Allenspach et al. 2006) in dogs and cats. Cyclosporine A is often used concurrently with corticosteroids to treat patients with IMHA or IMT, especially in cases with severe clinical presentations. In a small randomized controlled clinical trial, cyclosporine A alone appeared to have some efficacy when used as an alternative to prednisone in dogs with IMHA, thereby avoiding adverse effects of corticosteroids (Rhoades et al. 2016).

Cyclosporine A is considered the first-line agent for treating perianal fistulas in dogs (Patricelli et al. 2002) and is frequently used in veterinary dermatology (Chapter 18) for treating a variety of canine and feline allergic and inflammatory dermatoses (Kovalik et al. 2012).

Clinical controversy: To decrease the cost of cyclosporine A, some veterinarians sometimes exploit a drug–drug interaction to decrease the dose of cyclosporine A needed to achieve therapeutic plasma concentrations. The azole antifungal drug ketoconazole inhibits both P-glycoprotein and cytochrome P450 enzymes. Because cyclosporine A is a substrate for both, concurrent oral administration of ketoconazole (8 mg/kg once a day) (Patricelli et al. 2002) with cyclosporine A increases the oral bioavailability of cyclosporine A in dogs, enabling the dose of cyclosporine A to be decreased by 50–75%, which significantly reduces the cost of therapy, particularly for large- and giant-breed dogs. Use of both drugs in this manner constitutes extra-label drug use and might increase the risk of potential adverse events caused by ketoconazole. Pharmacists should ensure that the owner understands potential risks as well as potential cost savings.

Several veterinary clinical pharmacology laboratories offer therapeutic drug monitoring for cyclosporine A in veterinary patients (Appendix D). In veterinary patients, the therapeutic blood/plasma concentrations of cyclosporine A necessary for the effective treatment of immune-mediated diseases have not been as clearly established as they are for people (i.e. in transplant medicine or in the treatment of immune-mediated diseases) (Teramura et al. 2007). Extrapolated from transplant patients, trough whole-blood cyclosporine A concentrations between 400 and 600 ng/mL are sometimes used as the therapeutic target in veterinary medicine for efficacy and safety (Nam et al. 2008; Archer et al. 2011). However, because trough levels often do not reliably predict clinical response, one veterinary laboratory is offering pharmacodynamic assessment of cyclosporine A in canine blood samples. Whether or not this approach is superior, comparable, or inferior to therapeutic drug monitoring for accurately predicting drug efficacy and safety remains to be determined. Dosing information for cyclosporine A is provided in Table 14.1.

14.3.3 Azathioprine

In people, azathioprine is used to treat immune-mediated disease and to prevent rejection in organ transplant patients (Kruh and Foster 2012). Azathioprine is not labeled for use in any veterinary species but is sometimes used in dogs. Azathioprine should not be used in cats because that species is highly susceptible to adverse effects (discussed in detail in the "Adverse Drug Effects" section later in this chapter). Because its immuno-suppressive effects are delayed, based on its mechanism of action, azathioprine is not used as monotherapy in the treatment of acute immune-mediated disease (Cummings and Rizzo 2017). In dogs, azathioprine is often used for its corticosteroid "sparing effect," whereby adding azathioprine to the regimen enables the veterinarian to decrease the patient's corticosteroid dose with less risk of disease relapse. Few controlled studies have been published evaluating the efficacy of azathioprine for treating immune-medi-ated disease in dogs. Its use in this manner is supported by retrospective studies in which it was used to treat IMHA (Reimer et al. 1999; Weinkle et al. 2005; Piek et al. 2008). Azathioprine dosing information is listed in Table 14.1.

14.3.4   Chlorambucil

Chlorambucil does not have an FDA-approved indication for animals; therefore, the uses described are all extra-label. Because azathioprine is considered unsafe to use in cats, chlorambucil has been used to fill the role that azathioprine does for dogs, specifi-cally in conjunction with glucocorticoids. With regard to chlorambucil use in cats, the majority of published studies focus on its use as a chemotherapeutic agent for treating small-cell lymphoma (Kiselow et al. 2008; Lingard et al. 2009; Barrs and Beatty 2012) or as a second-line therapy for treating IBD (Willard 1999; Trepanier 2009; Jergens 2012). Despite the lack of prospective clinical trials evaluating the use of chlorambucil as an immunosuppressive agent, it is used as the cytotoxic drug of choice in cats. Only recently has a case series and retrospective study been published supporting the use of chlorambu-cil as a second-line agent for treating feline IMT (Wondratschek et al. 2010) and PRCA (Black et al. 2016), respectively. Other

immune-mediated diseases effectively treated with chlorambucil alone or chloram-bucil combined with corticosteroids include canine eosinophilic granuloma of the digits (Knight and Shipstone 2016), chronic inflam-matory enteropathies in dogs (Dandrieux et al. 2013), and dogs with slowly progressive immune-mediated glomerular disease (Segev et al. 2013). At the time of this writing, the price of the FDA-approved chlorambucil for-mulation had sharply increased to the point that it was no longer affordable for most pet owners. Consequently, pharmacists may receive prescriptions for compounded chlo-rambucil. Chlorambucil dosing information is provided in Table 14.1. The use of chlo-rambucil as an antineoplastic drug is dis-cussed in Chapter 20 ("Pharmacotherapeutics of Cancer").

14.3.5   Mycophenolate Mofetil

There are no FDA-approved indications for mycophenolate mofetil in veterinary species; therefore, all uses described here are extra-label. The use of mycophenolate mofetil in veterinary patients is extrapolated from its use in people for treating immune-mediated diseases, including SLE, IMHA, and IMT (Appel et al. 2005; Danovitch 2005). Mycophenolate mofetil should be reserved as either a second- or third-tier immunosuppressive agent when treating immune-mediated diseases in dogs and cats. This would include treatment of patients with refractory disease that had not responded sufficiently to glucocorti-coids alone or glucocorticoids combined with the more commonly used second-tier drugs (i.e. cyclosporine, azathioprine in dogs, or chlorambucil in cats). Another indication would be patients experiencing significant adverse effects to first- and sec-ond-tier drugs. Mycophenolate mofetil offers a potential advantage relative to aza-thioprine for treating acute immune-medi-ated diseases by virtue of its relatively rapid onset of action compared to azathioprine. In canine transplant models, the time to peak inhibition of inosine monophosphate dehydrogenase activity after oral administration is approximately two to four hours (Langman et al. 1996; Lupu et al. 2006). Currently recommended doses for mycophenolate mofetil are listed in Table 14.1. Limited evidence is available to support the clinical use of mycophenolate mofetil in veterinary medicine, so it is not widely used in dogs and cats with immune-mediated diseases. Recently, likely associated with a reduction in its cost, reports of the drug's use in dogs and cats have emerged (West and Hart 2014; Cummings and Rizzo 2017). One of these reports is a retrospective study of dogs with IMT in which a small number (≤20 per group) of dogs treated with mycophenolate and glucocorticoids were compared to a group treated with cyclosporine and glucocorticoids. The authors concluded that there was no difference between treatments, the dogs treated with the mycophenolate and glucocorticoid combination experienced fewer adverse effects, and that treatment cost less than the treatment in the cyclosporine and glucocorticoid group (Cummings and Rizzo 2017). A substantial number of flaws detract from the findings of this study, including the fact that it was statistically underpowered for a non-inferiority study and that dogs receiving corticosteroids did not all receive the same type or same dose. Pharmacists may be surprised that, based on this report, other veterinarians will prescribe mycophenolate mofetil for patients with IMT. This may be in stark contrast to the level of evidence required to support off-label drug use in human patients. However, it is important for pharmacists to understand that research funding available to support the rigorous clinical trials in human patients is simply not available for veterinary clinical trials. When there are no FDA-approved drugs to treat a disease (e.g. IMT or IMHA), veterinarians must make their best judgment with the available information and in accordance with what the owner can afford. Another report describes the use of mycophenolate mofetil in conjunction with corticosteroids in the treatment of immune-mediated skin disease in dogs (Ackermann et al. 2017). Information on the use of mycophenolate mofetil in cats is even more limited: One report describes its use in the treatment of primary IHMA in two cats (Bacek and Macintire 2011).

14.3.6 Leflunomide

As is the case for people with rheumatoid arthritis, the use of leflunomide was initially extrapolated to dogs with IMPA as a second- or third-tier drug often used in combination with other immunosuppressive therapies (Colopy et al. 2010). Reported uses of leflunomide in dogs with immune-mediated disease are limited. Published reports of its use include the treatment of canine IMPA (Colopy et al. 2010), treatment of a group of Miniature Dachshunds with inflammatory colorectal polyps refractory to prednisone and cyclosporine (Fukushima et al. 2016), and treatment of a diverse group of dogs ($n = 92$) diagnosed with immune-mediated or inflammatory diseases (i.e. IMPA [$n = 42$], IMT [$n = 17$], IMHA [$n = 17$], IBD [$n = 6$], IMHA/IMT [$n = 2$], pancytopenia [$n = 2$], vasculitis [$n = 1$], uveitis [$n = 1$], and chronic hepatitis [$n = 1$]) (Sato et al. 2017). Leflunomide dosing information is provided in Table 14.1.

14.4 Adverse Drug Effects of Immunosuppressive Drugs in Veterinary Species

This goal of this section is to provide information to pharmacy professionals about adverse drug effects that are more prone to occur in veterinary species as compared to people. Drug-induced adverse effects common to both people and veterinary species will be briefly reviewed. In those instances, when a physiological reason or theory for the species susceptibility is known, it will be provided.

14.4.1 Corticosteroids

Adverse effects of corticosteroids common to dogs, cats, and people include suppression of the hypothalamic-pituitary-adrenal axis, GI ulceration (dogs are particularly sensitive), insulin resistance and secondary diabetes mellitus (cats are particularly sensitive), skeletal muscle catabolism, delayed wound healing, opportunistic infections, and behavior changes (at higher dosages). Pharmacists should alert dog owners to expect the following clinical signs: polydipsia, polyuria, polyphagia, weight gain, and increased panting. These can be troublesome to owners, particularly for indoor dogs since dogs will need to be let outside to urinate frequently or have "accidents" in the house. Additionally, dogs are often ravenous, and their food-seeking behavior may become aggressive (e.g. begging for food, or seeking food off countertops or tables). Concurrent administration of corticosteroids with NSAIDs is contraindicated due to the significant risk of GI ulceration or even perforation (Boston et al. 2003).

Dramatic difference

Cats treated with corticosteroids may develop insulin-dependent diabetes mellitus requiring discontinuation of corticosteroids. Unique to cats, diabetes mellitus may be transient in some cats, especially if appropriate treatment is initiated early. Thus, while polyuria and polydipsia are expected to occur in dogs treated with corticosteroids, pharmacists should inform cat owners that if polyuria and polydipsia occur, the cat should be screened for diabetes mellitus (Sieber-Ruckstuhl et al. 2008).

Another interesting species difference is that dogs, but not cats or people, have a corticosteroid-inducible ALP isoenzyme. Serum biochemical profiles from dogs treated with corticosteroids can have ALP concentrations five-fold higher than baseline values with no evidence of liver disease. On the contrary, even mild elevations of ALP in a cat treated with corticosteroids would likely indicate hepatobiliary disease.

14.4.2 Cyclosporine A, Modified

The side effect profile of cyclosporine A is somewhat different from that reported in people. Vomiting associated with oral cyclosporine A dosing can limit its use in veterinary patients. Oral tolerability can be improved by freezing cyclosporine A capsules prior to oral administration. Freezing (−20 °C) the FDA-approved canine formulation of modified cyclosporine A (Atopica) for 28 days did not affect drug stability or oral absorption in dogs (Bachtel et al. 2015).

Adverse effects of cyclosporine A that are common to people and veterinary patients include opportunistic fungal infections (Dowling et al. 2016; Rhoades et al. 2016; McAtee et al. 2017), gingival hyperplasia, hepatotoxicity, thromboembolism, and lymphoproliferative disorders (Robson 2003; Schmiedt et al. 2009; Namikawa et al. 2012; Thomason et al. 2012). Nephrotoxicity, a major concern in people treated with cyclosporine A, is uncommon in veterinary species. Drugs that inhibit the cytochrome P450 enzymes system (CYP3A) and/or P-glycoprotein (Trepanier 2006) can increase cyclosporine A plasma concentrations. Examples include azole antifungals (McAnulty and Lensmeyer 1999; Patricelli et al. 2002; Katayama et al. 2010a, 2010b), clarithromycin (Katayama et al. 2012), and grapefruit juice (Amatori et al. 2004; Radwanski et al. 2011).

14.4.3 Azathioprine

The most common adverse effects associated with azathioprine reported in dogs include GI upset (i.e. diarrhea), hepatotoxicity (reported incidence of 15% within the first one to four weeks) resulting in increased ALT (great than twofold) responsive to dose reduction or drug withdrawal (Wallisch and Trepanier 2015), and myelosuppression (reported incidence of 13% within three months), including dose-dependent neutropenia and thrombocytopenia (Piek et al. 2008).

In people, thiopurine methyltransferase (TPMT), the enzyme responsible for metabolizing azathioprine's active metabolite 6-mercaptopurine to inactive metabolites, is polymorphic, resulting in variable TPMT activity and consequently variable clinical outcomes. Individuals with low TPMT activity have an increased risk of azathioprine-induced myelosuppression. In dogs, a nine-fold difference in TPMT activity has been reported. For example, Giant Schnauzers have low TPMT activity, while Alaskan malamutes have high TPMT activity (Kidd et al. 2004). Compared to dogs or people, cats have very low TPMT activity, and are therefore incredibly susceptible to myelosuppression (Beale et al. 1992; Salavaggione et al. 2004); therefore, azathioprine is rarely prescribed for cats. Horses also have very low TPMT activity.

14.4.4 Chlorambucil

Myelosuppression and GI toxicity are the most common adverse effects associated with chlorambucil in dogs and cats. Myelosuppression is considered mild relative to other alkylating agents and generally occurs 7–14 days after treatment begins. Chlorambucil-associated neurotoxicity has been reported in people (Salloum et al. 1997), and was recently in a cat (Benitah et al. 2003) and a dog (Giuliano 2013). Reversible myoclonus occurred in a cat that received an overdose of chlorambucil (Benitah et al. 2003), and a suspected chlorambucil-related seizure was recently reported in a dog with nephrotic syndrome (Giuliano 2013). Acquired Fanconi's syndrome was reported in four cats with immune-mediated GI disease that were treated with chlorambucil (Reinert and Feldman 2016). Within 2–26 months of introducing chlorambucil, routine serum biochemical panel and urinalysis identified glucosuria with normal blood glucose. Aminoaciduria was also identified, confirming the diagnosis of Fanconi's syndrome. Only one of the four cats had clinical signs (i.e. lethargy

and decreased appetite), and the acquired Fanconi's syndrome improved or resolved in three of the four cats within three months of discontinuing chlorambucil.

14.4.5 Mycophenolate Mofetil

GI signs, most commonly diarrhea, are the most common adverse effects associated with mycophenolate mofetil in dogs and cats. Other potential adverse effects reported in people include myelosuppression and neurotoxicity (i.e. progressive multifocal leukoencephalopathy) (Berger 2010).

While the disposition of mycophenolate mofetil in dogs and cats is not characterized, its disposition after oral administration to people is a complex process (Figure 14.2). Mycophenolate mofetil is a pro-drug that undergoes metabolic activation to mycophenolic acid, which is 99% bound to albumin in the circulation. Mycophenolic acid is metabolized to inactive metabolites via glucuronidation, with the glucuronide conjugate secreted in urine or bile by specific drug transporters. Enterohepatic recirculation occurs as a result of deconjugation reactions mediated by gut microflora. Tremendous species and even breed differences may exist at each of these steps that could impact the safety and efficacy of mycophenolate mofetil in dogs or cats compared to people. For example, conversion of mycophenolate mofetil to the active drug mycophenolic acid is slower in cats than people (Slovak et al. 2017), suggesting differences in esterase activity (Figure 14.4). Dogs have several polymorphic forms of albumin (Chapter 5), which might alter the ratio of bound to unbound mycophenolic acid in plasma. Even a small increase in the fraction of unbound mycophenolic acid would greatly increase the risk of adverse effects. Because cats lack several glucuronidation enzymes (Chapter 4), conjugation of mycophenolic acid to form inactive metabolites might involve alternative, potentially slower, pathways. Transporter defects or polymorphisms (Chapters 4 and 5) in dogs and cats may alter biliary or renal excretion; and, lastly, species differences

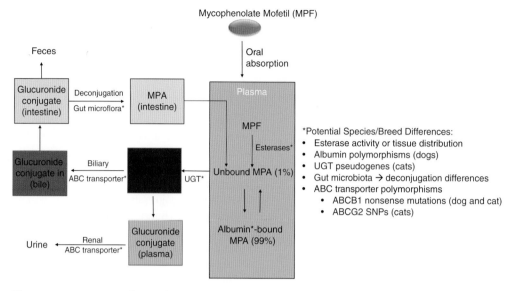

Figure 14.4 Disposition of mycophenolate mofetil (MPF), which is a pro-drug, and mycophenolic acid (MPA), which is the active drug. Asterisks indicate potential sites of species or breed variation in drug disposition. UGT, UDP glucuronyl transferase; ABC, ATP binding cassette transporter. *Source:* Courtesy of Dr. Katrina Mealey, Washington State University College of Veterinary Medicine.

between people and cat/dog gut microflora could impact enterohepatic circulation. Thus, extrapolating dosing regimens from one species (i.e. human beings) to another (i.e. dogs or cats) is inherently risky. By working together, pharmacists and veterinarians may be able to improve these extrapolations. The reports described further in this chapter illustrate how initial doses of mycophenolate mofetil in dogs and cats were likely too high.

In one of the first reports describing mycophenolate mofetil use in dogs, five IMHA patients were treated at a dose of 10–15 mg/kg every eight hours. Prednisone was administered concurrently. All dogs developed GI toxicity (i.e. decreased appetite, vomiting, and diarrhea) that was severe enough to require drug discontinuation. Because these signs are not typical of prednisone use in dogs, the adverse reaction was attributed to mycophenolate mofetil (West and Hart 2014). In another study, also involving dogs with IMHA treated with mycophenolate mofetil (median dose 21 mg/kg/day) and prednisone, severe diarrhea was reported (Wang et al. 2013). Clinical experience suggests it may be dose-related, as dose reduction (8 mg/kg/day) often resolves the diarrhea without disease relapse. It has been proposed that lower doses of mycophenolate mofetil may be effective for immune-mediated disease in dogs and cause fewer adverse effects; however, published evidence is lacking.

As part of a safety study, adverse clinical effects associated with oral mycophenolate in healthy cats included decreased appetite and diarrhea. GI signs appeared to be dose-dependent and occurred at doses >15 mg/kg PO every 12 hours (Slovak and Villarino 2017). Compared to people or dogs, less is known about the safety and adverse effects profile of mycophenolate mofetil in cats with immune-mediated disease. As discussed in this chapter, glucuronidation is the primary pathway involved in producing inactive drug metabolites. Because cats have a decreased capacity to conjugate drugs via glucuronidation, sulfation, and/or glycination (Court 2013) compared to other species (i.e. dogs or people), administration of mycophenolate mofetil to cats may be associated with a higher risk of adverse drug effects. Other potential reasons that cats may be more susceptible to adverse drug reactions caused by mycophenolate mofetil than dogs or people include: increased esterase activity relative to dogs/people, lower fraction of mycophenolic acid bound to plasma albumin, deconjugation reactions in the gut may be greater in cats due to microflora differences in carnivores compared to omnivores, and decreased transporter function at the biliary canaliculi or proximal tubule (Figure 14.4).

14.4.6 Leflunomide

Because leflunomide is not FDA approved for dogs or cats, there are no preclinical data to help veterinarians establish a safe and effective dose. Little is known about the side effect profile of leflunomide in dogs, which is very concerning since the leflunomide label has a boxed warning related to risks of severe liver injury, including fatal liver failure. In people with rheumatoid arthritis treated with leflunomide, approximately 40% of patients have to stop using the drug because of serious adverse effects (i.e. GI upset, hepatotoxicity, pancytopenia, and pneumonitis) (Osiri et al. 2002). Because of its complex disposition after oral administration, leflunomide has multiple steps where species and breed differences can manifest, resulting in highly variable plasma drug concentrations (Figure 14.5). Leflunomide is metabolized by CYP 1A2 (Bohanec Grabar et al. 2008) and CYP 2C19 (Wiese et al. 2012; Hopkins et al. 2016) to the active metabolite teriflunomide. Teriflunomide is highly bound (>99%) to albumin in the circulation. Elimination of teriflunomide via biliary excretion is dependent upon the transporter ABCG2; however, it can undergo enterohepatic recycling. This complex disposition makes extrapolations from people to dogs or cats quite challenging. Some pharmacokinetic parameters of leflunomide have been determined in dogs and are different compared to those in people (i.e. shorter terminal half-life and T_{max} and lower C_{max}) (Singer et al. 2011).

Adverse effects of leflunomide in dogs have been recently reported and include bone marrow suppression (i.e. leukopenia, thrombocytopenia, and anemia) and increased liver enzymes (Fukushima et al. 2016). These were apparently reversible after dose reduction or drug discontinuation. Similar adverse effects were recently reported in a retrospective study of 92 dogs diagnosed with immune-mediated disease and treated with leflunomide (Sato et al. 2017). Dogs that were treated with higher dosages (median 2.9 mg/kg/day; $n = 11$) were more likely to develop adverse effects, necessitating dose reduction or drug discontinuation compared to dogs treated with lower doses (median dosage 1.5 mg/kg/day; $n = 81$). Based on these results, the authors of this retrospective study suggested a starting leflunomide dose of 1–2 mg/kg/day instead of what has been recommended for dogs (3–4 mg/kg/day) in order to minimize the risk of adverse events. Anecdotally, clinical adverse effects suspected to be caused by leflunomide dosed at 3–4 mg/kg/day have included diarrhea, vasculitis of the skin and other organs (which can be severe), opportunistic infections, and myelosuppression (author's unpublished clinical experience). Because so little is known about the tolerability of leflunomide in dogs relative to other immunosuppressant drugs described in this chapter, it is preferable to use agents with better described and potentially less severe adverse effects.

Leflunomide pharmacokinetics have been described in cats. The mean (range) elimination half-life of teriflunomide in cats is 59 (44–101) hours (Mehl et al. 2011), compared to 21 (19–23) hours for dogs (Singer et al. 2011). These values represent the elimination half-life of the active drug teriflunomide after oral administration of the pro-drug leflunomide. The prolonged elimination half-life in cats may be due to the fact that ABCG2 is involved in biliary excretion of the active metabolite and ABCG2 function is defective in cats relative to people and dogs. Regardless of the mechanism, prolonged elimination of teriflunomide in cats indicates

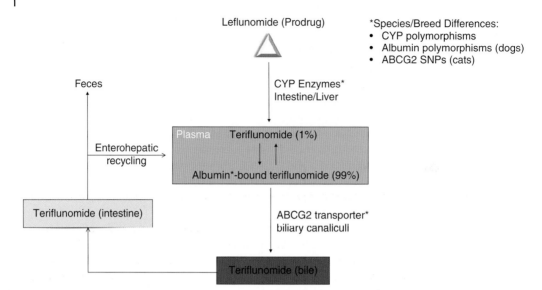

Figure 14.5 Disposition of leflunomide, which is a pro-drug, and teriflunomide, the active metabolite. Asterisks indicate potential sites of species or breed variation in drug disposition. CYP, cytochrome P450 enzymes; ABCG2, ATP binding cassette transporter subfamily G2. *Source:* Image courtesy of Dr. Katrina Mealey, Washington State University College of Veterinary Medicine.

that drug accumulation will occur if dosed at intervals similar to those used in other species.

14.5 Nutritional Supplements for Immune-Mediated Disease

It is easy for pet owners to find internet sites promoting nutritional supplements for a variety of diseases. For immune-mediated disease, melatonin is the current favorite among some veterinarians. This appears to be based on a publication describing three human patients with immune-mediated thrombocytopenia who were treated with melatonin (Todisco and Rossi 2002). This is certainly not enough evidence to support its use for IMT. Despite the fact that there is even less justification for its use to treat IMHA, there are internet sites promoting just that. What is particularly concerning is that melatonin is reported to promote glucocorticoid resistance (Konakchieva et al. 1998). Since glucocorticoids are often used in patients with immune-mediated diseases, concurrent use of melatonin may actually be contraindicated. Until there is evidence based on well-designed clinical trials, use of melatonin for immune-mediated disease should be considered questionable.

Abbreviations

ABCB1	ATP-binding cassette subfamily B member 1	IBD	Inflammatory bowel disease
DM	Diabetes mellitus	IMHA	Immune-mediated hemolytic anemia
GI	Gastrointestinal	IMPA	Immune-mediated polyarthritis
HPA axis	Hypothalamic-pituitary-adrenal axis	IMPDH	Inosine monophosphate dehydrogenase

IMT	Immune-mediated thrombocytopenia
ITP	Idiopathic thrombocytopenia purpura
6-MMP	6-Methylmercaptopurine

6-MP	6-Mercaptopurine
NSAIDs	Nonsteroidal anti-inflammatory drugs
PRCA	Pure red cell aplasia
TPMT	Thiopurine methyltransferase

References

Ackermann, A.L., May, E.R., and Frank, L.A. (2017). Use of mycophenolate mofetil to treat immune-mediated skin disease in 14 dogs – a retrospective evaluation. *Vet. Dermatol.* 28: 195–e144.

Allenspach, K., Rufenacht, S., Sauter, S. et al. (2006). Pharmacokinetics and clinical efficacy of cyclosporine treatment of dogs with steroid-refractory inflammatory bowel disease. *J. Vet. Intern. Med.* 20: 239–244.

Amatori, F.M., Meucci, V., Giusiani, M. et al. (2004). Effect of grapefruit juice on the pharmacokinetics of cyclosporine in dogs. *Vet. Rec.* 154: 180–181.

Appel, G.B., Radhakrishnan, J., and Ginzler, E.M. (2005). Use of mycophenolate mofetil in autoimmune and renal diseases. *Transplantation* 80: S265–S271.

Archer, T.M., Fellman, C.L., Stokes, J.V. et al. (2011). Pharmacodynamic monitoring of canine T-cell cytokine responses to oral cyclosporine. *J. Vet. Intern. Med.* 25: 1391–1397.

Bacek, L.M. and Macintire, D.K. (2011). Treatment of primary immune-mediated hemolytic anemia with mycophenolate in two cats. *J. Vet. Emerg. Crit. Care (San Antonio)* 21: 45–49.

Bachtel, J.C., Pendergraft, J.S., Rosychuk, R.A. et al. (2015). Comparison of the stability and pharmacokinetics in dogs of modified ciclosporin capsules stored at –20 degrees C and room temperature. *Vet. Dermatol.* 26: e228–e250.

Baker, K.F. and Isaacs, J.D. (2017). Novel therapies for immune-mediated inflammatory diseases: what can we learn from their use in rheumatoid arthritis, spondyloarthritis, systemic lupus erythematosus, psoriasis, Crohn's disease and ulcerative colitis? *Ann. Rheum. Dis.* 77 (2): http://dx.doi.org/10.1136/annrheumdis-2017-211555.

Ballard, P.L., Carter, J.P., Graham, B.S. et al. (1975). A radioreceptor assay for evaluation of the plasma glucocorticoid activity of natural and synthetic steroids in man. *J. Clin. Endocrinol. Metab.* 41: 290–304.

Barrs, V.R. and Beatty, J.A. (2012). Feline alimentary lymphoma: 2. Further diagnostics, therapy and prognosis. *J. Feline Med. Surg.* 14: 191–201.

Beale, K.M., Altman, D., Clemmons, R.R. et al. (1992). Systemic toxicosis associated with azathioprine administration in domestic cats. *Am. J. Vet. Res.* 53: 1236–1240.

Benitah, N., deLorimier, L.P., Gaspar, M. et al. (2003). Chlorambucil-induced mycoclonus in a cat with lymphoma. *J. Am. Anim. Hosp. Assoc.* 39 (3): 283–287.

Berger, J.R. (2010). Progressive multifocal leukoencephalopathy and newer biological agents. *Drug Saf.* 33: 969–983.

Black, V., Adamantos, S., Barfield, D. et al. (2016). Feline non-regenerative immune-mediated anaemia: features and outcome in 15 cases. *J. Feline Med. Surg.* 18: 597–602.

Boddu, P.C. and Kadia, T.M. (2017). Updates on the pathophysiology and treatment of aplastic anemia: a comprehensive review. *Expert. Rev. Hematol.* 10: 433–448.

Bohanec Grabar, P., Rozman, B., Tomsic, M. et al. (2008). Genetic polymorphism of CYP1A2 and the toxicity of leflunomide treatment in rheumatoid arthritis patients. *Eur. J. Clin. Pharmacol.* 64: 871–876.

Boston, S.E., Moens, N.M., Kruth, S.A. et al. (2003). Endoscopic evaluation of the gastroduodenal mucosa to determine the safety of short-term concurrent administration of meloxicam and dexamethasone in healthy dogs. *Am. J. Vet. Res.* 64: 1369–1375.

Brown, M.R. and Rogers, K.S. (2001). Neutropenia in dogs and cats: a retrospective study of 261 cases. *J. Am. Anim. Hosp. Assoc.* 37: 131–139.

Cantrill, H.L., Waltman, S.R., Palmberg, P.F. et al. (1975). In vitro determination of relative corticosteroid potency. *J. Clin. Endocrinol. Metab.* 40: 1073–1077.

Center, S.A., Randolph, J.F., Warner, K.L. et al. (2013). Influence of body condition on plasma prednisolone and prednisone concentrations in clinically healthy cats after single oral dose administration. *Res. Vet. Sci.* 95: 225–230.

Cerquetella, M., Spaterna, A., Laus, F. et al. (2010). Inflammatory bowel disease in the dog: differences and similarities with humans. *World J. Gastroenterol.* 16: 1050–1056.

Cines, D.B., Bussel, J.B., Liebman, H.A. et al. (2009). The ITP syndrome: pathogenic and clinical diversity. *Blood* 113: 6511–6521.

Colopy, S.A., Baker, T.A., and Muir, P. (2010). Efficacy of leflunomide for treatment of immune-mediated polyarthritis in dogs: 14 cases (2006–2008). *J. Am. Vet. Med. Assoc.* 236: 312–318.

Cooper, N. (2017). State of the art – how I manage immune thrombocytopenia. *Br. J. Haematol.* 177: 39–54.

Court, M.H. (2013). Feline drug metabolism and disposition: pharmacokinetic evidence for species differences and molecular mechanisms. *Vet. Clin. North Am. Small Anim. Pract.* 43: 1039–1054.

Cummings, F.O. and Rizzo, S.A. (2017). Treatment of presumptive primary immune-mediated thrombocytopenia with mycophenolate mofetil versus cyclosporine in dogs. *J. Small Anim. Pract.* 58: 96–102.

Dalal, R.L. and Schwartz, D.A. (2016). The Gastroenterologist's role in management of perianal fistula. *Gastrointest. Endosc. Clin. N. Am.* 26: 693–705.

Dale, D.C. and Bolyard, A.A. (2017). An update on the diagnosis and treatment of chronic idiopathic neutropenia. *Curr. Opin. Hematol.* 24: 46–53.

Dandrieux, J.R., Noble, P.J., Scase, T.J. et al. (2013). Comparison of a chlorambucil-prednisolone combination with an azathioprine-prednisolone combination for treatment of chronic enteropathy with concurrent protein-losing enteropathy in dogs: 27 cases (2007–2010). *J. Am. Vet. Med. Assoc.* 242: 1705–1714.

Danovitch, G.M. (2005). Mycophenolate mofetil: a decade of clinical experience. *Transplantation* 80: S272–S274.

Day MJ. (2013). Triggers of immune-mediated diseases. In World Small Animal Veterinary Association World Congress Proceedings, Auckland, New Zealand.

De Cassan, C., Fiorino, G., and Danese, S. (2012). Second-generation corticosteroids for the treatment of Crohn's disease and ulcerative colitis: more effective and less side effects? *Dig. Dis.* 30: 368–375.

Devine, L., Armstrong, P.J., Whittemore, J.C. et al. (2017). Presumed primary immune-mediated neutropenia in 35 dogs: a retrospective study. *J. Small Anim. Pract.* 58: 307–313.

Dowling, S.R., Webb, J., Foster, J.D. et al. (2016). Opportunistic fungal infections in dogs treated with ciclosporin and glucocorticoids: eight cases. *J. Small Anim. Pract.* 57: 105–109.

Ellison, G.W. (1995). Treatment of perianal fistulas in dogs. *J. Am. Vet. Med. Assoc.* 206: 1680–1682.

Fukushima, K., Eguchi, N., Ohno, K. et al. (2016). Efficacy of leflunomide for treatment of refractory inflammatory colorectal polyps in 15 miniature dachshunds. *J. Vet. Med. Sci.* 78: 265–269.

Gershwin, L.J. (2007). Veterinary autoimmunity: autoimmune diseases in domestic animals. *Ann. NY. Acad. Sci.* 1109: 109–116.

Giuliano, A. (2013). Suspected chlorambucil-related neurotoxicity with seizures in a dog. *J. Small Anim. Pract.* 54: 437.

Go, R.S., Winters, J.L., and Kay, N.E. (2017). How I treat autoimmune hemolytic anemia. *Blood* 129: 2971–2979.

Graham-Mize, C. and Rosser, E. (2004). Bioavailability and activity of prednisone and prednisolone in the feline patient [abstract]. *Vet. Dermatol.* 15: 7.

Hopkins, A.M., Wiese, M.D., Proudman, S.M. et al. (2016). Genetic polymorphism of CYP1A2 but not total or free teriflunomide concentrations is associated with leflunomide cessation in rheumatoid arthritis. *Br. J. Clin. Pharmacol.* 81: 113–123.

Huang, A.A., Moore, G.E., and Scott-Moncrieff, J.C. (2012). Idiopathic immune-mediated thrombocytopenia and recent vaccination in dogs. *J. Vet. Intern. Med.* 26: 142–148.

Jergens, A.E. (2012). Feline idiopathic inflammatory bowel disease: what we know and what remains to be unraveled. *J. Feline Med. Surg.* 14: 445–458.

Jergens, A.E. and Simpson, K.W. (2012). Inflammatory bowel disease in veterinary medicine. *Front. Biosci. (Elite Ed.)* 4: 1404–1419.

Jordan, H.L., Grindem, C.B., and Breitschwerdt, E.B. (1993). Thrombocytopenia in cats: a retrospective study of 41 cases. *J. Vet. Intern. Med.* 7: 261–265.

Katayama, M., Igarashi, H., Fukai, K. et al. (2010a). Fluconazole decreases cyclosporine dosage in renal transplanted dogs. *Res. Vet. Sci.* 89: 124–125.

Katayama, M., Katayama, R., and Kamishina, H. (2010b). Effects of multiple oral dosing of itraconazole on the pharmacokinetics of cyclosporine in cats. *J. Feline Med. Surg.* 12: 512–514.

Katayama, M., Nishijima, N., Okamura, Y. et al. (2012). Interaction of clarithromycin with cyclosporine in cats: pharmacokinetic study and case report. *J. Feline Med. Surg.* 14: 257–261.

Kidd, L.B., Salavaggione, O.E., Szumlanski, C.L. et al. (2004). Thiopurine methyltransferase activity in red blood cells of dogs. *J. Vet. Intern. Med.* 18: 214–218.

Kiselow, M.A., Rassnick, K.M., McDonough, S.P. et al. (2008). Outcome of cats with low-grade lymphocytic lymphoma: 41 cases (1995–2005). *J. Am. Vet. Med. Assoc.* 232 (3): 405–410.

Knight, E.C. and Shipstone, M.A. (2016). Canine eosinophilic granuloma of the digits treated with prednisolone and chlorambucil. *Vet. Dermatol.* 27: 446–e119.

Kohn, B., Engelbrecht, R., Leibold, W. et al. (2000). Clinical findings, diagnostics and treatment results in primary and secondary immune-mediated thrombocytopenia in the dog. *Kleintierpraxis* 45: 893–907.

Konakchieva, R., Mitev, Y., Almeida, O.F. et al. (1998). Chronic melatonin treatment counteracts glucocorticoid-induced dysregulation of the hypothalamic-pituitary-adrenal axis in the rat. *Neuroendocrinology* 67: 171–180.

Kovalik, M., Thoday, K.L., and van den Broek, A.H. (2012). The use of ciclosporin A in veterinary dermatology. *Vet. J.* 193: 317–325.

Kruh, J. and Foster, C.S. (2012). Corticosteroid-sparing agents: conventional systemic immunosuppressants. *Dev. Ophthalmol.* 51: 29–46.

Langman, L.J., Shapiro, A.M., Lakey, J.R. et al. (1996). Pharmacodynamic assessment of mycophenolic acid in a canine model. *Transplant. Proc.* 28: 934–936.

Liebman, H.A. and Weitz, I.C. (2017). Autoimmune hemolytic anemia. *Med. Clin. North Am.* 101: 351–359.

Lingard, A.E., Briscoe, K., Beatty, J.A. et al. (2009). Low-grade alimentary lymphoma: clinicopathological findings and response to treatment in 17 cases. *J. Feline Med. Surg.* 11 (8): 692–700.

Lucidi, C.A., de Rezende, C.L.E., Jutkowitz, L.A. et al. (2017). Histologic and cytologic bone marrow findings in dogs with suspected precursor-targeted immune-mediated anemia and associated phagocytosis of erythroid precursors. *Vet. Clin. Pathol.* 46: 401–415.

Lupu, M., McCune, J.S., Kuhr, C.S. et al. (2006). Pharmacokinetics of oral mycophenolate mofetil in dog:

bioavailability studies and the impact of antibiotic therapy. *Biol. Blood Marrow Transplant.* 12: 1352–1354.

McAnulty, J.F. and Lensmeyer, G.L. (1999). The effects of ketoconazole on the pharmacokinetics of cyclosporine A in cats. *Vet. Surg.* 28: 448–455.

McAtee, B.B., Cummings, K.J., Cook, A.K. et al. (2017). Opportunistic invasive cutaneous fungal infections associated with Administration of Cyclosporine to dogs with immune-mediated disease. *J. Vet. Intern. Med.* 31 (6): 1724–1729.

McCullough, S. (2003). Immune-mediated hemolytic anemia: understanding the nemesis. *Vet. Clin. North Am. Small Anim. Pract.* 33: 1295–1315.

Means, R.T. Jr. (2016a). Pure red cell aplasia. *Blood* 128: 2504–2509.

Means, R.T. Jr. (2016b). Pure red cell aplasia. *Hematology Am. Soc. Hematol. Educ. Program* 2016: 51–56.

Mehl, M.L., Tell, L., Kyles, A.E. et al. (2011). Pharmacokinetics and pharmacodynamics of A77 1726 and leflunomide in domestic cats. *J. Vet. Pharmacol. Ther.* 35: 139–146.

Mizuno, T. (2016). A brighter future for dogs with immune-mediated haemolytic anemia. *Vet. J.* 209: 1–2.

Nakamura, R.K., Tompkins, E., and Bianco, D. (2012). Therapeutic options for immune-mediated thrombocytopenia. *J. Vet. Emerg. Crit. Care (San Antonio)* 22: 59–72.

Nam, H.S., McAnulty, J.F., Kwak, H.H. et al. (2008). Gingival overgrowth in dogs associated with clinically relevant cyclosporine blood levels: observations in a canine renal transplantation model. *Vet. Surg.* 37: 247–253.

Namikawa, K., Maruo, T., Honda, M. et al. (2012). Gingival overgrowth in a dog that received long-term cyclosporine for immune-mediated hemolytic anemia. *Can. Vet. J.* 53: 67–70.

Oohashi, E., Yamada, K., Oohashi, M. et al. (2010). Chronic progressive polyarthritis in a female cat. *J. Vet. Med. Sci.* 72: 511–514.

Osiri, M., Shea, B., Welch, V. et al. (2002). *Leflunomide for the Treatment of*

Rheumatoid Arthritis. Chichester, UK: Wiley.

Palmeiro, B.S. (2013). Cyclosporine in veterinary dermatology. *Vet. Clin. North Am. Small Anim. Pract.* 43: 153–171.

Patricelli, A.J., Hardie, R.J., and McAnulty, J.E. (2002). Cyclosporine and ketoconazole for the treatment of perianal fistulas in dogs. *J. Am. Vet. Med. Assoc.* 220: 1009–1016.

Piek, C.J., Junius, G., Dekker, A. et al. (2008). Idiopathic immune-mediated hemolytic anemia: treatment outcome and prognostic factors in 149 dogs. *J. Vet. Intern. Med.* 22: 366–373.

Pietra, M., Fracassi, F., Diana, A. et al. (2013). Plasma concentrations and therapeutic effects of budesonide in dogs with inflammatory bowel disease. *Am. J. Vet. Res.* 74: 78–83.

Plumb, D.C. (2011). *Plumb's Veterinary Drug Handbook.* Ames, IA: Iowa State University Press.

Putsche, J.C. and Kohn, B. (2008). Primary immune-mediated thrombocytopenia in 30 dogs (1997–2003). *J. Am. Anim. Hosp. Assoc.* 44: 250–257.

Radwanski, N.E., Cerundolo, R., Shofer, F.S. et al. (2011). Effects of powdered whole grapefruit and metoclopramide on the pharmacokinetics of cyclosporine in dogs. *Am. J. Vet. Res.* 72: 687–693.

Reimer, M.E., Troy, G.C., and Warnick, L.D. (1999). Immune-mediated hemolytic anemia: 70 cases (1988–1996). *J. Am. Anim. Hosp. Assoc.* 35: 384–391.

Reinert, N.C. and Feldman, D.G. (2016). Acquired Fanconi syndrome in four cats treated with chlorambucil. *J. Feline Med. Surg.* 18: 1034–1040.

Rhoades, A.C., Vernau, W., Kass, P.H. et al. (2016). Comparison of the efficacy of prednisone and cyclosporine for treatment of dogs with primary immune-mediated polyarthritis. *J. Am. Vet. Med. Assoc.* 248: 395–404.

Robson, D. (2003). Review of the pharmacokinetics, interactions and adverse reactions of cyclosporine in people, dogs and cats. *Vet. Rec.* 152: 739–748.

Salavaggione, O.E., Yang, C., Kidd, L.B. et al. (2004). Cat red blood cell thiopurine S-methyltransferase: companion animal pharmacogenetics. *J. Pharmacol. Exp. Ther.* 308: 617–626.

Salloum, E., Khan, K.K., and Cooper, D.L. (1997). Chlorambucil-induced seizures. *Cancer* 79: 1009–1013.

Sato, M., Veir, J.K., Legare, M. et al. (2017). A retrospective study on the safety and efficacy of leflunomide in dogs. *J. Vet. Intern. Med.* 31 (5): https://doi.org/10.1111/jvim.14810.

Schmiedt, C.W., Grimes, J.A., Holzman, G. et al. (2009). Incidence and risk factors for development of malignant neoplasia after feline renal transplantation and cyclosporine-based immunosuppression. *Vet. Comp. Oncol.* 7: 45–53.

Scott, D.L., Wolfe, F., and Huizinga, T.W. (2010). Rheumatoid arthritis. *Lancet* 376: 1094–1108.

Segev, G., Cowgill, L.D., Heiene, R. et al. (2013). Consensus recommendations for immunosuppressive treatment of dogs with glomerular disease based on established pathology. *J. Vet. Intern. Med.* 27 (Suppl. 1): S44–S54.

Sieber-Ruckstuhl, N.S., Kley, S., Tschuor, F. et al. (2008). Remission of diabetes mellitus in cats with diabetic ketoacidosis. *J. Vet. Intern. Med.* 22: 1326–1332.

Singer, L.M., Cohn, L.A., Reinero, C.R. et al. (2011). Leflunomide pharmacokinetics after single oral administration to dogs. *J. Vet. Pharmacol. Ther.* 34: 609–611.

Slovak, J.E., Rivera, S.M., Hwang, J.K. et al. (2017). Pharmacokinetics of Mycophenolic acid after intravenous Administration of Mycophenolate Mofetil to healthy cats. *J. Vet. Intern. Med.* 31: 1827–1832.

Slovak, J.E. and Villarino, N.F. (2017). Safety of oral and intravenous mycophenolate mofetil in healthy cats. *J. Feline Med. Surg.* https://doi.org/10.1177/1098612X17693521.

Stroup, S.T., Behrend, E.N., Kemppainen, R.J. et al. (2006). Effects of oral administration of controlled-ileal-release budesonide and assessment of pituitary-adrenocortical axis suppression in clinically normal dogs. *Am. J. Vet. Res.* 67: 1173–1178.

Stull, J.W., Evason, M., Carr, A.P. et al. (2008). Canine immune-mediated polyarthritis: clinical and laboratory findings in 83 cases in western Canada (1991–2001). *Can. Vet. J.* 49: 1195–1203.

Swann, J.W. and Garden, O.A. (2015). Novel immunotherapies for immune-mediated haemolytic anaemia in dogs and people. *Vet. J.* 209: 1–2.

Swann, J.W. and Skelly, B.J. (2012). Systematic review of evidence relating to the treatment of immune-mediated hemolytic anemia in dogs. *J. Vet. Intern. Med.* 27: 1–9.

Teramura, M., Kimura, A., Iwase, S. et al. (2007). Treatment of severe aplastic anemia with antithymocyte globulin and cyclosporin A with or without G-CSF in adults: a multicenter randomized study in Japan. *Blood* 110: 1756–1761.

Thomason, J., Lunsford, K., Stokes, J. et al. (2012). The effects of cyclosporine on platelet function and cyclooxygenase expression in normal dogs. *J. Vet. Intern. Med.* 26: 1389–1401.

Todisco, M. and Rossi, N. (2002). Melatonin for refractory idiopathic thrombocytopenic purpura: a report of 3 cases. *Am. J. Ther.* 9: 524–526.

Trepanier, L. (2009). Idiopathic inflammatory bowel disease in cats. Rational treatment selection. *J. Feline Med. Surg.* 11: 32–38.

Trepanier, L.A. (2006). Cytochrome P450 and its role in veterinary drug interactions. *Vet. Clin. North Am. Small Anim. Pract.* 36: 975–985, v.

Tumulty, J.W., Broussard, J.D., Steiner, J.M. et al. (2004). Clinical effects of short-term oral budesonide on the hypothalamic-pituitary-adrenal axis in dogs with inflammatory bowel disease. *J. Am. Anim. Hosp. Assoc.* 40: 120–123.

Viviano, K.R. and Webb, J.L. (2011). Clinical use of cyclosporine as an adjunctive therapy in the management of feline idiopathic pure red cell aplasia. *J. Feline Med. Surg.* 13: 885–895.

Wahl, K. and Schuna, A. (2014). *Rheumatoid Arthritis*, 9e. New York: McGraw-Hill Education.

Wallisch, K. and Trepanier, L.A. (2015). Incidence, timing, and risk factors of azathioprine hepatotoxicosis in dogs. *J. Vet. Intern. Med.* 29: 513–518.

Wang, A., Smith, J.R., and Creevy, K.E. (2013). Treatment of canine idiopathic immune-mediated haemolytic anaemia with mycophenolate mofetil and glucocorticoids: 30 cases (2007 to 2011). *J. Small Anim. Pract.* 54: 399–404.

Waugh, C.E., Scott, K.D., and Bryan, L.K. (2014). Primary immune-mediated neutropenia in a cat. *Can. Vet. J.* 55: 1074–1078.

Weinkle, T.K., Center, S.A., Randolph, J.F. et al. (2005). Evaluation of prognostic factors, survival rates, and treatment protocols for immune-mediated hemolytic anemia in dogs: 151 cases (1993–2002). *J. Am. Vet. Med. Assoc.* 226: 1869–1880.

Weiss, D.J. (2002). Primary pure red cell aplasia in dogs: 13 cases (1996–2000). *J. Am. Vet. Med. Assoc.* 221: 93–95.

Weiss, D.J. (2003). New insights into the physiology and treatment of acquired myelodysplastic syndromes and aplastic pancytopenia. *Vet. Clin. North Am. Small Anim. Pract.* 33 (6): 1317–1334.

West, L.D. and Hart, J.R. (2014). Treatment of idiopathic immune-mediated hemolytic anemia with mycophenolate mofetil in five dogs. *J. Vet. Emerg. Crit. Care (San Antonio)* 24: 226–231.

Whalen, R.D., Tata, P.N., Burckart, G.J. et al. (1999). Species differences in the hepatic and intestinal metabolism of cyclosporine. *Xenobiotica* 29: 3–9.

Whitley, N.T. and Day, M.J. (2011). Immunomodulatory drugs and their application to the management of canine immune-mediated disease. *J. Small Anim. Pract.* 52: 70–85.

Wiese, M.D., Schnabl, M., O'Doherty, C. et al. (2012). Polymorphisms in cytochrome P450 2C19 enzyme and cessation of leflunomide in patients with rheumatoid arthritis. *Arthritis Res. Ther.* 14: R163.

Willard, M.D. (1999). Feline inflammatory bowel disease: a review. *J. Feline Med. Surg.* 1: 155–164.

Wondratschek, C., Weingart, C., and Kohn, B. (2010). Primary immune-mediated thrombocytopenia in cats. *J. Am. Anim. Hosp. Assoc.* 46: 12–19.

15

Endocrine Pharmacotherapeutics

Katrina L. Mealey

College of Veterinary Medicine, Washington State University, Pullman, WA, USA

Key Points

- Common endocrine disorders in dogs include hypothyroidism, diabetes mellitus (type 1), and hyperadrenocorticism (Cushing's syndrome).
- Common endocrine disorders in cats include hyperthyroidism and diabetes mellitus (type 1 > type 2).
- Pharmacotherapy of endocrine diseases often involves the same therapeutic class of drugs used in human patients, but

pharmacokinetic and pharmacodynamic species differences necessitate dose or formulation modifications for canine and feline patients.
- The most common cause of death in diabetic cats and dogs is owner-elected euthanasia. By incorporating pharmacists into diabetes education efforts, an owner's confidence in their ability to manage a diabetic pet can be enhanced, which might save the pet's life.

15.1 Comparative Aspects of Endocrine Disease

Many endocrine system disorders that adversely affect human health also occur in veterinary species. Among the most common endocrine disorders in people are diabetes mellitus, hyperthyroidism, hypothyroidism, and dysfunction of the hypothalamic-pituitary-adrenal axis resulting in cortisol excess or deficiency. Dysfunction of the thyroid gland and endocrine pancreas is common in both dogs and cats, while dysfunction of the hypothalamic-pituitary-adrenal axis is relatively common in dogs, ferrets, and horses but less common in cats. Despite the fact that dogs, cats, and even horses suffer from some of the

same endocrine diseases as people, the diseases themselves and aspects of their treatment can differ substantially between species. Additionally, even if pharmacotherapy of a particular endocrine disease involves the same therapeutic class of compounds used in human patients, there are often substantial pharmacokinetic and/or pharmacodynamic species differences that necessitate distinct dose rates or formulation modifications in dogs, cats, and other veterinary species. In fact, there are a number of US Food and Drug Administration (FDA)-approved veterinary formulations for treating endocrine disorders of dogs and cats because the human formulations are unsatisfactory. Other endocrine diseases that are diagnosed less frequently in dogs and cats include

Pharmacotherapeutics for Veterinary Dispensing, First Edition. Edited by Katrina L. Mealey.
© 2019 John Wiley & Sons, Inc. Published 2019 by John Wiley & Sons, Inc.

acromegaly (which can be a cause of diabetes mellitus in cats), hyperparathyroidism, hypoparathyroidism, insulinoma, hyperaldosteronism, and central diabetes insipidus. Pharmacotherapy of these endocrinopathies is beyond the scope of this textbook.

15.1.1 Diseases of the Thyroid Gland

Hyperthyroidism is a common disease of middle-aged to older cats but rarely occurs in dogs. It is predicted that over 10% of cats will develop the disorder in their lifetime (Peterson 2012). Hyperthyroidism is also diagnosed in human patients, but the pathophysiology of feline and human hyperthyroidism differs. The most common cause of hyperthyroidism in people is Grave's disease, which is an autoimmune syndrome in which thyroid-stimulating autoantibodies are produced. These antibodies bind to thyrotropin or thyroid-stimulating hormone (TSH) receptors located on thyroid epithelial cells. When these antibodies bind the TSH receptor, the receptor is activated, stimulating the same cascade of events that occur when TSH binds the receptor (Jonklaas and Kane 2017). The most common cause of hyperthyroidism in cats is adenomatous hyperplasia, usually involving both thyroid glands (van Hoek et al. 2015). This is most similar to toxic nodular goiter (toxic adenoma) in humans. Genetic, nutritional, and environmental factors are thought to be involved in the pathogenesis of feline hyperthyroidism, with exposure to environmental thyroid-disruptor compounds in food or water receiving a great deal of attention recently (Peterson 2014). Many of the clinical signs observed in hyperthyroidism in cats overlap with those of humans with thyrotoxicosis (weight loss despite a good appetite, hyperactivity/nervousness, tachycardia, etc.). Treatment options for human hyperthyroidism include surgical thyroidectomy, radioiodine treatment, and pharmacotherapy (methimazole). There is one additional option for treating hyperthyroid cats – a commercially available iodine-restricted diet – although long-term studies of safety and efficacy are not yet available. Treatment of hyperthyroidism in cats depends on owner finances, owner motivation, concurrent disease conditions (renal dysfunction and cardiac disease are common), and availability of special handling facilities for radioiodine (^{131}I) therapy.

Dramatic difference

Cats treated with ^{131}I are required to undergo posttreatment isolation for several days to weeks to minimize radiation exposure risk to individuals that might come in contact with the treated cat. The length of isolation depends on state radiation regulations. Human patients treated with ^{131}I are not required to undergo isolation.

Hypothyroidism occurs in roughly 2% of the human population (Jonklaas and Kane 2017). It is considered a common endocrinopathy in dogs but rarely occurs spontaneously in cats. When it is diagnosed in cats, it is almost uniformly iatrogenic, resulting from "overtreatment" of hyperthyroidism. In both humans and dogs, the most common cause of hypothyroidism is lymphocytic (chronic autoimmune) thyroiditis. Many clinical signs of hypothyroidism are common to both humans and dogs, including weight gain, lethargy, exercise intolerance, and muscle weakness. Clinical signs that are unique to dogs, and often troublesome to owners, are the dermatologic abnormalities that occur in hypothyroid dogs: bilateral symmetrical alopecia or thinning hair coat, seborrhea, hyperpigmentation, and pyoderma. The tail is frequently affected by thinning hair, giving the dog a "rat tail" appearance. Levothyroxine is the treatment of choice for hypothyroidism in both dogs and people.

15.1.2 Diseases of the Adrenal Gland

In both dogs and humans, adrenal gland hyperfunction is more common than hypofunction. Adrenal disorders are uncommon in cats. Hyperfunction results in clinical signs related to excess cortisol synthesis and secretion (i.e. Cushing's syndrome), while hypofunction most commonly involves deficient synthesis and secretion of both cortisol and aldosterone. Hyperadrenocorticism in both dogs (Hill 2015) and people (Hwang et al. 2017) can be primary, caused by unregulated production of cortisol by an adrenal tumor, or secondary, caused by excess adrenocorticotropic hormone (ACTH) production by a pituitary adenoma stimulating the adrenal glands to secrete cortisol. Secondary hyperadrenocorticism (Cushing's syndrome) is more common than primary hyperadrenocorticism in both dogs and people. There is less overlap in clinical signs of hyperadrenocorticism than one might expect between dogs and humans. Among the most common findings in people are central obesity, facial rounding, osteoporosis, and hypertension (Hwang et al. 2017), while dogs are presented to veterinarians for excessive thirst and urination (polydipsia and polyuria [PU/PD]), ravenous appetite, a "pot belly" (Figure 15.1), alopecia, and muscle wasting (Hill 2015). Cats rarely develop hyperadrenocorticism, but when they do it is characterized by PU/PD as well as a very unusual clinical sign – fragile, easily torn skin. Hyperadrenocorticism in dogs can be treated either surgically or pharmacologically. Surgery is the treatment of choice for adrenal tumors (primary hyperadrenocorticism),

while pharmacological management is currently the treatment of choice for secondary (pituitary-dependent) hyperadrenocorticism. Dogs may be treated with the human drug mitotane or the veterinary drug trilostane, which is FDA approved for treating pituitary-dependent hyperadrenocorticism in dogs.

Hypofunction of the adrenal gland (Addison's disease) is a less common adrenal disorder in both dogs and people. Both species develop fairly vague clinical signs, including weakness, inappetence, hypotension, and general malaise. Pharmacological treatment of dogs with hypoadrenocorticism most often includes both mineralocorticoid supplementation and glucocorticoid supplementation. Either the human drug fludrocortisone, available in tablet form for daily oral administration, or the veterinary drug desoxycorticosterone pivalate (DOCP) suspension, available as an injection to be administered at 25-day intervals, can be used for mineralocorticoid replacement. Glucocorticoid replacement generally consists of prednisone administered daily at physiologic doses.

15.1.3 Diseases of the Endocrine Pancreas

Diabetes mellitus, a metabolic disorder consisting of insulin resistance and/or insufficient insulin secretion, is estimated to affect more

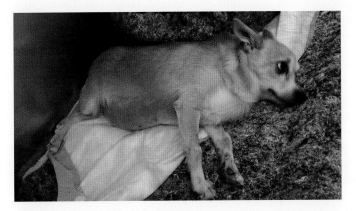

Figure 15.1 Nine-year-old Chihuahua with "pot belly" appearance commonly seen as a consequence of metabolic changes in dogs with hyperadrenocorticism. This is a result of abdominal muscle weakness and hepatomegaly due to glycogen accumulation. *Source:* Photo courtesy of Dr. Jillian Haines, Washington State University.

than 10% of people in the USA (Triplitt et al. 2017). It is estimated to affect less than 1% of cats, with greater frequency in certain breeds such as Burmese, Russian Blue, and Abyssinian (Ohlund et al. 2015). Similarly, diabetes mellitus affects less than 1% of all dogs, but breed predilection has been documented in Miniature Schnauzers and Yorkshire Terriers (Mattin et al. 2014). The clinical presentation of diabetes mellitus in dogs and cats is similar to that in people. Common signs include polydipsia, polyuria, lethargy, and weight loss despite polyphagia. Diabetes mellitus can be classified as type 1 or type 2, depending on whether or not there is an absolute (type 1) or relative (type 2) insulin deficiency. The vast majority of human diabetics fall into the latter category. Conversely, dogs develop type 1 diabetes exclusively, while cats may develop type 1 or type 2 diabetes mellitus. Therefore, all dogs and most cats with diabetes require insulin.

Optimal management of diabetes in people incorporates dietary measures and regular physical activity. The same is true for veterinary patients. Dietary recommendations for dogs are similar to those for people with diabetes – to increase the fiber (complex carbohydrate) content of the diet while limiting simple carbohydrates. Cats are slightly different. As true carnivores, a high protein content along with low simple carbohydrates have been shown to be beneficial. There are numerous commercially available dog and cat foods that have been formulated specifically for diabetic patients. Weight control through both dietary measures and moderate physical activity is important for limiting insulin resistance. Getting a dog to exercise is generally not a problem, since most dogs seem to enjoy going for walks, playing fetch, or getting a chance to run around at a dog park. Cats are not small dogs. Most cats don't enjoy leash-walks, playing fetch, or going to dog parks. There are no established methods for getting a cat to exercise.

Pharmacological management of diabetes in all dogs and the vast majority of cats requires insulin (Sparkes et al. 2015). The specifics regarding differences in insulin pharmacokinetics and pharmacodynamics in dogs, cats, and humans will be discussed further in this chapter. Most human diabetics receive oral hypoglycemic drugs such as sulfonylureas, glinides, biguanides, alpha-glucosidase inhibitors, and others (Triplitt et al. 2017). Despite their widespread use and proven efficacy for type 2 human diabetics, oral hypoglycemics are ineffective in dogs, and only glipizide has ample evidence to support its use in cats (and even then is rarely recommended). The primary indication for using glipizide is in a newly diagnosed diabetic cat if the owner refuses insulin treatment. Many owners initially refuse to consider daily insulin injections for their cat. The efficacy of glipizide in controlling hyperglycemia usually wanes within a few weeks, and some owners will then agree to try managing their diabetic cat with insulin.

Managing a diabetic pet requires a great deal of effort on the part of the pet owner. Imagine trying to manage an infant with diabetes mellitus – an infant can't communicate the early warning signs of hypoglycemia. The same is true for pets. Because there is a higher risk of death from hypoglycemia than from hyperglycemia, at least in the short term, the general treatment philosophy for diabetic pets is to err on the side of caution. In human patients, the goal is to try to maintain plasma glucose concentrations within the normal range (80–130 mg/dL). This often involves monitoring blood glucose levels multiple times per day with frequent insulin dose adjustments. In dogs and cats, intensive blood glucose monitoring schemes are the exception rather than the norm for a variety of reasons: (i) Dogs and cats develop an aversion to the individual "poking" them for blood glucose determinations; (ii) owners' work schedules and/or lifestyles don't permit intensive blood glucose monitoring; and (iii) technology for continuous blood glucose monitoring or insulin pumps is not routinely available, economically feasible, or practical for veterinary patients at the current time.

For veterinary patients, therefore, the goal is to keep the blood glucose below the renal threshold (~ 250 mg/dL), which prevents the clinical signs associated with osmotic diuresis (frequent drinking and urination). These are the clinical signs most troubling to pet owners, particularly dog owners. Essentially, owners notice that the dog is either soiling the house or "asking" to go outside to urinate repeatedly, including at night when the owner prefers to be sleeping.

Now that justification for the upper range of acceptable blood glucose values has been established, it is important for the pharmacist to understand the rationale for the lowest acceptable blood glucose concentration for diabetic dogs and cats. Even though normal blood glucose concentrations in dogs and cats range from approximately 80 to 110 mg/dL, it is too risky to allow the blood glucose to drop below 100 mg/dL in diabetic patients treated with insulin. If the dog or cat expends more calories (exercise) or consumes fewer calories from one day to the next, hypoglycemia might occur. To avoid hypoglycemia, when a blood glucose value below 100 mg/dL is detected in a diabetic patient, it generally indicates that a decrease in insulin dose is necessary. Thus, the acceptable blood glucose range in diabetic dogs and cats (100–250 mg/dL) is much wider than would be desirable in diabetic human patients. Less stringent glycemic control in diabetic pets may increase the risk of long-term hyperglycemic complications, but it decreases the risk of life-threatening hypoglycemia, which is difficult to detect in dogs and cats. This can't be overstated, especially for pets that are not monitored for 8–10 hours per day while the owner is at work or school. A hypoglycemic episode during this time period could be fatal.

Long-term complications from diabetes mellitus that occur in people, including diabetic retinopathy, nephropathy, and vascular disease (atherosclerosis and calcification), are rare in dogs and cats, probably because these conditions develop after decades of hyperglycemia and its associated metabolic abnormalities. Few diabetic dogs and cats experience even one decade of hyperglycemia. This is because dogs and cats have much shorter lifespans than humans and because diabetes tends to develop in older animals. Susceptibility to infections and diabetic ketoacidosis are common complications in both dogs and cats, while cataracts are a common complication in dogs but not cats. It has been proposed that low activity of aldose reductase in the cat may be responsible for this species difference in susceptibility to diabetic cataracts (Richter et al. 2002). Diabetic cats can develop a neuropathy that manifests most commonly as a plantigrade stance (Figure 15.2) when standing or walking (Mizisin et al. 2002). This may have some similarities to diabetic neuropathy in humans.

The most important "complication" of diabetes in dogs and cats, however, is euthanasia. Many animals are euthanized immediately after they are diagnosed because the owner does not feel they have the time, skill, or resources necessary to manage a diabetic patient. Other owners believe it is inhumane to inject their pet with insulin twice a day. Pharmacists that have been trained as diabetes educators for human patients can play a key role in educating and supporting owners of diabetic dogs and cats by learning about species differences in insulin structure, potency, and duration of action (discussed further in this chapter).

One last interspecies comparison with respect to diabetes mellitus deserves mention. A "transient" diabetes state has been described in cats that is thought to be similar to what has been described in human medicine (Gostelow et al. 2014). The mechanism likely involves curtailing glucotoxicity via diet (decreased carbohydrates and increased protein), stress management (cortisol released as a result of stress causes insulin resistance), and other factors. It has been proposed that initial treatment of diabetic cats with insulin glargine is more likely to induce remission, but this has not been definitively demonstrated (Gostelow et al. 2014).

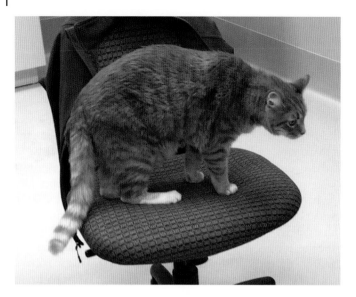

Figure 15.2 Plantigrade stance in a cat (note rear limbs). *Source:* Image courtesy of Dr. Amanda Taylor, Auburn University College of Veterinary Medicine.

15.1.4 Drug-Induced Endocrine Disease

Transient hypothyroidism can be caused by drugs used to treat hyperthyroidism (e.g. methimazole and iodides). Many other drugs can decrease basal thyroid hormone concentrations. The most common of these are furosemide, glucocorticoids, phenobarbital, phenothiazines, sulfonamides, and some nonsteroidal anti-inflammatory drugs (NSAIDs) (Feldman and Nelson 2004). Treatment with any form of corticosteroid drug carries the risk of causing clinical signs of hyperadrenocorticism. For very small dogs and cats, even certain forms of "topical" therapy, particularly with highly potent corticosteroids, result in sufficient systemic exposure to cause clinical signs consistent with cortisol excess. Even more dangerous is acute withdrawal of corticosteroid therapy in patients that have been receiving corticosteroids chronically. This can cause an adrenal (Addisonian) crisis. Other drugs that can suppress cortisol synthesis include mitotane, ketoconazole, and etomidate. Drug-induced diabetes mellitus can occur with drugs that are cytotoxic to pancreatic beta cells, such as streptozotocin and alloxan. Glucocorticoids, beta adrenergic agonists, progestagens, and diazoxide can cause insulin resistance and predispose cats, in particular, to diabetes.

15.2 Diagnostic Testing

Definitive diagnosis of the more common canine and feline endocrine diseases is relatively straightforward and involves measuring endogenous hormone levels or measuring hormone levels after administration of provocative or suppressive agents. Veterinarians tend to have a high index of suspicion of common endocrine diseases after taking a thorough history and performing a thorough physical examination.

- Physical examination
- Radiography
- Complete blood count
- Biochemical profile (glucose, liver and kidney parameters, and electrolytes)
- Urinalysis
- Plasma and/or urine endogenous hormone concentrations (cortisol, adrenocorticotropic hormone [ACTH], and thyroid hormones)

- Endocrine stimulation or suppression testing (ACTH stimulation, dexamethasone suppression, etc.)
- Plasma concentrations of antibodies directed against endocrine tissues
- Glycated proteins (diagnosis and monitoring of diabetes mellitus)
- Advanced imaging, such as computerized tomography (CT) or magnetic resonance imaging (MRI).

15.3 Pharmacological Treatment of Common Diseases

15.3.1 Canine Hypothyroidism

By the time hypothyroidism is diagnosed in dogs, the thyroid gland has undergone permanent damage. Because residual thyroid tissue is insufficient to maintain a euthyroid state, an exogenous source of thyroid hormone is necessary. Synthetic levothyroxine is the treatment of choice for canine hypothyroidism. There are many veterinary formulations (e.g. Soloxine® and Laventa®) available, as well as human formulations (Synthroid®). However, the tablet strengths of human levothyroxine formulations routinely stocked by most community pharmacies are sufficient for dosing only small and toy breed dogs.

Dramatic difference

Because oral bioavailability of levothyroxine is lower and its clearance is faster, dosage rates are much higher in hypothyroid dogs than their human counterparts. The total daily dose for a 10–20-pound dog is equivalent to that for an adult human.

It is strongly recommended that the same brand-name levothyroxine veterinary product be used consistently because of the overall low oral bioavailability of levothyroxine in dogs and overall lack of bioequivalence between different brands (Plumb 2015). Additionally, adverse events have been associated with specific formulations of levothyroxine.

A veterinary product from a less established manufacturer as well as the human product have been reported to cause severe cutaneous hypersensitivity in a dog. However, the reaction did not recur when the dog was treated with the veterinary brand name product Laventa (Lavergne et al. 2015). There are several other thyroid preparations sometimes used for treating hypothyroidism in people, including thyroid USP, liothyronine, and liotrix. These are all considered less suitable than synthetic levothyroxine for canine hypothyroid patients. Thyroid USP contains desiccated pork thyroid gland. Some veterinarians and owners believe that because this product is "natural," it is superior and safer than synthetic levothyroxine. There is no evidence to substantiate that claim. The bioequivalence of levothyroxine delivered by animal-derived desiccated thyroid gland products is highly variable, making them less desirable than synthetic levothyroxine (Behrend et al. 2012). Use of liothyronine (T3) and liotrix (a combination of T3 and T4) is discouraged because these products contain synthetic T3, the active form of thyroid hormone. Although levothyroxine (T4) is the predominant thyroid hormone secreted by the thyroid gland, it is not the active form of the hormone. Individual tissues are thought to convert T4 to T3 on an "as-needed" basis. Thus, provision of T3 does not replicate the normal physiologic condition.

15.3.1.1 Drugs Most Likely to Be Prescribed for Hypothyroidism

Levothyroxine: 0.02 milligrams/kg PO every 12 hours. The dose should be titrated based on plasma concentrations of thyroid hormone and patient response. For large dogs, a maximum dose of 0.8 milligrams per dog is recommended for initial treatment, with the dose adjusted accordingly.

15.3.2 Feline Hyperthyroidism

Treatment of hyperthyroidism can be accomplished with surgery, with radioactive iodine, or pharmacologically. Methimazole is FDA approved for treating hyperthyroidism in both human and feline patients. Methimazole functions by blocking enzymes responsible for thyroid hormone synthesis. The FDA-approved formulation for cats (Felimazole®) is available in more feline-friendly tablet strengths (2.5 and 5 mg) compared to human formulations (5 and 10 mg). It is important to distinguish the treatment strategy for hyperthyroid cats versus hyperthyroid human patients. Recall that hyperthyroidism in cats is a result of adenomatous hyperplasia of the thyroid gland(s), whereas the most common cause in people is production of autoantibodies that stimulate thyroid hormone production (Grave's disease). Hyperthyroid cats will require lifelong treatment with methimazole, while most human patients will undergo remission allowing methimazole treatment to be withdrawn after 12–24 months (Jonklaas and Kane 2017). The pharmacotherapeutic goal in cats is to suppress thyroid hormone production, such that plasma thyroxine levels are within the normal range. Thus, cats treated with methimazole will require monitoring of plasma thyroid hormone concentrations at three- to six-month intervals. Since methimazole does not suppress growth of adenomatous thyroid tissue, it is possible that the methimazole dose required to maintain plasma thyroid hormone levels within the normal range will increase over time as adenomatous tissue enlarges. Methimazole has numerous adverse effects in cats, affecting roughly 20% of treated cats (Behrend 2006). These are discussed in detail in the "Adverse Drug Effects" section in this chapter. However, it is important to mention one particularly common adverse effect in this section because it influences a number of prescribing decisions by veterinarians. Anorexia and vomiting are the most common adverse effects of methimazole in cats (Behrend 2006). To circumvent this adverse effect, the daily methimazole dose can be divided twice or three times daily. Unfortunately, it is difficult to "pill" a cat even once per day – two or three times per day for the lifetime of the cat is a very high burden for both owner and cat. Another option that veterinarians have turned to is the drug carbimazole. Carbimazole is a pro-drug that is rapidly metabolized to methimazole. It is much less likely to cause gastrointestinal disturbances than methimazole. Unfortunately, carbimazole is not FDA approved and is therefore not available in the USA. Last but not least, veterinarians rely on pharmacists to compound transdermal formulations of methimazole. Methimazole is one of the very few drugs where there is evidence to support its use as a compounded transdermal formulation. Methimazole compounded in pluronic lecithin organogel has shown efficacy in the treatment of hyperthyroid cats when applied to the inner pinna (Sartor et al. 2004). Transdermal methimazole causes fewer gastrointestinal adverse effects in cats, but the overall efficacy of transdermal methimazole is less than that of oral methimazole. Additionally, the stability of methimazole in the transdermal preparations is low – two months after methimazole is compounded in a transdermal formulation, the potency is less than 90% (Pignato et al. 2010). Pharmacists can play a key role in educating veterinarians that transdermal methimazole should not be prescribed for amounts exceeding a two-month supply.

15.3.2.1 Drugs Most Likely to Be Prescribed for Hyperthyroidism

Methimazole (oral): 2.5 milligrams per cat (not per kg) PO every 12 hours. Doses may be adjusted based on plasma thyroid hormone concentrations.

Methimazole (transdermal): A methimazole preparation that has become standard for compounding is 5 milligrams/0.1 mL in pluronic lecithin organogel. An initial dose of 2.5 milligrams per cat (not per kg) is applied to the inner pinna, and dose adjustments should be made based on plasma thyroid hormone concentrations. Owners must use nonpermeable gloves or finger cots to apply. Transdermal methimazole should be avoided if the cat may come in contact with small children.

15.3.3 Canine Hyperadrenocorticism

Successful pharmacological management of primary (adrenal) hyperadrenocorticism in dogs is not a reasonable expectation. It should be considered palliative therapy at best. Successful pharmacological management of pituitary-dependent hyperadrenocorticism in dogs is a reasonable expectation. Median survival of dogs treated with either trilostane or mitotane is roughly two years. From the perspective of human medicine, this may seem like a poor prognosis, but when one considers the lifespan of dogs relative to humans together with the fact that hyperadrenocorticism occurs in middle-aged to older dogs, a two-year median survival time seems more reasonable. Canine hyperadrenocorticism can be treated with the adrenolytic agent mitotane (extra-label use of a human drug) or with the steroidogenesis inhibitor trilostane (FDA approved for dogs). Although trilostane is classified as a steroidogenesis inhibitor, it has caused destruction of the adrenal gland in some dogs. Therefore, both drugs can induce an adrenal (Addisonian) crisis. Monitoring parameters for mitotane and trilostane differ because they are based on each drug's mechanism of action. ACTH stimulation testing can be performed anytime during the dosing interval for mitotane, but should be performed four hours after dosing for trilostane.

Selegiline (L-deprenyl), although FDA approved for treating pituitary-dependent hyperadrenocorticism in dogs, is not recommended by most veterinary endocrinologists. This apparent contradiction (not to prescribe an FDA-approved drug for the indication printed on the drug label) deserves an explanation. Selegiline, as a monoamine oxidase type B inhibitor, inhibits metabolic deactivation of dopamine. Dopamine plays a key role in suppressing ACTH secretion from the intermediate lobe of the pituitary gland (pars intermedia). Treatment with selegiline blocks dopamine degradation, leading to higher levels of dopamine, which subsequently decrease ACTH secretion from the pars intermedia. Thus, it would *seem* that selegiline would be effective for treating canine pituitary-dependent hyperadrenocorticism. The problem with selegiline lies in the fact that

unregulated production of ACTH in most dogs with pituitary-dependent hyperadrenocorticism originates not from the pars intermedia, but from the anterior pituitary (Behrend 2006). Since dopamine does not play a role in regulating ACTH production from the anterior pituitary, selegiline is ineffectual in these patients (Reusch et al. 1999; Braddock et al. 2004). Figure 15.3 summarizes results from studies evaluating the efficacy of selegiline, mitotane, and trilostane for treating dogs with pituitary-dependent hyperadrenocorticism as evaluated by ACTH-stimulated plasma cortisol concentrations.

15.3.3.1 Drugs Most Likely to Be Prescribed for Pituitary-Dependent Hyperadrenocorticism

Mandatory monitoring
Patients treated with mitotane or trilostane should be monitored for hypocortisolism and treated accordingly. Hypocortisolism can be life-threatening. Signs of hypocortisolism include inappetence, vomiting, diarrhea, lethargy, and, in severe cases, hypovolemia and collapse.

Mitotane: The dosing regimen involves judicious monitoring with dose adjustments based on ACTH-stimulated plasma cortisol concentrations; it is beyond the scope of this book. To provide a general idea for the pharmacist, protocols include an induction phase (daily doses in the range of 20–25 milligrams/kg PO every 12 hours) and maintenance phase (approximately 12.5 milligrams/kg PO every other day).

Trilostane: A consensus has not been reached on the optimal dosing of trilostane. Some protocols involve once-daily dosing (1.0–6.6 milligrams/kg PO every 24 hours), and others involve twice-daily dosing (1.5–2.75 milligrams/kg PO every 12 hours) (Arenas et al. 2013). As for mitotane, patients treated with trilostane must be monitored and dosed based on ACTH stimulation testing and plasma cortisol concentrations.

(a)

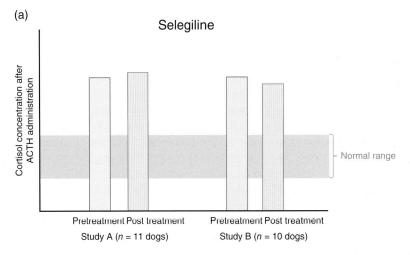

(b)

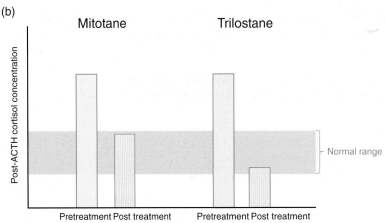

Figure 15.3 (a) Depiction of results from two separate clinical trials (Reusch et al. 1999; Braddock et al. 2004) of selegiline for treatment of pituitary-dependent hyperadrenocorticism in dogs. The small number of dogs in each trial can be explained by the fact that the studies were suspended for lack of efficacy. (b) Depiction of results from clinical trials of mitotane and trilostane for treatment of pituitary-dependent hyperadrenocorticism in dogs (Kintzer and Peterson 1991; Arenas et al. 2013).

Prednisone: 0.25 milligrams/kg PO once daily or divided *as needed*. Prednisone should be dispensed with trilostane or mitotane in the event of iatrogenic hypocortisolism. Owners should be instructed to administer prednisone if clinical signs of hypocortisolism occur.

15.3.4 Canine Hypoadrenocorticism

Treatment of an Addisonian crisis is a medical emergency, so drugs used to manage an acute presentation would not be dispensed by a community pharmacist. For chronic treatment of hypoadrenocorticism, most dogs require both mineralocorticoid and glucocorticoid replacement (Lathan 2015). Mineralocorticoid replacement needs can be met by either oral fludrocortisone or intramuscular injection of desoxycorticosterone pivalate (DOCP). Fludrocortisone is a human-approved formulation that is used in an extra-label manner in dogs, while DOCP is FDA approved for use in dogs with hypoadrenocorticism. There are important differences between the two drugs. The first is that even though fludrocortisone is classified as a mineralocorticoid, it also has some glucocorticoid activity. What this means for the patient is that glucocorticoid replacement may not be necessary in some dogs treated with fludrocortisone, or that a lower glucocorticoid replacement dose might be necessary compared to dogs treated with DOCP. DOCP has no glucocorticoid activity; therefore, all dogs treated with DOCP will require glucocorticoid replacement therapy. The other difference between the two drugs is the route of administration. Fludrocortisone is administered orally, while DOCP must be injected intramuscularly once every 25 days or so (dosing interval is determined by patient response). Although DOCP is labeled for intramuscular injection, some veterinarians may prescribe DOCP for subcutaneous injection, since this route of injection is tolerated better by most dogs. It is important for the pharmacist to inform the owner that DOCP may not be as effective if administered subcutaneously, or it may have to be administered more frequently than when injected intramuscularly. Information on injection techniques can be found in Chapter 24. Hydrocortisone is an inexpensive corticosteroid with both mineralocorticoid and glucocorticoid actions but unfortunately has not been effective for chronic management of hypoadrenocorticism in dogs. Glucocorticoid replacement needs can be met by prednisone administered at physiologic doses.

15.3.4.1 Drugs Most Likely to Be Prescribed for Hypoadrenocorticism

Mineralocorticoid replacement:

Fludrocortisone acetate: 0.01 mg/kg PO every 12 hours (dose usually needs to be increased over the first year of treatment).

Dramatic difference

Oral bioavailability of fludrocortisone is lower in dogs than in people. The dose for an adult human is roughly the same as what would be prescribed for a 25-pound dog.

Desoxycorticosterone pivalate (DOCP): 2.2 mg/kg by intramuscular injection every 25 days. Dosing interval may be shorter or longer for some dogs as determined by plasma electrolyte concentrations. Subcutaneous injection has been used successfully in some, but not all, patients.

Glucocorticoid replacement:

Prednisone: 0.25 mg/kg PO once daily or divided. The dose should be doubled in "stressful" situations such as illness, boarding, or strenuous exercise.

15.3.5 Diabetes Mellitus

Oral hypoglycemics are ineffective for treating diabetic dogs and are also ineffective for most diabetic cats. Despite the plethora of oral hypoglycemic agents available for treating human diabetics, glipizide is the only agent that is used for diabetic cats (Palm and Feldman 2012). While most cats won't respond to oral hypoglycemics, a subset of diabetic cats, roughly 30%, will show improvement in clinical signs with glipizide. Newer oral hypoglycemics have thus far not shown consistent efficacy in diabetic cats.

Insulin is the mainstay for managing canine and feline diabetes. While the general principles of insulin treatment in companion animals and people are similar, there are physiologic, pharmacokinetic, pharmacodynamic, and pragmatic differences that the pharmacist should understand. First, insulin secreted by the human pancreas is different than insulin secreted by the canine and feline pancreas. There are four amino acid differences between human and feline insulin and one amino acid difference between human and canine insulin. To prevent antibody production to a foreign protein, it has been suggested that insulin preparations for a dog or cat should take into account insulin amino acid sequence differences. This would mean that bovine insulin would be best for cats because there is only one amino acid difference between feline and bovine insulins. Dogs and pigs share the exact same insulin amino acid sequence, so pork insulin would be best for dogs if all other considerations were equal. Although animal-origin insulin products are no longer on the market for people, there are veterinary formulations containing pork or beef insulins. Some human insulin formulations are also used in diabetic dogs and cats.

An interesting species difference is the duration of action of insulin. Insulin's duration of action is substantially shorter in cats than in dogs or humans. The "once-a-day" human insulins such as insulin glargine or insulin detemir are predominantly administered twice daily in diabetic cats. These are used less frequently in dogs because other, less expensive insulin products seem to have better efficacy (Hess and Drobatz 2013; Fracassi et al. 2015).

The concentration of insulin supplied in human versus veterinary formulations is different. The pharmacist can play a key role in educating the owner about the difference in concentrations, and therefore the volume of insulin per dose. The two currently available veterinary insulin formulations are U40 and U100. If an owner doesn't understand the difference between U40 and U100 insulin, the pet might die as a result. Administering the same volume of U100 insulin under the assumption that it was U40 insulin would likely cause severe hypoglycemia. Equally important is the fact that U40 insulin must be administered with 40 U/mL syringes (red cap), whereas U100 insulin must be administered with 100 U/mL syringes (orange cap). For all but the largest of dogs, a low-dose (0.5 mL) syringe rather than a 1 mL syringe should be used for administering insulin. This allows more accurate dosing (Figure 15.4).

15.3.5.1 Drugs Most Likely to Be Prescribed for Diabetes Mellitus

Glipizide: Cats: 2.5 milligrams per cat PO every 12 hours.

NPH insulin, human recombinant: Dogs: 0.25 IU/kg by subcutaneous injection every 12 hours; adjust as appropriate. Available at a concentration of 100 IU/mL.

Lente insulin: Dogs: 0.25 IU/kg by subcutaneous injection every 12 hours; adjust as appropriate. Available as a veterinary formulation at a concentration of 40 IU/mL.

Porcine insulin zinc suspension: Dogs and cats: The veterinary formulation (Vetsulin), unlike most insulins, which should be gently rolled for mixing, requires thorough shaking.

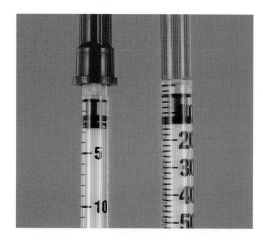

Figure 15.4 Two types of insulin syringes. The red cap indicates that the syringe is used for 40 U/mL insulin products, while the orange cap indicates the syringe is used for 100 U/mL insulin products. Notice how difficult it would be for an owner to accurately measure small doses (<20 units) of insulin using the orange-capped syringe, which is the standard size for human adults. The low-dose syringe is preferred for most veterinary diabetic patients to ensure that an accurate dose is administered. *Source:* Photo courtesy of Henry Moore Jr., Washington State University College of Veterinary Medicine, Biomedical Communications Unit.

Protamine zinc insulin: Cats: Starting dose is 0.2–0.7 IU/kg by subcutaneous injection every 12 hours. Available as a veterinary formulation at a concentration of 40 IU/mL.

Glargine insulin: Cats: 0.25 IU/kg lean body weight by subcutaneous injection every 12 hours up to a maximum dose of 3 IU per cat; adjust as appropriate. Available as a human formulation at a concentration of 100 IU/mL.

Detemir insulin: Cats: 1–2 IU per cat by subcutaneous injection every 12 hours; adjust as appropriate.

15.4 Adverse Drug Effects in Veterinary Species

Drugs for thyroid diseases: Levothyroxine adverse effects in dogs are similar to those described in human patients (signs of hyperthyroidism). Cats are at risk for several adverse effects of methimazole that are generally not a problem in people. Agranulocytosis and thrombocytopenia, which are rare complications in people treated with methimazole, occur more frequently in cats and tend to be more severe.

Mandatory monitoring

Cats can experience severe pruritis of the head and neck, which can result in vigorous scratching and self-trauma. Owners should be instructed to discontinue methimazole and seek veterinary care if this occurs.

Drugs for adrenal disease: Adverse effects of mitotane in dogs are similar to those that occur in people. Acute hypocortisolemia is arguably the most severe adverse event. This can be avoided by careful monitoring of the patient's clinical signs, particularly during the induction phase, and co-dispensing prednisone. Key monitoring parameters for dogs receiving mitotane include gastrointestinal signs (vomiting and diarrhea), decreased appetite, and a drop in energy level. A physiologic dose of prednisone should be administered if any of these occur, and the veterinarian should be contacted.

The same adverse event risks (and monitoring parameters) are true for trilostane. The primary mechanism of action of trilostane is reported to be inhibition of 3-beta hydroxysteroid dehydrogenase (Ouschan et al. 2012). However, a number of dogs treated with trilostane have developed adrenal necrosis, suggesting an adrenolytic effect, at least in some dogs (Chapman et al. 2004; Reusch et al. 2007).

Drugs for diabetes mellitus: The most common adverse effect of glipizide in diabetic cats is lack of efficacy. In these nonresponders, insulin is required for effective blood glucose control. Almost 20% of cats receiving glipizide will develop gastrointestinal signs (vomiting and anorexia) that will require dose reduction or discontinuation of the drug. A smaller percentage of cats may develop severe liver disease. Monitoring of liver enzymes is recommended.

The most common adverse effect of insulin is hypoglycemia. In veterinary patients, clinical signs of hypoglycemia include hunger, weakness, trembling, muscle twitching, lethargy, ataxia, seizures, blindness, behavior changes, coma, and death. Patients with mild signs of hypoglycemia can be treated by offering food. Patients with more severe signs of hypoglycemia, for example if the patient is too disoriented to eat, should be treated with oral dextrose solutions (Karo syrup) rubbed on the gums and immediately seen by a veterinarian. Exogenous insulin that is not identical to a patient's own insulin may result in the production of insulin antibodies, since it is a foreign protein. In some feline patients, insulin antibodies are thought to be a cause of insulin resistance whereby the cat's insulin requirement becomes quite high. Other causes of insulin resistance, including concurrent disease (infection, acromegaly, and hyperthyroidism), should be ruled out before attributing the high insulin requirement to insulin antibodies.

15.5 Nutritional Supplements for Veterinary Endocrine Diseases

Thyroid: An iodine-limited cat food has been recently introduced commercially and is being promoted for nutritional management of hyperthyroid cats (Van der Kooij et al. 2014). The product is relatively new, but early results indicate a high level of safety (at least in the short term) and moderate to good efficacy, with efficacy defined as returning thyroxine concentrations to the normal range.

Adrenal: Advertisements for herbal and nutritional products to treat Cushing's disease (hyperadrenocorticism) in dogs are abundant on the internet. Owners who are more comfortable with natural remedies may seek advice from the pharmacist. Currently, there are absolutely no data to support the use of any of these advertised products. Similarly, there are advertisements touting natural products for treating hypoadrenocorticism (Addison's disease) in dogs. One of the most common ingredients contained in these products is licorice (*Glycyrrhiza glabra*). Licorice inhibits 11 beta-hydroxysteroid dehydrogenase type 2, an enzyme that normally metabolizes cortisol to inactive metabolites. At high enough doses, licorice prolongs the plasma half-life of cortisol in individuals with functional adrenal glands (zona fasciculata). However, dogs with hypoadrenocorticism do not have functional adrenal glands and therefore have extremely low, often undetectable, plasma cortisol concentrations. Thus, there is insufficient substrate for 11 beta-hydroxysteroid dehydrogenase to act upon. However, there is one report of licorice as an adjunct to fludrocortisone treatment in a dog with hypoadrenocorticism (Jarett et al. 2005). In this report, licorice added to the dog's diet resulted in improved plasma sodium and potassium concentrations. Salt (table salt, sodium chloride) can also be added to the dog's food, but *not water*, to help increase plasma sodium concentrations as an adjunct to exogenous mineralocorticoid treatment. Salting the water is contraindicated, as this may deter the dog from drinking, which can be fatal since dogs with hypoadrenocortism are prone to hypovolemia and circulatory shock.

Diabetes: A number of dog and cat foods are marketed for diabetics. In general, these contain higher fiber (dogs and cats) and higher protein (cats) than standard pet foods. Some may also contain other ingredients such as chromium or vanadium that have been promoted as natural treatments for diabetes. Chromium supplementation, as an adjunct to insulin in 13 diabetic dogs, did not improve glycemic control compared to insulin treatment alone but caused no identifiable adverse effects (Schachter et al. 2001). The author was unable to find peer-reviewed publications reporting efficacy of chromium supplementation in diabetic cats. Vanadium was studied in a small number of diabetic cats (Martin and Rand 2000). It appears to decrease the insulin requirements of diabetic cats when administered concurrently but was ineffective as a stand-alone treatment.

15.6 FDA-Approved Veterinary Drug Products with No Human Drug Equivalent

See Table 15.1.

Abbreviations

ACTH	Adrenocorticotropic hormone
CT	Computed tomography
MRI	Magnetic resonance imaging
FDA	US Food and Drug Administration
NSAIDs	Nonsteroidal anti-inflammatory drugs
PO	Per os ("orally")
T3	Liothyronine (active form of thyroid hormone)
T4	Thyroxine (thyroid hormone that must be activated to T3)
TSH	Thyroid-stimulating hormone

Table 15.1 Drugs that are FDA approved for endocrine disease in a veterinary species but are not available in a human formulation.

Brand name	Active ingredient(s)	Drug class	Rationale/notes
Vetoryl®	Trilostane	Steroidogenesis inhibitor	Indicated for pituitary-dependent hyperadrenocorticism in dogs
Percorten-V®	DOCP	Mineralocorticoid	Some dogs with hypoadrenocorticism are inadequately controlled with fludrocortisone.
Vetsulin®, VetPen®	Porcine insulin zinc suspension	Intermediate-acting insulin	The amino acid sequence of pork and canine insulin is identical; 40 IU/mL concentration allows more accurate dosing for dogs and cats than most human insulin products.
ProZinc®	Recombinant human protamine zinc insulin	Long-acting insulin	40 IU/mL concentration allows more accurate dosing for dogs and cats than most human insulin products.

References

Arenas, C., Melian, C., and Perez-Alenza, M.D. (2013). Evaluation of 2 trilostane protocols for the treatment of canine pituitary-dependent hyperadrenocorticism: twice daily versus once daily. *J. Vet. Intern. Med.* 27: 1478–1485.

Behrend, E.N. (2006). Drugs used to treat endocrine disease. *Vet. Clin. North Amer. Sm. An. Pract.* 36: 1087–1105.

Behrend, E.N., Civco, T.D., and Boothe, D.M. (2012). Drug therapy for endocrinopathies. In: *Small Animal Clinical Pharmacology and Therapeutics*, 2e (ed. D.M. Boothe), 783–847. St. Louis, MO: Elsevier.

Braddock, J.A., Church, D.B., Robertson, I.D. et al. (2004). Inefficacy of selegiline in treatment of canine pituitary-dependent hyperadrenocorticism. *Aust. Vet. J.* 82: 272–277.

Chapmen, P.S., Kelly, D.F., Archer, J. et al. (2004). Adrenal necrosis in a dog receiving trilostane for the treatment of hyperadrenocorticism. *J. Small Anim. Pract.* 45: 307–310.

Feldman, E.C. and Nelson, R.W. (2004). Hypothyroidism. In: *Canine and Feline Endocrinology and Reproduction*, 3e (ed. E.C. Feldman and R.W. Nelson), 86–151. St. Louis, MO: Saunders.

Fracassi, F., Corradini, S., Hafner, M. et al. (2015). Detemir insulin for the treatment of diabetes mellitus in dogs. *J. Am. Vet. Med. Assoc.* 247: 73–38.

Gostelow, R., Forcada, Y., Graves, T. et al. (2014). Systematic review of feline diabetic remission: separating fact from opinion. *Vet. J.* 202: 208–221.

Hess, R.S. and Drobatz, K.J. (2013). Glargine insulin for treatment of naturally occurring diabetes mellitus in dogs. *J. Am. Vet. Med. Assoc.* 243 (8): 1154–1161.

Hill, K. (2015). Hyperadrenocorticism. In: *Clinical Veterinary Advisor: Dogs and Cats*, 3e (ed. E. Cote), 502–504. St Louis, MO: Elsevier.

Hwang, A.Y., Smith, S.M., and Gums, J.G. (2017). Adrenal gland disorders. In: *Pharmacotherapy: A Pathophysiologic Approach*, 10e (ed. J.T. DiPiro, R.L. Talbert, G.C. Yee, et al.), 1207–1226. New York: McGraw-Hill.

Jarrett, R.H., Norman, E.J., and Squires, R.A. (2005). Licorice and canine Addison's disease. *N.Z. Vet. J.* 53: 214.

Jonklaas, J. and Kane, M.P. (2017). Thyroid disorders. In: *Pharmacotherapy: A Pathophysiologic Approach*, 10e (ed. J.T. DiPiro, R.L. Talbert, G.C. Yee, et al.), 1183–1205. New York: McGraw-Hill.

Kintzer, P.P. and Peterson, M.E. (1991). Mitotane (o,p'-DDD) treatment of 200 dogs with pituitary-dependent hyperadrenocorticism. *J. Vet. Intern. Med.* 5 (3): 182–190.

Lathan, P. (2015). Hypoadrenocorticism. In: *Clinical Veterinary Advisor: Dogs and Cats*, 3e (ed. E. Cote), 525–527. St Louis, MO: Elsevier.

Lavergne, S.N., Fosset, F.T.J., Kennedy, P. et al. (2015). Potential cutaneous hypersensitivity reaction to an inactive ingredient of thyroid hormone supplements in a dog. *Vet. Derm.* 27: 53–e16.

Martin, G. and Rand, J. (2000). Current understanding of feline diabetes: part 2, treatment. *J. Fel. Med. Surg.* 2: 3–17.

Mattin, M., O'Neill, D., Church, J.D. et al. (2014). An epidemiological study of diabetes mellitus in dogs attending first opinion practice in the UK. *Vet. Rec.* 174 (14): 349.

Mizisin, A.P., Shelton, G.D., Burgers, M.L. et al. (2002). Neurological complications associated with spontaneously occurring feline diabetes mellitus. *J. Neuropathol. Exp. Neurol.* 61: 872–884.

Ohlund, M., Fail, T., Strom Holst, B. et al. (2015). Incidence of diabetes mellitus in insured Swedish cats in relation to age, breed and sex. *J. Vet. Intern. Med.* 29 (5): 1342–1347.

Ouschan, C., Lepschy, M., Zeugswether, F. et al. (2012). The influence of trilostane on steroid hormone metabolism in canine adrenal glands and corpora lutea: an in vitro study. *Vet. Res. Commun.* 36: 35–40.

Palm, C.A. and Feldman, E.C. (2012). Oral hypoglycemics in cats with diabetes mellitus. *Vet. Clin. North Am. Sm. An. Pract.* 43: 407–415.

Peterson, M. (2012). Hyperthyroidism in cats: what's causing this epidemic of thyroid disease and can we prevent it? *J. Feline Med. Surg.* 14: 804–818.

Peterson, M.E. (2014). Animal models of disease: feline hyperthyroidism an animal model for toxic nodular goiter. *J. Endocrinol.* 223 (2): T97–T114.

Pignato, A., Pankaskie, M., and Birnie, C. (2010). Stability of methimazole in poloxamer lecithin organogel to determine beyond-use date. *Int. J. Pharm. Compd.* 14: 522–525.

Plumb, D.C. (2015). Levothyroxicine sodium. In: *Plumb's Veterinary Drug Handbook*, 8e (ed. D.C. Plumb), 619–623. Ames, IA: Wiley-Blackwell.

Reusch, C.E., Sieber-Ruckstuhl, N., Wenger, M. et al. (2007). Histological evaluation of the adrenal glands of seven dogs with hyperadrenocorticism treated with trilostane. *Vet. Rec.* 160: 219–224.

Reusch, C.E., Steffen, T., and Hoerauf, A. (1999). The efficacy of L-deprenyl in dogs with pituitary-dependent hyperadrenocorticism. *J. Vet. Intern. Med.* 13: 291–301.

Richter, M., Guscetti, F., and Spiess, B. (2002). Aldose reductase activity and glucose-related opacities in incubated lenses from dogs and cats. *Am. J. Vet. Res.* 63: 1591–1597.

Sartor, L.L., Trepanier, L.A., Kroll, M.M. et al. (2004). Efficacy and safety of transdermal methimazole in the treatment of cats with hyperthyroidism. *J. Vet. Intern. Med.* 18: 651–655.

Schachter, S., Nelson, R.W., and Kirk, C.A. (2001). Oral chromium picolinate and control of glycemia in insulin-treated diabetic dogs. *J. Vet. Intern. Med.* 15: 379–384.

Sparkes, A.H., Cannon, M., Church, D. et al. (2015). ISFM consensus guidelines on the practical management of diabetes mellitus in cats. *J. Feline Med. Surg.* 17: 235–250.

Triplett, C.L., Repas, T., and Alvarez, C. (2017). Diabetes mellitus. In: *Pharmacotherapy: A Pathophysiologic Approach*, 10e (ed. J.T. DiPiro, R.L. Talbert, G.C. Yee, et al.), 1139–1181. New York: McGraw-Hill.

Van der Kooij, M., Becvarova, I., Meyer, H.P. et al. (2014). Effects of an iodine-restricted food on client-owned cats with hyperthyroidism. *J. Fel. Med. Surg.* 16: 491–498.

Van Hoek, I., Hesta, M., and Biourge, V. (2015). A critical review of food-associated factors proposed in the etiology of feline hyperparathyroidism. *J. Feline Med. Surg.* 17 (10): 837–847.

16

Behavioral Pharmacotherapeutics

Karen L. Overall

Department of Biology, University of Pennsylvania, Philadelphia, PA, USA
Department of Health Management, Atlantic Veterinary College, UPEI, Charlottetown, PE, Canada

---

Key Points

- The use of behavioral medication is essential for veterinary patients with behavioral pathology.
- The most common canine behavioral conditions for which medication will be of benefit include: separation anxiety, generalized anxiety disorder, noise phobias, aggression, and profound fears in dogs.
- The most common feline behavioral conditions for which medication will be of benefit include: profound fears, aggression, and anxiety affecting various types of inappropriate urination.

- The key to successful pharmacological therapy in patients with behavioral conditions is to couple its use to plans for modifying behavior by learning new and more appropriate responses, since most of the medications used help to facilitate learning.
- Because veterinary patients cannot explain how medication makes them feel, it is critical that owners have an understanding of how the medication works, what the specific expected behavioral changes might be, and how to monitor for adverse effects.

16.1 Comparative Aspects of Behavior Disorders

The most common behavioral conditions seen in veterinary medicine vary by species and the individual species' evolutionary history. Accordingly, when considering horses, it is clear that many anxiety-related conditions that are recognized are associated with the absence of what would be the normal social group of a herd, and with lack of access to spaces over which travel and foraging otherwise would be almost continuous. For cats, recognized behavioral conditions almost always reflect the presence of some social stressor, best understood within the evolutionary history of cats. Cats are born into extended matrilineal family groups, and mixing of families is rare in the natural setting. Unfortunately, mixing of families tends to be the usual pattern for multicat households, contributing to feline behavioral disorders (Figure 16.1) that require pharmacological treatment. By nature, cats also have activity and foraging behaviors that are quite different from those that most households impose on them. Accordingly, anxieties and aggressions that are rooted in unmet or disrupted social and environmental needs are common in both cats and hoofed stock.

Pharmacotherapeutics for Veterinary Dispensing, First Edition. Edited by Katrina L. Mealey.
© 2019 John Wiley & Sons, Inc. Published 2019 by John Wiley & Sons, Inc.

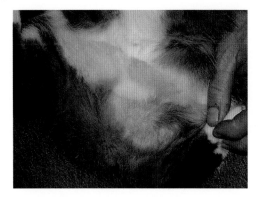

Figure 16.1 Cat with alopecia caused by overgrooming. This behavior was temporally associated with the addition of a new cat to the household.

The evolutionary history of dogs is different from that of cats or horses. Dogs share an extended evolutionary history with modern humans based on collaborative and cooperative work, and convergent patterns of social interaction, communication, and parental care. Accordingly, when dogs develop mental health conditions, these conditions parallel and may be excellent models for those in humans. Among the most common and easily recognizable of these similar conditions are obsessive-compulsive disorder (Figure 16.2), separation anxiety (Figure 16.3),

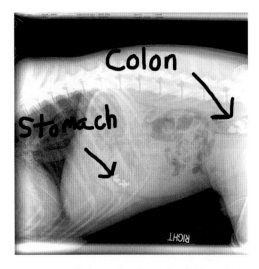

Figure 16.2 Abdominal radiograph of a dog with obsessive-compulsive disorder who seeks and ingests rocks.

phobic reactions to noise (Figure 16.4), fear of novel places and experiences, and generalized anxiety.

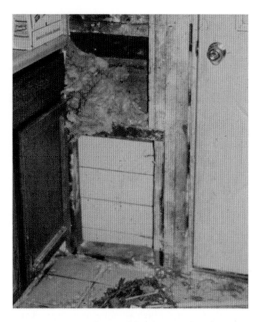

Figure 16.3 A small part of the damage done by a dog (Shar Pei) who had been left alone for two hours and who was profoundly afflicted with separation anxiety.

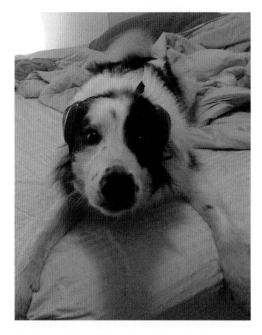

Figure 16.4 A Border Collie with noise phobia wearing noise-blocking earphones during a storm.

16.2   Diagnostic Testing

Specific diagnostic tests for most mental health conditions are lacking in veterinary medicine. Instead, it is most common to rule out putative somatic reasons for behavioral change with routine and specialized diagnostic testing, as is also done in humans. Once somatic disease is ruled out, patterns of behavior are assessed to see if they meet published diagnostic criteria and whether the pattern of behavior is consistent with the context in which such criteria might occur. Veterinary behavioral medicine is a relatively new field, and veterinary behavioral specialists are only now beginning discrete assessments of changes in physiology and patterns of behaviors, coupled occasionally with imaging studies that, when combined, may be diagnostic for a particular condition.

16.3   Pharmacological Treatment of Common Behavioral Disorders

The use of medication is essential for effective treatment of many behavioral problems in veterinary patients. While medication is most commonly recommended for ongoing or severe behavioral problems, it may be even more effectively used *early* in the course of the condition.

The one common and outstanding finding from placebo-controlled, double-blind studies is that the addition of psychotherapeutic agents to behavioral and environmental modification leads to faster and better treatment outcomes (King et al. 2000a,b; Landsberg et al. 2008; Sherman and Mills 2008). The reason for the enhanced efficacy of treatment approaches that combine medication with behavioral work and environmental change lies in the effects of these medications on neurons: Both learning and behavioral medications rely on the same molecular changes, and serotonergic neurons, which are affected by many of

the medications routinely used, are most dense in the frontal cortex and hippocampus, the parts of the brain primarily involved in learning. Accordingly, use of psychopharmaceuticals, especially for canine and feline patients, is becoming widespread, with new medications, supplements, and diets continually being developed.

16.3.1   Medications Used Most Frequently to Treat Behavioral Conditions

Medications most commonly used to treat behavioral conditions in dogs and cats are antidepressants and anxiolytics, which fall into three main classes (Overall 2001; Simpson and Papich 2003):

- Benzodiazepines (alprazolam, clorazepate, diazepam, midazolam, oxazepam, clonazepam, lorazepam, and temazepam)
- Tricyclic antidepressants (TCAs; amitriptyline, nortriptyline, clomipramine, imipramine, and doxepin)
- Selective serotonin reuptake inhibitors (SSRIs; fluoxetine, paroxetine, sertaline, fluvoxamine, citalopram, and escitalopram).

Increasingly, veterinary behaviorists are starting to treat patients with:

- Noradrenergic reuptake inhibitors (reboxetine)
- Dual serotonin–norepinephrine reuptake inhibitors (venlafaxine and duloxetine)
- Dual serotonin 2A agonist–serotonin reuptake inhibitors (trazodone and nefazaodone)
- Noradrenergic and specific serotonergic antidepressants (mirtazapine)
- Centrally acting alpha-adrenergic receptor agonists (clonidine, guanfacine, medetomidine, and dexmedetomidine; dexmedetomidine also affects alpha$_{1A}$-receptors).

Less commonly used medications include:

- Monoamine oxidase inhibitors (selegiline)
- Azapirones (buspirone)
- N-methyl-ᴅ-aspartate (NMDA) antagonists (memantine)

- Sympathomimetics (dextroamphetamine and methyphenidate)
- Hormonal agents.

Behavior-modifying medications exert their effects primarily through modulation of the neurotransmitters serotonin (5-HT), dopamine, noradrenaline/norepinephrine, gamma amino butyric acid (GABA), and their related metabolites (e.g. the excitatory amino acid glutamate, which becomes GABA). Accordingly, any medication, supplement, or dietary constituent that shares a metabolic or synthetic pathway with any of these neurotransmitters can cause a drug interaction. There are now a number of veterinary diets that act in such ways, including Royal Canin's CALM diet, which uses alpha casozepine, a benzodiazepine mimic, to affect GABA$_A$ receptors. Pharmacists should therefore question owners about an animal's diet prior to dispensing behavior-modifying drugs to prevent drug–diet interactions.

The vast majority of medications prescribed to treat behavioral disorders in veterinary patients are used in an extra-label manner. While such use is legal in the USA, it should be explained to the owner. Published data on safety and efficacy for medications used in an extra-label manner may or may not exist for the species treated, but all FDA-approved medications are required to undergo toxicology studies in dogs and so may have canine pharmacokinetic and toxicology data available.

As of this writing, clomipramine (Clomicalm°, Novartis), fluoxetine (Reconcile°, Elanco), selegiline (Anipryl°, Zoetis), oral transmucosal dexmedetomidine (dexmedetomidine OTM; Sileo°, Orion), and imepitoin (Pexion, Boehringer Ingelheim Vetmedica) are all FDA veterinary drug products.

16.3.1.1 Benzodiazepines

Benzodiazepines easily cross the blood–brain barrier and are lipophilic. The rate at which they diffuse through the brain is dependent on the individual benzodiazepine and largely controlled by its lipophilicity. The faster the diffusion rate, the quicker the onset of action. Distribution half-lives of intravenously administered benzodiazepines can be on the order of minutes. Orally administered benzodiazepines reach their maximum plasma concentrations in as little as 30 minutes or as long as several hours in humans (Riss et al. 2008), which is likely the case in domestic species also (see Tables 16.1 and 16.2).

Benzodiazepines can be classified as low-, moderate-, or high-potency compounds based on the *in vivo* affinity of the parent compound and any active metabolites for the receptor. Clonazepam and lorazepam are considered high-potency benzodiazepines with concomitantly long elimination half-lives, while clorazepate and diazepam are considered moderate-potency benzodiazepines (Riss et al. 2008).

Table 16.1 Elimination half-lives of benzodiazepine parent compounds and intermediate metabolites in humans.

Parent compound	t$_{1/2}$ parent compound (hours)	t$_{1/2}$ active metabolite (hours)	Overall duration of action (hours)
Triazolam	2–4	2	Ultra-short: 6
Oxazepam	8–12		Short: 12–18
Alprazolam	6–12	6	Medium: 24
Diazepam	24–40	60	Long: 24–48
Clonazepam	50 19–60[a]		Long: 24–48

[a] Riss et al. (2008).
Source: Greenblatt et al. (1981, 1983).

Table 16.2 Duration of action of diazepam and its intermediate metabolite, nordiazepam (N-desmethyl diazepam), in selected domestic animals.

Species	Diazepam $t_{1/2}$ (hours)	N-desmethyl diazepam $t_{1/2}$ (hours)
Horse	24–48	51–120
Cat	5.5	21
Dog	3.2	3–6

Source: Schwartz et al. (1965).

Benzodiazepines decrease muscle tone by a central action that is independent of the sedative effect, but may function as a nonspecific anxiolytic effect since many distressed animals have increased muscle tone. Clonazepam has muscle relaxation effects at lower dosages than those needed for behavioral effects, a beneficial therapeutic effect for distressed dogs and cats.

Benzodiazepines are essential for treatment of sporadic events involving profound anxiety or panic, such as storms (Crowell-Davis et al. 2003), fireworks, and panic associated with departure of their human companions signaled by an outside indicator like an alarm clock. For these drugs to be efficacious, based on predicted maximal plasma concentrations, they should be administered to the patient *at least one hour before the anticipated stimulus, and preferably before the patient exhibits any anticipatory signs of distress.*

Benzodiazepines can also be used as interventional drugs, and can be used with daily TCAs or SSRIs. For dogs that are easily scared or aroused by numerous stimuli throughout the day, benzodiazepines can be given two to three times per day when the owner knows that the dog will be exposed to such stimuli. Repeat dosing allows the dog to benefit from active intermediate metabolites that have different half-lives than do the parent compounds. In this case, owners need not give the benzodiazepine on days when the stimuli are not expected. Finally, if the

dog does experience profound fear or panic, benzodiazepines administered at the time when or shortly after the animal becomes distressed can decrease the fear, shorten the recovery period, and prevent the patient from developing a learned response associated with their fear. Alprazolam is actually considered panicolytic.

Amnestic effects are associated with most benzodiazepines at clinically relevant concentrations. These effects are beneficial when benzodiazepines are a component of preoperative sedative protocols or when used immediately after a profoundly distressing event (e.g. a storm, entrapment, or a fight with another dog or cat). However, if benzodiazepines are to be used as part of a treatment plan that requires active learning, the pharmacist should recommend to pet owners that some assessment of whether the patient is learning is helpful. At lower concentrations, benzodiazepines will facilitate learning by decreasing anxiety and muscular tension. At higher concentrations, they can interfere with complex learning through sedative and anamnestic effects. Owners can become quite adept at noting when their dog or cat is able to acquire and use new information, versus situations where the animal seems sedated or just not able to learn.

The benzodiazepines currently and commonly used in dogs and cats are listed in Table 16.3, along with their major properties, extrapolated from human and rodent literature.

While many benzodiazepines can cause sedation, the benzodiazepines that are currently used most commonly (e.g. alprazolam, oxazepam, and clonazepam) are less sedating than diazepam and clorazepate. Because dogs and cats, like humans, can experience a wide range of effects when treated with benzodiazepines, owners should be advised to initially administer benzodiazepines when they can monitor the patient. This means that the first dose or two should be given when the owner is home and can monitor the animal.

Table 16.3 Characterization of and potential therapeutic uses for select benzodiazepines commonly used to treat behavioral disorders in dogs and cats.

Benzodiazepine	Pharmacokinetic characteristics (human and rodent data)	Potential therapeutic use for behavioral disorders
Alprazolam	<ul><li>Intermediate acting</li><li>Extended-release form available</li><li>Absorption delayed by food</li><li>Substrate of CYP450 enzyme 3A4</li><li>No interactions between alprazolam and sertraline or paroxetine</li><li>Fluoxetine prolongs $t_{1/2}$ and increases AUC of alprazolam</li><li>Fluvoxamine increases alprazolam concentrations (up to 100%)</li><li>Venlafaxine lowers the AUC by ~30%</li></ul>	Panic and panic disorder Short-term treatment of acute and severe anxiety
Clonazepam	<ul><li>Long acting</li><li>High (90%) oral bioavailability</li><li>Biotransformation possibly involving CYP3A</li><li>Undergoes extensive metabolism, but no active intermediate metabolites are formed</li></ul>	Muscle relaxant Anxiety
Clorazepate	<ul><li>Undergoes complete conversion to N-desmethyl diazepam in GI tract</li><li>Effects almost entirely due to concentrations of N-desmethyl diazepam</li></ul>	Panic Profound anxiety
Diazepam	<ul><li>Action primarily due to N-desmethyl diazepam, especially with repeat dosing</li><li>Temazepam and oxazepam are relatively minor metabolites</li><li>Phenobarbital decreases AUC and oral bioavailability</li><li>Omeprazole inhibits the formation of the 3 main metabolites: nordiazepam, temazepam, and 4'-hydroxydiazepam</li><li>Readily absorbed orally, rectally, and intranasally</li></ul>	Anxiolytic Preoperative anesthesia
Lorazepam	<ul><li>Premedication for general anesthesia</li><li>Metabolism impaired by CYP enzyme inhibitors (e.g. ketoconazole or fluconazole)</li></ul>	Anxiolytic Sedative Amnestic agent (possible use for panic associated with highly unpleasant experience)
Midazolam	<ul><li>Short acting</li><li>Effects dose-dependent and even with CYP3A induction $t_{1/2}$ increases with high dosages because of a concomitant increase in volume of distribution</li><li>Can be administered by mouth, sublingually, or IV</li></ul>	Sedative Premed for anxiety and induction prior to anesthesia
Oxazepam	<ul><li>Intermediate acting</li><li>Less likely to accumulate in patients with hepatic impairment than other benzodiazepines</li></ul>	Anxiolytic Anorexia in cats

AUC, Area under the curve; IV, intravenous.
Source: Mandrioli et al. (2008).

Some dogs and cats experience excitement when treated with benzodiazepines. The excitement will resolve in a few hours, during which time the animal should be prevented from causing harm to itself. If necessary, the benzodiazepine antagonist flumazenil can be used to reverse the excitatory effects.

Undesirable excitement and sedation in dogs and cats can be a function of dose and/or the specific benzodiazepine chosen. Owners should be encouraged to try at least three dosages (at the low, median, and high ends of the dose range) before concluding that the particular benzodiazepine either excites or sedates their dog or cat. Patients who respond to one benzodiazepine in this manner may not do so to another. Unfortunately, trial and error is currently the only means available to determine if an animal can tolerate a particular benzodiazepine. Anecdotal reports indicate that geographical and family groups of dogs have no apparent response to some or all benzodiazepines, suggesting that there may be a genetic mechanism interfering with benzodiazepine action (e.g. cytochrome P450 [CYP] enzymes, benzodiazepine receptor, etc.) in these patients. Specific polymorphisms have not yet been reported but if identified could become the basis of a test for benzodiazepine sensitivity. Human drug-metabolizing enzymes (and their canine orthologs) involved in benzodiazepine metabolism include CYP3A4 (CYP3A12, CYP3A26), CYP3A5, CYP2C19 (CYP2D6, CYP2D41), and uridine diphosphate (UDP) glucuronyltransferases. While polymorphisms are known to exist for canine CYP3A12, it is not yet known how the polymorphisms affect benzodiazepine metabolism. Table 16.4 lists medications that may affect the action of benzodiazepines through induction or inhibition of human drug-metabolizing enzymes. However, it is important to note that CYP enzyme inducers and inhibitors can differ dramatically between species.

Some veterinarians hesitate to prescribe benzodiazepines for animals because of the concern that the animal's behaviors will become "disinhibited." The particular concern is for disinhibition of aggression in animals being treated for problematic aggressive behavior. For example, one might be concerned that if benzodiazepines were used at

Table 16.4 Inhibitors and inducers of human drug-metabolizing enzymes involved in the metabolism of various benzodiazepines.

CYP450 enzyme	Benzodiazepine substrate	Inhibitors	Inducers
CYP2C19	Diazepam	Fluvoxamine Omeprazole Oxcarbazepine	Dexamethazone Phenobarbital Phenytoin St. John's wort
CYP3A4	Clonazepam Diazepam Midazolam	Azole antifungals (e.g. ketoconazole) Cimetidine Clarithromycin Diltiazem Erythromycin Fluoxetine Nefazodone Sertraline	Carbamazepine Phenobarbital Phenytoin St. John's wort
UDP Glucuronyl transferase	Lorazepam Oxazepam	Valproate	Carbamazepine Phenobarbital Phenytoin

Source: Adapted from Riss et al. (2008).

anti-anxiety levels, some behaviors that a dog was suppressing because of its anxiety may suddenly emerge. That said, while only truly inhibited aggressions might be at risk for dis-inhibition after benzodiazepine treatment, the risk is likely offset by the improvement in pathology that would make expression of aggression less likely.

Data from the literature on human responses to benzodiazepines suggest that concerns about disinhibition are overblown, and that there is no direct evidence for benzodiazepines engendering disinhibition. Rothschild et al. (2000) found no evidence for disinhibition in a human population based on occurrence of acts of self-injury, assaults on staff or other patients, need for seclusion or restraints, increased need for observation while hospitalized, or decreases in patient privileges (which would result from behavioral disinhibition) for patients treated with alprazolam or diazepam when compared with patients not treated with a benzodiazepine. This finding is consistent with other reviews and meta-analyses when these used controlled, blinded studies (Rothschild 1992; Jonas and Hearron 1996).

Many of the behaviors attributed to disin-hibition may actually be due to the sedating properties of benzodiazepines since this affects memory and cognition. Adverse effects on cognition appear to parallel the sedative properties of particular benzodiazepines. There is evidence that sedation may be more likely with benzodiazepines that go through the N-desmethyldiazepam pathway (Riss et al. 2008). Many of the long-term and adverse effects of benzodiazepines are caused by intermediate metabolites. N-desmethyldi-azepam (nordiazpepam), the intermediate metabolite produced from first-pass metabo-lism of diazepam, is heavily sedative. At high concentrations, it causes confusion, ataxia, and apparent amnesia. These conditions are noted in humans, with the elderly at higher risk. There are little to no data on effects for elderly cats and dogs.

The long half-life of nordiazepam may also be relevant for an idiosyncratic hepatic necrosis reported with oral diazepam administration in cats (Center et al. 1996; Hughes et al. 1996). In dogs, diazepam has an elimination half-life of 3.2 hours, while nordiazepam has an elimination half-life of 3–6 hours. For cats, the corresponding half-lives are 5.5 hours and 21 hours, respectively. This means that an extremely sedating intermediate metabolite (nordiaz-epam), plus the parent compound (diaze-pam), now must be metabolized through a glucuronidation pathway in a species (the cat) that lacks several UDP glucuronyl transferase enzymes relative to dogs and humans. While hepatic necrosis is rare, sedation can be a real concern in cats. Use of benzodiazepines that do not involve the nordiazepam intermediate metabolite and are less affected by glucuronidation (e.g. oxazepam and alprazolam) may be more desirable for use in cats.

Pet owners often ask about two specific potential side effects of continued benzodiaz-epine use: tolerance and dependence. The term "dependence" is used in human medi-cine to describe the desire/compulsion to take the medication to achieve a desired effect or to avoid the lack of the drug's effect when not taking the medication (Riss et al. 2008). As such, the ability to become dependent relies on the presence of opposable thumbs and access to the medication at will. Canine and feline patients do not have such access. However, it is important to note that because of the concern for human dependence, cer-tain households should not have access to benzodiazepines. The pharmacist can play a key role in preventing drug diversion.

Physiological "tolerance" can occur with benzodiazepines regardless of species. Cross-tolerance is possible with benzodiazepines and may be specific to the compound used. Oddly, in humans, the tendency to develop physiological tolerance does not depend on the chemistry or pharmacokinetics, but it may be a pharmacodynamic function of a particular benzodiazepine in an individual patient. While dependence is associated in humans with high dosages of benzodiazepines, high potency, short duration of action, and long duration of treatment, these factors appear to be only partially involved in physiological tolerance.

Rebound and withdrawal phenomena/syndromes are well known for benzodiazepines but also occur with TCAs, SSRIs, and other drugs that modify neurotransmission. With rebound syndrome, the patient's original signs reappear once medication is discontinued. With withdrawal syndrome, new signs accompanied by distress appear once medication is discontinued. Gradual weaning (over a period of weeks) to the lowest effective level of medication usually prevents occurrence of these phenomena, while abrupt withdrawal, especially with shorter acting compounds, may increase the risk of these phenomena.

16.3.1.2 Gabapentinoids

Gabapentin is a synthetic GABA analog, but it is not active at GABA receptors, not regulated at the neurochemical somatodendritic autoreceptor level, and not biotransformed (in humans), so there are no pharmacologically active intermediate metabolites. Current thought is that gabapentin binds to an auxiliary subunit of voltage-gated calcium channels, which stimulates a range of other actions that result in membrane depolarization. Gabapentin also affects the amino acid active transporter by increasing the concentration of brain and intracellular GABA, increases nonsynaptic GABA release from glia, modulates glutamate metabolism (possibly very important for conditions involving impulsivity), and modulates sodium and calcium ion channels (which subsequently increases blood serotonin concentrations).

Dramatic difference
Gabapentin is available as an oral solution for human patients. ***This should NOT be used in dogs*** because it contains xylitol, which is highly toxic to dogs.

Common therapeutic uses for gabapentin in veterinary patients include:

- Myogenic and neurogenic pain
- Anxiety disorders, including panic

- Generalized anxiety disorder and social phobias
- Adjuvant to other treatments for obsessive-compulsive disorder.

Because human studies have shown that gabapentin has no active metabolites, is not highly bound to plasma proteins, and does not induce CYP450 enzymes, it is considered a relatively safe medication to use, especially in animals with hepatic compromise. However, because gabapentin relies almost exclusively on renal excretion, it should be used cautiously in patients with renal compromise. Side effects in humans have been reported to include "psychosis," so pet owners should be counseled to watch for "personality changes," but the most commonly reported side effect is sedation.

16.3.1.3 Tricyclic Antidepressants

TCAs are structurally related to the phenothiazine antipsychotics and are used in humans to treat endogenous depression, panic attacks, phobic and obsessive states, neuropathic pain states, and pediatric enuresis. While TCAs have a number of pharmacological actions, their ability to inhibit presynaptic reuptake of NE and 5-HT is responsible for the antidepressant effect. With long-term use, TCAs may cause downregulation of beta-adrenergic and 5-HT_2 receptors. Many TCAs can block muscarinic, alpha-1 adrenergic, and H_1 and H_2 receptors, which account for common undesired effects reported in humans (e.g. dry mouth, sedation, and hypotension). In veterinary medicine, however, the antihistaminergic effects may be useful in treating pruritic conditions and those involving excess salivation and urination as nonspecific signs of distress. In companion animals, the primary use of the TCA doxepin, which is 800 times more potent than diphendramine as an H_1 antagonist, is for pruritic conditions, particularly those with concurrent behavioral foci. Cats are extremely sensitive to doxepin and can become heavily sedated or ataxic, so close monitoring, low starting dosages, and gradual dose increases are essential.

Despite the frequent use of TCAs in companion animals, there is only one TCA that is FDA approved for veterinary use. Clomipramine (Clomicalm) is indicated for treating separation anxiety in dogs six months of age or older. The pharmacokinetics of clomipramine in dogs are as follows: Steady-state levels after oral administration are reached in three to five days, with C_{max} occurring one to three hours after an oral dose. The elimination $t_{1/2}$ of the parent compound and active metabolite are 1–16 hours and 1–2 hours, respectively (Hewson et al. 1998; King et al. 2000a,b). The disposition of clomipramine is reported to differ in cats. The C_{max} of clomipramine is three hours, while that of its active metabolite, desmethyl-clomipramine, is seven hours (Lainesse et al. 2006, 2007a,b). It has been suggested that cats may have a lower capacity to hydroxylate metabolites of clomipramine, compared to dogs and humans, so cats undergoing chronic dosing should be monitored closely for adverse effects (Lainesse et al. 2007b).

Even before the introduction of clomipramine to the veterinary drug market, TCAs have been extremely successful in treating many canine and feline behavior disorders, including separation anxiety, generalized anxiety that may be a precursor to some elimination (urinating or defecating in inappropriate locations), or aggressive behaviors. They are also used for treating pruritic conditions that may be involved in, or precursors to, self-mutilation (repeated licking or biting of an area of the body when no underlying disease process can be identified) or compulsive grooming (Figure 16.1). Additionally, TCAs have been used to treat narcolepsy in a number of species, including horses. Amitriptyline, an older TCA, has been used successfully for treating separation anxiety and generalized anxiety. Imipramine has been useful for treating mild attention deficit disorders in people, and it may be useful for similar disorders in dogs, since it has been used to treat mild narcolepsy. Clomipramine has been successful in the treatment of human and canine obsessive-compulsive disorders (Overall and Dunham 2002) in addition to separation anxiety. Whether this is due to the parent compound's TCA effects or the actions of the active metabolite, n-desmethyl serotonin, as an SSRI is not known.

Knowledge of whether or not a particular TCA has an active metabolite can be important: Cats and dogs experiencing sedation or other side effects with a particular TCA may do quite well if treated with the active metabolite instead (Table 16.5). For example, cats that become sedated or nauseous when treated

Table 16.5 Relative activity of TCA parent compounds and active metabolites on NE and 5-HT reuptake and muscarinic receptors.

Parent compound	Active metabolite	NE	5-HT	Potential for sedation[a]	Potential for anticholinergic effects
Desipramine		++	+	Low	Low
Imipramine	Desipramine	+++	++	Moderate	Moderate
Amitriptyline	Nortriptyline	++	++	High	High
Nortriptyline		+	+	Moderate	Moderate
Clomipramine	n-Desmethyl clomipramine + clomipramine[b]	++	+++	High	High

+, Mild effect; ++, moderate effect; +++, large effect.
[a] At therapeutic concentrations in dogs and cats, sedative effects are transient. Dogs and cats may sleep more deeply and soundly but should not be groggy. If the patient is groggy or sedated after three to four days of treatment, this should be considered a true side effect, prompting a medication and/or dose modification.
[b] Does not include the specific effect of the intermediate metabolite as a selective serotonin reuptake inhibitor (SSRI).

with amitriptyline may respond well when treated with nortriptyline at the same dose.

Many adverse effects of TCAs reported in humans are mediated by their anticholinergic effects. These include dry mouth, constipation, urinary retention, tachycardia, and other arrhythmias. Other adverse effects, such as orthostatic hypotension, syncope, disorientation, generalized lethargy, and inappetence, may be associated with alpha-1 adrenergic receptor blockade. TCA-induced adverse effects seem to be rare and less diverse in dogs. Reported adverse effects in dogs include gastrointestinal distress, changes in appetite, occasional serious sedation, and distress/discomfort associated with unremitting tachycardia. These resolve when the drug is withdrawn.

Many of the contraindications for use of TCAs in human patients are similar for veterinary patients, including animals with a history of urinary retention, glaucoma, and uncontrolled cardiac arrhythmias (Reich et al. 2000). TCA-induced cardiac changes manifest on electrocardiogram (ECG) as flattened T waves, prolonged Q-T intervals, and depressed S-T segments. At high doses, TCAs have been implicated in euthyroid sick syndrome. For patients undergoing thyroid function testing, measured thyroid hormone concentrations should be interpreted with caution, since TCAs (and SSRIs) can cause artifactual decreases in thyroid hormone concentrations.

In older animals or those with compromised liver or kidney function, complete serum biochemical evaluations are urged since high concentrations of TCAs may cause liver damage. Extremely high concentrations are associated with convulsions, cardiac abnormalities, and hepatotoxicity.

Dramatic difference

Cats may be at greater risk for TCA-induced adverse effects than dogs or humans because TCAs are metabolized through glucuronidation. Cats lack several UDP glururonyl transferase enzymes compared to most other species. Cats are also much more sensitive to the potential arrhythmogenic effects of this and related classes of medications.

16.3.1.4 Selective Serotonin Reuptake Inhibitors

The effects of SSRIs (fluoxetine, paroxetine, sertraline, and fluvoxamine) are due to highly selective blockade of the reuptake of 5-HT1A into presynaptic neurons. Because SSRIs do not have major effects on NE, dopamine, acetylcholine, histaminic, and alpha-adrenergic receptors, their safety profile is generally considered superior to TCAs. SSRIs and any of their active metabolites typically have longer elimination half-lives than TCAs. Because fluoxetine (Reconcile) is FDA approved for treating separation anxiety in dogs, it is the SSRI for which pharmacokinetics in veterinary species are most well characterized. The C_{max} for fluoxetine and its active metabolite norfluoxetine are achieved about 2 and 12 hours after oral dosing in dogs. The elimination half-life of fluoxetine and norfluoxetine in dogs is 6 and 49 hours, respectively; therefore, steady state is not achieved until about two weeks after treatment is initiated. However, there is a delay in onset of activity beyond that. Treatment must continue for a minimum of six to eight weeks before a determination about SSRI efficacy can be made for behavioral disorders. The precise reason for the delay in SSRI efficacy has not been definitively determined. One proposed reason for this is that SSRIs induce receptor conformation changes that require the production of new protein – an action that can take several weeks. Regardless of the mechanism, it is widely accepted that a minimum treatment period of eight weeks is required before a treatment "failure" can be pronounced.

Fluoxetine is efficacious in the treatment of profound aggressions, separation anxiety (Landsberg et al. 2008; Sherman and Mills 2008), panic, and obsessive-compulsive disorders. Paroxetine is efficacious in the treatment of depression, social anxiety, and agitation associated with depression.

Sertraline is thought to be useful particularly for generalized anxiety and panic disorder in humans, and these same patterns have been thought, anecdotally, to pertain in veterinary medicine.

The SSRIs, while considered safer than TCAs, can participate in serious drug–drug interactions. SSRIs should not be used with monoamine oxidase inhibitors (MAOIs) because that greatly increases the risk of serotonin syndrome (Brown et al. 1996). While many MAOIs have few to no effects on serotonin directly, dopamine is converted to norepinephrine, so co-administration may cause an undesirable stimulatory synergy with far-reaching effects. Serotonin syndrome is covered in more depth further in this chapter.

There are two MAOIs that are licensed for use in veterinary patients that pharmacists may not be familiar with. Selegilene (Anipryl) is a MAOI labeled for treating canine cognitive dysfunction or pituitary-dependent Cushing's disease. Amitraz (Mitaban®) is a MAOI that is formulated as a dip indicated for treating generalized demodicosis in dogs. Despite the fact that it is applied topically, there may be enough absorbed transdermally or the dog may ingest a sufficient amount of the compound while grooming to achieve pharmacologically relevant systemic concentrations. Additionally, the active compound in many tick collars (Preventic®) is amitraz. Such collars deliver a steady stream of this compound and so are not recommended for use with TCAs, SSRIs, or related compounds. The pharmacist can play a key role in owner education regarding the risk of MAOIs for animals being treated with SSRIs.

Several other drugs can interact with SSRIs, including buspirone, TCAs, and benzodiazepines. Co-administration of buspirone with SSRIs may decrease the efficacy of buspirone and potentiate extrapyramidal symptoms. However, there have also been reports of synergistic effects between buspirone and SSRIs. SSRIs can inhibit CYP enzymes, but the particular CYP enzyme inhibited and the degree of inhibition vary dramatically between the different SSRIs.

Drugs that rely on CYP enzymes for metabolic activation (e.g. concomitant use of TCAs or benzodiazepines with SSRIs) can have complex effects on all drugs involved, particularly if CYP enzymes mediate the formation of active metabolites. While polypharmacy can be safe and rational, and can save animals' lives, an understanding of how each drug influences the other is required. Drug interactions involving CYP enzymes and behavior-modifying drugs are discussed in more detail further in this chapter.

16.3.1.5 Serotonin–Norepinephrine Reuptake Inhibitors

No serotonin–norepinephrine reuptake inhibitors are FDA approved for use in veterinary patients. Despite little data being available on the usage of these agents in veterinary patients, they seem to be used extensively. In particular, these medications may be used to treat patients who are experiencing an incomplete response to SSRIs or when administration of both a TCA and an SSRI is undesirable. Venlafaxine has a short elimination half-life in dogs (two to four hours) (Howell et al. 1994). That, and the fact that the active metabolite (formed in abundance in humans) was nondetectable in dogs, may render venlafaxine much less effective for dogs than for people.

16.3.1.6 Serotonin 2A Antagonist/ Reuptake Inhibitors (SARIs)

Recent attention has been given to the SARI trazodone, which may be useful for panic disorders and phobias as an adjuvant to benzodiazepine, TCA, and/or SSRI treatment. The primary actions of SARIs are to antagonize 5-HT2$_A$ receptors and to inhibit 5-HT reuptake.

Trazodone is not FDA approved for use in veterinary patients, so established dosages based on extensive pharmacokinetic data are not available, but a wide range of doses for trazodone have been used in dogs and cats (1.7–9.5 mg/kg/day) (Gruen and Sherman 2008; Gruen et al. 2014; Gilbert-Gregory et al. 2016). Among the most common reasons for trazodone use, particularly for cats, is to ease the distress of veterinary visits (Orlando et al. 2016). Because veterinarians have perceived that trazodone is "mild" and "safe," it is now commonly given for many forms of distress (both in-hospital and outpatient), often in high dosages and in combination with other medications. Unfortunately, the veterinarian often fails to discuss the potential (albeit low) risks of serotonin syndrome. However, there are anecdotal and increasingly frequent reports of tachycardia and enhanced anxiety, especially in patients treated with trazodone at high doses and/or frequent dosing intervals. This is ironic given that the only placebo-controlled, double-blind study evaluating trazodone to facilitate calming in dogs undergoing veterinary procedures showed no significant difference between trazodone and placebo (Gruen et al. 2017).

While G-coupled protein systems like those involved in the effects of TCAs, SSRIs, serotonin–norepinephrine reuptake inhibitors, and SARIs can respond almost instantly, the more long-term effects on molecular transcription and translation are believed to underlie the efficacy of these medications for behavior disorders (Duman 1998). Thus, "as-needed" usage of these compounds is simply not likely to be effective. The scientifically accepted way to evaluate drug efficacy is through placebo-controlled, double-blind clinical trials (Overall and Dunham 2009), so that placebo effects can also be assessed.

16.3.1.7 Drugs Used as First- or Second-Line Medications or in Combination with Benzodiazepines, TCAs, and SSRIs

16.3.1.7.1 *Beta-Adrenergic Receptor Antagonists*
Beta-adrenergic receptor antagonists (beta blockers) are used in humans to treat self-injurious behavior, intermittent explosive disorder, conduct disorders, dementia, brain disease and injury, autism, and schizophrenia. Older beta blockers, like propranolol (a nonselective beta blocker), have not been as successful as hoped for treating canine or feline aggression as sole therapy.

Dramatic difference
Dogs do not respond as well as humans to beta-adrenoreceptor antagonists because, at rest, dogs lack adrenergic tone relative to humans (Kantelip et al. 1982).

Conversely, beta blockers have been used with some success in combination with TCAs or SSRIs to treat some anxieties and noise phobias. Pindolol, a nonselective beta blocker, has been used successfully to augment the actions of TCAs and SSRIs by blocking the presynaptic $5HT1_A$ autoreceptor. This blockade is thought to abrogate the initial "downregulation" phase of monoamine release: The relevant monoamine continues to be produced despite accumulation in the synaptic cleft resulting from SSRI- or TCA-induced presynaptic reuptake inhibition (Duman 1998). Beta blockers are used in an extra-label manner for veterinary patients.

16.3.1.7.2 *Alpha-Adrenergic Agonists*
Clonidine, a centrally acting, alpha-adrenergic agonist that lowers heart rate and blood pressure, has been used in the treatment of noise reactivity and panic disorder in dogs (Ogata and Dodman 2010). Dogs appear to be less sensitive to the hypotensive effects than do many other species (Murrell and Hellebreker 2005), but they do exhibit sedation across a range of dosages. Clonidine and guanfacine decrease cardiac output and peripheral vascular resistance by extremely efficient binding of alpha-adrenergic receptors in the vasomotor center, the locus coeruleus, in the brainstem. The result is decreased presynaptic calcium release, and so adrenergic receptors don't fire, which subsequently inhibits adrenal release of norepinephrine. Consequently, one potential side effect is sedation, but decreased arousal below the level of sedation is considered a desired effect.

Dexmedetomidine oral mucosal gel (Sileo) is an alpha-2 adrenoceptor agonist that is FDA approved for treatment of canine noise aversion. It is intended to be administered using a specially designed syringe for placement of the gel between the dog's cheek and gum. Dexmedetomide has anxiolytic and sedative/hypnotic actions that are mediated through inhibition of locus coeruleus firing. The locus coeruleus nucleus contains one of the highest densities of alpha-2 adrenoceptors and is a key source of noradrenergic innervation of the forebrain. The locus coeruleus modulates sympathetic tone, vigilance, and attention. There is abundant evidence to show that overactivation of the noradrenergic neurotransmission, with increased release of noradrenaline in the locus coeruleus, induces fear and anxiety in animals exposed to stress (Tanaka et al. 2000). In a placebo-controlled, double-blind study (Korpivaara et al. 2017), Sileo (125 micrograms per square meter body surface area) reduced or abated signs of distress associated with fear or phobia of fireworks in pet dogs. Extra-label uses of the formulation may include treatment of fears governed by profound arousal such as fear of veterinary visits, other noise fears and phobias, fears involved in meeting novel humans or dogs, and others.

Because neurons from the locus coeruleus project to limbic structures (e.g. the amygdala) and the forebrain, the use of alpha-adrenergic agonists for treating anxiety-related conditions is logical. Clonidine has been used to treat autonomic hyperarousal in human posttraumatic stress disorder; therefore, it stands to reason that it may be useful for treating conditions in dogs involving hyperarousal and hyperreactivity. Guanfacine appears to be less sedating than clonidine, although it has a longer duration of action (Scahill et al. 2001). Guanfacine improves precortical function in nonhuman primates and so may be promising for use in dogs where anxiety affects cognitive performance. Guanfacine is not widely used in dogs. Drug interactions involving all alpha-adrenergic agonists are possible with TCAs, since TCAs block alpha$_1$-adrenergic receptors. Compared with guanfacine and dexmedetomidine, clonidine has weaker but measurable effects on alpha$_1$-adrenergic receptors, possibly permitting informed use, but the effects of TCAs and alpha-agonists may be incompatible. In humans treated with both classes of drugs, hypertensive crises have been reported.

16.3.1.7.3 *Partial Serotonin Agonists*

Partial 5-HT$_{1A/B}$ agonists (e.g. buspirone) have few adverse effects; do not negatively affect cognition; allow rehabilitation by influencing cognition, attention, arousal, and mood regulation; and may aid in treating aggression associated with impaired social interaction. Buspirone is the most commonly used partial serotonin agonist in veterinary behavioral medicine, although it is not labeled for veterinary use. It has been used with varying, but overall unimpressive, success in the treatment of canine aggression, canine and feline ritualistic or stereotypic behaviors, self-mutilation, possible obsessive-compulsive disorders, thunderstorm phobias, and feline spraying. Buspirone may be most effective when used in combination with other medications for most canine behavioral disorders. As a solitary agent, buspirone may be effective for treating intercat aggression. It is important to note that buspirone is intended to modify the behavior of the victim, rather than the aggressor, of intercat aggression. Cat owners should understand that buspirone's desired effect on the victim is to make that cat less anxious and more interactive/assertive, even though this might lead to more confrontations between cats in the household. Anecdotal reports of buspirone causing animals to be more aggressive are misleading. In the wild, the victim of intercat aggression would simply flee the aggressor's territory. This is not possible for victim cats living within a household environment with an aggressor. Cats treated with buspirone may alter their former response to the aggressor, which could lead to an agonistic encounter. This example highlights how pharmacological changes do not occur in a vacuum and behavioral and environmental changes – including those in the social environment – are important to monitor and consider modifying.

16.3.1.8 Miscellaneous

16.3.1.8.1 Memantine

Memantine is sometimes used to treat conditions in which glutamate is implicated, including obsessive-compulsive disorder, a common canine and feline behavioral concern. Memantine blocks NMDA glutamate receptors and is thought to have a positive effect on cognition, mood, and behavior. Because of its expense, it is currently not used frequently for companion animals.

16.3.1.8.2 Sympathomimetics and Stimulants

There are few treatment and diagnostic situations that have been more misunderstood than those involving stimulants and "hyperactivity." The original literature on "hyperkinesis/hyperactivity" in dogs actually focused on laboratory dogs as a potential animal model for a very restrictive variant of hyperactivity in humans ("hyperkinesis") (Corson et al. 1971). However, it is important to note that *truly hyperactive states that meet specific definitions of hyperkinesis are rare in canine and feline patients*. Therefore, there are few true indications for the use of this class of drugs in companion animal behavioral therapy. Potential adverse effects of stimulants can include increased heart and respiratory rates, possible anorexia, and tremors with possible hyperthermia. Stimulants are contraindicated in animals with cardiovascular disease, glaucoma, concurrent MAO therapy, and hyperthyroidism.

16.3.1.9 Hormonal Therapy

The use of progestins and estrogens has appropriately been superseded by the drug classes discussed in this chapter. Not only are hormonal therapies such as progestins less effective, but also they can cause numerous severe adverse effects, including diabetes, acromegaly, polyphagia, polyuria, jaundice, mammary gland hyperplasia, endometrial hyperplasia, pyometra, adrenal cortical suppression, and myelosuppression (Eigenmann and Eigenmann 1981a,b).

16.4 Use of Behavior-Modifying Drugs in Animals with Concurrent Disease Processes

16.4.1 Thyroid Disease

TCAs, SSRIs, and related compounds cause an artifactual decrease in measured thyroid hormone (T_3 and T_4) plasma concentrations using standard thyroid panels for both cats and dogs. Although thyroid dysfunction can affect behavior, there is now evidence that most behavioral concerns in dogs are not directly associated with hypothroidism. Conversely, behavioral complaints may be the first sign of hyperthyroidism for cats (Peterson et al. 1997, 2001; Kemppainen and Birchfield 2006). The effects of TCAs, SSRIs, and other behavioral drugs on lowering measured thyroid hormone concentrations are sufficient enough to mask a diagnosis of hyperthyroidism (cats treated with these compounds may appear to have thyroid hormone concentrations within the reference range, even though the cat has hyperthyroidism). In people, high doses of TCAs have been implicated in sick euthyroid syndrome, now more commonly called nonthyroidal illness syndrome (Warner and Beckett 2010). Whether or not this can be caused in dogs or cats treated with TCAs has not yet been documented.

16.4.2 Pain Management

Quality of life matters for dogs and cats, and pain takes a toll on quality of life. Pain management may involve treatment with tramadol (not FDA approved for veterinary use) and/or nonsteroidal anti-inflammatory drugs (NSAIDs; several NSAIDs are FDA approved for veterinary use). Potential drug interactions exist for both of these analgesic classes if used in combination with common behavior-modifying drugs. Drug interactions involving tramadol pose an increased risk of toxicity, while drug interactions involving NSAIDs potentially involve decreased efficacy of the behavior-modifying drug.

Tramadol is a prodrug that requires metabolism to an active metabolite (M1). The M1 metabolite, not tramadol itself, binds to mu opioid receptors and is responsible for the vast majority of tramadol's analgesic effects. In humans, CYP2D6 is responsible for M1 formation. Despite the fact that veterinarians frequently use tramadol for pain management in dogs, there are conflicting reports on its efficacy, and recent pharmacokinetic studies suggest this is because many, if not most, dogs do not metabolize tramadol to its active metabolite (mediated by canine CYP2D15), and the mu opioid effects are small in dogs (KuKanich and Papich 2004). Tramadol in the immediate-release form has been shown to increase nociceptive thresholds in dogs (Kongara et al. 2009; KuKanich and Papich 2011), with peak effects seen ~6 hours after treatment with 9.9 mg/kg.

An important concern is that tramadol has the potential to increase the risk of serotonin syndrome when used concurrently with TCAs, SSRIs, serotonin–norepinephrine reuptake inhibitors, and SARIs. In experiments with synaptosomes in rodent brains, tramadol acts as a 5-HT reuptake inhibitor (Gobbi and Mennini 1999). It is important to note that it is thought to be tramadol, not the M1 metabolite, that inhibits serotonin reuptake. Currently, there is insufficient understanding of which serotonergic drugs (TCAs, SSRIs, etc.) inhibit canine CYP2D15 to confidently predict the drug interaction potential for tramadol. To further complicate matters, CYP2D15 is polymorphic in dogs, so individual animals may react differently to drug combinations. Cat liver microsomes convert tramadol to its active metabolite to a greater extent than dog liver microsomes do, but it is not known which feline CYP enzyme is responsible. Thus, with respect to drug interactions, there are no data to suggest that one particular TCA or SSRI is safer than another in dogs or cats.

NSAIDs are also frequently used for pain management in dogs and cats. There is a mechanism whereby NSAIDs interfere with behavior-modifying drugs that rely on serotonergic receptors. Specifically, NSAIDs decrease expression of a small, acidic protein (p11) that is responsible for facilitating the movement and attachment of serotonin receptors at the cell surface, enhancing the excitability of neurons (Svenningsson et al. 2006). The primary effect of p11 appears to be on 5-HT$_{1B}$ receptors, but TCAs and SSRIs that primarily affect other receptors appear to interact with p11 (Warner-Schmidt et al. 2011). NSAIDs appear to inhibit antidepressant-induced increases in p11 and may interfere with behavior-modifying drugs that act primarily by affecting serotonergic receptors (Warner-Schmidt et al. 2011). This effect is not seen with the TCAs, which primarily affect norepinephrine. Initiating NSAID therapy in a patient undergoing successful treatment with an SSRI for behavioral conditions may cause a relapse. Pharmacists can help ensure that owners monitor their pet carefully if NSAIDs are given with SSRIs.

These findings do not mean that tramadol or NSAIDs cannot be used to mitigate pain in veterinary patients treated with behavior-modifying drugs. Instead, starting with lower dosages of each therapeutic agent may be necessary. Owners must be instructed to monitor the patient for early signs of serotonin syndrome, especially in the early phases of treatment, since this is when it is most likely to occur. Balancing the patient's needs often involves risk–benefit assessments and must include input from well-informed owners, careful dosing, and objective monitoring by all parties (owner, veterinarian, and pharmacist). Anxiety and pain constitute a mutual positive-feedback loop. Rational treatment strategies mandate that the healthcare team address both, with the understanding that decreasing pain likely also decreases anxiety.

16.4.3 Seizures

Many serotonergic agents are thought to lower seizure thresholds, and so their use is cautioned in patients with seizure disorders. However, there is now evidence that anxiety itself may lower seizure thresholds in both humans and dogs, *so treatment of the anxiety may actually raise the seizure threshold.* For some patients, this may allow dose reductions of antiepileptic drugs.

16.4.4 Drug Interactions Involving Canine and Feline Cytochrome P450 (CYP) Enzymes

Pharmacists are well aware of drug interactions that involve the human CYP enzyme system. Behavior-modifying drugs can be "victims" of drug interactions by virtue of the fact that they are substrates for CYP enzymes (e.g. alprazolam, amitriptyline, carbamazepine, diazepam, fluoxetine, imipramine, nefazodone, sertaline, traszoldon, triazolam, and venlafaxine). Thus, drugs that inhibit CYP enzymes (Table 16.6) can increase the plasma concentration and therefore the pharmacological effect of drugs that are CYP substrates. However, it is important to note that in the case of prodrugs or drugs with active metabolites (some benzodiazepines, TCAs, and SSRIs), inhibition of CYP enzymes may actually *decrease* the pharmacological effect by inhibiting formation of the active metabolite. Drugs that induce CYP enzymes (Table 16.6) would have the opposite effect as CYP inhibitors.

Behavior-modifying drugs can also be the "perpetrator" in drug–drug interactions. Table 16.7 lists behavior-modifying drugs that are inhibitors or inducers of human CYP enzymes. Currently, there are little data on which behavior-modifying drugs inhibit and

Table 16.6 Commonly used drugs that are thought to inhibit or induce canine and feline CYP enzymes.

CYP Inhibitors	CYP Inducers
Fluoroquinolones	Phenobarbital
Azole antifungals	Omeprazole
Cimetidine	Rifampin
Omeprazole	Corticosteroids
Clarithromycin	
Erythromycin	

Source: Adapted from Schatzberg and Nemeroff (2017).

Table 16.7 Behavior-modifying drugs that are substrates for, or inhibitors or inducers of, human CYP enzymes.

P450 enzyme	Substrate	Inhibitor	Inducer
CYP1A2	TCAs Fluvoxamine Mirtazapine Duloxetine	Fluvoxamine Fluoxetine Paroxetine Sertraline Some TCAs	Phenobarbital Carbamazepine Phenytoin
CYP2C9/10	Sertraline Fluoxetine Amitriptyline	Fluvoxamine Fluoxetine Sertraline	Carbamazepine
CYP2C19	Citalopram Sertaline Clomipramine Imipramine	Fluvoxamine Fluoxetine Sertraline	Carbamazepine
CYP2D6	Fluoxetine Fluvoxamine Citalopram Duloxetine Paroxetine Venlafaxine Trazodone Nefazodone TCAs	Duloxetine Fluoxetine Paroxetine Norfluoxetine Citalopram Sertaline Some TCAs	
CYP3A4	Nefazodone Sertaline Venlafaxine Trazodone TCAs	Fluvoxamine Norfluoxetine TCAs Nefazadone	Carbamazepine

induce canine or feline CYP enzyme families. Pharmacists should use drug interaction data from humans as a guide for veterinary patients, but they should not assume that CYP-mediated drug interaction information derived from one species applies to all species.

In humans, the most important CYP subfamilies for drug metabolism are CYP1A, CYP2C, CYP2D, CYP2E, and CYP3A (van Beusekom et al. 2010). However, tremendous species differences exist in isoform composition, isoform expression, and even naming of CYP enzymes (Martignoni and de Kanter 2006). More importantly, drugs that are substrates for a particular CYP subfamily in one species are often not the same for a different species. For example, the CYP3A family is responsible for metabolizing roughly 50% of drugs used in people, while the canine CYP3A family contributes minimally to drug metabolism (see Chapter 4 for more information on CYP species differences).

In humans, a number of genetic variants of the CYP450 system have been identified. Many of these can have dramatic clinical consequences for patients treated with drugs that are substrates for that particular CYP enzyme. More information on pharmacogenetic effects in veterinary species can be found in Chapter 5.

16.5 Adverse Effects of Behavior-Modifying Drugs in Veterinary Species

Common adverse effects of psychotherapeutic drugs are usually caused by blockade of muscarinic acetylcholine receptors, which have diffuse connections throughout the brain. These "common" side effects are actually not very common and generally manifest themselves as *transient* changes. The most common complaints are related to gastrointestinal function, appetite change, sedation, or alterations – usually increases – in heart rate. For the overwhelming majority of patients, side effects will truly be transient, occurring only within the first week. However, if any side effect is *not* transient, owners need

to understand that their pet may be experiencing a serious problem. Pharmacists should encourage owners to help monitor both their animal's response to the medication and any side effects the animal may experience.

16.5.1 Serotonin Syndrome

Serotonin syndrome – which may better be described as serotonin toxicity – is the most severe side effect that can occur with any medication affecting the neurotransmitter serotonin. Untreated, serotonin syndrome can be fatal. While rare, when it does occur serotonin syndrome occurs most commonly within the first week or so of treatment and/or when switching or adding other medications that affect serotonin. Serotonin concentrations 10–50 times above baseline are generally required for a toxic effect to be experienced (Gillman 2006, 2010). The nonspecific signs for serotonin syndrome can be grouped by system: cognitive alterations (disorientation and confusion), behavior (agitation and restlessness), autonomic nervous system (fever, shivering, diaphoresis, and diarrhea), and neuromuscular (ataxia, hyperreflexia, and myoclonus) (Lane and Baldwin 1997). It has been suggested that a diagnosis of serotonin syndrome can be confirmed *only* when three of the following signs occur, coincident with the addition, or increased dosage, of a known serotonergic agent and only in the absence of another etiologic agent: *agitation, mental system changes* (*confusion* and *hypomania*), *myoclonus, hyperreflexia, diaphoresis, shivering, tremor, diarrhea, incoordination,* and *fever.* Additionally, the signs must not have predated when the serotonergic drug was initiated or the dose increased. Canine – and one would assume feline – patients experiencing serotonin syndrome become anxious, agitated, anorectic, and unfocused and are often tachycardic and tachypneic. Patients don't sleep, cannot calm, may seizure, and (whether or not they seizure) can become hyperthermic, and it is the hyperthermia that poses the largest risk of death, even more so than seizures.

Serotonin syndrome, while rare, can occur when a patient is given one medication affecting serotonin or a combination of them. The pharmacist can be instrumental in monitoring drug–drug interactions for patients on serotonergic drugs, many of which are used for treating behavioral disorders.

Cyproheptadine is a nonspecific serotonin antagonist that can be used at 1.1 mg/kg PO as an aid in combating serotonin syndrome (Wismer 2000). Cyproheptadine is antiserotonergic, antihistaminic, anticholinergic, and a 5-HT_2 antagonist that is most commonly used to stimulate appetite in cats and dogs and to control incompletely controlled asthma in cats. In some cases, cyproheptadine has been helpful in treating otherwise nonresponsive urinary spraying in cats.

Because the most severe side effects of TCAs, SSRIs, and the more recently popular SARIs can involve cardiac effects, *owners should and can easily be taught to take pulse rates, which may be the first sign of developing serotonin syndrome.* Slight increases in pulse rate are not worrisome. Huge, sustained increases in heart rate *are* problematic. For example, if owners know that their dog's resting heart rate is 65 beats per minute (bpm) and that with medication this changes to 150 bpm, they should immediately contact their veterinarian. If the increase in heart rate is minor (65–75 bpm), the owner can take notes and not worry. *Because cardiac adverse effects can be severe, baseline ECGs are recommended for any patient with a history of any cardiac arrhythmia, heart disease, or prior drug reaction; who is on more than one medication; and who may be undergoing anesthesia or sedation* (Reich et al. 2000). Cats may be more sensitive to cardiac side effects than are dogs, and, minimally, a lead II ECG evaluation for any arrhythmias should be done before treating cats with agents that may affect serotonin.

16.5.2   Liver and Kidney Function

Most behavioral drugs are eliminated through renal and hepatic pathways, so knowledge of baseline, pre-medication renal and liver function is essential. Liver or renal abnormalities may not rule out the use of a drug, but knowing that they exist can serve as a guide to dosage

and help owners anticipate side effects. Annual laboratory evaluation can help monitor changes in renal or hepatic function that may affect excretion or metabolism of behavioral medications. Should changes occur, their magnitude can guide alterations (usually decreases) in the dosages of behavioral medication.

Atypical reactions can occur, so for any unexplained or sudden illness, laboratory evaluation is essential. If any rare but profound alteration in hepatic function occurs, immediate withdrawal from behavioral medicine is an option while the patient receives supportive care. While dogs have been known to die of toxic overdose of their owners' medication (TCAs, SSRIs, etc.), there have been few confirmed cases of death due to behavioral medication prescribed for the dog at therapeutic dosages.

16.5.3   Benzodiazepines and Excessive Sedation

Compared with barbiturates, cortical function is relatively unimpaired by benzodiazepines. All benzodiazepines potentiate the effects of GABA by increasing binding affinity of the GABA receptor for GABA and by increasing the flow of chloride ions into the neuron, primarily affecting the $GABA_A$ receptors. $GABA_A$ receptors are ionotropic, transmembrane receptors. Barbiturates also affect the $GABA_A$ receptor's benzodiazepine receptor–chloride ion channel complex by using a slightly different mechanism than do benzodiazepines, but because of detrimental effects on cognition, barbiturates have been superseded by benzodiazepines and TCAs in the treatment of anxiety and aggression.

- Benzodiazepine effects are dose dependent.
- At low dosages, benzodiazepines act as calming agents or mild sedatives, facilitating calmer activity by tempering excitement and engendering muscle relaxation.
- At moderate dosages, they act as anti-anxiety agents, facilitating social interaction in a more proactive manner.
- At high dosages, they act as hypnotics, facilitating sleep.

Ataxia and profound sedation usually only occur at dosages beyond those needed for anxiolytic effects.

16.6   Nutritional Supplements for Behavioral Disorders

Nutritional supplements (sometimes called "nutraceuticals") and specialty diets are now all popular interventions for behavioral disorders in veterinary patients. Unfortunately, the quality of data regarding efficacy of these products is generally not comparable to that for pharmaceutical products, although there are some exceptions.

A "nutraceutical" is generally defined as a food product that is purported to provide health and medical benefits by affecting physiology, and that is marketed in forms not packaged or marketed as food. Nutraceuticals can be herbal, isolated from nutrients, derivatives of food products, or manufactured as dietary supplements. It is important to note that the word "nutraceutical" is not specifically recognized by the FDA. The FDA considers nutraceuticals nutritional supplements and, by extension, food. The nutraceuticals that are being and have been investigated for effects in veterinary behavioral medicine include alpha-casozepine (Zylkene®), L-theanine (Anxitane®), Harmonease®, and Calmex® (VetPlus), which contains a combination of L-theanine, L-tryptophan, an array of B vitamins, and *Piper methysticum.*

Alpha-casozepine (Zylkene), an alpha casein derivative, has been used to treat nonspecific anxiety in cats and dogs (Beata et al. 2007). In a blinded, controlled study, dogs with a variety of anxiety-related conditions improved when treated with alpha-casozepine to the same extent as those treated with selegiline using a standardized, scored assessment. However, the conditions varied considerably, and outcomes were based on client scores, so it is unlikely that this study could be replicated or that a placebo effect of simply participating in a study could be ruled out.

Palestrini et al. (2010) conducted a placebo-controlled, double-blind study on the effects of a diet containing caseinate hydrolysate using both behavioral and physiological assays in anxious and non-anxious laboratory Beagles. Anxiety scores were not affected by diet, and behavioral scores were only mildly affected. A large and statistically significant effect was found for decreased serum cortisol for anxious dogs fed a diet with caseinate hydrolysate, but not for non-anxious dogs, suggesting that such diets may play a role in alleviating some aspects of distress.

Alpha-casozepine is also one of the main ingredients in the CALM Diet formulated by Royal Canin. This diet, which also contains an anti-oxidant complex of vitamin E, vitamin C, taurine, and lutein, is intended to be fed to a dog 10 days before an expected stressful event and then for an additional two to three months. Kato et al. (2012) examined the effect of the CALM Diet compared with a control diet (both with ~25% protein) on behavior and urinary cortisol-to-creatinine ratios (UCCRs) in anxious pet dogs. They found a small but statistically significant effect on UCCR for the dogs eating the CALM Diet: Their UCCR increased less in response to a stressor than did that of dogs fed a control diet. However, this effect could have been confounded by the casozepine or slightly higher fat and protein (in g/kg) in the CALM Diet. The study design used also did not control for effects of habituation, a common design flaw in many behavioral studies.

Harmonease (Veterinary Products Laboratories) is a proprietary blend of extract of *Magnolia officinalis* and *Phellodendron amurense* extracts. These compounds have been reported to decrease mild, transient stress (Kalman et al. 2008) in healthy women. In one crossover study of laboratory Beagles who were mildly reactive when subjected to a compact disc recording of thunderstorms, but who did not show clinical signs of noise phobia, there was a mild but significant effect of Harmonease on activity level (DePorter et al. 2012).

L-theanine (Anxitane; Virbac Animal Health) is the levorotatory isomer of theanine. It is naturally occurring in the tea plant and has been proposed to lessen stress and mild anxiety-related problems in pets

(Araujo et al. 2010). L-theanine is an analog of glutamic acid. As such, it may inhibit reuptake of glutamate by the glutamate transporter (Sadzuka et al. 2001), thereby increasing GABA concentrations. Because high glutamate levels have been associated with neurocytotoxicity, L-theanine may also have a neuroprotectant effect and may modulate neurotransmitters that interact with glutamate receptor subtypes (e.g. serotonin and dopamine). Side effects tend to be inapparent, even at dosages in excess of recommended doses. Clinical trials are lacking.

The nutritional supplements discussed and some prescription diets (e.g. Hill's B/D®) contain bioactive compounds that may act as precursors or enhancers for some neurochemicals. While side effects are rare, attention should be paid when concurrently treating these patients with behavioral medications. While no dosage adjustments will be necessary in the vast majority of cases, there are reports of fatal drug–herbal and drug–nutritional supplement interactions.

In addition to the CALM Diet (Royal Canin), there are two other strategies for behavioral improvement found in commercial diets. Hill's B/D is a diet enriched with neuroprotective substances, including DHA, EPA, taurine, vitamin E, L-carnitine, and choline.

In controlled studies in laboratory dogs, learning was enhanced and maintained better in aging dogs fed B/D compared to a control diet, a pattern replicated in a study of young dogs (Zicker et al. 2012). Interestingly, young pups fed this diet not only had improved scores on a problem-solving test, but also had a better and earlier immune response to vaccination. Similar cognitive results have been documented for middle-aged and old cats fed a similarly supplemented diet (Landsberg et al. 2017). The Purina line of products (e.g. Purina EN, Bright Minds, and Purina Neurocare) use medium-chain triglycerides to create ketogenic diets, which promote energy storage in astrocytes. The results are purported to be neuroprotective and support behavioral health in dogs (Studzinski et al. 2008; Taha et al. 2009; Pan et al. 2010). These diets appear to enhance cognition and decrease anxiety by facilitating learning and decreasing central nervous system concentrations of neurocytotoxic amino acids like glutamate (see review in Overall 2011).

16.7 FDA-Approved Veterinary Drug Products for Treating Behavioral Disorders

Brand name (manufacturer)	Active ingredient(s)	Drug class	Rationale/notes
Anipryl® (Zoetis)	Selegiline	Monoamine oxidase inhibitor	Indicated for canine cognitive dysfunction and pituitary-dependent hyperadrenocorticism in dogs
Clomicalm® (Novartis)	Clomipramine	Tricyclic antidepressant	Indicated for separation anxiety in dogs Flavored tablet – keep container inaccessible to dogs
Reconcile® (Elanco)	Fluoxetine	Selective serotonin reuptake inhibitor	Indicated for separation anxiety in dogs Flavored tablet – keep container inaccessible to dogs
Sileo® (Zoetis)	Dexmedetomidine	Selective alpha-2 adrenoreceptor agonist	Indicated for noise aversion/phobias in dogs Oromucosal gel – anyone handling the drug or syringe should wear impermeable gloves; pregnant women should not handle drug or syringe

Abbreviations

5-HT	Serotonin
bpm	Beats per minute
C_{max}	Maximum plasma concentration after one oral dose
ECG	Electrocardiogram
GABA	Gamma aminobutyric acid
H_1	Histamine 1
H_2	Histamine 2
MAO-I	Monoamine oxidase inhibitor
NSAID	Nonsteroidal anti-inflammatory drug
NaSSA	Noradrenergic and specific serotonergic antidepressant
NE	Norepinephrine
NMDA	N-methyl-D-aspartate
SARI	Serotonin 2A antagonist/reuptake inhibitor
SSRI	Selective serotonin reuptake inhibitor
TCA	Tricyclic antidepressant

References

Araujo, J.A., de Rivera, C., Ethier, J.L. et al. (2010). Anxitane tablets reduce fear of human beings in a laboratory model of anxiety-related behavior. *J. Vet. Behavior* 5 (5): 268–275.

Beata, C., Beaumont-Graff, E., Diaz, C. et al. (2007). Effects of alpha-casozepine (Zylkene) versus selegiline hydrochloride (Selgian, Anipryl) on anxiety disorders in dogs. *J. Vet. Behavior* 2 (5): 175–183.

Brown, T.M., Skop, B.P., and Mareth, T.R. (1996). Pathophysiology and management of the serotonin syndrome. *Ann. Pharmcother.* 30: 527–533.

Center SA, Elston TH, Rowland PH, et al. (1996). Fulminant hepatic association associated with oral administration of diazepam in 11 cats. *J. Am. Vet. Med. Assoc.* 209:618–625.

Corson, S.A., Corson, E.O., and Kirilcuk, V. (1971). Tranquilizing effects of D-amphetamine on hyperkinetic untrainable dogs. *Fed. Proc.* 30: 206.

Crowell-Davis, S.L., Seibert, L.M., Sung, W. et al. (2003). Use of clomipramine, alprazolam, and behavior modification for treatment of storm phobia in dogs. *J. Am. Vet. Med. Assoc.* 222: 744–748.

DePorter, T.L., Landsberg, G.M., Araujo, J.A. et al. (2012). Harmonease chewable tablets reduces noise-induced fear and anxiety in a laboratory canine thunderstorm simulation: a blinded and placebo controlled study. *J. Vet. Behavior* 7 (4): 225–232.

Duman, R.S. (1998). Novel therapeutic approaches beyond the serotonin receptor. *Biol. Psychiatry* 44: 324–335.

Eigenmann, J.E. and Eigenmann, R.Y. (1981a). Influence of medroxyprogesterone acetate (provera) on plasma growth hormone levels and on carbohydrate metabolism, part II. *Acta Endocrinol.* 98: 602–608.

Eigenmann, J.E. and Eigenmann, R.Y. (1981b). Influence of medroxyprogesterone acetate (provera) on plasma growth hormone levels and on carbohydrate metabolism, part I. *Acta Endocrinol.* 98: 599–602.

Gilbert-Gregory, S.E., Stull, J.W., Rice, M.R. et al. (2016). Effects of trazodone on behavioral signs of stress in hospitalized dogs. *J. Am. Vet. Med. Assoc.* 249: 1281–1291.

Gillman, P.K. (2006). A review of serotonin toxicity data: implications for the mechanisms of antidepressant drug action. *Biol. Psychiatry* 59: 1046–1051.

Gillman, P.K. (2010). Triptans, serotonin agonists, and serotonin syndrome (serotonin toxicity): a review. *Headache* 50: 264–272.

Gobbi, M. and Mennini, T. (1999). Release studies with rat brain cortical synaptosomes indicate that tramadol is a 5-hydroxytraptamine uptake blocker and not a

5-hyrdroxytraptamine releaser. *Eur. J. Pharmacol.* 370: 23–26.

Greenblatt, D.J., Shader, R.I., Divoll, M. et al. (1981). Benzodiazepines: a summary of pharmacokinetic properties. *Br. J. Pharmacol.* 11 (Suppl 1): 11S–16S.

Greenblatt, D.J., Shader, R.I., and Abernethy, D.R. (1983). Drug-therapy: current status of benzodiazepines. *NEJM* 309: 344–358.

Gruen, M.E., Roe, S.C., Griffith, E. et al. (2014). Use of trazodone to facilitate postsurgical confinement in dogs. *J. Am. Vet. Med. Assoc.* 245: 296–301.

Gruen, M.E., Roe, S.C., Griffith, E. et al. (2017). The use of trazodone to facilitate calm behavior after elective orthopedic surgery in dogs: results and lessons learned from a clinical trial. *J. Vet. Behav. Clin. Appl. Res.* 22: 41–45. doi: 10.1016/j.jveb.2017.09.008.

Gruen, M.E. and Sherman, B.L. (2008). Use of trazodone as an adjunctive agent in the treatment of canine anxiety disorders: 56 cases (1995–1997). *J. Am. Vet. Med. Assoc.* 233: 1902–1907.

Hewson, C.J., Conlon, P.D., Luescher, U.A. et al. (1998). The pharmacokinetics of clomipramine and desmethylclomipramine in dogs: parameter estimates following a single oral dose and 28 consecutive daily oral doses of clomipramine. *J. Vet. Pharmcol. Ther.* 21: 214–222.

Howell, S.R., Hicks, D.R., Scatina, J.A. et al. (1994). Pharmacokinetics of venlafaxine and O-desmethylvenlafaxine in laboratory animals. *Xenobiotica* 24: 315–327.

Hughes, D., Moreau, R.E., Overall, K.L. et al. (1996). Acute hepatic necrosis and liver failure associated with benzodiazepine therapy in six cats: 1986–1995. *J. Vet. Emerg. Crit. Care* 6: 13–20.

Jonas, J.M. and Hearron, A.E. Jr. (1996). Alprazolam and suicidal ideation: a meta-analysis of controlled trials in the treatment of depression. *J. Clin. Psychopharmacol.* 16: 208–211.

Kalman, D.S., Feldman, S., Feldman, R. et al. (2008). Effect of a proprietary Magnolia and Phellodendron extract on stress levels in healthy women: a pilot double-blind placebo-controlled clinical trial. *Nutr. J.* 7: 11–14.

Kantelip, J.P., Duchene-Marullaz, P., Delaigue-Farbry, R. et al. (1982). Comparison of the effects of propranolol, pindolol, oxprenolol and acebutolol on atrioventircular conduction in unanesthetized dogs. *Br. J. Clin. Pharmacol.* 13 (Suppl. 2): 159S–166S.

Kato, M., Miyaji, K., Ohtani, N. et al. (2012). Effects of prescription diet on dealing with stressful situations and performance of anxiety-related behaviors in privately owned anxious dogs. *J. Vet. Behavior* 7 (1): 21–26.

Kemppainen, R.J. and Birchfield, J.R. (2006). Measurement of total thyroxine concentration in serum from dogs and cats by use of various methods. *Am. J. Vet. Res.* 67: 259–265.

King, J., Simpson, B., Overall, K.L. et al. (2000a). Treatment of separation anxiety in dogs with clomipramine. Results from a prospective, randomized, double-blinded, placebo-controlled clinical trial. *J. Appl. Anim. Behav. Sci.* 67: 255–275.

King, J.N., Maurer, M.P., Altman, B. et al. (2000b). Pharmacokinetics of clomipramine in dogs following single-dose and repeated-dose oral administration. *Am. J. Vet. Res.* 61: 80–85.

Kongara, K., Chambers, P., and Johnson, C.B. (2009). Glomerular filtration rate after tramadol, parecoxib and pindolol following anesthesia and analgesia in comparison with morphine in dogs. *Vet. Anaesth. Analg.* 36: 86–94.

Korpivaara, M., Laapa, K., Huhtinen, M. et al. (2017). Dexmedetomidine oromucosal gel for noise-associated acute anxiety and fear in dogs – a randomized, double-blind, placebo-controlled clinical study. *Vet. Rec.* doi:10.1136/vr.104045.

KuKanich, B. and Papich, M.G. (2004). Pharmacokinetics of tramadol and the metabolite O-desmethyltramadol in dogs. *J. Vet. Pharmacolo. Ther.* 27: 239–246.

KuKanich, B. and Papich, M.G. (2011). Pharmacokinetics and antinociceptive effects of oral tramadol hydrochloride administration in Greyhounds. *Am. J. Vet. Res.* 72: 256–162.

Lainesse, C., Frank, D., Beaudry, F. et al. (2007a). Effects of physiological covariables on pharmacokinetic parameters of clomipramine in a large population of cats after a single oral administration. *J. Vet. Pharmacol. Ther.* 30: 116–126.

Lainesse, C., Frank, D., Beaudry, F. et al. (2007b). Comparative oxidative metabolic profiles of clomipramine in cats, rats and dogs: preliminary results from an *in vitro* study. *J. Vet. Pharm. Therapeutics* 30: 387–393.

Lainesse, C., Frank, D., Meucci, V. et al. (2006). Pharmacokinetics of clomipramine and desmethylclomipramine after single-dose intravenous and oral administration in cats. *J. Vet. Pharmacol. Ther.* 29: 271–278.

Landsberg, G.M., Melese, P., Sherman, B.L. et al. (2008). Effectiveness of fluoxetine chewable tablets in the treatment of canine separation anxiety. *J. Vet. Behav. Clin. Appl. Res.* 3: 12–19.

Landsberg, G., Milgram, B., Mougeot, L. et al. (2017). Therapeutic effects of an alpha-casozepine and L-tryptophan supplemented diet on fear and anxiety in the cat. *J. Fel. Med. Surg.* 19 (6): 594–602.

Lane, R. and Baldwin, D. (1997). Selective serotonin reuptake inhibitor-induced serotonin syndrome: review. *J. Clin. Psychopharmacol.* 17: 208–221.

Mandrioli, R., Mercolini, L., and Raggi, M.A. (2008). Benzodiazepine metabolism: an analytical perspective. *Curr. Drug Metab.* 9: 827–844.

Martignoni, M. and de Kanter, R. (2006). Species differences between mouse, rat, dog, monkey and human CYP-mediated drug metabolism, inhibition and induction. *Expert Opin. Drug Metab. Toxicol.* 2 (6): 875–894.

Murrell, J.C. and Hellebrekers, L.J. (2005). Medetomidine and dexmedetomidine: a review of cardiovascular effects and antinociceptive properties in the dog. *Vet. Anaesth. Analg.* 32: 117–127.

Ogata, N. and Dodman, N.H. (2010). The use of clonidine in the treatment of fear-based behavior problems in dogs: an open trial. *J. Vet. Behav.: Clin. Appl. Res.* 6: 130–137.

Orlando, J.M., Case, B.C., Thomson, A.E. et al. (2016). Use of oral trazodone for sedation in cats: a pilot study. *J. Feline Med. Surg.* 18: 476–482.

Overall, K.L. (2001). Pharmacological treatment in behavioral medicine: the importance of neurochemistry, molecular biology, and mechanistic hypotheses. *Vet. J.* 162: 9–23.

Overall, K.L. (2011). Caring for the brains of young pups. *Vet. Rec.* 169 (18): 465–466.

Overall, K.L. and Dunham, A.E. (2002). Clinical features and outcome in dogs and cats with obsessive-compulsive disorder: 126 cases (1989–2000). *J. Am. Vet. Med. Assoc.* 221: 1445–1452.

Overall, K.L. and Dunham, A.E. (2009). Homeopathy and the curse of the scientific method. *Vet. J.* 180: 140–148.

Palestrini, C., Minero, M., Cannas, S. et al. (2010). Efficacy of a diet containing caseinate hydrolysate on signs of stress in dogs. *J. Vet. Behavior* 5 (6): 309–317.

Pan, Y., Larson, B., Araujo, J.A. et al. (2010). Dietary supplementation with medium-chain TAG has long-lasting cognition-enhancing effects in aged dogs. *Br. J. Nutr.* 103: 1746–1754.

Peterson, M.E., Melián, C., and Nichols, R. (1997). Meaurement of serum total thyroxine, triiodothyronine, free thyroxine, and thyrotropin concentrations for diagnosis of hypothyroidism in dogs. *J. Am. Vet. Med. Assoc.* 211: 1396–1402.

Peterson, M.E., Melián, C., and Nichols, R. (2001). Measurement of serum concentrations of free thyroxine, total thyroxine, and total triiodothyronine in cats with hyperthyroidism and cats with nonthyroidal disease. *J. Am. Vet. Med. Assoc.* 218: 529–536.

Reich, M.R., Ohad, D.B., Overall, K.L. et al. (2000). Electrocardiographic assessment of antianxiety medication in dogs and correlation with drug serum concentration. *J. Am. Vet. Med. Assoc.* 216: 1571–1575.

Riss, J., Cloyd, J., Gates, J. et al. (2008). Benzodiazepines in epilepsy: pharmacology and pharmacokinetics. *Acta Neurol. Scand.* 118: 69–86.

Rothschild, A.J. (1992). Disinhibition, amnestic reactions, and other adverse reactions secondary to triazolam: a review of the literature. *J. Clin. Psychiatry* 53 (Suppl.): 69–79.

Rothschild, A.J., Shindul-Rothschild, J.A., Viguera, A. et al. (2000). Comparison of the frequency of behavioral disinhibition on alprazolam, clonazepam, or no benzodiazepine in hospitalized psychiatric patients. *J. Clin. Psychopharmacol.* 20: 7–11.

Sadzuka, Y., Sugiyama, T., Suzuki, T. et al. (2001). Enhancement of doxorubicin by inhibition of glutamate transporter. *Toxicol. Lett.* 123 (2–3): 159–167.

Scahill, L., Chappell, P.B., Kim, Y.S. et al. (2001). A placebo-controlled study of guanfacine in the treatment of children with tic disorders and attention deficit hyperactivity disorder. *Am. J. Psychiatry* 158: 1067–1074.

Schatzberg, A.F. and Nemeroff, C.B. (2017). *APA Textbook of Psychopharmacology*, 5e. Washington, DC: APA Press.

Schwartz, M.A., Koechlin, B.A., Postma, E. et al. (1965). Metabolism of diazepam in rat, dog, and man. *J. Pharm. Exper. Ther.* 149: 423–435.

Sherman, B.L. and Mills, D.S. (2008). Canine anxieties and phobias: an update on separation anxiety and noise aversions. *Vet. Clin. North Am. Small Anim. Pract.* 38 (5): 1081–1106.

Simpson, B.S. and Papich, M.G. (2003). Pharmacologic management in veterinary behavioral medicine. *Vet. Clin. North Am. Small Anim. Pract.* 33: 365–404.

Studzinski, C.M., MacKay, W.A., Beckett, T.L. et al. (2008). Induction of ketosis may improve mitochondrial function and decrease steady-state amyloid beta precursor protein (APP) levels in the aged dog. *Brain Res.* 1226: 209–217.

Svenningsson, P., Chergui, K., Rachleff, I. et al. (2006). Alterations in 5-HT1B receptor function by p11 in depression-like states. *Science* 311: 77–80.

Taha, A.Y., Henderson, S.T., and Burnham, W.M. (2009). Dietary enrichment with medium chain triglycerides (AC-1203) elevates polyunsaturated fatty acids in the parietal cortex of aged dogs: implications for treating age-related cognitive decline. *Neurochem. Res.* 34: 1619–1625.

Tanaka, M., Yoshida, M., Emoto, H. et al. (2000). Noradrenaline systems in the hypothalamus, amygdala and locus coeruleus are involved in the provocation of anxiety: basic studies. *Eur. J. Pharmacol.* 405: 397–406.

van Beusekom, C.D., Schipper, L., and Fink-Gremmels, J. (2010). Cytochrome P450-mediated hepatic metabolism of new fluorescent substrates in cats and dogs. *J. Vet. Pharm. Ther.* 33 (6): 519–527.

Warner, M.H. and Beckett, G.J. (2010). Mechanisms behind the non-thyroidal illness syndrome: an update. *J. Endocrinol.* 205: 1–13.

Warner-Schmidt, J.L., Vanover, K.E., Chen, E.Y. et al. (2011). Antidepressant effects of selective serotonin reuptake inhibitors (SSRIs) are attenuated by antiinflammatory drugs in mice and humans. *PNAS* 108: 9262–9267.

Wismer, T.A. (2000). Antidpressant drug overdoses in dogs. *Vet. Med.* 95: 520–525.

Zicker, S.C., Jewell, D.E., Yamka, R.M. et al. (2012). Evaluation of cognitive learning, memory, psychomotor, immunologic, and retinal functions in healthy puppies fed foods fortified with docosahexaenoic acid-rich fish oil from 8 to 52 weeks of age. *J. Am. Vet. Med. Assoc.* 241 (5): 583–594.

17

Pharmacotherapeutics of Neurological Disorders

Annie Chen-Allen

Neurology and Neurosurgery, College of Veterinary Medicine, Washington State University, Pullman, WA, USA

Key Points

- Although dogs and cats can be afflicted by neurological disorders similar to those that affect humans, effective pharmacological therapy may not be as readily available for veterinary patients.
- The goal of seizure management is to reduce the frequency and severity of seizures while minimizing adverse drug effects. Long-term seizure freedom is not commonly achieved in veterinary patients.
- Antiepileptic drug (AED) therapy is initiated when the risks of seizures outweigh the risks of treatment.
- Choosing the appropriate AED is often based on the pet owner's compliance and financial capabilities rather than the specific seizure type or classification, as is often the case for human patients.

- Monotherapy is preferred over polytherapy when initiating AED therapy. Due to pharmacokinetic variability and sensitivity to adverse drug effects, most veterinary patients are started at the lower end of the dose range initially. Doses will need to be titrated based on seizure frequency, drug tolerance, and therapeutic drug monitoring.
- Despite the availability of multiple AEDs, 25–30% of epileptic dogs are refractory to treatment.
- For many pet owners, the cost and emotional toll of managing a poorly controlled epileptic dog lead them to consider euthanasia.

17.1 Comparative Aspects of Neurological Disorders

Many neurological disorders that require pharmacotherapy in human patients are similar to those that require pharmacotherapy in veterinary patients. These include epilepsy, pain (Chapter 6), infections or neoplasia of the central nervous system (Chapters 9 and 20, respectively), and inflammatory/ immune-mediated disorders (Chapter 14). Other neurological disorders in human patients either do not have a recognized corresponding condition in veterinary patients (e.g. Parkinson's disease), or pharmacotherapy is not available for the corresponding condition in veterinary patients (e.g. amyotrophic lateral sclerosis and Alzheimer's disease). Therefore, this chapter

Pharmacotherapeutics for Veterinary Dispensing, First Edition. Edited by Katrina L. Mealey.
© 2019 John Wiley & Sons, Inc. Published 2019 by John Wiley & Sons, Inc.

will focus on the most common veterinary neurological disorder that requires pharmacological treatment: epilepsy.

Neurological disorders can have devastating consequences in both human and veterinary patients, often requiring long-term intensive care and rehabilitation. Because most veterinary patients in the USA do not have insurance or other third-party payment options like most human patients do, financial constraints of the owner often dictate whether or not the dog or cat will be treated. In many cases, veterinary patients are euthanized.

Seizures are a common neurological disorder in dogs and cats. The incidence of idiopathic epilepsy has been reported to be between 0.5% and 5.0% of the pet dog population, with some breeds having a much higher incidence. The prevalence of seizures in people ranges from 1 to 3% worldwide and is estimated to be 1% in the USA.

A seizure is the clinical manifestation of abnormal electrical activity in the brain. Epilepsy refers to multiple seizures occurring over a period of time. Some veterinarians define that as two or more seizures occurring over a period of at least one month.

A refractory epileptic is a patient who has poor seizure control despite documented evidence of plasma drug concentrations within the therapeutic range for two or more AEDs. Refractory cases account for 25–30% of all epileptic dogs. Similarly, 20–35% of human patients will have unsatisfactory control with AEDs. The most common reason why epileptic dogs are euthanized is inadequate seizure control, followed by adverse effects of AEDs.

A responder is a patient who has experienced at least a 50% reduction in seizure frequency following the addition of a specific AED. This is often the definition of success in veterinary seizure studies.

Dramatic difference

The goal of seizure management in veterinary patients is to reduce the frequency and severity of seizures while minimizing adverse effects associated with AEDs. In people, the goal of seizure management is to eliminate all seizures while minimizing side effects of AEDs. Only a small percentage of canine epileptics become seizure-free with drug therapy, while this is achieved in 70–80% of human epileptics. Pharmacists can play an important role in managing the expectations of pet owners when dispensing AEDs. Similar to human patients, evidence indicates that there is no benefit to starting treatment after a single unprovoked event. However, the earlier an AED is started, the better chance for control because recurrent seizures can increase epileptogenesis and drug resistance, which can lead to increased morbidity and cost due to prolonged hospitalization.

In 2015, the American College of Veterinary Internal Medicine established a consensus statement on seizure management in dogs based on current literature and a panel of clinical experts. The goal was to establish concise guidelines for an approach to seizure management. Based on this consensus statement, the current recommendations for initiating an AED are when there are (i) an identifiable structural lesion or prior history of brain disease or injury, (ii) cluster seizures (>2 seizures in a 24-hour period) or status epilepticus (ictus >5 minutes), (iii) ≥2 seizure events in a six-month period, and (iv) prolonged, severe, or unusual post-ictal periods. In general, an AED is started when the risks of further seizures outweigh the risks of treatment. The risks of seizures include not only the seizures themselves but also the emotional effects of these seizures on the pet owner/family (Figure 17.1). The risks of treatment include adverse drug effects and the associated cost both for the drug and for long-term drug monitoring. In people, AED therapy is highly recommended once a patient experiences two or more unprovoked seizures, regardless of the time period between seizures. However, the decision to start AED therapy in veterinary patients is ultimately based on the pet owner's lifestyle and preferences.

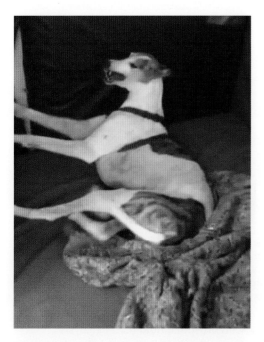

Figure 17.1 Image obtained from a video of an 11-year-old greyhound with idiopathic epilepsy during a generalized seizure. Generalized seizures in dogs are characterized by paddling and extensor rigidity of all four limbs, along with facial contracture (appearance of growling) and vocalization. To prevent injury during seizures, the dog was housed in a padded cage area until seizure frequency was improved.

Survivability of seizures in veterinary patients depends on many factors, including the underlying cause, the patient's quality of life, the emotional strain on the owner, drug compliance, and the financial burden associated with seizure management. Similar to people, lack of drug compliance is often the single most common reason for treatment failure. As a result, the pressure is on both the pharmacist and veterinarian to clearly communicate and balance both the patient's and owner's interests and needs when making recommendations for AED therapy. For example, if the patient is a service animal, severe epilepsy or high doses of some AEDs might adversely impact the animal's cognitive abilities.

17.2 Diagnostic Testing

Diagnostic testing is dependent on the cause of the seizure. Similar to people, seizures can result from structural diseases of the brain, metabolic diseases, or exposure to toxins, or they can be idiopathic in origin. Common structural causes include brain tumors, encephalitis/meningitis (which can be infectious or non-infectious), hydrocephalus, head trauma, and ischemic/vascular disorders. Common metabolic conditions that can lead to seizures include hepatic encephalopathy, electrolyte disturbances, and hypoglycemia. Numerous toxins, such as ethylene glycol, lead, strychnine, and mycotoxins, can lead to seizures. These are more common potential causes of seizures in veterinary patients than human patients.

Idiopathic epilepsy is the most common cause of epilepsy in dogs. Cats can have idiopathic epilepsy as well, but it is more common to have an underlying cause for their seizures. A diagnosis of idiopathic epilepsy can only be made once structural and metabolic causes have been ruled out. The age of onset for idiopathic epilepsy in dogs is usually between one and five years of age. Although idiopathic epilepsy has been documented to be inherited in many breeds, it can occur in any breed of dog or cat.

Working up a seizure disorder starts with a good history and a thorough physical and neurological exam. A veterinary neurological examination differs from those performed on humans because veterinarians can't ask the patient how they feel or request that the patient perform certain tasks. Because neurological examinations in veterinary patients involve physical manipulations of the patient, the veterinary neurological exam is often very concise (a dog, cat, or horse will tolerate only so many physical manipulations) and requires subjective interpretation by the veterinarian (Figure 17.2). The main components of the neurological exam are evaluation of mental status and behavior, gait and postural reactions, cranial nerves, spinal reflexes, and pain perception. Often, the information gathered initially can help prioritize the differential list. Here is a list of diagnostics that

(a)

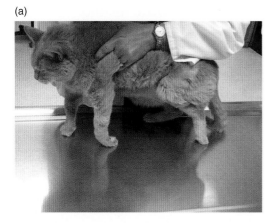

(b)

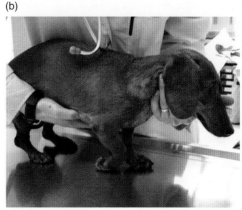

Figure 17.2 Neurological examination of animals involves assessing postural reactions. This is accomplished by placing the animal in a standing position and turning the paw over such that the dorsal surface contacts the floor or table. A neurologically normal animal will immediately flip its paw back into the normal position (<1 second). A delay or inability to return the paw to the normal position (the cat in image A and the dog in image B) indicates a neurological problem involving the proprioceptive pathway of that limb.

are commonly performed when working up a seizure patient:

- Complete blood count
- Serum chemistry panel
- Serum pre- and post bile acid to rule out liver dysfunction
- Toxicology screen if possible exposure
- Brain imaging: magnetic resonance imaging or computed tomography (Figure 17.3)

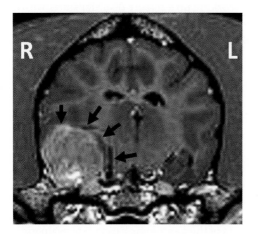

Figure 17.3 A magnetic resonance imaging (MRI) image of the brain of a nine-year-old Corgi with a one-month history of seizures and no other neurological abnormalities. A large contrast-enhancing mass (arrows) was identified at the level of the right pyriform lobe. Stereotactic biopsy and histopathology indicated a diagnosis of histiocytic sarcoma.

- Cerebrospinal fluid (CSF) analysis
- Serum and CSF titers and cultures for infectious diseases
- Serial blood pressures if ischemic/vascular brain disorder is suspected
- Electroencephalogram (EEG), but this is less commonly performed in veterinary medicine due to lack of accessibility. Video EEG is the gold standard for diagnosing epilepsy in people.
- Therapeutic drug monitoring is performed in veterinary patients treated with AEDs (Table 17.1 lists therapeutic drug concentrations for commonly used AEDs).

17.3 Pharmacotherapy of Epilepsy

Similar to human patients, monotherapy is preferred when initiating AED therapy. Polytherapy is considered when seizure control and quality of life are not achieved with monotherapy. In people, the classification and diagnosis of seizure type are critical to selection of the specific AED. In veterinary medicine, there is less sophistication and fewer specific guidelines when selecting the appropriate AED. Most AEDs used in veterinary medicine are not US Food and Drug

Table 17.1 Therapeutic range and drug monitoring for AEDs in dogs and cats.

Drug	Therapeutic range	Drug monitoring
Phenobarbital	15–35 microgram/mL	2 weeks, then every 6 months; 2 weeks after a dose change and if toxicity noted
Primidone	Same as phenobarbital	Same as phenobarbital
Potassium bromide	810–2500 microgram/mL when used with phenobarbital; up to 3000 microgram/mL when used alone	12 weeks, then every year; 12 weeks after a dose change and if toxicity noted
Levetiracetam	5–45 microgram/mL in people – use as a guidance in dogs	Not routinely performed
Zonisamide	10–40 microgram/mL in people – use as a guidance in dogs	2 weeks, 3 months, then every 6 months; 2 weeks after a dose change and if toxicity noted
Imepitoin	Unknown	Not commercially available

Administration (FDA) approved for treating seizures in dogs or cats, so extra-label drug use is the rule rather than the exception. Also, there is no specific classification system for seizure types in veterinary patients. Additionally, the decision regarding the most appropriate AED to use is often based on the owner's financial means and availability to administer the drug once, twice, or three times a day.

The dose recommendations in the remainder of this section are a general guide only. Because of the variability in pharmacokinetics in patients and sensitivity to side effects, most newly diagnosed patients are started at the lower end of the dose range initially. Doses will need to be titrated based on seizure frequency, drug tolerance, and therapeutic drug monitoring. Autoinduction of metabolism for certain drugs will often require an increase in dose in the weeks to months after initiating treatment.

17.3.1 Phenobarbital

Phenobarbital is one of the two traditional first-choice AEDs for dogs and the first AED of choice for cats. It is a Schedule IV controlled substance and the only US Drug Enforcement Agency (DEA)-scheduled commonly used maintenance AED for veterinary patients. It has high oral bioavailability and

achieves maximal plasma concentration within four to eight hours after oral administration in dogs. The majority of the drug is metabolized by the liver, with one-third excreted unchanged in the urine. The elimination half-life for phenobarbital is 40–90 hours in dogs and 40–50 hours in cats after oral administration. Steady state is reached after 10–15 days of drug administration. Phenobarbital induces the hepatic microsomal cytochrome P450 (CYP450, or CYP) enzymes (in veterinary patients as well as human patients), which can progressively increase metabolic clearance of other AEDs, including levetiracetam and zonisamide. Over time, this may lower plasma concentrations of AEDs and cause breakthrough seizures. Phenobarbital monotherapy had a success rate (i.e. >50% seizure reduction) of 82%, a seizure-free rate of 31%, and a failure rate (no improvements seen) of 15% in 311 epileptic dogs. Reported clinical experiences with phenobarbital in cats resulted in a seizure-free rate of 40–50%.

Phenobarbital starting dosage: 2.5 mg/kg PO (orally) every 12 hours in both dogs and cats.

Therapeutic drug monitoring should be performed when the drug achieves steady-state concentrations after about two weeks of dosing, and at six-month intervals thereafter. Therapeutic drug monitoring should also be performed two weeks after a dosage change and if signs of toxicity are noted. The target therapeutic range in veterinary patients is 15–35 microgram/mL.

17.3.2 Primidone

Primidone is the only FDA-approved AED for dogs in the USA. In Europe, phenobarbital, imepitoin, and potassium bromide are approved for treatment of epilepsy in dogs. When given orally, primidone is quickly metabolized into phenobarbital, which contributes to >85% of the anticonvulsant effect, and phenylethylmalonamide (PEMA), a metabolite that provides minimal anticonvulsant effects but contributes to hepatotoxicity. In multiple studies, phenobarbital has been shown to be more effective than primidone in seizure reduction and attaining a seizure-free period. Therefore, there are no benefits to switching a phenobarbital-resistant dog to primidone. Primidone is not recommended in cats by most clinicians due to increased risk of toxicity.

Therapeutic drug monitoring is similar to phenobarbital, since phenobarbital is the active metabolite.

17.3.3 Potassium Bromide (KBr)

Potassium bromide is the other traditional first-choice AED in dogs. It is used only in severe, refractory epilepsy in cats because of serious adverse effects. This AED has been regarded as the first effective medication for epilepsy in people, with its use starting as early as the 1850s. Because KBr causes profound sedation in people, its use waned when phenobarbital was introduced in the early 1900s. The sedation associated with KBr poses less of a problem for veterinary patients, with some exceptions (i.e. service or working dogs).

KBr is excreted in the urine, undergoing no liver metabolism. KBr has an elimination half-life of 24 days (yes, *days* – this is not a typo) in dogs and 11 days in cats. It takes about 80–120 days in dogs to achieve steady-state

levels of KBr. High-chloride (salt) diets can increase renal excretion and lower serum concentrations, which can cause breakthrough seizures. Drug clearance can be decreased in dogs with renal dysfunction, resulting in higher serum drug concentrations. KBr monotherapy achieved a >50% seizure reduction in 74% and a seizure-free rate of 52% in 23 epileptic dogs over a six-month treatment period. *Potassium bromide starting dosage:* 30–40 mg/kg PO every 24 hours. If more rapid seizure control is needed, a total loading dose of 400–600 mg/kg is administered orally over 24–72 hours, divided into multiple small doses to avoid gastrointestinal upset.

Therapeutic drug monitoring should be performed when steady state is achieved at about 12 weeks, on an annual basis thereafter, and if signs of toxicity are noted. KBr serum concentrations between 810 and 2500 micrograms/mL have been shown to be effective when concurrently using phenobarbital. When KBr is administered as monotherapy, target KBr serum concentrations are up to 3000 micrograms/mL.

17.3.4 Levetiracetam

Levetiracetam is almost 100% orally bioavailable in dogs and cats, with an elimination half-life of approximately four hours in dogs and three hours in cats. In humans, approximately 70–90% of the parent drug is excreted unchanged in the urine, with the remainder undergoing CYP-independent metabolism. While the exact mechanism of drug clearance has not been determined for dogs or cats, there is clinical evidence that levetiracetam metabolism is accelerated over time when the drug is used concurrently with phenobarbital in dogs. No other known drug–drug interactions have been reported for levetiracetam. Because of its wide safety margin, it has gained popularity in veterinary medicine. However, there are no published reports on its efficacy as a monotherapy drug for canine or feline epilepsy. Levetiracetam as an add-on therapy in 52 dogs resulted in

69% having a 50% or greater reduction of seizures and a seizure-free rate of 15% with a follow-up time of 1.2 years. Other reports have found the efficacy of levetiracetam questionable as an add-on AED and have reported a "honeymoon" effect in dogs, suggesting the drug works well initially but loses its efficacy over time. This honeymoon effect has not been reported in cats. A published study on levetiracetam as an add-on therapy to phenobarbital reported a 70% responder rate and 25–30% seizure-free rate in cats. Injectable levetiracetam has also been shown to be an effective emergency AED for control of cluster seizures and status epilepticus.

Levetiracetam starting dosage: 20 mg/kg PO every eight hours for both dogs and cats. Extended-release levetiracetam can be used at 30 mg/kg PO every 12 hours in dogs.

Therapeutic drug monitoring is not routinely performed due to levetiracetam's wide therapeutic index and lack of established therapeutic range in dogs. The therapeutic range in people is 5–45 microgram/mL, and this is often extrapolated for use in dogs. Because phenobarbital appears to alter the pharmacokinetics of levetiracetam in dogs, there is justification for monitoring levetiracetam serum concentrations when these drugs are used concurrently in an effort to optimize drug efficacy on an individual basis.

17.3.5 Zonisamide

Zonisamide has an elimination half-life of approximately 15 hours in dogs and 33 hours in cats. It is metabolized predominately by hepatic CYP450 enzymes. Co-administration with phenobarbital increases the clearance of zonisamide by 50%, consequently shortening the elimination half-life. Zonisamide does not affect its own metabolism or the disposition of other drugs because it has not been shown to inhibit or induce hepatic CYP450 enzymes. Zonisamide as monotherapy for idiopathic epilepsy in 10 dogs had a >50% seizure reduction success rate of 60% with a follow-up of 12–36 months. There are limited clinical data regarding the efficacy of zonisamide in cats, although anecdotal successes have been reported.

Zonisamide starting dosage (dogs): 5 mg/kg PO every 12 hours as monotherapy; 10 mg/kg PO every 24 hours when using concurrently with phenobarbital in dogs.

Zonisamide starting dosage (cats): 10 mg/kg PO every 24 hours.

Therapeutic drug monitoring should be done at two weeks, three months, every six months thereafter, two weeks after a dose change, and if signs of toxicity are noted. The therapeutic range in people is 10–40 micrograms/mL and can be used as a guidance of drug efficacy in dogs.

17.3.6 Imepitoin

Imepitoin was approved in Europe for the treatment of idiopathic epilepsy in dogs in 2012 and was approved in Australia in 2015. It is currently unavailable in the USA. It was originally developed to treat epilepsy in humans, but clinical trials were terminated upon findings of unfavorable metabolic differences in smokers versus nonsmokers. Whether or not dogs exposed to secondhand smoke experience similar metabolic alterations is not known. Imepitoin is a low-affinity partial agonist on the benzodiazepine site of the GABAA receptor, thereby potentiating GABAergic inhibitory actions. Despite binding to the benzodiazepine receptor, it differs in chemical structure from benzodiazepines. Imepitoin is the first partial agonist approved for the treatment of epilepsy. In a dose-dependent manner, imepitoin also blocks voltage-gated calcium channels. It is an imidazolone, and it has some structural similarities to hydrantoin anticonvulsants like ethotoin and phenytoin.

Imepitoin has high oral bioavailability and a short (two-hour) elimination half-life in dogs, such that no clinically relevant drug accumulation occurs even during chronic treatment. Imepitoin does not appear to affect hepatic CYP450 enzymes and does not cause elevations in liver enzymes. It is excreted primarily in the feces, suggestive of biliary elimination. Imepitoin has not been reported to alter the metabolism of other drugs. Drug interactions have not been reported when using imepitoin. When compared to phenobarbital in 266 epileptic dogs, imepitoin was as effective as phenobarbital in seizure control and was associated with fewer adverse effects. In the only feline clinical trial ($n = 8$), seizure freedom was achieved in 50% of cats with a follow-up of only eight weeks.

Imepitoin starting dosage (dogs): 15 mg/kg PO every 12 hours

Imepitoin starting dosage (cats): 30 mg/kg PO every 12 hours.

Therapeutic drug monitoring is not needed and currently not commercially available.

17.4 Adverse Drug Effects in Veterinary Species

17.4.1 Phenobarbital

During the first few weeks after initiation of phenobarbital, restlessness and/or sedation often occur, but they typically resolve within one to two weeks. Pharmacists can be helpful in convincing owners to be patient through the first few weeks of phenobarbital therapy. Adverse effects that are seen with chronic administration can result in polydipsia, polyuria, and polyphagia. These can be frustrating for pet owners. Serum alkaline phosphatase (ALP) activity can increase as early as two weeks after initiation of treatment in dogs. This does not necessarily indicate clinically significant liver disease or the need to discontinue therapy. Drug-induced hepatotoxicity happens most commonly with a serum phenobarbital concentration >35 microgram/mL. Therefore, liver values including bile acids should be monitored every six months concurrently with therapeutic drug monitoring. Serum total and free thyroxine (T4) concentrations may be low and thyroid-stimulating hormone may be high in dogs treated with phenobarbital mimicking subclinical hypothyroidism. Idiosyncratic reactions such as immune-mediated anemia, neutropenia, and thrombocytopenia can develop with a reported prevalence of 4.2% in dogs. These reactions occur typically within the first six months of treatment and are reversible when phenobarbital is discontinued. Superficial necrolytic dermatitis has also been reported in dogs as a rare idiosyncratic reaction.

Adverse effects of phenobarbital in cats can be quite different from those in humans. Uncommon phenobarbital-related side effects reported in cats include facial pruritus, generalized pruritus with distal limb edema, cutaneous eruptions, and lymphadenopathy. These suspected hypersensitivity reactions resolved shortly after discontinuing phenobarbital.

17.4.2 Primidone

Primidone causes side effects similar to those reported for phenobarbital. Hepatic enzyme increases are more severe when using primidone than with phenobarbital because both primidone and phenobarbital (the active metabolite) can adversely affect the liver. Primidone carries a greater risk of liver disease when compared to phenobarbital. Therefore, liver values including bile acids should be monitored every three to six months to monitor for hepatotoxicity in dogs. Primidone is not recommended for use in cats because this species has an even greater risk for developing toxicity.

17.4.3 Potassium Bromide

KBr can cause dose-dependent sedation, polydipsia, polyuria, polyphagia, and mild ataxia. Since it is a salt, it can cause gastric mucosal irritation, which can lead to inappetence and vomiting. KBr should be administered with food to avoid gastrointestinal intolerance. Additionally, KBr solution (rather than capsules) is less likely to cause gastric irritation. Pancreatitis has also been linked to KBr usage – whether this is a direct effect or is secondary to polyphagia has not been determined. At serum concentrations >3000 mg/L, severe mental alteration, ataxia, and weakness can occur. Animals receiving KBr will have an artifactual increase of chloride on serum chemistry panels because some assays cannot distinguish chloride from bromide ions. Between 34 and 42% of cats taking KBr develop pneumonitis characterized by coughing, dyspnea, and a bronchial pattern on chest radiographs that is typically reversible after stopping bromide but has also been fatal. For this reason, most veterinarians do not recommend using KBr in cats. Dogs have also been rarely reported to develop a persistent cough while on KBr, which resolves after KBr discontinuation, but fatalities have not been reported.

17.4.3.1 Levetiracetam

Levetiracetam has a wide safety margin in both dogs and cats and is well tolerated. Experimental studies in dogs have shown ataxia, salivation, vomiting, restlessness, and sedation with doses 5–20 times greater than the recommended dosage. These side effects typically resolve within 24 hours of drug discontinuation. Clinically, most dogs and cats experience no apparent side effects from levetiracetam, but there have been infrequent reports of mild ataxia, sedation, and inappetence.

17.4.4 Zonisamide

Zonisamide can cause sedation, generalized ataxia, vomiting, and inappetence, with a prevalence of 10–55% in dogs. Most of these side effects are transient but sometimes may warrant dose reduction. Idiosyncratic reactions such as keratoconjunctivitis sicca, polyarthropathy, acute hepatic necrosis, and renal tubular acidosis have been reported but are rare in dogs. Chronic use of zonisamide can increase ALP activity and decrease serum albumin concentration, demonstrating a potential for hepatotoxicity in dogs. A decreased total T4 (thyroxine) concentration has also been reported in healthy dogs given zonisamide for eight weeks. In a chronic-dosing pharmacokinetic study in cats, three of six cats developed somnolence, ataxia, vomiting, and diarrhea when given a 20 mg/kg/day oral dose (i.e. twice the recommended dose) for nine weeks. A case of zonisamide-related lymphadenopathy, hyperglobulinemia, and cytopenia was reported in a cat. These resolved with discontinuation of zonisamide.

17.4.5 Imepitoin

Imepitoin has a wide safety margin and is well tolerated in dogs and cats. Experimental studies have shown no adverse side effects with doses well above the recommended doses for clinical use in dogs and cats. In clinical studies, imepitoin was associated with mild sedation and transient polyphagia, polyuria, polydipsia, and hyperactivity in dogs. In cats, lethargy, decreased appetite, and vomiting were noted clinically but were often mild and transient. Chronic use of imepitoin does not result in tolerance or dependence, and it should not result in withdrawal effects with abrupt termination of treatment.

17.5 Nutritional Supplements for Epilepsy in Veterinary Species

Ketogenic diets have been used for managing epilepsy in people for decades. In the 1920s, Wilder discovered that the ketosis and acidosis resulting from minimal caloric intake produced an anti-seizure effect. This is a high-fat, low-protein, low-carbohydrate diet thought to simulate a fasted state that is used to potentiate mitochondrial-dependent energy metabolism in neurons and inhibit glutamatergic metabolic pathways and synaptic transmission. Ketogenic diets are used primarily in children with medically refractory epilepsy. Long-term use in people can lead to kidney stones, increased incidence of bone fractures, and adverse effects on growth.

In the one and only study in 10 dogs, a ketogenic diet failed to improve seizure control compared to a control diet and led to pancreatitis in three dogs. The major drawback of the ketogenic diet is compliance, as the diet is typically unpalatable, making it difficult to maintain animal patients on this strict diet. A medium-chain triglyceride–based diet decreased seizure frequency in 21 dogs with idiopathic epilepsy for 12 weeks compared to those on the placebo diet. Omega-3 fatty acid supplementation in 15 dogs with idiopathic epilepsy did not decrease the seizure frequency and severity when compared to the placebo group. Homeopathic remedies such as silicea, cuprum, and causticum have been used in people with epilepsy.

Evidence to support homeopathic remedies for seizure management in veterinary medicine is currently lacking. More studies are needed to clarify the benefits of these supplementations to justify their usage for seizure management.

Abbreviations

AED	Antiepileptic drug
CSF	Cerebrospinal fluid
EEG	Electroencephalogram
IV	Intravenous
KBr	Potassium bromide
PO	Per os ("by mouth," or orally)
T4	Thyroxine

Further Reading

Avanzini, G., Beghi, E., de Boer, H. et al. (2012). Neurological disorders: a public health approach. In: *Neurological Disorders: Public Health Challenges*, 41–110. Geneva: World Health Organization.

Bailey, K.S., Dewey, C.W., Boothe, D.M. et al. (2008). Levetiracetam as an adjunct to phenobarbital treatment in cats with suspected idiopathic epilepsy. *J. Am. Vet. Med. Assoc.* 232 (6): 867–872.

Baird-Heinz, H.E., Van Schoick, A.L., Pelsor, F.R. et al. (2012). A systematic review of the safety of potassium bromide in dogs. *J. Am. Vet. Med. Assoc.* 240: 705–715.

Berendt, M., Gredal, H., Ersboll, A. et al. (2007). Premature death, risk factors, and life patterns in dogs with epilepsy. *J. Vet. Intern. Med.* 21: 754–759.

Bersan, E., Volk, H.A., Ros, C. et al. (2014). Phenobarbitone-induced haematological abnormalities in idiopathic epileptic dogs: prevalence, risk factors, clinical presentation and outcome. *Vet. Rec.* 175: 247.

Bertolani, C., Hernandez, J., Gomes, E. et al. (2012). Bromide-associated lower airway disease: a retrospective study of seven cats. *J. Feline Med. Surg.* 14: 591–597.

Bhatti, S.F., De Risio, L., Munana, K. et al. (2015). International veterinary task force recommendations for a veterinary epilepsy-specific MRI protocol. *BMC Vet. Res.* 11: 194.

Boothe, D.M. (2001). Anticonvulsants and other neurologic therapies. In: *Small Animal Clinical Pharmacology and Therapeutics* (ed. D.M. Boothe), 431–456. Philadelphia: W.B. Saunders.

Boothe, D.M., Dewey, C., and Carpenter, D.M. (2012). Comparison of phenobarbital with bromide as a first choice antiepileptic drug for treatment of epilepsy in dog. *J. Am. Vet. Med. Assoc.* 240: 1073–1083.

Boothe, D.M., George, K.L., and Couch, P. (2002). Disposition and clinical use of bromide in cats. *J. Am. Vet. Med. Assoc.* 221: 1131–1135.

Boothe, D.M. and Perkins, J. (2008). Disposition and safety of zonisamide after intravenous and oral single dose and oral multiple dosing in normal hound dogs. *J. Vet. Pharmacol. Ther.* 31: 544–553.

Brodie, M.J., Barry, S.J., Bamagous, G.A. et al. (2012). Patterns of treatment response in newly diagnosed epilepsy. *Neurology* 78: 1548–1554.

Brodie, M.J., Barry, S.J., Bamagous, G.A. et al. (2013). Effect of dosage failed of first antiepileptic drug on subsequent outcome. *Epilepsia* 54: 194–198.

Carnes, M.B., Axlund, T.W., and Boothe, D.M. (2011). Pharmacokinetics of levetiracetam after oral and intravenous administration of a single dose to clinically normal cats. *Am. J. Vet. Res.* 72 (9): 1247–1252.

Chandler, K.C. (2006). Canine epilepsy: what can we learn from human seizure disorders? *Vet. J.* 172: 207–217.

Chang, Y., Mellor, D.J., and Anderson, T.J. (2006). Idiopathic epilepsy in dogs: owners' perspectives on management on phenobarbitone and/or potassium bromide. *J. Small Anim. Pract.* 47: 574–581.

Charalambous, M., Pakozdy, A., Bhatti, S.F.M. et al. (2018). Systematic review of antiepileptic drugs' safety and effectiveness in feline epilepsy. *BMC Vet. Res.* 14 (1): 64.

Chung, J.Y., Hwang, C.Y., Chae, J.S. et al. (2012). Zonisamide monotherapy for idiopathic epilepsy in dogs. *N.Z. Vet. J.* 60: 357–359.

Cochrane, S.M., Parent, J.M., Black, W.D. et al. (1990). Pharmacokinetics of phenobarbital in the cat following multiple oral administration. *Can. J. Vet. Res.* 54: 309–312.

Cook, A.K., Allen, A.K., Espinosa, D. et al. (2011). Renal tubular acidosis associated with zonisamide therapy in a dog. *J. Vet. Intern. Med.* 25: 1454–1457.

Danial, N.N., Hartman, A.L., Stafstrom, C.E. et al. (2013). How does the ketogenic diet work? Four potential mechanisms. *J. Child Neurol.* 28: 1027–1033.

Dayrell-Hart, B., Steinberg, S.A., VanWinkle, T.J. et al. (1991). Hepatotoxicity of phenobarbital in dogs: 18 cases (1985–1989). *J. Am. Vet. Med. Assoc.* 199: 1060–1066.

Dewey, C.W. (2006). Anticonvulsant therapy in dogs and cats. *Vet. Clin. North Am. Small Anim. Pract.* 36: 1107–1127.

Engel, J. (2006). Report of the ILAE classification core group. *Epilepsia* 47: 1558–1568.

Engel, O., von Klopmann, T., Maiolini, A. et al. (2017). Imepitoin is well tolerated in healthy and epileptic cats. *BMC Vet. Res.* 13: 172–178.

England, M.J., Liverman, C.T., Schultz, A.M. et al. (2012). A summary of the Institute of Medicine report: epilepsy across the spectrum: promoting health and understanding. *Epilepsy Behav.* 25 (2): 266–276.

Farnbach, G.C. (1984). Efficacy of primidone in dogs with seizures unresponsive to phenobarbital. *J. Am. Med. Assoc.* 185: 867–868.

Finnerty, K.E., Barnes-Heller, H.L., Mercier, M.N. et al. (2014). Evaluation of therapeutic phenobarbital concentrations and application of a classification system for seizures in cats: 30 cases (2004–2013). *J. Am. Vet. Med. Assoc.* 244 (2): 195–199.

Frey, H.H., Gobel, W., and Loscher, W. (1979). Pharmacokinetics of primidone and its active metabolites in the dog. *Arch. Int. Pharmacodyn. Ther.* 242: 14–30.

Garnet, W.R. (2000). Antiepileptic drug treatment: outcomes and adherence. *Pharmacotherapy* 20: 191s–199s.

Gaskill, C.L., Burton, S.A., Gelens, H.C. et al. (1999). Effects of phenobarbital treatment on serum thyroxine and thyroid-stimulating hormone concentrations in epileptic dogs. *J. Am. Vet. Med. Assoc.* 215: 489–496.

Gaskill, C.L. and Cribb, A.E. (2000). Pancreatitis associated with potassium bromide/phenobarbital combination therapy in epileptic dogs. *Can. Vet. J.* 41: 555–558.

Hasegawa, D., Kobayashi, M., Kuwabara, T. et al. (2009). Pharmacokinetics and toxicity of zonisamide in cats. *J. Feline Med. Surg.* 10 (4): 418–421.

Hojo, T., Ohno, R., Schimoda, M. et al. (2002). Enzyme and plasma protein induction by multiple oral administrations of phenobarbital at a therapeutic dosage regiment in dogs. *J. Vet. Pharmacol. Ther.* 25: 121–127.

Jacobs, G., Calvert, C., and Kaufman, A. (1998). Neutropenia and thrombocytopenia in three dogs treated with anticonvulsants. *J. Am. Vet. Med. Assoc.* 212: 681–684.

Kantrowitz, L.B., Peterson, M.E., Trepanier, L.A. et al. (1999). Serum total thyroxine, total triiodothyronine, free thyroxine, and thyrotropin concentrations in epileptic dogs treated with anticonvulsants. *J. Am. Vet. Med. Assoc.* 214: 1804–1808.

Kelley, S.A. and Hartman, A.L. (2011). Metabolic treatments for intractable epilepsy. *Semin. Pediatr. Neurol.* 18: 179–185.

Krumholz, A., Wiebe, S., Gronseth, G. et al. (2015). Evidence-based guidelines: management of an unprovoked first seizure in adults. *Neurology* 84: 1705–1713.

Law, T.H., Davies, E.S., Pan, Y. et al. (2015). A randomized trial of a medium chain TAG diet as treatment for dogs with idiopathic epilepsy. *Br. J. Nutr.* 114: 1438–1447.

Louis, E.K., Rosenfeld, W.E., and Bramley, T. (2009). Antiepileptic drug monotherapy: the initial approach in epilepsy management. *Current Neuropharm* 7: 77–82.

Marsh, P.A., Hillier, A., Weisbrode, S.E. et al. (2004). Superficial necrolytic dermatitis in 11 dogs with history of phenobarbital administration (1995–2002). *J. Vet. Med.* 18: 65–74.

Miller, M.L., Center, S.A., Randolph, J.F. et al. (2011). Apparent acute idiosyncratic hepatic necrosis associated with zonisamide administration in a dog. *J. Vet. Intern. Med.* 25: 1156–1160.

Moore, S.A., Munana, K.R., Papich, M.G. et al. (2011). The pharmacokinetics of levetiracetam in healthy dogs concurrently receiving phenobarbital. *J. Vet. Pharmacol. Ther.* 34: 31–34.

Munana, K.R., Nettifee-Osborne, J.A., and Papich, M.G. (2015). Effect of chronic administration of phenobarbital, or bromide, on pharmacokinetics of levetiracetam in dogs with epilepsy. *J. Vet. Intern. Med.* 29: 614–619.

Munana, K.R., Thomas, W.B., Inzana, K.D. et al. (2012). Evaluation of levetiracetam as adjunctive treatment for refractory canine epilepsy: a randomized, placebo-controlled, crossover trial. *J. Vet. Intern. Med.* 26: 341–348.

Nguyen, V.V., Baca, C.B., Chen, J.J. et al. (2017). Epilepsy. In: *Pharmacotherapy: A Pathophysiologic Approach*, 10e (ed. J.T. Dipiro, R.L. Talbert, G.C. Yee, et al.), 837–866. New York: McGraw-Hill Education.

Orito, K., Saito, M., Fukunaga, K. et al. (2008). Pharmacokinetics of zonisamide and drug interaction with phenobarbital in dogs. *J. Vet. Pharmacol. Ther.* 31: 259–264.

Packer, R.M. and Volk, H.A. (2015). Study on the effects of imepitoin on the behavior of dogs with epilepsy. *Vet. Rec.* 177: 132.

Pan, Y., Larson, B., Arujo, J.C. et al. (2010). Dietary supplementation with median chain TAG has long-lasting cognition-enhancing effects in aged dogs. *Br. J. Nutr.* 103: 1746–1754.

Patterson, E., Munana, K., Kirk, C. et al. (2005). Results of ketogenic food trial for dogs with idiopathic epilepsy. *J. Vet. Intern. Med.* 19: 421.

Patterson, E.E., Goel, V., Coyd, J.C. et al. (2008). Intramuscular, intravenous and oral levetiracetam in dogs: safety and pharmacokinetics. *J. Vet. Pharmacol. Ther.* 31: 253–258.

Podell, M. (2013). Antiepileptic drug therapy and monitoring. *Top. Companion. Anim. Med.* 28: 59–66.

Podell, M., Volk, H., Berendt, M. et al. (2016). ACVIM Small Animal Consensus Statement on Seizure Management in Dogs. *J. Vet. Intern. Med.* 30: 477–490.

Ravis, W.R., Pedersoli, W.M., and Wike, J.S. (1989). Pharmacokinetics of phenobarbital in dogs given multiple doses. *Am. J. Vet. Res.* 50: 1343–1347.

Ricotti, V. and Delanty, N. (2006). Use of complementary and alternative medicine in epilepsy. *Curr. Neurol. Neurosci. Rep.* 6: 347–353.

Rossmeisl, J.H. and Inzana, K.D. (2009). Clinical signs, risk factors, and outcomes associated with bromide toxicosis (bromism) in dogs with idiopathic epilepsy. *J. Am. Vet. Med. Assoc.* 234: 1425–1431.

Rundfeldt, C., Gasparic, A., and Wlaz, P. (2014). Imepitoin as novel treatment option for canine idiopathic epilepsy: pharmacokinetics, distribution, and metabolism in dogs. *J. Vet. Pharmacol. Ther.* 37: 421–434.

Rundfeldt, C. and Loscher, W. (2014). The pharmacology of imepitoin: the first partial benzodiazepine receptor agonist developed for treatment for epilepsy. *CNS Drugs* 28: 29–43.

Schwartz, M., Munana, K.R., and Olby, N.J. (2011). Possible drug-induced hepatopathy in a dog receiving zonisamide monotherapy for treatment of cryptogenic epilepsy. *J. Vet. Med. Sci.* 73: 1505–1508.

Schwartz-Porsche, D., Loscher, W., and Frey, H.H. (1982). Treatment of canine epilepsy with primidone. *J. Am. Vet. Med. Assoc.* 181: 592–595.

Schwartz-Porsche, D., Loscher, W., and Frey, H.H. (1985). Therapeutic efficacy of phenobarbital and primidone in canine epilepsy: a comparison. *J. Vet. Pharmacol. Therap.* 8: 113–119.

Tellez-Zenteno, J.F., Hernandez-Ronquillo, L., Bucey, S. et al. (2014). A validation of the new definition of drug-resistant epilepsy by the International League Against Epilepsy. *Epilepsia* 55: 829–834.

Thomas, W.B. (2010). Idiopathic epilepsy in dogs and cats. *Vet. Clin. North Am. Small Anim. Pract.* 40: 161–179.

Thomas, W.B. and Dewey, C.W. (2016). Seizures and narcolepsy. In: *Practical Guide to Canine and Feline Neurology*, 3e (ed. C.W. Dewey and R.C. da Costa), 249–267. Hoboken, NJ: Wiley Blackwell.

Tipold, A., Keefe, T.J., Loscher, W. et al. (2015). Clinical efficacy of safety of imepitoin in comparison with phenobarbital for control of idiopathic epilepsy in dogs. *J. Vet. Pharmacol. Ther.* 38: 160–168.

Trepanier, L.A. (1995). Use of bromide as an anticonvulsant for dogs with epilepsy. *J. Am. Vet. Med. Assoc.* 207: 163–166.

Trepanier, L.A. and Babish, J.G. (1995). Effect of dietary chloride content on the elimination of bromide by dogs. *Res. Vet. Sci.* 58: 252–255.

Trepanier, L.A., Van Schoick, A., Schwark, W.S. et al. (1998). Therapeutic serum drug concentrations in epileptic dogs treated with potassium bromide alone or in combination with other anticonvulsants: 122 cases (1992–1996). *J. Am. Vet. Med. Assoc.* 213: 1449–1453.

Volk, H.A., Matiasek, L.A., Lujan Feliu-Pascual, A. et al. (2008). The efficacy and tolerability of levetiracetam in pharmacoresistant epileptic dogs. *Vet. J.* 176: 310–319.

von Klopmann, T., Rambeck, B., and Tipold, A. (2007). Prospective study of zonisamide therapy for refractory idiopathic epilepsy in dogs. *J. Small Anim. Pract.* 48: 134–138.

Walker, R.M., DiFonzo, C.J., Barsoum, N.J. et al. (1988). Chronic toxicity of the anticonvulsant zonisamide in beagle dogs. *Fundam. Appl. Toxicol.* 11: 333–342.

18

Dermatologic Pharmacotherapeutics

Alice M. Jeromin

Private practice, Richfield, OH, USA

Key Points

- Inhalant allergy (atopic dermatitis [AD]) is a genetic disease that can affect dogs and cats with similarities and differences to human AD.
- Treatment for AD is aimed at controlling symptoms by addressing the underlying immune dysfunction and defective skin barrier.

- With the discovery of the pathogenesis of AD in dogs and cats, FDA-approved drugs addressing disease pathogenesis are now emerging.
- Over-the-counter medications to alleviate symptoms are sometimes used by owners and can potentially cause harm to their pets.

18.1 Comparative Aspects of Atopic Dermatitis

Inhalant allergy, or atopic dermatitis (AD), in humans is described as an immune-mediated inflammation of the skin arising from a combination of genetic and environmental factors. It manifests as an exaggerated response to a substance (allergen) that non-atopics tolerate without reactivity (Marsella et al. 2012). It is the most common inflammatory skin disorder diagnosed in humans (Rodrigues Hoffmann 2017). The same exaggerated response to an allergen exists in dogs and cats as AD. Canine AD is an inflammatory pruritic skin disease for which affected dogs have a genetic predisposition (Verde 2016). The same is true for atopy in cats, although a genetic predisposition has not been proven (Reinero 2009). Similarities between AD in dogs and humans include genetic predisposition, early age of onset, similar areas of the body affected, and association of epidermal barrier defects (Asahina and Maeda 2017). The major difference between AD in humans compared to dogs and cats is that humans tend to outgrow their allergies. In dogs and cats, clinical manifestations evolve and worsen throughout the life of the pet if not managed.

More is known about the pathophysiology of AD in the dog as opposed to the cat. AD in dogs is a complex multifactorial disease, with genetic and environmental factors playing a fundamental role (Verde 2016). In both canine and feline AD, abnormalities of the skin barrier exist, allowing percutaneous absorption of potential allergens. The allergen is then processed and presented to dendritic cells in the dermis, inciting an inappropriate immune response. Therapies, therefore, should be multifaceted and involve

Pharmacotherapeutics for Veterinary Dispensing, First Edition. Edited by Katrina L. Mealey.
© 2019 John Wiley & Sons, Inc. Published 2019 by John Wiley & Sons, Inc.

both modulation of the immune response and repair of the defective skin barrier. Drug actions should thus include blocking the synthesis and release of inflammatory products such as histamine, leukotrienes, and other inflammatory cytokines.

The onset of AD in dogs can range from six months to six years of age, depending upon the breed and environment. Clinical signs begin before three years of age in 68% of cases (Verde 2016). Breed predisposition includes, but is not limited to, retrievers, herding breeds, bulldogs, terriers, dachshunds, poodles, and mixes thereof. Initially, pruritus is the presenting sign, followed by secondary bacterial or yeast overgrowth that tends to exacerbate the pruritus. Pruritic skin changes occur in areas where potential allergens enter the body, such as the skin over the abdomen, feet, rectal area, and face/ears (Figure 18.1). Because allergic disease in dogs and cats affects the skin (unlike allergic symptoms in humans, which are mainly respiratory), pets lick and scratch affected areas, often causing tissue trauma. Chronic skin manifestations due to pruritus include hyperpigmentation, lichenification, erythema, and acral lick granulomas (Figure 18.2). All of these skin changes may be difficult to "reverse," which is why early diagnosis and treatment of AD are important (Figure 18.3). Some atopic dogs and cats manifest with seasonal symptoms attributed to pollens, while others are affected nonseasonally. House dust mite is the most

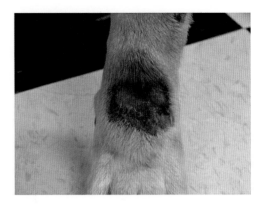

Figure 18.2 Atopic dermatitis in a dog. This is an acral lick granuloma, a lesion that can result when pruritus triggers an intense drive to repeatedly lick the itch. The rough surface of the animal's tongue eventually damages cutaneous and subcutaneous tissues.

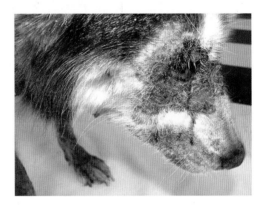

Figure 18.3 Chronic changes of the skin in a long-standing atopic dog (face and feet).

common nonseasonal allergen affecting dogs, cats, and humans (Loft and Rosser 2014).

Unlike dogs, cats with AD can manifest symptoms at *any* age. While it would be unusual to see the initial presentation of AD in an older dog, it frequently occurs in elderly cats. Cats also differ from dogs in their presentation of symptoms. Any area of the body may be affected, and atopic lesions may include alopecia of the ventral abdomen due to licking, tiny crusty lesions (miliary dermatitis), or raised erythemic plaques (eosinophilic granuloma complex) on the legs (Figure 18.4), trunk, or in the oral cavity (Figure 18.5). There appears to be no sex predisposition. In terms of breed disposition, Devon Rex, Sphinx, and possibly gold-colored cats may be predisposed (Philippa 2014).

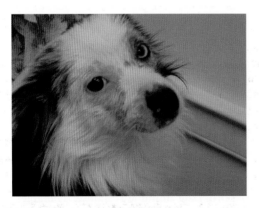

Figure 18.1 Atopic dermatitis in a dog. Face-rubbing in early atopy resulting in alopecia and erythema of the muzzle and periocular area.

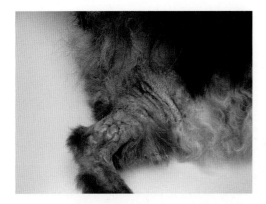

Figure 18.4 Eosinophilic granuloma complex on the inner thigh of an atopic cat.

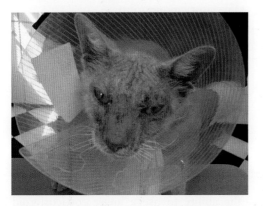

Figure 18.5 Facial excoriation in an atopic cat.

18.2   Diagnostic Testing

Intradermal skin testing (IDST) or serum testing for AD can be performed for human, canine, and feline patients. Both types of tests are designed to identify allergen-specific immunoglobulin-E (IgE) that can then be used to determine patient-specific allergens. These allergens may then be avoided if possible or used in formulating injectable or sublingual allergy immunotherapy solutions (Novak et al. 2011). Because canine and feline AD have so many "look-alike" diseases, it is important to diagnostically rule out or control those diseases before confirming a diagnosis of atopy. Serum allergy testing is not a reliable standalone diagnostic test for AD. In one study, up to 25% of clinically atopic dogs did not have allergen-specific serum IgE elevations. Conversely, some dogs without AD symptoms may have detectable allergen-specific IgE elevations using serum testing (Marsella et al. 2012). Diseases in the dog that may be mistaken for AD include flea allergy dermatitis, scabies (sarcoptic mange), *Cheyletiella* mites, bacterial pyoderma, food allergy, demodicosis (demodectic mange), and dermatophytosis. In cats, flea allergy dermatitis, *Cheyletiella* mites, dermatophytosis, hyperthyroidism, pemphigus foliaceus, and food allergy all need to be ruled out before a diagnosis of atopy can be confirmed. Because AD requires lifelong treatment for affected dogs and cats, the veterinarian must be confident of the diagnosis.

Common diagnostic procedures in dogs and cats suspected to have atopic dermatitis:

- A thorough history, including age of onset of clinical signs, areas of the body affected, seasonality of flare-ups, and response to prior medications
- Cytology
- Food trial (prescription or home-cooked food consisting of a novel protein source)
- Histopathology
- Bacterial and/or fungal cultures
- Intradermal or serum allergen testing
- Skin scrapings and fur combings (to identify ectoparasites such as fleas, scabies, and *Cheyletiella* mites).

18.3   Pharmacological Treatment of Atopic Dermatitis

Treatment of AD in the dog and cat is multimodal and aimed at modulating the immune response and improving the defective skin barrier. Addressing the accompanying bacterial and/or yeast overgrowth also may alleviate some of the pet's symptoms. Whereas in human AD, the majority of symptoms are respiratory – runny eyes, nose, and congestion – in the dog and cat, symptoms are confined to the skin, with upper respiratory symptoms being rare (Rosser 1999). The main goal in dog and cat AD is to control the itch!

18.3.1 Corticosteroids: Canine AD

Corticosteroids have been effective in the management of AD for decades (Fadok 2016). However, their long-term use is not advised due to adverse effects. If used, short-term, short-acting corticosteroids are preferred such as prednisone or methylprednisolone rather than dexamethasone, which is longer acting.

Adverse effects: Adverse effects of corticosteroids in dogs include (Fadok 2016) polyuria, polydipsia, polyphagia, muscle weakness, delayed wound healing, thinning of the skin, weakened ligaments, cataracts, calcinosis cutis, iatrogenic Cushing's disease, increased susceptibility to urinary tract and skin infections, and personality changes (aggression or apparent depression).

Contraindications: Contraindications to the use of corticosteroids in dogs include Cushing's disease, diabetes mellitus, and concurrent use of nonsteroidal anti-inflammatory drugs (NSAIDs).

If the dog's skin condition is worsening on corticosteroids, the veterinarian should be contacted.

18.3.2 Corticosteroids: Feline AD

Cats seem to be more tolerant of corticosteroids than dogs, but adverse effects include diabetes, heart disease, and skin fragility syndrome (hair loss, thin skin that is easily torn, bruising, and medially curled ear pinnae), which may occur with short-term or chronic use (Lowe 2008).

18.3.3 Corticosteroid Dosing Guidelines

Prednisone and prednisolone:

- *Dogs:* 0.25–0.5 mg/kg PO every 12 hours, and slowly taper to every other day (preferred over continuous daily dosing)
- *Cats:* Prednisolone (prednisone is not orally bioavailable in cats) 0.5–1 mg/kg PO every 12 hours (Lowe 2010).

Methylprednisolone:

- May be less likely to cause polyuria and polydipsia than prednisone and prednisolone in dogs

- *Dogs:* 0.4–0.5 mg/kg PO every 12–24 hours, tapering to lowest effective dose every other day
- *Cats:* 4 mg PO every 24 hours, tapering to every other day or less frequently.

Dexamethasone:

- Not preferred in dogs due to its longer duration of action and increased risk for gastrointestinal ulceration
- *Dogs:* 0.1–0.3 mg/kg PO every 24 hours and taper to two to three times weekly or less
- *Cats:* 0.1–0.3 mg/kg every 24 hours and taper to two to three times weekly.

Mandatory monitoring
Because cats treated with corticosteroids are at increased risk for developing diabetes mellitus, blood glucose should be monitored during treatment.

Combination antihistamine (trimeprazine 5 mg) and corticosteroid (prednisolone 2 mg) – Temaril P tablets:

- The potential advantage of using combination antihistamine and corticosteroid is the ability to use a lower corticosteroid dose to relieve pruritus.
- *Dogs:* 1 tablet/4.5 kg body weight PO every 12 hours and taper
- *Cats:* 1 tablet PO every 12–24 hours and taper (extra-label).

18.4 Antihistamines (H1)

Histamine blockers work by competitively antagonizing histamine receptors on cell membranes. They also appear to decrease histamine release from basophils and mast cells *in vitro* (Ferrer 2016). Antihistamines are not effective in *acute* flare-ups (Olivry et al. 2010). They are best used prophylactically when administered 10–14 days prior to an allergic event. The main adverse effect of antihistamines in dogs and cats is drowsiness, which may actually be desirable in pruritic pets! There is some evidence that combining antihistamines with essential fatty acids achieves greater efficacy than when each is used separately (Verde 2016). There may be variability between pets of individual responses to antihistamines, requiring a trial of more than one antihistamine to see which works for that patient. **Do not use combination (usually over-the-counter [OTC]) antihistamine products in dogs or cats, as they may contain acetaminophen, aspirin, or decongestants (vasoconstrictors) such as phenylephrine, which can cause severe, even fatal, adverse reactions.**

Use with caution in dogs or cats with:

- Glaucoma
- A current pregnancy, or animals intended for breeding
- Cardiac disease
- Seizures
- Keratoconjunctivitis sicca (KCS).

Antihistamines – dogs:

- *Cetirizine:* 0.5–1 mg/kg PO every 12–24 hours
- *Chlorpheniramine:* 0.4 mg/kg PO every 12 hours
- *Clemastine:* 0.05–0.1 mg/kg PO every 12 hours
- *Cyproheptadine:* 1–2 mg/kg PO every 12 hours
- *Diphenhydramine:* 2.2 mg/kg PO every 8–12 hours
- *Hydroxyzine:* 2.2 mg/kg PO every 8–12 hours
- *Loratadine:* 1 mg/kg PO every 12–24 hours.

Antihistamines – cats (note that some drug dose rates are indicated PER CAT, while others are per kilogram of body weight):

- *Cetirizine:* 2.5–5 mg/cat PO every 24 hours
- *Chlorpheniramine:* 2–4 mg/cat PO every 12–24 hours
- *Clemastine:* 0.67 mg/cat PO every 12 hours
- *Cyproheptadine:* 2–4 mg/cat PO every 12–24 hours
- *Hydroxyzine:* 2.2 mg/kg PO every 12 hours
- *Loratadine:* 2.5–5 mg/cat PO every 24 hours.

It can be challenging to administer oral antihistamines to cats because of their bitter taste, which is difficult to mask and may cause excessive drooling!

18.5 Tricyclic Antidepressants

The exact mode of action of tricyclic antidepressants with respect to treatment of AD is unknown, but they bind with varying affinity to a number of different receptors, including histamine (H1 and H2), muscarinic, noradrenergic, and serotonin receptors. The affinity of tricyclic antidepressants for H1 and H2 receptors is marked, making them some of the most potent histamine blockers known (Reedy et al. 1997). Although they are prescribed to both dogs and cats for their antihistaminic effects, their use has been more widely investigated in dogs rather than cats. Doxepin and amitriptyline are the two most commonly used tricyclic antidepressants used for dermatologic reasons in veterinary patients. One study demonstrated that pruritus either complete or partially resolved in 30% of atopic dogs treated with amitriptyline.

Doxepin:

- *Dogs:* 1 mg/kg PO every eight hours (rarely used in cats)
- *Adverse effects:* Vomiting, sleepiness, panting, trembling.

Amitriptyline:

- *Dogs:* 1–2 mg/kg PO every 12 hours
- *Cats:* 0.5–1 mg/kg PO every 24 hours
- *Adverse effects in dogs:* Sedation, vomiting, bizarre behavior, and liver enzyme elevations
- *Adverse effects in cats:* Sedation, hyperactivity, and drooling.

Prescribing tricyclic antidepressants for pets with allergies may create concern for some pet owners who fear that their dog or cat is "depressed"! Most veterinarians prescribing this class of medication explain to the owner why this is being used, but the pharmacist may be questioned as well.

18.6 Immunosuppressants

18.6.1 Modified Cyclosporine

Modified cyclosporine is US Food and Drug Administration (FDA) approved for use in dogs and cats as a primary treatment for AD. It is useful as an alternative to corticosteroids, particularly when corticosteroids are contraindicated (e.g. for diabetes mellitus, NSAID therapy, and Cushing's disease). It appears to be a much safer drug for treating AD in the dog and cat than as a transplant anti-rejection drug in humans.

Significant points to remember when dispensing:

- Modified cyclosporine has better oral bioavailability than cyclosporine – the two are NOT interchangeable.
- Compounding modified cyclosporine is not advised due to lack of stability and sterility, and variable potency (Umstead et al. 2012).
- Do not open or crush capsules.
- Concurrent administration of ketoconazole can increase blood concentrations of modified cyclosporine and is often prescribed concurrently for that purpose (a lower dose of modified cyclosporine provides a cost savings for the owner).

Adverse effects in dogs and cats include anorexia, vomiting, and gingival hyperplasia.
Modified cyclosporine dosing – dogs:

- 5–7 mg/kg PO every 24 hours and tapered to every other day or two times per week
- When used with ketoconazole: Both drugs are used at a dose of 2.5 mg/kg PO every 24 hours.
- Do not use in dogs fed a raw diet due to inherent risks of pathogen contamination in raw diets (Freeman et al. 2013).

Modified cyclosporine dosing – cats:

- 5–7 mg/kg PO every 24 hours and tapered to every other day or two times per week
- Not to be used in outdoor cats that hunt or if fed a raw diet, due to possible recrudescence of toxoplasmosis.

18.7 Oclacitinib

Oclacitinib is an FDA-approved drug indicated for control of pruritus associated with allergic dermatitis and control of AD in dogs older than one year of age (Falk and Ferrer 2015). Oclacitinib is a Janus kinase enzyme (JAK) inhibitor that inhibits JAK1 and, to a lesser degree, JAK3. JAK1 is involved in signaling pathways for cytokines that mediate allergy and inflammation, including interleukins (IL2, IL4, IL6, IL13, and IL31). IL31 is considered to have a major role in the pathophysiology of canine and human pruritus (Falk and Ferrer 2015; Ruzicka 2017). Similar JAK inhibitors in humans include tofacitinib and ruxolitinib, with many others currently in clinical trials. These agents are used in humans for inflammatory diseases such as rheumatoid arthritis, psoriasis, ankylosing spondylitis, ulcerative colitis, and Crohn's disease (Clark et al. 2014). Oclacitinib has been shown to be as effective for canine AD as cyclosporine or corticosteroids (Little et al. 2015), with dogs typically responding within the first week of treatment.

Adverse effects: Gastrointestinal disturbances, lethargy, increased incidence of skin lesions (nodules, cysts, and sebaceous adenomas), interdigital lesions, and increased susceptibility to mange (Cosgrove et al. 2013)

Contraindications: Dogs with serious infections, neoplasia or history of neoplasia, and concurrent use of corticosteroids (Zoetis 2013)

Ocalacitinib dosing:

Dogs: 0.4–0.6 mg/kg every 12 hours for up to 14 days, then once daily if used long term
Cats (extra-label): Not FDA approved for use in cats, as there are insufficient safety and efficacy data.

18.8 Monoclonal Antibody (mAb) Therapy

The goal of mAb therapy is to exploit their specificity target (a particular cell or protein) to selectively control a key factor contributing to disease pathogenesis. The potential advantage of targeted mAb therapy over traditional pharmacological agents is fewer side effects (Olivry et al. 2015). Omalizumab for asthma, dupilumab for AD, and rituximab for non-Hodgkin's lymphoma are three examples of mAb therapies used in human medicine. Possible future application of mAb for dogs and cats ranges from allergies to osteoarthritis, autoimmune diseases, and neoplasia; currently, a caninized mAb targeting IL31 is licensed by the US Department of Agriculture (USDA) for the control of clinical signs associated with AD in dogs (Gearing 2013). IL31 is a key mediator of inflammation and pruritus in canine AD.

Cytopoint (canine atopic dermatitis immunotherapeutic):

- Caninized monoclonal antibody (mAb) against IL31 for administration by or under the supervision of a veterinarian
- Eliminated via normal protein degradation pathways
- **Specific for use in dogs only**
- Subcutaneous injection that can be repeated at four- to eight-week intervals (Zoetis 2016)
- According to the label, it can be used in conjunction with other medications, including parasiticides, antibiotics, corticosteroids, vaccines, immunotherapy, antihistamines, oclacitinib, and cyclosporine.

18.9 Immunotherapy (Hyposensitization)

Injectable immunotherapy, often called "hyposensitization," exposes the patient to ultralow doses of offending allergens that have been identified via intradermal or serum testing. It is an effective treatment method for allergic respiratory disease in humans when symptomatic treatment has failed or cannot be used (Zur et al. 2002). Hyposensitization is thought to enhance immunoglobulin-G (IgG) production while suppressing IgE production by the patient. The IgG molecules act to block the allergic reaction. Other theories include induction of suppressor T cells or alteration in the balance of TH1 and TH2 cells. In people undergoing hyposensitization, an increase in serum concentrations of allergen-specific IgG is well correlated with improvement of symptoms (Herrmann et al. 1995).

Injectable immunotherapy in dogs with AD has been used since the late 1960s. As is the case in people, allergen-specific hyposensitization also increases serum concentrations of allergen-specific IgG in dogs (Hites et al. 1989). The success rate of hyposensitizaton for canine AD ranges from 64% to 72% after 6–12 months of treatment (Schnabl et al. 2006). It is currently the only treatment for AD that is disease modifying rather than merely addressing the symptoms of AD, and it may actually prevent progression of the disease (Jacobsen et al. 2007). Intradermal skin testing in conjunction with allergen-specific immunotherapy has also achieved good results for feline AD (Halliwell 1997).

Sublingual immunotherapy for humans was designed as an alternative to injections. Sublingual allergy drops containing patient-specific allergens are self-administered at home. Sublingual immunotherapy is mainly used in dogs; results in cats and horses have not been reported (DeBoer et al. 2013). Sublingual immunotherapy solutions are available in metered-dose dispensing bottles and are administered twice daily. The dog should not be allowed to eat or drink for 15 minutes after administration.

Immunotherapy – injectable:

- Requires intradermal skin testing and/or serum testing to identify the offending allergens. Results should concur with the time of year the patient is affected to achieve treatment success.
- Injections are given subcutaneously for the life of the pet at weekly or biweekly intervals.
- Injectable immunotherapy solutions lose efficacy (shelf life) on average after one year.
- Injectable immunotherapy solutions must be refrigerated, not frozen, and may darken with age.
- Disposable (single-use) tuberculin syringes (1 cc) with 25 gauge, 5/8 in. needles are required. **Syringes larger than 1 cc should not be dispensed, nor should insulin syringes.**
- The pharmacist can play a key role in training the owner to properly and accurately

use syringes to deliver the appropriate dose.

- *Adverse effects:* The most common side effect is increased pruritus after an injection (the veterinarian should be contacted before proceeding further). Anaphylaxis is rare (<1% of dogs) and consists of vomiting, diarrhea, and/or collapse.

Dramatic difference

Early signs of anaphylaxis in dogs (gastrointestinal) tend to differ from those in humans (respiratory) because the "shock organ" in dogs is the liver, while in humans it is the lungs.

Immunotherapy – sublingual drops:

- Requires intradermal skin testing and/or serum testing to identify the offending allergens. Results should concur with the time of year the patient is affected to achieve treatment success.
- Sublingual immunotherapy solutions are supplied in a metered-dose bottle and are administered twice daily to the buccal mucosa.
- Sublingual immunotherapy solutions do not require refrigeration.
- The patient should not eat or drink for 15 minutes after administration.
- Anaphylactic reactions are rare. The most common side effect is face rubbing or increased pruritus after a dose – the prescribing veterinarian should be consulted if this occurs.
- Most dogs respond within three to six months, but the treatment is long term.
- Dogs that do not respond to injectable immunotherapy may respond to sublingual immunotherapy.

18.10 Topical Medications

Since a dysfunctional skin barrier is present in AD, topical therapy serves to prevent percutaneous absorption of the allergen and prevent secondary bacterial and yeast overgrowth. In humans with AD, moisturizers

and topical steroids may aid in treating eczematous dermatitis. In dogs and cats, physical removal of offending allergens by frequent bathing in hypoallergenic shampoos and/or by rinsing or wiping the fur and feet after the animal has been outside can be helpful. Foot soaks are contraindicated because excessive moisture further compromises the skin barrier. Topical glucocorticoids and tacrolimus effectively reduce clinical signs of canine AD, but there is a risk of skin atrophy with prolonged use of the former (Olivry et al. 2010).

- The pH of canine skin is basic, whereas human skin pH is acidic (Matousek and Campbell 2002). This is of unknown clinical significance.
- Hypoallergenic shampoos or shampoos with phytosphingosine, ceramides, or fatty acids may be helpful in repairing the skin barrier.
- **CAUTION FOR OWNERS: Phytosphingosine shampoo was believed to have caused a fatal asthma attack in a woman after using it to bathe her pet** (FDA 2015).
- Shampoos containing tar or selenium sulfide are contraindicated in cats due to their irritant properties.

18.10.1 Topical Corticosteroids

- Short-acting topical corticosteroids are useful for controlling focal areas of pruritis but should not be used chronically.
- Betamethasone-containing products should be restricted to <14 days duration of application due to cutaneous adverse effects (DeBoer et al. 2002).
- Should not be used over weight-bearing areas such as the elbows and hocks; on thin-skinned areas such as the scrotum, groin, and axillae; or on areas of cutaneous ulcers.
- Some pets will show signs of iatrogenic Cushing's disease after topical corticosteroid use, as they can be absorbed systemically.
- Side effects of topical corticosteroids include thinning of the skin, peeling of the skin, comedones, and calcinosis cutis. Owners will see the skin "getting worse" and tend to use MORE of the steroid, when

in fact they are exacerbating the problem and need to consult with the veterinarian.

- Topical corticosteroids in cats are difficult to restrict to topical use, as "what's on the cat, is in the cat" (cats are notoriously fastidious in their grooming and licking and may ingest topical products).

18.10.2 Tacrolimus 0.1% Topical Ointment

- Effective for pruritic feet when applied to the feet twice daily for one week, then as needed (Bensignor and Olivry 2005).
- Too expensive for many pet owners. Compounded preparations may be more affordable.
- Topical cyclosporine is not effective due to its large molecular size (does not adequately penetrate the skin).

18.11 Nutritional Supplements for Veterinary Atopic Dermatitis

In humans with AD, polyunsaturated fatty acids (PUFAs) have been reported to modulate the inflammatory response (Glos et al. 2007). Similarly, oral PUFAs decrease inflammation and pruritus in atopic dogs (Glos et al. 2007). The use of dietary omega-3 fatty acids as adjunctive treatment for several clinical disorders has been evaluated to a greater extent in dogs than in cats (Bauer 2011). Less is known about appropriate dosing for treating inflammatory disorders in cats. One study, using a mixture of omega-6 and omega-3 essential fatty acids in cats, demonstrated efficacy in reducing inflammation in feline dermatoses such as flea allergy dermatitis and feline atopy (Harvey 1993). In dogs, supplementation with omega-6 fatty acids such as gamma-linoleic acid (GLA), omega-3 fatty acids such as eicosapentanoic acid (EPA), and combinations of GLA and EPA have been reported to be beneficial (Glos et al. 2007). Commercially available diets

formulated for allergic dogs, particularly prescription diets such as Hill's D/D, J/D, Blue Buffalo HF, and Royal Canin PW, are supplemented with PUFAs, and studies show they are helpful in treating symptoms of canine AD (Vetri-Science 2010). In general, EFA-enriched diets provide higher amounts of EFA than when EFA is administered as an oral supplement (Roudebush et al. 1997). In dogs, it appears that marine-derived omega-3 fatty acids are more potent than plant-derived omega-3 fatty acids (flax seed oil), as dogs required 2.3 times more flax seed oil than marine-based supplements to achieve similar improvements (Bauer 2011). Whichever essential fatty acid supplement is used, it may take 60–90 days of treatment before benefits become evident. The approximate dose of combined EPA and DHA recommended as adjunctive dietary treatment for atopy in the dog is 125 mg/kg daily (Bauer 2011). However, it must be noted that not all fish oil supplements are equivalent with respect to the source of the fatty acids, and since these products are nutritional supplements rather than drugs, there is limited FDA regulation as to product content. For cats, low doses are likely safe for dermatitis-related disorders, given that such doses have been used in some open-label studies. Doses of >75 mg of combined EPA and DHA per kg body weight should be used with caution in the cat and only under veterinary supervision (Bauer 2011).

Other dietary supplements such as pantothenate, choline, nicotinamide, histadine, and inositol have been shown to increase the production of ceramide skin lipids *in vitro* and to reduce transepidermal water loss *in vivo* in HEALTHY dogs, but additional studies are needed to see if these compounds benefit dogs with AD (Olivry et al. 2010). Increasing ceramide and reducing transepidermal water loss help repair the skin barrier and keep it intact. It is important to note that there are species differences not only with prescription medications but also with supplements. The fact that a dietary supplement has been used safely in people does not mean these products have been evaluated adequately to be deemed safe for pets.

18.12 Pharmacotherapeutics of "Autoimmune" Dermatologic Disease

Key points to remember:

- Pemphigus foliaceus (PF) is the most common autoimmune skin disease diagnosed in dogs and cats.
- Discoid lupus erythematosus (DLE) and dermatomyositis (DMS) are commonly diagnosed in people, less so in dogs, and rarely in cats.
- PF, DLE, and DMS share some of the same clinical manifestations, genetic predispositions, and treatment modalities in all three species.
- Ultraviolet (UV) light is a potential trigger for immune-mediated skin diseases, and sunlight avoidance is advised.
- Vitamin E is used in canine immune-mediated skin diseases as an immune modulator.

18.12.1 Comparative Aspects of Pemphigus Foliaceus

The term *pemphigus* (Latin for "blister") is used for an entire group of autoimmune blistering diseases in which intraepithelial separation occurs (acantholysis) (Tater and Olivry 2010). PF is a more superficial form of the pemphigus complex, which includes pemphigus vulgaris, paraneoplastic pemphigus, and bullous pemphigoid – all three affecting deeper layers of the skin and manifesting as ulcerations. Autoantibodies attack intercellular connections between epithelial cells and cause "rounding up" (acantholysis) of normally stellate keratinocytes, which are under tension, resulting in blisters. These "blisters" appear clinically as pustules, crusts, or erosions and may or may not be pruritic.

In dogs, genetics may play a role in disease pathogenesis, as it is seen most frequently within certain breeds, such as Akitas and Chows. However, Dachshunds, Schipperkes, herding breeds, and Shih Tzus are among some of the many breeds affected. There is no sex or age predilection. Lesions may be present on the face, trunk (Figure 18.6), foot pads (Figure 18.7), ear pinnae, and (rarely) the nailbeds. In dogs with footpad involvement only, "punched-out" lesions can be seen on the pads, resulting in lameness. Lymph nodes may be enlarged, and the dog may be depressed and febrile. The cause of PF is unknown in dogs. It is unknown if diet plays a role, but in rare cases of PF in dogs, a prescription hypoallergenic diet has resulted

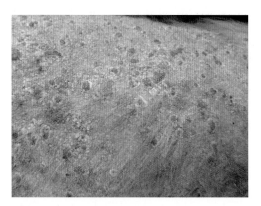

Figure 18.6 Crusting on the skin overlying the trunk of a dog with pemphigus foliaceus.

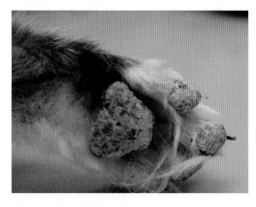

Figure 18.7 Pemphigus foliaceus in a dog. Crusting on the footpads makes it painful to walk.

in remission. Canine PF has been reported in patients with other conditions such as hypothyroidism, leishmaniasis, thymoma, and systemic lupus erythematosus (SLE) (Tater and Olivry 2010). PF may also be drug-induced in any species and has been associated with penicillamine, penicillins, cephalosporins, enalapril, cimetidine, amoxicillin/clavulanic acid, ampicillin, sulfa drugs, and (in dogs) topical amitraz-containing products. In humans, a form of PF known as "fogo selvagem" is endemic in Brazil; the disease is a result of a suspected arthropod bite.

PF in cats may consist of erosions and yellow crusts affecting the face (Figure 18.8), ear pinnae, nailbeds, and/or abdomen, including nipples (Figure 18.9). Affected cats may be febrile and sometimes pruritic, especially if crusts are present. There is no sex or age predilection. Lesions may be mistaken for allergy, dermatophytosis ("ringworm"), or a bacterial skin infection.

18.12.1.1 Diagnostic Testing

Skin biopsies or cytology of an intact pustule yield acantholytic cells (the keratinocytes that have lost their attachment to one another and have "rounded up") in dogs or cats with PF. However, this is not 100% diagnostic for PF, as acantholytic cells may also be present

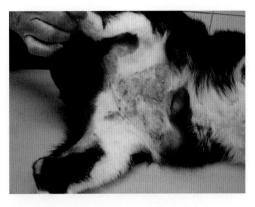

Figure 18.9 Pemphigus foliaceus in a cat manifesting as "blisters" or crusts on the ventral abdomen.

in dermatophytosis or severe bacterial infections. A fungal culture, therefore, is needed to rule out fungal disease since therapeutics for PF would exacerbate a fungal infection. Clinically, the lesions of PF and dermatophytosis can appear similar, and occasionally this is true histopathologically. Periodic acid Schiff (PAS) staining of biopsy samples may help differentiate PF and dermatophytosis. Bacterial culture of a PF pustule is sterile, whereas that of a true bacterial pyoderma will yield growth of excessive bacterial numbers. Testing includes:

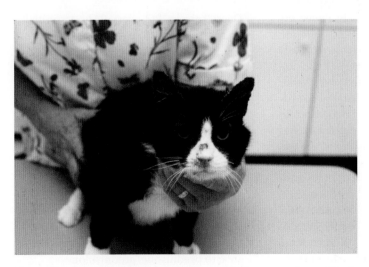

Figure 18.8 Pemphigus foliaceus in a cat manifesting as crusting on the dorsum of the nose.

- Thorough history and physical examination
- Cytology
- Histopathology
- Complete blood count (CBC)
- Bacterial and/or fungal culture.

18.12.1.2 Pharmacological Treatment of Pemphigus Foliaceus

PF is a chronic manageable disease, with remission being the goal. The disease can wax and wane with or without treatment. Unless owners' expectations are managed through appropriate education regarding the chronicity of the disease, frustration can result. Therapy varies for each patient, as there are no "set" pharmacological protocols for PF in dogs and cats. Factors that are considered include age, condition of the patient, expenses that will be incurred, ability of the owners to administer medications, and availability for periodic recheck appointments. For all dogs and cats with PF, minimizing exposure to UV light is a key component of disease management.

18.12.1.2.1 Corticosteroids: Canine PF

Systemic corticosteroids are the initial drug of choice for achieving remission, as they are fast-acting compared to many other immunosuppressants. The ultimate goal is to induce remission via immunosuppression with corticosteroids, then slowly lower the dose and replace corticosteroids with an alternate therapy for long-term control. Daily doses of a short-acting corticosteroid are used initially, then tapered to every other day, twice weekly, and potentially even discontinued altogether. Because corticosteroid resistance can develop, if the patient comes out of remission the dose must be increased, and even then may not be as effective. One potential option for patients that have relapsed is to use a different corticosteroid (i.e. from prednisone to methylprednisolone or triamcinolone). Topical corticosteroids such as triamcinolone 0.1% or fluocinonide 0.05% can be used for focal lesions or combined with systemic corticosteroids in an effort to decrease the systemic dose.

Long-acting injectable corticosteroids ("depo" formulations) are not recommended for treatment of autoimmune diseases, including PF, because they are inconsistently absorbed. Rarely can corticosteroid monotherapy maintain canine PF patients in remission long term – hence, the need for accompanying medications.

Adverse effects of glucocorticoids have been discussed previously in this chapter.

18.12.1.2.2 Corticosteroids: Feline PF

It is sometimes tempting to use long-acting depo formulations for cats because they are notoriously difficult to "pill" (medicate orally). Oral corticosteroids are preferred for treating feline PF. Short-acting prednisolone generally achieves remission within one to two weeks. Since cats seem to be more tolerant of corticosteroid side effects than dogs (still no reason not to be glucocorticoid-stingy!), some cats can be maintained in remission on twice-weekly oral corticosteroid doses.

Adverse effects of corticosteroids in cats have been discussed previously in this chapter.

18.12.1.2.3 Corticosteroid Dosing for PF
Prednisone and prednisolone:

- *Dogs:* 2 mg/kg PO every 24 hours initially, then tapered slowly over several weeks depending upon the patient's response
- *Cats:* Prednisolone, rather than prednisone, should be used in cats because oral bioavailability of the active drug (prednisolone) is low in cats after oral dosing of prednisone. 2–4 mg/kg PO every 24 hours, then tapered slowly over several weeks depending upon the patient's response.

Methylprednisolone:

- May be less likely to cause polyuria and polydipsia than prednisone in the dog
- May be used if the patient develops resistance to prednisone/prednisolone
- *Dogs:* 4 mg methylprednisolone = 5 mg prednisone

- *Cats:* 4–8 mg per cat PO every 24 hours, then tapered over several weeks.

Triamcinolone:

- *Cats:* 0.2–0.6 mg/kg PO every 24 hours, then tapered over several weeks.

Dexamethasone:

- *Dogs:* Not recommended due to its long duration of action and greater risk of adverse effects such as gastrointestinal ulceration
- *Cats:* 0.3–0.6 mg/kg PO every 24 hours until remission, then gradually tapered to every other day or every third day. As stated previously, cats should be aggressively monitored for the development of diabetes mellitus.

18.12.1.2.4 Adjuvant Therapy for Canine PF

Studies indicate that corticosteroid monotherapy results in acceptable management of PF in only 35–39% of dogs (Ihrke et al. 1985). Most dogs will achieve remission but will either relapse or develop intolerable adverse effects. Co-treatment with an adjuvant immunomodulating drug is advised because most adjuvant immunomodulating drugs used in veterinary patients are not quick-acting. By doing so, full pharmacological activity of the adjuvant immunomodulating drug can be realized at the same time the corticosteroid dose is decreased or discontinued. Adjuvant immunomodulating drugs used for PF include drugs that interfere with nucleic acid synthesis (azathioprine), cross-link DNA (chlorambucil), block transcription of genes in activated T-lymphocytes (cyclosporine), and modulate the immune system by inhibiting neutrophil chemotaxis (doxycycline and niacinamide).

Azathioprine:

- *Dose:* Dogs – 2–2.5 mg/kg PO every 24 or 48 hours. *Not* recommended in cats because they lack the enzyme responsible for metabolic conversion of azathioprine to inactive metabolites.

- *Adverse effects:* Vomiting, diarrhea, myelosuppression, pancreatitis, hepatotoxicity (rare)
- Obtain baseline CBC, then monitor every two to three months; monitor serum chemistry profiles every six months (liver enzymes and pancreatic enzymes).
- Occasionally, a patient may respond to the brand-name formulation (Imuran, Promethius Labs) and not to generic azathioprine (Cuffari et al. 2000).

Chlorambucil:

- *Dose:* 0.1–0.2 mg/kg PO every 24 or 48 hours; it is sometimes tapered to one to two doses per week.
- *Adverse effects:* Myelosuppression, hepatopathy (rare), vomiting, anorexia, diarrhea. Generally well tolerated in dogs. A recent price increase may make the drug unaffordable for some owners (it is more expensive than using azathioprine).
- Can decompose rapidly in compounded aqueous formulations that contain simple syrup (Papich 2016).
- Obtain baseline CBC, then monitor every two to three months, eventually every six months.

Cyclosporine (modified):

- 5–10 mg/kg PO every 24 hours. Use of modified cyclosporine (microemulsion) is advised instead of cyclosporine because of better oral bioavailability.
- An FDA-approved formulation for dogs is available (Table 18.1).
- *Adverse effects:* Anorexia, vomiting, diarrhea, gingival hyperplasia, hair growth, psoriasiform lichenoid dermatosis (an atypical presentation of bacterial skin infection), and papillomas
- Capsule may be placed in freezer for up to 48 hours before administration to reduce incidence of vomiting (Bachtel et al. 2015).
- Usually effective in conjunction with corticosteroids, but rarely effective as single-drug therapy for PF.
- May take several weeks to achieve full efficacy.

Table 18.1 Drugs that are FDA approved for dermatologic disease in dogs and/or cats but are not available in equivalent human formulations.

Brand name (manufacturer)	Active ingredient(s)	Drug class	Rationale/notes
Apoquel (Zoetis)	Oclacitinib maleate	Janus kinase (JAK) inhibitor	Inhibits primarily JAK1 and JAK3, but limited effect on JAK2. At the time of this writing, there are no JAK inhibitors approved for dermatologic diseases in people, but there are some approved for other inflammatory diseases in people.
Atopica (Elanco)	Modified cyclosporine	Immune-modulating agent (calcineurin inhibitor)	FDA approved for both dogs and cats; human products may not be bioequivalent.
Cytopoint (Zoetis)	Monoclonal antibody to canine IL31	Monoclonal antibody	IL31 is a cytokine involved in the "itch pathway." USDA approved for dog with atopic dermatitis (FDA does not regulate veterinary biologicals).
Temaril-P (Zoetis)	Trimeprazine, prednisolone	Antihistamine/ phenothiazine and corticosteroid	Trimeprazine-containing products labeled for human use may be available outside the USA. Approved for use in dogs.

FDA, US Food and Drug Administration; IL31, interleukin-31; USDA, US Department of Agriculture.

- Cimetidine, itraconazole, fluconazole, or ketoconazole may increase oral bioavailability of cyclosporine when used concomitantly (Papich 2016). This drug interaction is used intentionally in some cases to reduce the expense of cyclosporine. Ketoconazole at 2.5–5 mg/kg PO every 24 hours is administered concurrently with modified cyclosporine.

Niacinamide and tetracycline combination:

- Dose:
  - Dogs weighing <10 kg: 250 mg each of tetracycline and niacinamide PO every eight hours
  - Dogs weighing > 10 kg: 500 mg each of tetracycline and niacinamide PO every eight hours
- This dose may be decreased in "lean" dogs or dogs with a sensitive gastrointestinal tract. Doxycycline or minocycline may be substituted for tetracycline at 3–5 mg/kg

PO every 12–24 hours. Both niacinamide and tetracyclines should be administered with food.
- *Adverse effects:* Anorexia, vomiting, diarrhea, depression, and elevated liver enzymes
- May be used as sole therapy in mild PF cases or when corticosteroids are contraindicated (i.e. in dogs with diabetes, cardiomyopathy, and pancreatitis).
- Niacinamide should not be confused with niacin. DO NOT DISPENSE NIACIN, as it causes hepatotoxicosis in dogs.

18.12.1.2.5 Adjuvant Therapy for Feline PF

Cats with PF may be successfully managed long term with low-dose corticosteroid therapy as long as the patient is diligently monitored for adverse effects. Diabetes, thinning of the skin, and cardiac disease may be consequences of long-term corticosteroid use in cats. There is wide individual variation in the ability of cats to tolerate corticosteroids:

Some tolerate glucocorticoids for a long period of time, while others exhibit side effects rapidly. This author prefers to use corticosteroids for immediate remission of PF, then use an adjuvant immunomodulating drug such as chlorambucil, or modified cyclosporine for long-term maintenance.

Chlorambucil:

- *Dose:* 0.1–0.2 mg/kg PO every 24–48 hours, with goal of tapering to once weekly
- Generally well tolerated in cats
- Monitoring for myelosuppression (i.e. CBC) is done initially every three to four weeks, then every six months.
- Other adverse effects are rare but include hepatotoxicosis, anorexia, vomiting, and diarrhea.
- Once corticosteroid treatment has induced remission, most cats can be successfully managed with chlorambucil alone.
- May take two to six weeks to achieve efficacy.

Cyclosporine (modified):

- *Dose:* 5–10 mg/kg PO every 24 hours or 2.5–5 mg kg^{-1} PO every 12 hours
- Adverse effects include vomiting, diarrhea, and recrudescence of toxoplasmosis – not advisable to use in cats eating a raw diet or in cats that go outdoors (hunting).
- An FDA-approved oral solution (Atopica) is available for cats (Table 18.1).
- Once opened, the oral solution should be used within 60 days (5 mL container) or 11 weeks (17 mL container).
- When dispensing Atopica oral solution, owner education should include instructions for administering the correct dose (Elanco n.d.), as the syringes included with the product are marked for the cat's weight, not by volume or drug quantity (milligrams).
- If using the canine capsule formulation and vomiting occurs, capsules may be placed in a freezer for up to 48 hours before administration to decrease gastric irritation (Bachtel et al. 2015).
- Compounded modified cyclosporine is not advised due to reports of instability, inaccurate concentrations, and undesirable products (Umstead et al. 2012).

Doxycycline:

- Not recommended in cats. Tablet and capsule formulations can cause esophageal strictures in cats when administered orally, and the compounded suspension doxycycline products have low stability (shelf life of one week) (Papich et al. 2013).

18.12.2 Comparative Aspects of Discoid Lupus Erythematosus (DLE)

DLE is thought to be a more benign variant of SLE, confined solely to the skin. In humans, the lymphocytes infiltrating skin lesions of discoid and SLE are primarily T cells, with T helper cells predominating in DLE and T suppressor cells common in SLE (Muller et al. 1989). Common to both humans and dogs, DLE is exacerbated by exposure to ultraviolet light. In fact, most cases of DLE in dogs are diagnosed after a summer of sun exposure. Also common to both dogs and humans with DLE are the areas of the body affected, including the face (Figure 18.10), nose, ears, and (in dogs) sometimes the genital area. DLE can occur at any age in the dog, with certain breeds more frequently affected, including German Shepherds, Collies, Siberian Huskies, Shetland Sheepdogs, Chow Chows, and mixes of these breeds. The lesions can be chronic and persist for months to years (Fitzpatrick 1987). DLE is generally not seen in cats, although a study conducted in Europe described four cases (Willemse and Koeman 1990). Lesions in dogs consist of depigmentation, crusting, scaling, and ulceration of the nose. Conditions previously called "collie nose" or "nasal solar dermatitis" probably were, in fact, DLE.

18.12.2.1 Diagnostic Testing

- History and physical examination
- Histopathology, including immunohisto-pathology
- CBC and serum chemistry profile.

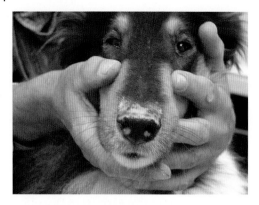

Figure 18.10 Discoid lupus erythematosus in a dog manifesting as ulceration and depigmentation of the nose and periocular area.

18.12.2.2 Pharmacological Treatment of DLE

Perhaps the single most important factor in treating dogs with DLE is eliminating sun exposure. Owners often ask about using sunblock topically or wearing cute visors, but complete avoidance of sun exposure is most helpful. Early-morning or late-evening (dusk or later) walks are advised. Affected dogs should receive little to no sun exposure during peak UV exposure hours of the day. With regard to pharmacological therapy, immunomodulating drugs are the mainstay for DLE. Therapy is continued for the life of the dog and may include topical and/or systemic medications. Most often, topicals are the initial mode of therapy, as they are most innocuous, with systemic medications being reserved for patients that fail to respond to topicals. Systemic medications may include oral corticosteroids, the combination of niacinamide and a tetracycline, modified cyclosporine, or azathioprine.

18.12.2.2.1 *Topical Medications for Canine DLE*

- *Glucocorticoids:* Triamcinolone 0.1% ointment, fluocinonide 0.05% ointment, or Panalog (a veterinary product containing nystatin-neomycin, thiostrepton, and triamcinolone) applied once daily, then tapered as needed. Since the dog can lick the ointment off, it helps to have the dog hold something in its mouth after application of the topical to allow it to "soak in."
- *Tacrolimus 0.1%:* Apply once or twice daily to the affected area.
- *Sunblock:* Not advised when the area is ulcerated, as contact allergy may occur when a non-intact skin barrier is present.

18.12.2.2.2 *Systemic Medications for Canine DLE*
Niacinamide in combination with a tetracycline:
- Dosing and adverse effects as described for pemphigus foliaceus

Modified cyclosporine:

- Dosing and adverse effects as described for pemphigus foliaceus

Systemic glucocorticoids:

- Not recommended due to lifelong nature of the disease

Azathioprine:

- Used only in cases of DLE where other more innocuous treatments have failed
- Dosing and adverse effects as described for pemphigus foliaceus.

18.12.3 Comparative Aspects of Dermatomyositis (DMS)

Dermatomyositis (DMS) is an uncommon condition in dogs that predominantly affects the skin and, to a lesser extent, striated muscle (Berger 2016). Affected dogs are suspected to be genetically predisposed (autosomal dominant with incomplete penetrance) to an immune-mediated vasculitis. Collies and Shetland Sheepdogs are the predominant breeds affected, and symptoms usually appear before six months of age. Lesions, including alopecia, blistering, and scarring, occur on the tail tip (Figure 18.11), face (Figures 18.12 and 18.13), ears, and distal limbs. Because symptoms occur in puppies, the facial lesions are often mistakenly explained by the breeder as excoriations from the puppies playing together. Affected dogs should not be bred. In humans, DMS is one of the major systemic inflammatory

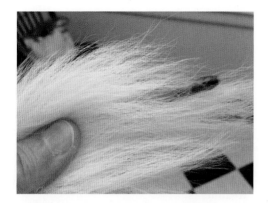

Figure 18.11 Tail-tip alopecia in a dog with dermatomyositis.

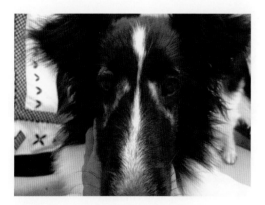

Figure 18.12 Facial alopecia in a dog with dermatomyositis.

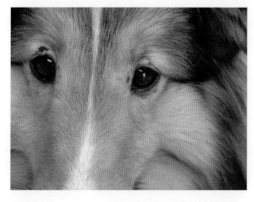

Figure 18.13 Early, subtle areas of alopecia in a dog with dermatomyositis (DMS). DMS usually results in scarring.

diseases of connective tissue (Mills 1990). Dermatitis occurs in about half of the human cases (the majority present with muscle weakness), whereas in dogs, dermatitis is the main presenting sign, with muscle involvement usually not clinically apparent. Interestingly, the lesions in humans occur in the same areas as in dogs: face, knuckles, elbows, and knees. Since sunlight activation may play a role, avoidance of sun exposure is advised. DMS has not been described in cats.

18.12.3.1   Diagnostic Testing

The diagnosis is made by skin biopsy and consideration of the age and breed of the dog and the anatomic areas affected. Diseases that clinically mimic DMS include demodicosis, bacterial pyoderma, dermatophytosis, allergic dermatitis, and DLE.

18.12.3.2   Pharmacological Treatment of DMS

The severity of the disease dictates the most appropriate therapy for individual patients. The waxing and waning course of DMS make it difficult to determine the efficacy of any given treatment. In recurrent moderate-to-severe disease, pentoxifylline has historically been the drug of choice (Berger 2016). Niacinamide with a tetracycline may be added for long-term control. Modified cyclosporine or azathioprine have also been employed. In severe cases, systemic corticosteroids are used short term to induce a response, while topical glucocorticoids or tacrolimus are employed once in remission. Even though affected dogs will experience flare-ups periodically, long-term use of systemic corticosteroids is not advised for the disease.

18.12.3.2.1   Systemic Medications for Canine DMS

Pentoxifylline:

- *Dose:* 15–25 mg/kg PO every 8–12 hours. May take many months to achieve efficacy.
- *Adverse effects:* These include anorexia, vomiting, and diarrhea. Gastrointestinal adverse

effects may be exacerbated if the tablet is crushed or split prior to administration.

- If compounded, aqueous solubility is limited (77 mg/ml); therefore, suspension formulations rather than solutions are often prepared. Suspensions may be stable for up to 90 days and require shaking before administration (Papich et al. 2013).

Niacinamide in combination with tetracycline, doxycycline, or minocycline:

- Dosing and adverse effects as described for pemphigus foliaceus

Glucocorticoids:

- May be used initially in moderate to severe cases to reduce inflammation, but long-term use is discouraged as other (safer) drug options are available.
- *Dose:* Prednisone 1–2 mg/kg every 24 hours until remission achieved, then taper to every 48 or 72 hours using the lowest effective possible.
- *Adverse effects:* As described for pemphigus foliaceus.

Azathioprine:

- Dose and adverse effects as described for pemphigus foliaceus. May be used for its "corticosteroid-sparing" effects when pentoxifylline or niacinamide/tetracycline therapy is insufficient to control the disease.

18.12.3.2.2 *Topical Medications for Canine DMS*
- *Glucocorticoids:* Triamcinolone 0.1% or fluocinonide 0.05% can be applied once daily on focally affected areas, such as facial lesions, pinnal lesions, or carpal or tail-tip lesions. Some dogs may display systemic signs of corticosteroid exposure, either because they are exquisitely sensitive to corticosteroids or because of excessive systemic absorption through debrided skin.
- *Tacrolimus 0.1%:* Used once or twice daily to focally affected areas. Most useful for patients in remission to replace systemic treatments.
- For all topical medications, owners should be advised to wear nonpermeable gloves while applying, and avoid contact with treated areas.

18.13 FDA-Approved Veterinary Drug Products with No Human Drug Equivalent

See Table 18.1.

Abbreviations

AD	Atopic dermatitis
IDST	Intradermal skin testing
NSAIDS	Nonsteroidal anti-inflammatory drugs
JAK	Janus kinase enzymes
Mab	Monoclonal antibody
PF	Pemphigus foliaceus
DLE	Discoid lupus erythematosus
DMS	Dermatomyositis

References

Asahina, R. and Maeda, S. (2017). A Review of the roles of keratinocyte-derived cytokines and chemokines in the pathogenesis of atopic dermatitis in humans and dogs. *Vet. Dermatol.* 28 (1): 16–24.

Bachtel, J.C., Pendergraft, J.S., Rosychuk, R.A. et al. (2015). Comparison of the stability and pharmacokinetics in dogs of modified ciclosporin capsules stored at −20′ and room temperature. *Vet. Dermatol.* 26 (4): 228–e50.

Bauer, J. (2011). Therapeutic use of fish oils in companion animals. *J. Amer. Med. Assoc.* 239 (11): 1441–1451.

Bensignor, E. and Olivry, T. (2005). Treatment of localized lesions of canine atopic dermatitis with tacrolimus ointment: a blinded randomized controlled trial. *Vet. Dermatol.* 16: 52–60.

Berger D. (2016). Canine dermatomyositis. Clinicians' Brief, June. https://www.cliniciansbrief.com/article/canine-dermatomyositis (subscription required).

Clark, J., Flanagan, M.E., and Telliez, J.B. (2014). Discovery and development of Janus kinase (JAK) inhibitors for inflammatory diseases. *J. Med. Chem.* 57 (12): 5023–5038.

Cosgrove, S.B., Wren, J.A., Cleaver, D.M. et al. (2013). Efficacy and safety of oclacitinib for the control of pruritus and associated skin lesions in dogs with canine allergic dermatitis. *Vet. Dermatol.* 24 (6): 587–597.

Cuffari, C., Hunt, S., and Bayless, T.M. (2000). Enhanced bioavailability of azathioprine compared to 6-mercaptopurine therapy in inflammatory bowel disease: correlation with treatment efficacy. *Alim. Pharmacol. Ther.* 14: 1009–1014.

DeBoer DJ. (2013). Sublingual immunotherapy for atopic dermatitis. Clinician's Brief, June. https://www.cliniciansbrief.com/article/sublingual-immunotherapy-atopic-dermatitis (subscription required).

DeBoer, D.J., Schafer, J.H., Salsbury, D.S. et al. (2002). Multiple center study of reduced concentration triamcinolone topical solution for the treatment of dogs with known or suspected allergic pruritus. *Amer. J. Vet. Res.* 63 (3): 408–413.

Elanco. (n.d.). Atopica 100 mg/ml oral solution for cats [package insert]. Elanco, Greenfield, IN.

Fadok V. (2016). Which drugs are most effective in managing atopic dermatitis? Plumb's Therapeutic Brief, January. https://www.cliniciansbrief.com/article/which-drugs-are-most-effective-managing-atopic-dermatitis-part-2 (subscription required).

Falk E, Ferrer L. (2015). Oclacitinib. Clinician's Brief, December. https://www.cliniciansbrief.com/article/oclacitinib (subscription required).

Ferrer L. (2016). Second-generation H1 antihistamines. Plumb's Therapeutics Brief. June. https://www.cliniciansbrief.com/article/second-generation-h1-antihistamines (subscription required).

Fitzpatrick, T.B., Eisen, A.Z., Wolff, K. et al. (1987). *Dermatology in General Medicine*, 3e, 1816–1833. New York: McGraw-Hill.

Food and Drug Administration (FDA). (2015). FDA issues caution to pet owners with the use of unapproved pet shampoo product. Office of the Commissioner, FDA External Affairs, FDA, Washington, DC, March.

Freeman, L.M., Chandler, M.L., Hamper, B.A. et al. (2013). Current knowledge about the risks and benefits of raw meat-based diets for dogs and cats. *J. Amer. Med. Assoc.* 243 (11): 1549–1558.

Gearing, D.P., Virtue, E.R., Gearing, R.P. et al. (2013). A fully caninized anti-ngf monoclonal antibody for pain relief in dogs. *BMC Vet. Res.* 9: 226.

Glos, K., Linek, M., Loewenstein, C. et al. (2007). The efficacy of commercially available veterinary diets recommended for dogs with atopic dermatitis. *Vet. Dermatol.* 181 (17): 280–287.

Halliwell, R. (1997). Efficacy of hyposensitization in feline allergic diseases based on results of *in vitro* testing for allergen-specific immunoglobulin E. *J. Amer. Anim. Hosp. Assoc.* 33: 282–288.

Harvey, R. (1993). Essential fatty acids and the cat. *Vet. Dermatol.* 4 (4): 175–179.

Herrmann, D., Henzgen, M., Frank, E. et al. (1995). Effect of hyposensitization for tree pollenosis on associated apple allergy. *J. Invest. Allergy Clin. Immunol.* 5: 259–267.

Hites, M.J., Kleinbeck, M.L., Loker, J.L. et al. (1989). Effect of immunotherapy on the serum concentration of allergen-specific IgG antibodies in the dog sera. *Vet. Immune Immunopathol.* 222: 39–51.

Ihrke, P.J., Stannard, A.A., Ardans, A.A. et al. (1985). Pemphigus foliaceus in dogs: a review of 37 cases. *J. Amer. Vet. Med. Assoc.* 186 (1): 59–66.

Jacobsen, L., Niggemann, B., Dreborg, S. et al. (2007). How strong is the evidence that immunotherapy in children prevents the progression of allergy and asthma? *Curr. Opin Allergy Clin. Immunol.* 7: 560–566.

Little, P., King, V.L., Davis, K.R. et al. (2015). A blinded, randomized clinical trial comparing the efficacy and safety of oclacitinib and cyclosporine for the control of atopic dermatitis in client-owned dogs. *Vet. Dermatol.* 26 (1): 23–30, e7–e8.

Loft, K. and Rosser, E. (2014). Group 1 and 2 *Dermatophagoides* house dust mite allergens in the microenvironment of cats. *Vet. Dermatol.* 21 (2): 152–158.

Lowe, A. (2008). Glucocorticoid use in cats. *Vet. Dermatol.* 19 (6): 340–347.

Lowe, A. (2010). Glucocorticoid use in cats. *Vet. Med.* 105 (2): 56–62.

Marsella, R., Sousa, C.A., Gonzales, A.J. et al. (2012). Current understanding of the pathophysiologic mechanisms of canine atopic dermatitis. *J. Amer. Med. Assoc.* 241 (2): 194–207.

Matousek, J. and Campbell, K. (2002). A comparative review of cutaneous pH. *Vet. Dermatol.* 13 (6): 293–300.

Mills JA. (1990). Dermatomyositis. In *Dermatology in General Medicine*, 3., Fitzpatrick TB, Eisen AZ, Wolff K, et al. (eds), pp. 1834–1841. McGraw-Hill, New York.

Muller, G.H., Kirk, R.W., and Scott, D.W. (1989). *Small Animal Dermatology*, 4e. Philadelphia: WB Saunders.

Novak, N., Bieber, T., and Allam, J.P. (2011). Immunological mechanisms of sublingual allergen-specific immunotherapy. *Allergy* 68: 733–739.

Olivry T, Bainbridge G. (2015). Clinical notes: advances in veterinary medicine: therapeutic monoclonal antibodies for companion animals. Clinician's Brief, March. https://www.zoetis.com/conditions/dogs/itchcycle/downloads/resources/publications/zoetiscn_mar_fnl.pdf.

Olivry, T., DeBoer, D.J., Favrot, C. et al. (2010). Treatment of canine atopic dermatitis: 2010 clinical practice guidelines from the international task force on canine atopic dermatitis. *Vet. Dermatol.* 21: 233–248.

Papich MG. (2016). *Saunders Handbook of Veterinary Drugs*, 4, 147–148, 193–196, 620–622, Small and Large Animal series. Elsevier, Philadelphia.

Papich, M.G., Davidson, G.S., and Fortier, L.A. (2013). Doxycycline concentration over time after storage in a compounded veterinary preparation. *J. Amer. Vet. Med. Assoc.* 242 (12): 1674–1678.

Ravens, P.A. (2014). Feline atopic dermatitis: a retrospective of 45 cases (2001–12). *Vet. Dermatol.* 25 (2): 95–e28.

Reedy, L., Miller, W.H., and Willemse, T. (1997). *Allergic Skin Diseases of Dogs and Cats*, Medical Management of Allergic Diseases series., 2e, 150–172. Philadelphia: Saunders.

Reinero, C.R. (2009). Feline Immunoglobulin E: historical perspective, diagnostics, and clinical relevance. *Vet. Immunol. Immunopathol.* 132: 13–20.

Rodrigues Hoffman, A. (2017). The cutaneous ecosystem: the roles of the skin microbiome in health and its association with inflammatory skin conditions in humans and animals. *Vet. Dermatol.* 28 (1): 60–70.

Rosser, E.J. (1999). Advances in the diagnosis and treatment of atopy. *Vet. Clin. North Am. Small Anim. Pract.* 29 (6): 1437–1447.

Roudebush P, Bloom P, Jewell D. (1997). Consumption of essential fatty acids in selected commercial dog foods compared to dietary supplementation. In Proceedings of ACVD/AAVD Meeting, pp. 10–11. AAVD and ACVD, Nashville, TN.

Ruzicka, T. (2017). Anti-interleukin 31 receptor a antibody for atopic dermatitis. *New Engl. J. Med.* 376 (9): 826–835.

Schnabl, B., Bettenay, S.V., and Graham, K.J. (2006). Results of allergen-specific immunotherapy in 117 dogs with atopic dermatitis. *Vet. Record* 21: 81–85.

Tater, K.C. and Olivry, T. (2010). Canine and feline pemphigus foliaceus: improving your chances of a successful outcome. *Vet. Med.* 105 (1): 18–30.

Umstead, M., Boothe, D.M., Cruz-Espindola, C. et al. (2012). Accuracy and precision of compounded ciclosporin capsules and solution. *Vet. Dermatol.* 23 (5): 431–e82.

Verde M. (2016). Canine atopic dermatitis. Clinician's Brief, March. https://www. cliniciansbrief.com/article/canine-atopic-dermatitis (subscription required).

Vetri-Science. (2010). Omega-3, 6, 9. Vetri-Science Laboratories. http://www. vetriscience.com.

Willemse, T. and Koeman, J.P. (1990). Discoid lupus erythematosus in cats. *Vet. Dermatol.* 1 (1): 19–24.

Zoetis (2013). *Apoquel [package insert]*. Kalamazoo, MI: Zoetis.

Zoetis (2016). *Canine atopic dermatitis immunotherapeutic [package insert]*. Kalamazoo, MI: Zoetis.

Zur, G., White, S., Ihrke, P.J. et al. (2002). Canine atopic dermatitis: a retrospective study of 169 cases examined at the University of California, Davis, 1992–1998. Part II. response to hyposensitization. *Vet. Dermatol.* 13: 103–111.

19

Ophthalmic Pharmacotherapeutics

Terri L. Alessio[1] and Katrina L. Mealey[2]

[1] *Veterinary Medical Teaching Hospital, College of Veterinary Medicine, Washington State University, Pullman, WA, USA*
[2] *College of Veterinary Medicine, Washington State University, Pullman, WA, USA*

Key Points

- Numerous differences exist in ocular anatomy and physiology in humans compared with veterinary species and even among different veterinary species.
- Ophthalmic diseases common in both humans and companion animals include glaucoma, conjunctivitis, cataracts, trauma to the eye, blepharitis, and uveitis.

- Veterinary patients can experience severe local and systemic adverse drug reactions after topical (ophthalmic) drug administration.
- Cats are particularly susceptible to fluoroquinolone-induced acute retinal degeneration and blindness.

19.1 Comparative Aspects of Ophthalmic Disease

Veterinary species suffer from many of the same ophthalmic conditions that people do (conjunctivitis, glaucoma, corneal ulcers, anterior uveitis, and cataracts), but because of species differences, there are some aspects of these conditions that are unique to animals. There are also some diseases that are unique to particular veterinary species and even breeds. The anatomy and physiology of the eye and visual system vary tremendously between species. This is not surprising when one considers how individual species have evolved. Is the animal prey or a predator? Nocturnal or diurnal? The eye has adapted to the evolutionary needs of the animal, resulting in some interesting species differences

(pupil shape, the presence and extent of *tapeta lucida*, and even the position of the eyes on the head). Predators tend to have eyes that face forward on the skull for binocular vision that allows them to focus on their prey. The eyes of prey animals tend to be located laterally, one on each side of the skull, for an extremely wide visual field (>180°) allowing them to spot predators without having to turn their heads. Many animals have better night vision than people do. The *tapetum lucidum* is a reflective layer of tissue that reflects light back through the retina and greatly enhances night vision. Humans lack a *tapetum lucidum*. Pupil shape is thought to be another adaptation to night vision. For example, animals that have vertical slit pupils in bright light (e.g. cats and foxes) can change the surface area of their pupil by a factor of

>100, while animals with circular pupils (e.g. dogs and humans) can change the surface area of their pupil by a factor of 15. Avian species have circular pupils, but the constrictor and dilator muscles are composed primarily of striated rather than smooth muscle as found in mammalian species. From a pharmacological standpoint, this means that the traditional agents used to dilate the pupil for ophthalmic examinations are not effective for avian species. The information presented in this chapter represents only a fraction of the array of fascinating differences in ophthalmic physiology (and by extent pharmacology) between species.

Most domestic animal species have three eyelids – the superior and inferior lids, like humans, and the nictitans (called the nictitating membrane or third eyelid) as well (Figure 19.1). The nictitating membrane, which moves medial to lateral (perpendicularly to the upper and lower lids), helps protect the conjunctiva and cornea. Birds actually "blink" with their third eyelids. The third eyelid contains additional glands that are not present in people. The lacrimal gland of the third eyelid contributes about 25–35% of the aqueous tear film in animals. Prolapse of the third eyelid (called "cherry eye") can occur in dogs, and occasionally cats, and causes inflammation of the glands of the third eyelid. If the prolapsed is not surgically

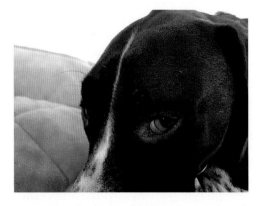

Figure 19.1 The third eyelid (nicitating membrane) in a German Shorthair Pointer. *Source:* Photo courtesy of Dr. Katrina Mealey, Washington State University.

corrected, chronic conjunctivitis and ocular discharge occur. Blepharitis, or inflammation of the eyelids, can have similar etiologies in companion animals and humans (allergies, infectious agents, immune-mediated, and glandular abnormalities).

The most common causes of disease affecting the cornea and conjunctiva in both humans and domestic species include trauma, infection (viral, bacterial, fungal, and parasitic), allergy, and defective tear composition or production. The latter can be drug-induced. The most common cause of feline conjunctivitis and keratitis is feline herpesvirus type 1 (Stiles 2014), while the most common cause of canine conjunctivitis is keratoconjunctivitis sicca, also called KCS or dry eye (Williams 2008). While advanced disease may require surgical intervention, pharmacological treatment is almost always indicated in the form of topical ophthalmic formulations. With few exceptions, most drugs used to treat corneal/conjunctival disease in companion animals are human formulations that are used in an extra-label manner. KCS is seen frequently enough in dogs that a US Food and Drug Administration (FDA)-approved drug (0.2% cyclosporine ophthalmic ointment) is commercially available specifically indicated for management of KCS in dogs.

Canine corneal diseases that are relatively common in dogs but less so in humans include endothelial dystrophy (similar to Fuchs dystrophy in humans) and chronic superficial keratitis (pannus). Endothelial dystrophy is commonly seen in middle-aged to older dogs, especially Boston Terriers and Chihuahuas. The pathogenesis involves failure of the endothelial Na/K pump, resulting in endothelial cell death and progressive corneal edema. Chronic superficial keratitis is a progressive and potentially blinding disease seen most frequently in German Shepherd dogs, other herding breeds, and Greyhounds. The cornea becomes progressively covered with blood vessels, inflammatory cell infiltrate, and pigmentation (Figure 19.2), interfering with vision. Dogs living at higher

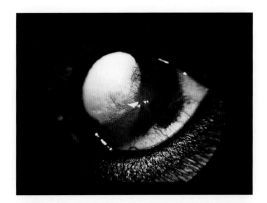

Figure 19.2 "Pannus" or chronic superficial keratitis in a dog. Vascularization and pigmentation invade the cornea in a progressive manner that, in severe cases, can cause blindness. *Source:* Photo courtesy of Dr. T Alessio, Washington State University.

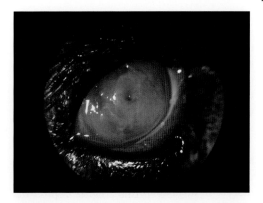

Figure 19.3 Melting ulcer in a dog. Melting ulcers can be a complication of bacterial keratitis. *Source:* Photo courtesy of Dr. T Alessio, Washington State University.

altitudes (>4000 ft. above sea level) are more likely to be affected. Exposure to sunlight exacerbates the disease, so owners are encouraged to walk their dogs before sunrise or after sunset or use ultraviolet (UV)-protective eyewear such as "doggles" or "Rex specs" (sunglasses for dogs). Although ingrowth of blood vessels along the cornea can occur in people, the etiology is different: The most common cause of corneal pannus in humans is ill-fitting contact lenses.

Corneal ulceration can be seen in dogs, cats, horses, and other veterinary species. A corneal ulcer is defined as a break in the corneal epithelium that exposes corneal stroma. Corneal ulcers can be caused by trauma, infection, KCS, and other factors. Infectious causes of ulcerative keratitis are common in the cat (feline herpes virus type 1) and horse (equine herpes virus), but less common in the dog. Complicated corneal ulcers are those that have not healed within 72 hours, have a mechanical obstruction to healing such as a foreign body, are infected, or have an excessive collagenase component (also known as a melting ulcer; Figure 19.3). During the normal healing process of the cornea, proteases and collagenases remove devitalized cells and debris. However, in some patients, excessive proteases and collagenases are produced, resulting in excessive

breakdown (melting) or the corneal stroma (Gelatt 2014a). Because inpatient treatment is essential for animals with complicated corneal ulcers, pharmacists are not likely to dispense collagenase inhibitors, the drugs typically used to treat melting ulcers. However, pharmacists might receive prescriptions for ethylenediaminetetraacetic acid (EDTA), acetylcysteine, and doxycycline for at-home treatment of melting ulcers after the animal has received acute treatment.

Aqueous humor formation, aqueous outflow, and intraocular pressure (IOP) vary somewhat between species. For example, normal IOP in horses can range from 17 to 28 mmHg, while that in humans is 12–22 mmHg, and that of cats and dogs is somewhat lower (approximately 10–20 mmHg). Similar to humans, glaucoma can threaten vision in domestic animal species. It can be primary (i.e. inherited) or secondary to disease, drugs, or trauma. While the overall prevalence of glaucoma in humans and dogs is similar (1–2%), the type of glaucoma most likely to affect these species is different. In North America, primary open-angle glaucoma is the most frequent type of glaucoma in humans, while in dogs primary narrow (closed) angle glaucoma is more prevalent (Gelatt 2014b). Glaucoma occurs less frequently in cats and horses, and tends to be secondary rather than primary.

Pharmacological therapy for primary open-angle glaucoma is generally more rewarding than for closed-angle glaucoma in both humans and companion animals. Because glaucoma in humans is much more responsive to medical and surgical treatments than it is in veterinary patients, therapeutic outcomes in veterinary patients are often less successful.

Some diseases of the lens and retina are similar between humans and domestic species. Cataracts are a common ophthalmic disease in dogs and often lead to vision loss. The most common cause of cataracts in dogs is diabetes mellitus.

Dramatic difference

Dogs are highly susceptible to diabetic cataracts because of the presence of aldose reductase within the lens. Aldose reductase converts glucose to sorbitol, which is osmotically active, altering the hydration status of lens fibers. Relative to adults of other species (humans and cats), dogs have much higher concentrations of aldose reductase. There are currently no drugs available for treating cataracts; however, surgical treatment is an option for dogs. Aldose reductase inhibitors may be commercially available in the future.

Diseases of the uvea (iris, choroid, and ciliary body) can be primary or secondary in both humans and companion animals. Uveitis is common and can be associated with many ocular diseases as well as systemic disease (infection, autoimmune, and neoplasia) (Gelatt 2014d). Ocular disorders that can cause uveitis include disruption of the lens (subluxation/luxation, cataract, and lens capsule rupture), glaucoma, ocular neoplasia, retinal detachment, intraocular hemorrhage, and genetic diseases that tend to be breed-specific (e.g. cystic uveitis/glaucoma in American Bulldogs). To avoid secondary ocular complications of uveitis, topical anti-inflammatory treatment is initiated, even in patients with systemic disease. For severe uveitis, systemic anti-inflammatory therapy may be needed.

One key characteristic of many ocular diseases is pain. If a condition is known to cause eye pain in humans, it should be assumed that it is causing pain in animals as well. Analgesia, either local or systemic, should be a component of treatment for ocular diseases that are painful in humans. Animals with eye pain may keep their eyes closed, exhibit photophobia, paw or rub their eye, rub their face, or simply withdraw from their usual activities (playing, socializing, and eating). Pharmacists can help educate owners to monitor eye pain to assess treatment efficacy.

19.1.1 Drug-Induced Ophthalmic Disease

A surprising number of drugs can cause severe adverse reactions that involve the eye, ranging from transient irritation to permanent blindness. Adverse drug reactions involving the eye are not limited to drugs that are administered directly to the eye – even drugs that are administered orally or by injection can cause ocular toxicity. Since veterinary patients are unable to convey their experiences to owners or veterinarians, drug-induced visual disturbances are often identified at a more advanced stage than in human patients. The pharmacist can improve detection of ocular adverse drug reactions in veterinary patients by helping pet owners proactively monitor their animal.

19.1.1.1 Fluoroquinolones

One of the most devastating adverse drug reactions involving the eye is fluoroquinolone-induced retinal degeneration in cats (Weibe and Hamilton 2002). Compared to other species, all cats have a deficiency in the blood–retina barrier, allowing fluoroquinolones to accumulate within the retina (Ramirez et al. 2011). When exposed to UV light, fluoroquinolones generate reactive oxygen species that damage sensitive retinal tissue, causing acute, irreversible retinal degeneration and blindness (Figure 4.3; see Chapter 4 for additional information). Fluoroquinolone-induced retinal degeneration has been reported with several different fluoroquinolones administered orally and parenterally. Cats that have delayed clearance (i.e. impaired renal function) or that receive high doses are more likely to develop retinal degeneration. Recently, the FDA reported that human patients treated with a compounded ocular product containing the fluoroquinolone moxifloxacin developed retinal degeneration (see https://www.fda.gov/Drugs/DrugSafety/ucm569114.htm). Because this compounded product was administered by intravitreal injection, the blood–retina barrier was bypassed, resulting in high concentrations of moxifloxacin.

19.1.1.2 Ivermectin

Ivermectin is a macrocyclic lactone anthelmintic (antiparasitic) used in dogs, cats, and livestock (Chapter 7). It is available commercially in several heartworm preventive products for dogs and cats at an ultra-low dose (6 micrograms per kg per month) that is quite safe. There are also commercially available products for livestock that are highly concentrated (10 000 microgram/mL). These products are sometimes obtained by kennel owners or breeders in an effort to treat their dogs "on the cheap." Obviously, the average owner would not be able to deliver an appropriate dose of ivermectin to a dog or cat using the livestock product (one would need a calibrated pipette or perhaps volumetric flasks to perform serial dilutions!). Accidental exposures to large-animal formulations of ivermectin also occur when horses are treated with an oral paste formulation and dogs or cats consume the medication that drips out of the horse's mouth. Consequently, dogs and cats can receive tremendous overdoses of ivermectin; and one of the complications, in addition to neurologic signs, is reversible central blindness that may be accompanied by reversible retinal changes (Kenny et al. 2008). Owners may notice dilated pupils and the animal's inability to navigate its environment. Approximately 1% of dogs and 4% of cats have a defective blood–brain barrier due to polymorphisms in the ABCB1 (MDR1) gene (see Chapter 5 for additional information). Dogs and cats with these defects develop signs of ivermectin toxicity at much lower doses (50–100-fold lower) than dogs or cats without ABCB1 polymorphisms.

19.1.1.3 Griseofulvin

Grisefulvin is FDA approved for treating dermatophytosis (ring worm) in dogs, cats, and horses. It is a teratogen in many species, but has been documented to cause ocular anomalies in cats (Gelatt 2014c) and horses (Schutte and van den Ingh 1997), particularly if used in early pregnancy. The gestation period of cats is 60–70 days, while that of horses is approximately 340 days. Severe microphthalmia, cyclopia, anophthalmia, and other ocular anomalies have been described in both species as a teratogenic consequence of griseofulvin treatment during pregnancy.

19.1.1.4 Drug-Induced Keratoconjunctivitis Sicca

Dogs appear to be more likely to develop drug-induced tear deficiency that results in KCS than other species. While sulfonamides are the drug class most likely to be associated with KCS, other drugs have been documented to cause it as well. The mechanism responsible for sulfonamide-associated KCS is not completely understood but is thought to involve an immune response to proteins haptenated by sulfonamide metabolites. Table 19.1 lists the drugs that have been associated with KCS in dogs (primarily) but also lists drugs that can decrease tear production in other species. Dogs that require sulfonamide treatment, particularly high-dose sulfonamides as indicated for treating *Nocardia* infections, should receive a baseline Schirmer tear test and follow-up Schirmer tear tests two to three times weekly. If tear production decreases, the sulfonamide should be discontinued and an alternative drug substituted for the sulfonamide.

19.2 Diagnostic Testing

A thorough history and general physical examination can provide important information to help diagnose ophthalmic disease. Since veterinary patients are unable to

Table 19.1 Drugs that decrease tear production after topical or systemic use.

Drug class	Examples	Onset	Topical or systemic
Sulfonamides[a]	Sulfamethoxazole, Sulfadiazine, Sulfasalazine,	Days to weeks, but can be permanent if drug is not discontinued	Systemic
NSAIDs[a]	Etodolac	Days to weeks	Systemic
Anesthetics	Topical and general: isoflurane, opioids, ketamine, acepromazine, α_2-drenergic agonists	Immediate	Both
Anticholinergics	Atropine	Immediate but can last for days to weeks	Both
Phenazopyridine[a]		Days to weeks	Systemic

Note: Some drug classes cause short-term decreases in tear production, but other drug classes can cause permanent decreases in tear production.
[a] Documented to decrease tear production in some dogs but not in other species (Bryan and Slatter 1973; Morgan and Bachrach 1982; Arnett et al. 1984; Hollingsworth et al. 1992; Dodam et al. 1998; Sanchez et al. 2006; Klauss et al. 2007; Meredith et al. 2011).

describe disturbances in visual acuity or the presence of eye pain, the veterinary patient often has more advanced disease than human patients at the time of diagnosis. The ophthalmic examination for a veterinary patient incorporates many of the same diagnostic tests as those performed for a human patient, but often the veterinary patient must be restrained or sedated. General veterinary practitioners are capable of performing many aspects of an ophthalmic examination, but specialized equipment may be available only at practices with a boarded veterinary ophthalmologist.

- Schirmer tear test
- Neurologic/ophthalmic assessment (pupillary light responses, corneal reflex, etc.)
- Tonometry
- Gonioscopy
- Ophthalmoscopy of posterior segment and slit-lamp biomicroscopy of anterior segment
- High-resolution ultrasonography
- Anterior segment optical coherence tomography (very limited availability)
- Culture and cytology of cornea/conjunctiva
- Fluorescein staining to identify corneal lesions, particularly ulceration
- Electroretinography

- Aqueous or vitreous paracentesis primary
- Biopsy.

19.3 Pharmacological Treatment of Common Eye Diseases

19.3.1 Glaucoma

The goal of pharmacological treatment of glaucoma is to sufficiently lower IOP to a level that substantially decreases the risk of optic nerve damage. Emergency treatment is not likely to involve drugs dispensed from a retail pharmacy, but outpatient management certainly will. Since there are no veterinary-approved drugs for treating glaucoma, veterinarians use human drugs in an extra-label manner. Thus, the pharmacist should be familiar with these agents. Carbonic anhydrase inhibitors, beta adrenergic receptor antagonists (β blockers), and prostaglandins are the most frequently prescribed pharmacological agents used to control IOP in veterinary patients (dogs, cats, and horses) with primary glaucoma. There is evidence that combining a carbonic anhydrase inhibitor with a β blocker is superior to monotherapy in glaucomatous dogs (Plummer et al. 2006). Long-term medical management of primary glaucoma in veterinary patients is generally less successful than for human patients, primarily because the disease is more advanced (more vision is lost) at diagnosis. Primary glaucoma in the cat and horse are usually associated with senile changes. Secondary glaucoma is a common sequelae to uveitis, which can result from disorders of the lens, systemic immune-mediated disease, neoplasia, and so on. There is a key difference between treatment for primary glaucoma compared to treatment of glaucoma secondary to uveitis. Prostaglandins (e.g. latanoprost) can actually increase IOP in patients with glaucoma caused by uveitis or anterior lens luxation. In these situations, prostaglandins are contraindicated. Thus, it is important for the pharmacist to ensure that the dog has had a thorough ophthalmic examination by a veterinary ophthalmologist to rule out uveitis or anterior lens displacement prior to dispensing prostaglandins.

Dramatic difference

Prostaglandins (e.g. latanoprost) are not as effective for decreasing IOP in cats in the long term potentially, because the feline iris lacks prostaglandin $F_2\alpha$ receptors relative to other species.

Miotics (parasympathomimetic agents) are sometimes prescribed to treat glaucoma in humans, dogs, cats, and horses. For veterinary species, miotics (e.g. a sterile compounded demecarium solution) are used in the healthy eye when primary glaucoma has been diagnosed in the opposite eye in order to delay the development of glaucoma in the unaffected eye. See the "Adverse Drug Effects" section later in this chapter for a discussion on veterinary-specific adverse reactions that can occur with ophthalmic pilocarpine.

19.3.1.1 Drugs Most Likely to Be Prescribed for Glaucoma

Timolol: 0.25 or 0.5% ophthalmic solution (1 drop every 12 hours). Used for primary or secondary glaucoma in dogs, cats, and horses. Systemic bioavailability of ophthalmically applied timolol can result in systemic effects, particularly for cats and small dogs. See the "Adverse Drug Effects" section later in this chapter for contraindications and patient (owner) counseling information for pharmacists.

Topical carbonic anhydrase inhibitors: Brinzolamide 1% or dorzolamide 2% ophthalmic suspensions – 1 drop every 6–12 hours. Used for primary or secondary glaucoma in dogs, cats, and horses.

Systemic carbonic anhydrase inhibitors: Methazolamide tablets: Dogs: 2–3 mg/kg PO every 8–12 hours.

Topical prostaglandin: Latanoprost 0.005% ophthalmic solution: Dogs: 1 drop every 12–24 hours. Contraindicated if anterior lens luxation or uveitis is present.

19.3.2 Conjunctivitis

Treatment of conjunctivitis depends on the underlying cause, which can vary depending on the species. In dogs, conjunctivitis is most commonly caused by KCS, environmental irritants, and allergies. Primary bacterial infections are not a common cause of conjunctivitis in dogs, but bacterial infections are often a secondary complication that may require treatment. However, treatment for KCS should be specific. KCS in dogs (Figure 19.4) is most commonly an immune-mediated

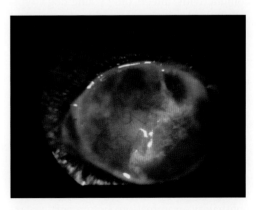

Figure 19.4 Severe keratoconjunctivitis sicca (KCS) in a dog. Note the heavy mucoid discharge that obscures the eye. *Source:* Photo courtesy of Dr. T Alessio, Washington State University.

Table 19.2 Drugs that are FDA approved for ocular disease in a veterinary species.

Brand name	Active ingredient(s)	Drug class	Rationale/notes
Optimmune®	Cyclosporine 0.2%	Immunosuppressant	Ophthalmic ointment indicated for management of chronic KCS in dogs

disease; therefore, treatment with an ophthalmic immunosuppressant is indicated. An FDA-approved ophthalmic formulation containing cyclosporine is commercially available and is specifically indicated for treating canine KCS (Table 19.2). It generally takes several weeks before tear production increases; therefore, tear substitutes can be used to provide lubrication and improve comfort. Military or police working dogs can be exposed to environmental irritants, such as smoke, particulate matter, and toxic chemical fumes. Conjunctival irrigation as soon as possible after exposure is indicated. Dogs with allergic conjunctivitis are often the same dogs that experience atopic dermatitis (Chapter 18). Symptomatic treatment with ophthalmic corticosteroid drops on a short-term basis can help relieve clinical signs when exposure to the allergen is unavoidable. Corneal ulcers must be ruled out before treating with corticosteroids, as discussed in this chapter (see Section 19.1.1, "Drug-Induced Ophthalmic Disease"). Alternatively, mast cell stabilizers such as ketotifen may be helpful.

A specific form of conjunctivitis, follicular conjunctivitis, affects only young dogs, typically less than two years old. Conjunctival hyperemia with variable degrees of discomfort and ocular discharge present bilaterally. The characteristic feature of the disease is lymphoid hyperplasia on the bulbar aspect of the third eyelid (Figure 19.5). Clinical signs resolve with ophthalmic corticosteroids. Dogs generally "outgrow" this condition by 18–24 months of age. In some cases, the hyperplastic follicles are rough enough to cause corneal ulceration. This must be ruled out (negative fluorescein staining during ophthalmic examination) before corticosteroid treatment is initiated. If corneal ulcers are identified, topical ketotifen (mast cell

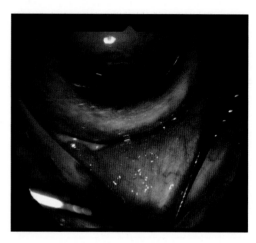

Figure 19.5 Follicular conjunctivitis in a young dog. Note the typical "cobblestone" appearance of the conjunctiva (arrow). *Source:* Photo courtesy of Dr. T Alessio, Washington State University.

stabilizer) and/or cyclosporine (Optimmune®) may be tried instead.

Conjunctivitis in cats is usually infectious in nature, with feline herpes virus type 1 (FHV1), *Chlamydia felis, Calici virus*, mycoplasma, and *Bartonella* being the most common pathogens. Occasionally, a parasitic organism (cuterebra) can cause conjunctivitis in cats. Herpes conjunctivitis is probably the most common eye disease in cats, particularly in shelters and catteries. Conjunctivitis in cats can be severe, of long duration, and quite painful. It may consist of chemosis (conjunctival edema; Figure 19.6), blepharospasm, ocular discharge, and, in severe cases, conjunctival ulceration. Many cats will be anorexic and listless. Once a cat is infected with FHV, it becomes a latent carrier, and the disease can recur. In many instances, a stressor (systemic illness, trauma, environmental change, or ocular or systemic corticosteroid treatment) may precipitate

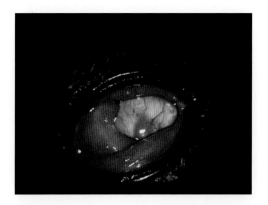

Figure 19.6 Severe conjunctivitis and keratitis in a cat caused by feline herpes virus type 1 (FHV1). *Source:* Photo courtesy of Dr. T Alessio, Washington State University.

recrudescence of latent virus. Because corticosteroids are almost uniformly contraindicated for infectious diseases of the eye, the pharmacist should question a prescription for ophthalmic corticosteroids in a feline patient. For cats with conjunctivitis caused by *C. felis*, mycoplasma, or *Bartonella*, ophthalmic erythromycin or oxytetracycline ophthalmic ointment (Terramycin˚) is most likely to be effective.

Conjunctivitis in horses can be caused by environmental irritants (e.g. dusty stalls). However, an unusual cause, at least from the perspective of human medicine, is parasites. Nematode parasites such as *Thelazia*, *Habronema*, and *Onchocerca* are common causes of conjunctivitis in horses. These should be treated with systemic anthelmintics specific for the parasite (Chapter 7).

19.3.2.1 Drugs Most Likely to Be Prescribed for Conjunctivitis

Cyclosporine 0.2% ophthalmic ointment (Optimmune): FDA approved for treating KCS in dogs. Excessive mucus should be cleared with gentle irrigation with suitable nonirritating solutions. A 1/8 in. strip of ointment should be applied to the affected eye(s) every 12 hours. The ointment may be placed directly on the cornea or into the conjunctival sac.

Artificial tears or natural tear replacement solutions: Indicated for all KCS patients. Use is similar to that in human patients.

Ophthalmic antibiotic solutions and ointments: Indicated for secondary bacterial infections. Use is similar to that in human patients.

Ophthalmic corticosteroids (prednisolone acetate 1% or dexamethasone 0.1%): Indicated for follicular conjunctivitis. One drop in each eye every eight hours initially, then tapered to the lowest dosing frequency that controls clinical signs.

19.3.3 Corneal Diseases

Although it has been stated multiple times in this chapter, it bears repeating that the presence of corneal ulcers is a contraindication to the use of ophthalmic corticosteroids. Corticosteroids not only delay wound healing by their actions on fibroblasts and epithelial cells, but, by enhancing the lytic activity of corneal collagenase, corticosteroids can actually promote stromal melting and corneal perforation. Similarly, the fact that corneal ulcers are painful cannot be overstated. Analgesia should be a part of the treatment plan for all veterinary patients with corneal ulcers. The cornea itself is richly innervated, making it exquisitely sensitive. In addition, disorders that affect the cornea can also cause pain by causing ciliary muscle spasm. Painful ciliary spasms are intensified in bright light. Atropine (classified as a cycloplegic) is used to prevent ciliary spasm in patients with corneal ulcers. Thus, atropine indirectly provides analgesia. Atropine is contraindicated in several ophthalmic diseases and can cause numerous species-specific adverse effects (see the "Adverse Drug Effects" section later in this chapter). Additional analgesia should be provided to address corneal pain and may be provided topically (compounded morphine 0.5% solution) or systemically (opioids are preferred since nonsteroidal anti-inflammatory drugs [NSAIDs] can delay healing).

Superficial uncomplicated corneal ulcers are treated with topical antibiotics to prevent infection. For dogs and horses, triple-antibiotic ophthalmic ointment (neomycin, polymyxin, and bacitractin) is a frequent choice, while oxytetratcycline or erythromycin is more frequently used for cats.

Feline herpes keratitis is treated with a multitude of drugs, with the most common denominator being topical (ophthalmic) antivirals. The pharmacist is likely to see prescriptions for trifluridine (FDA-approved human product) or requests to compound idoxuridine and cidoflovir as ophthalmic drops. Obviously, these must be compounded in appropriate sterile facilities.

19.3.3.1 Drugs Most Likely to Be Prescribed for Feline Herpes Keratitis

Trifluoridine 1% ophthalmic solution: One drop in each eye every four hours.

Famcyclovir: 15 mg/kg PO every eight hours (do not substitute acyclovir – it is toxic to cats).

Ophthalmic antibiotic solutions and ointments: Indicated for secondary bacterial infections. Use is similar to that in human patients, but for feline pathogens, ophthalmic erythromycin or oxytetracycline ophthalmic ointment (Terramycin) is most likely to be effective.

Atropine 1% ophthalmic ointment: For prevention of pain caused by ciliary spasm. Ointment is preferred to drops in cats. Drainage of the solution (drops) through the nasolacrimal duct can cause profuse salivation and foaming at the mouth.

Systemic and topical analgesics: Compounded morphine 0.5% ophthalmic solution. See Chapter 8 for systemic analgesics for cats.

L-*lysine:* See the "Nutritional Supplements for Ophthalmic Disease" section later in this chapter.

19.3.3.2 Drugs Most Likely to Be Prescribed for Chronic Superficial Keratitis (Pannus)

Cyclosporine 0.2% ophthalmic ointment (Optimmune): A 1/4 in. strip of ointment should be applied to the affected eye(s) every 12 hours. The ointment may be placed directly on the cornea or into the conjunctival sac.

Neomyin, polymixin, dexamethasone ophthalmic drops, or ointment: One drop in each eye every eight hours, then tapered to the least frequent dose that controls vessel growth and inflammatory cell infiltrate. Contraindicated if a corneal ulcer is present.

19.3.3.3 Drugs Most Likely to Be Prescribed for Corneal Edema (Dogs with Endothelial Dystrophy and Some Patients with Corneal Ulcers)

NaCl 5% ophthalmic ointment: Optimally, this is applied three to four times per day if the owner's schedule permits. Treatment with hyperosmotic medications (5% NaCl ointment) will dehydrate the epithelial surface but is considered palliative for dogs with endothelial dystrophy. Although a 5% NaCl ophthalmic solution is available, it is highly irritating and should not be substituted for the ointment.

19.3.4 Uveitis

Reducing inflammation is the therapeutic objective for treating uveitis in dogs, cats, and horses. Topical anti-inflammatory therapy is often sufficient for mild anterior uveitis, but systemic treatment is indicated for posterior uveitis, moderate and severe anterior uveitis, and uveitis due to systemic disease (in conjunction with treatment for the underlying disease). Topical corticosteroids that penetrate the cornea are prednisolone acetate and dexamethasone. In cats, or in patients with corneal ulcers or ocular infections, topical NSAIDs should be used instead of corticosteroids. However, NSAIDs are contraindicated in patients with active hemorrhage associated with uveitis because of their antiplatelet effect. Information regarding systemic anti-inflammatory drug therapy with corticosteroids and NSAIDs can be found in Chapters 8 and 14, respectively.

Mydriatics/cycloplegics (i.e. atropine) are used to decrease ocular pain associated with ciliary spasm as well as to decrease complications (synechia) associated with protracted pupillary constriction that can occur in patients with uveitis. However, these are contraindicated in patients with elevated IOP.

Information regarding systemic analgesic therapy can be found in Chapter 8.

19.3.4.1   Drugs Most Likely to Be Prescribed for Uveitis

Atropine 1% ophthalmic drops or ointment: For prevention of pain caused by ciliary spasm. Ointment is preferred to drops in cats due to excessive salivation caused by bitter taste; drops can be used for dogs and horses (see the "Adverse Drug Effects" section for feline-specific and equine-specific adverse drug reactions related to atropine).

Dramatic difference
The duration of mydriasis after topical application of atropine is 5–7 days for dogs, 3–5 days for cats, and 14 days for horses. Inflammation interferes with efficacy, so atropine is usually dosed once daily or to effect in patients with uveitis.

Ophthalmic corticosteroids (prednisolone acetate 1% suspension or dexamethasone 0.1% ointment): One drop or 1/8 in. strip in affected eye(s) every eight hours initially, then tapered to the lowest dosing frequency that controls clinical signs.

NSAID ophthalmic drops: NSAIDs are not contraindicated in patients with corneal ulceration or infectious disease. They are preferred to corticosteroids for uveitis in cats because NSAIDs will not activate latent herpes virus. NSAIDs are contraindicated in patients with active hemorrhage associated with uveitis, as they can interfere with clotting, thereby worsening hemorrhage.

1) *Flurbiprofen 0.03% ophthalmic solution:* Doses can range from one drop in affected eye once daily to every four hours based on severity of uveitis.
2) *Diclofenac 0.1% ophthalmic solution:* Doses can range from one drop in affected eye once daily to every four hours based on severity of uveitis.
3) *Ketorolac 0.5% ophthalmic solution:* Doses can range from one drop in affected

eye once daily to every four hours based on severity of uveitis. Can cause conjunctival irritation/inflammation, so other NSAIDs are preferred.

19.4   Adverse Drug Effects in Veterinary Species

Unless otherwise noted, the pharmacist should assume that adverse drug effects seen in human patients are also possible in veterinary patients. However, this section of the chapter will focus primarily on adverse drug effects that are unique to veterinary species or are more likely to affect veterinary patients as compared to human patients.

19.4.1   Systemic Absorption of Topically Administered Drugs

Systemic absorption of drugs administered topically to the eye, particularly in the form of drops, can result in systemic adverse drug effects. The volume of medication delivered by most ophthalmic dropper bottles greatly exceeds the volume of fluid that can be retained on the ocular surface, so excess fluid drains into the nasolacrimal system, where it can be absorbed systemically via the rich capillary system. Drugs absorbed through nasolacrimal mucosa do not undergo first-pass hepatic metabolism. Because most dogs and all cats weigh substantially less than adult humans, this route of administration can result in pharmacologic concentrations of drug in the systemic circulation. In particular, the pharmacist should assume that topical beta adrenergic antagonists and NSAIDs will be absorbed in sufficient quantities to achieve pharmacological concentrations if administered to cats and small dogs. See the remainder of this chapter for details regarding contraindications to individual drug classes.

Even large animals can experience systemic adverse effects after ocular drug administration. Horses can develop ileus (intestinal stasis) after atropine drops (or ointment) are administered due to systemic anticholinergic effects. Because the equine gastrointestinal tract is exquisitely sensitive to peristaltic disruption, atropine can cause severe, potentially fatal, colic in horses.

Drops versus ointment: Drugs administered topically to the eye can also reach the nasopharynx by way of the nasolacrimal system, where the drug can stimulate chemoreceptors (taste buds). Cats are particularly sensitive to unpleasant tastes and will salivate profusely if their taste buds are confronted with a noxious taste. This may cause anorexia and treatment aversion in a species that is notoriously difficult to treat to begin with. For this reason, ophthalmic ointments are often preferred to ophthalmic drops for cats. Atropine appears to be particularly distasteful to cats.

19.4.2 Topical Ophthalmic Drugs and Visual Disturbances

Most topical ocular drugs have the potential to interfere with vision (blurred vision, photophobia, double vision, etc.). Because animals are unable to communicate this, owners must be counseled to monitor their pet while it is receiving ocular drug therapy, so that the animal does not injure itself. Stairways, ledges, swimming pools, and even furniture present potential hazards for an animal with impaired vision.

19.4.3 Topical Corticosteroids

Veterinary species may be more susceptible to adverse effects associated with topical corticosteroid use. Susceptibility to infection is one major complication that can occur, with corticosteroids capable of activating or exacerbating viral, bacterial, or fungal ocular infections. Corticosteroid use is a contributing factor in the majority of cases of fungal keratitis in horses and has been documented to cause FHV1-associated keratitis in cats. Topical corticosteroids should be avoided in veterinary patients if infection has been ruled out. Another contraindication to topical corticosteroids in veterinary patients is the presence of a corneal ulcer due to the risk of corneal perforation. It is important for the pharmacist to be aware of these risks when dispensing topical corticosteroids for veterinary patients, particularly if the prescribing veterinarian is not a boarded veterinary ophthalmologist.

19.4.4 Topical Carbonic Anhydrase Inhibitors

Dogs have been reported to develop an immune-mediated keratitis that is not responsive to corticosteroids. Fortunately, it is rapidly responsive to drug cessation (Beckwith-Cohen et al. 2015). Hypersensitivity can be seen with dorzolamide.

19.4.5 Topical Prostaglandins

Ocular prostaglandins cause severe pain that is presumed to be caused by miosis. Cats and horses seem to be more susceptible than dogs or humans. This may be a result of physiologic differences since cats and horses have vertical and ovoid pupils, respectively, while dogs and humans have circular pupils. Miosis in the former species results in a greater surface area change than the latter species. In horses, pain associated with topical prostaglandin administration has been shown to be mitigated with concurrent topical administration of diclofenac, apparently without affecting efficacy (Tofflemire et al. 2017). Uveitis must be ruled out before administering latanoprost, since prostaglandins can actually exacerbate uveitis.

19.4.6 Topical Beta Adrenergic Antagonists

The nonselective beta adrenergic antagonist timolol (which has oral bioavailability of only 50%) can cause life-threatening bronchoconstriction in asthmatic cats because it is systemically absorbed through the nasolacrimal system. It should also be avoided in animals with cardiac diseases that would be adversely impacted by negative inotropic or chronotropic effects. Even in apparently healthy animals, if a dog or cat weighs less than 20 pounds, the lower strength formulation of timolol should be used (0.25% instead of 0.5%).

19.4.7 Topical NSAIDs

Ophthalmic NSAIDs should be used cautiously in cats with renal compromise, hypovolemia, or hypotension. Cats seem to be exquisitely sensitive to NSAID-induced renal toxicity, particularly in states of low renal perfusion. Topically, diclofenac can cause keratitis and blepharitis.

19.5 Nutritional Supplements for Veterinary Ophthalmic Diseases

The amino acid L-lysine may be recommended for treating feline herpes conjunctivitis or keratitis. In cell culture studies, L-lysine at concentrations of 200–300 micrograms per mL decreased FHV1 numbers relative to controls. *In vivo* studies with orally administered L-lysine at 500 mg per cat twice daily have shown inconsistent results. Even when L-lysine was administered six hours prior to inoculation of experimental cats with FHV1, clinical signs were decreased but not abolished.

19.6 FDA-Approved Veterinary Drug Products for Ophthalmic Diseases

See Table 19.2.

References

Arnett, B.D., Brightman, A.H., and Musselman, E.E. (1984). Effect of atropine sulfate on tear production in the cat when used with ketamine hydrochloride and acetylpromazine maleate. *J. Am. Vet. Med. Assoc.* 185: 214–215.

Beckwith-Cohen, B., Bentley, E., Gasper, D.J. et al. (2015). Keratitis in six dogs after topical treatment with carbonic anhydrase inhibitors for glaucoma. *J. Am. Vet. Med. Assoc.* 247 (12): 1419–1426.

Bryan, G.M. and Slatter, D.H. (1973). Keratoconjunctivitis sicca induced by phenazopyridinein dogs. *Arch. Ophthalmol.* 90 (4): 310–311.

Dodam, J.R., Branson, K.R., and Martin, D.D. (1998). Effects of intramuscular sedative and opioid combinations on tear production in dogs. *Vet. Ophthalmol.* 1: 57–59.

Gelatt, K.N. (2014a). Canine cornea: diseases and surgery. In: *Essentials of Veterinary Ophthalmology*, 3e (ed. K.N. Gelatt), 216–248. Ames, IA: Wiley Blackwell.

Gelatt, K.N. (2014b). Canine glaucomas. In: *Essentials of Veterinary Ophthalmology*, 3e (ed. K.N. Gelatt), 249–275. Ames, IA: Wiley Blackwell.

Gelatt, K.N. (2014c). Feline ophthalmology. In: *Essentials of Veterinary Ophthalmology*, 3e (ed. K.N. Gelatt), 379–417. Ames, IA: Wiley Blackwell.

Gelatt, K.N. (2014d). Systemic disease and the eye. In: *Essentials of Veterinary Ophthalmology*, 3e (ed. K.N. Gelatt), 545–614. Ames, IA: Wiley Blackwell.

Hollingsworth, S.R., Canton, D.D., Buyuknichi, N.C. et al. (1992). Effect of topically administered atropine on tear production in dogs. *J. Am. Vet. Med. Assoc.* 200 (10): 1481–1484.

Kenny, P.J., Vernau, K.M., Puschner, B. et al. (2008). Retinopathy associated with ivermectin toxicosis in two dogs. *J. Am. Vet. Med. Assoc.* 233 (2): 279–284.

Klauss, G., Giuliano, E., Moore, C.P. et al. (2007). Keratoconjunctivitis sicca associated with administration of etodolac in dogs: 211 cases (1992–2002). *J. Am. Vet. Med. Assoc.* 230 (4): 541–547.

Meredith, M.C., Accola, P.J., Cremer, J. et al. (2011). Effects of acepromazine maleate or morphine on tear production before, during, and after sevoflurane anesthesia in dogs. *Am. J. Vet. Res.* 72 (11): 1427–1430.

Morgan, R.V. and Bachrach, A. (1982). Keratoconjunctivitis sicca associated with sulfonamide therapy in dogs. *J. Am. Vet. Med. Assoc.* 180: 432–434.

Plummer, C.E., MacKay, E.O., and Gelatt, K.N. (2006). Comparison of the effects of topical administration of a fixed combination of dorzolamide-timolol to monotherapy with timolol or dorzolamide alone on IOP, pupil size and heart rate in glaucomatous dogs. *Vet. Ophthalmol.* 9 (4): 245–249.

Ramirez, C.J., Minch, J.D., Gay, J.M. et al. (2011). Molecular genetic basis for fluoroquinolone-induced retinal degeneration in cats. *Pharmacogenet. Genomics* 21 (2): 66–75.

Sanchez, R.F., Mellor, D., and Mould, J. (2006). Effects of medetomidine and medetomidine-butorphanol combination on Schirmer tear test 1 readings in dogs. *Vet. Ophthalmol.* 9: 33–37.

Schutte, J.G. and van den Ingh, T.S. (1997). Microphthalmia, brachygnathia superior and palatocheiloschisis ina foal associated with griseofulvin administration to the mare during early pregnancy. *Vet. Q.* 19 (2): 58–61.

Stiles, J. (2014). Ocular manifestations of feline viral diseases. *Vet. J.* 201 (2): 166–173.

Tofflemire, K., Whitley, E.M., Allbaugh, R. et al. (2017). Effect of topical ophthalmic latanoprost 0.005% solution alone and in combination with diclofenac 0.1% solution in healthy horses: a pilot study. *Vet. Ophthalmol.* 20 (5): 398–404.

Weibe, V. and Hamilton, P. (2002). Fluoroquinolone-induced retinal degeneration in cats. *J. Am. Vet. Med. Assoc.* 221 (11): 1568–1571.

Williams, D.L. (2008). Immunopathogenesis of keratoconjunctivitis sicca in the dog. *Vet. Clin. North Am. Small Anim. Pract.* 38 (2): 233–249.

20

Pharmacotherapeutics of Cancer

Katrina R. Viviano

Department of Medical Sciences, School of Veterinary Medicine, University of Wisconsin, Madison, WI, USA

Key Points

- Many cancers that affect people can also affect dogs and/or cats.
- Despite the recent US Food and Drug Administration (FDA) approval of antineoplastic drugs/biologics for veterinary species, the majority of anticancer drugs in veterinary patients are human products used in an extra-label manner.
- Most chemotherapy is administered to veterinary patients by infusion at the veterinary hospital (not at home). Oral chemotherapeutic protocols for dogs and cats may involve metronomic chemotherapy or FDA-approved veterinary tyrosine kinase inhibitors.
- Adverse effects of chemotherapeutic drugs in veterinary patients have some similarities to those in people (e.g. bone marrow suppression; nausea and vomiting) but some differences as well (e.g. hair loss is not common in veterinary patients).
- Pharmacogenetic testing is recommended for dogs and cats in order to determine appropriate doses for some antineoplastic drugs.

20.1 Comparative Aspects of Cancer

The fields of human and comparative oncology have improved our understanding and treatment of cancer in dogs and cats (Withrow and Vail 2007). Many cancers in dogs and cats share important characteristics with cancers in people (i.e. tumor genetics, histopathology, and biological behavior) to the point that veterinary oncologists can use information regarding treatment targets to improve clinical outcome in veterinary patients (Paoloni and Khanna 2007). The converse is also true. Some types of spontaneous tumors in veterinary species serve as clinical trial models for cancers in people (Gordon et al. 2009). For example, tumors with comparative attributes between dogs and people include osteosarcoma, malignant melanoma, non-Hodgkin's lymphoma, leukemia, carcinomas (i.e. prostatic, mammary, lung, head and neck, and bladder), mast cell tumor (called mast cell sarcoma or histiocytic mastocytoma in humans), and soft tissue sarcomas (Paoloni and Khanna 2007). Feline tumors that serve as models for the corresponding neoplasias in people include feline cutaneous or oral squamous cell carcinoma (Figure 20.1) for cutaneous or head and neck cancer, feline mammary tumors for "triple negative" breast cancer, and feline injection site sarcomas for inflammation-driven tumorigenesis (Cannon 2015).

Pharmacotherapeutics for Veterinary Dispensing, First Edition. Edited by Katrina L. Mealey.
© 2019 John Wiley & Sons, Inc. Published 2019 by John Wiley & Sons, Inc.

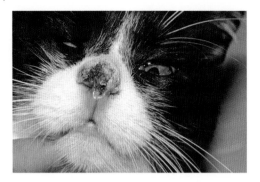

Figure 20.1 Cat with squamous cell carcinoma of the nasal planum. This is most typically diagnosed in cats with white noses that are chronically exposed to sunlight. As is the case in humans, there is typically progression from actinic keratitis to carcinoma *in situ* to invasive carcinoma. *Source:* Photo courtesy of Dr. Janean Fidel, Washington State University.

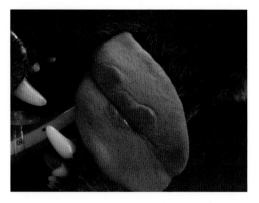

Figure 20.2 Transmissible venereal tumor (TVT) on the tongue of a dog. *Source:* Photo courtesy of Dr. Janean Fidel, Washington State University.

Among these common tumor types, there are differences in their frequency across species. For example, osteosarcoma is more commonly diagnosed in dogs relative to cats or people. Because of the relative frequency with which osteosarcoma occurs in dogs, and its similar biological behavior to osteosarcoma in people, numerous novel therapies have evolved through the use of this canine model (dogs with spontaneously occurring osteosarcoma). Examples include limb-sparing techniques, novel chemotherapeutic agents, gene therapy, and biologics. In fact, one of the most promising treatments for osteosarcoma in people at the current time is an immunotherapeutic that was first studied in canine osteosarcoma patients (Mason et al. 2016). Most dogs succumb to the disease within six months to one year of diagnosis, regardless of treatment. Canine osteosarcoma is arguably the most well-known spontaneous companion animal cancer model, but many others exist. Breast cancer is common in women as are mammary tumors in dogs and to some degree in cats. Lymphoma, a heterogeneous hematopoietic malignancy, is common in dogs, cats, and people.

Two types of cancer that occur in dogs but do not occur, or are extremely rare, in people are hemangiosarcoma and transmissible venereal tumor. Hemangiosarcoma is a highly metastatic malignant tumor arising from blood vessels. The tumors tend to occur on the spleen, liver, and/or heart. As the tumor grows, the disorganized blood vessels rupture, and extensive hemorrhage occurs. Prognosis is poor, with most dogs surviving only a few months after diagnosis even with surgery and chemotherapy. Identifying a successful treatment protocol is an area of intensive research in veterinary oncology. A transmissible venereal tumor is, as the name implies, a tumor that is sexually transmitted. The genitals are the most common location, but the tumor can also be transmitted to the nasal cavity, oral cavity (Figure 20.2), or skin surrounding the prepuce or vulva as a result of direct contact of these tissues with tumor cells. Transmissible venereal tumors tend to be easily treated (curable) with chemotherapy or radiation therapy.

20.2 Diagnostic Testing

Definitive diagnosis of neoplastic disease in veterinary patients, as in people generally, requires a biopsy with histopathologic assessment of tissue. Another step is usually necessary prior to determining the most appropriate treatment strategy, and that is staging. The goal of cancer staging is to determine how much cancer is present in the patient and where it is located. The diagnostic testing described here includes steps that may be undertaken to diagnose, grade, and stage cancer in veterinary patients. It is important to note that not every diagnostic test is necessary for every patient, but is highly dependent on the tumor type.

- Thorough history and physical examination
- Complete blood count
- Serum biochemical profile
- Urinalysis
- Bone marrow aspiration/core biopsy, if indicated
- Aspirates or biopsies of suspected masses/ sites of neoplasia
- Imaging, if indicated (radiographs, advanced imaging such as ultrasonography, computed tomography [CT], or magnetic resonance imaging [MRI])
- Histopathology of accessible lesions (may include special stains or immunohistochemistry)
- Serology.

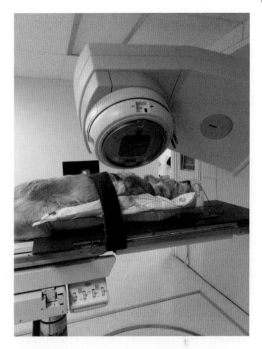

Figure 20.3 Dog under general anesthesia positioned for external beam radiation therapy of a tumor using a linear accelerator. *Source:* Photo courtesy of Dr. Janean Fidel, Washington State University.

20.3 Pharmacotherapy of Cancer

The treatment approach to cancer in dogs and cats (and even horses and ferrets) often incorporates a multimodal approach, which may include surgery, chemotherapy, radiotherapy (Figure 20.3), and even immunotherapy. However, even with multimodal therapy, survival times in veterinary cancer patients are often measured in months rather than years. When one considers that the life expectancy for a Golden Retriever is 10–12 years, then increasing survival time by six months is similar to increasing the survival time of a human cancer patient by about four years (assuming a lifespan of 80 years). Another important consideration is quality of life versus quantity – something that a veterinary patient cannot weigh in on. Many pet owners have low tolerance for chemotherapy-induced adverse effects or for procedures (i.e. surgery or radiation therapy) that require hospitalization because time spent in the hospital is not quality time.

The traditional approach to chemotherapy in veterinary patients has been high-dose (maximum-tolerated [or cytotoxic] dose, or MTD), intermittent, and most commonly parenterally administered drug administered in the hospital. Pharmacists working at veterinary hospitals would be highly involved in preparing these drugs for veterinary patients. Conversely, community pharmacists would have limited involvement with preparing or dispensing injectable chemotherapeutic agents commonly used in veterinary medicine (i.e. doxorubicin, cisplatin, carboplatin, vincristine, vinblastine, vinorelbine, and cyclophosphamide). Some orally administered high-dose chemotherapeutic drugs would be dispensed by community pharmacists to owners of veterinary cancer patients (i.e. cyclophosphamide, chlorambucil, methotrexate, and veterinary tyrosine kinase inhibitors). As is the case with MTD intermittent chemotherapy in people, limitations include the associated adverse drug reactions, which can be severe, and the development of drug resistance ultimately leading to treatment failure. It is worth noting that the MTD for an individual veterinary cancer patient should include considerations such as the pet owner's philosophy (quality of life versus quantity of life) and financial inclination (does the owner have the resources/willingness to pay for hospitalization in the event of a serious adverse drug reaction or complication?).

Low-dose metronomic chemotherapy (LDMC) has been used to treat some forms of cancer in people for several decades. More recently, LDMC has been and is currently being investigated in veterinary cancer patients and is an area of intense research. Community pharmacists are likely to receive prescriptions for oral chemotherapeutic agents as LDMC. Metronomic chemotherapy has the potential for a lower frequency of side effects (Bracha et al. 2014; Elmslie et al. 2008; Harper and Blackwood 2017; Tripp et al. 2011). LDMC is thought to target the vascular endothelium of the tumor and stimulate anti-angiogenic factors, and it may also trigger an immunomodulatory response (immune stimulation) that contributes to its antitumor effects. In some clinical situations, LDMC may have a palliative role in treating cancer patients, especially those with metastatic disease (Schmidt 2016).

The chemotherapeutic drugs most often used as part of a metronomic protocol in veterinary patients include the oral alkylating agents that are US Food and Drug Administration (FDA) approved for people (i.e. chlorambucil, cyclophosphamide, and lomustine). Other drugs sometimes used as part of LDMC protocols include antibiotics (i.e. doxycycline, used for its anti-collagenase activity to minimize the breakdown of the extracellular matrix) and nonsteroidal anti-inflammatory drugs (NSAIDs) used to inhibit the cyclooxygenase-1 and -2 (COX1/COX2) enzymes, as cyclooxygenase (COX) overexpression has been associated with increases in angiogenic growth factors and tumorigenesis. Because chlorambucil, cyclophosphamide, and lomustine are not FDA approved for veterinary species, the tablet/capsule strengths that are commercially available often exceed the dose required for metronomic chemotherapy in a dog or cat. Pharmacists, therefore, will likely receive prescriptions requesting compounded formulations of these drugs for dog- and cat-sized doses.

Many anticancer drugs, in both people and veterinary patients, are dosed based on body surface area (units of meters squared $[m^2]$). Body surface area dosing was originally derived to adapt laboratory animal drug doses to people based on basal metabolic rate, often for Phase I clinical trials (Beumer et al. 2012). Although there are a number of limitations to body surface area dosing, it is still widely used for chemotherapeutic drugs in dogs and cats. However, it is vital for pharmacists to understand that formulae for calculating body surface area differ between species. Do not use body surface area conversion charts, tables, or mobile device apps for any species other than the intended one. The appropriate conversion coefficient is different for dogs, cats, human beings, and so on, so dosing will not be correct. Appendix E lists body surface area conversions for cats and dogs based on body weight.

This chapter will limit the scope of the discussion to include the more common oral chemotherapeutic agents (i.e. alkylating agents) that pharmacists might dispense as well as FDA-approved veterinary anticancer drugs and biologics. Table 20.1 summarizes the reported metronomic oral chemotherapeutic dosages used in dogs and cats, while Table 20.2 summarizes the traditional (cytotoxic) doses of oral chemotherapeutic drugs. Adverse effects of these and other chemotherapeutic drugs are discussed in detail in the "Adverse Effects of Anticancer Drugs in Veterinary Species" section of the chapter.

Table 20.1 Metronomic doses for common oral chemotherapeutic drugs used in canine cancer patients.

Drug	Dosage(s)
Chlorambucil	Dogs: $4\,mg/m^2$ PO every 24 hours (Schrempp et al. 2013)
Cyclophosphamide	Dogs: $15\,mg/m^2$ PO every 24 hours (Setyo et al. 2017)
Lomustine (CCNU)	Dogs: $2.84\,mg/m^2$ PO every 24 hours (Tripp et al. 2011)
Piroxicam	Dogs: $0.3\,mg/kg$ PO every 24 hours (Knapp et al. 1994)

PO, Orally ("per os").

Table 20.2 Doses for common anticancer drugs (cytotoxic doses) used in canine and feline cancer patients.

Drug	Dosage(s)
Chlorambucil	*Dogs:* $3–6\,mg/m^2$ PO every 24 hours × 1–2 weeks, then $3–6\,mg/m^2$ PO every 48 hours, determined by individual patient response (Withrow et al. 2013) *Cats:* $20\,mg/m^2$ PO once every 2 weeks *OR* 2 mg PO every 2–3 days (Kent 2013)
Cyclophosphamide	*Dogs:* $250–300\,mg/m^2$ PO or IV every 3 weeks *OR* $50\,mg/m^2$ for 3–5 consecutive days (Withrow et al. 2013) *Cats:* $300\,mg/m^2$ IV every 1 week *OR* 50 mg PER CAT PO divided over 2–4 days (Kent 2013)
Lomustine (CCNU)	*Dogs:* $70–80\,mg/m^2$ PO every 3 weeks (Withrow et al. 2013) *Cats:* $50–60\,mg/m^2$ PO every 4–6 weeks (Kent 2013)
Toceranib	*Dogs:* $2.75\,mg/kg$ PO every other day *OR* Mon., Wed., and Fri. (Bernabe et al. 2013) *Cats:* $2.7\,mg/kg$ PO Mon., Wed., and Fri. (Merrick et al. 2017)

IV, Intravenously; PO, orally ("per os").

20.3.1 Alkylating Agents

20.3.1.1 Chlorambucil

Chlorambucil is used at cytotoxic antineoplastic doses for treating small-cell gastrointestinal (GI) lymphoma in cats (Barrs and Beatty 2012; Kiselow et al. 2008; Lingard et al. 2009; Stein et al. 2010) and chronic lymphoid leukemias in dogs (Lautscham et al. 2017). Additionally, it may be used in veterinary patients that are unable to tolerate cyclophosphamide due to either myelosuppression or sterile hemorrhagic cystitis. Table 20.2 lists doses of chlorambucil when used for its cytotoxic effects. Chlorambucil has also been used recently as a metronomic chemotherapeutic drug in dogs (Leach et al.

2012; Schrempp et al. 2013), including reports of its use to treat primary nodal hemangiosarcoma (Chan et al. 2016) and urinary bladder transitional cell carcinoma (Schrempp et al. 2013). Table 20.1 lists metronomic doses of chlorambucil.

20.3.1.2 Cyclophosphamide

Cyclophosphamide is one of the most common orally administered antineoplastic agents used in veterinary medicine, particularly for dogs, despite the fact that it is not FDA approved for any veterinary species. Cyclophosphamide is a component of several chemotherapy protocols, including COP (cyclophosphamide, vincristine, and prednisone), CHOP (cyclophosphamide, prednisone,

L-asparaginase, vincristine, and doxorubicin), and several others that are employed to treat canine and feline lymphoma. Lymphoma is the most common hematopoietic neoplasm in both dogs and cats. In fact, lymphoma is more common in dogs than it is in people (~100 cases per 100 000 dogs). Cyclophosphamide may also be used in other chemotherapy protocols to treat carcinomas in dogs and cats, but this is less common. Pharmacists are likely to see prescriptions for cyclophosphamide to treat veterinary patients and may be asked to compound the commercially available tablets into lower strength capsule form for cats and small dogs. As is the case in people, cyclophosphamide can cause serious adverse effects (see the "Adverse Effects of Anticancer Drugs in Veterinary Species" section).

Because cyclophosphamide has immunomodulatory and anti-angiogenic effects, it is one of the more studied chemotherapeutic agents used in metronomic protocols (Penel et al. 2012). Cyclophosphamide may be used alone or as part of multidrug metronomic protocols to treat a variety of malignancies. The metronomic cyclophosphamide protocols developed for dogs parallel those used in people and used as adjuvant chemotherapy to treat hemangiosarcoma (Lana et al. 2007; Wendelburg et al. 2015), soft tissue sarcomas (Burton et al. 2011; Cancedda et al. 2016; Elmslie et al. 2008), and osteosarcoma (London et al. 2015).

20.3.1.3 Lomustine (CCNU)

In people, lomustine is used to treat brain tumors, lymphoma, melanoma, and carcinomas (kidney and pulmonary). In dogs, lomustine has been used to treat brain tumors (Fulton and Steinberg 1990), mast cell tumors (Rassnick et al. 1999), and cutaneous lymphoma (Graham and Myers 1999). Relative to cyclophosphamide, less has been reported on the use of lomustine as part of metronomic chemotherapeutic protocols in dogs. In a prospective study using a metronomic protocol in tumor-bearing dogs with limited treatment options (i.e. dogs with incompletely

resected or unresectable tumors, tumors refractory to standard chemotherapy protocols, or dogs with metastatic disease), once-a-day lomustine was well tolerated in some dogs, but had to be discontinued in 22 of 81 dogs because of toxicosis (Tripp et al. 2011). Additional research is needed to evaluate the efficacy of lomustine as a primary metronomic therapy in specific tumor types in dogs.

20.3.1.4 Nonsteroidal Anti-inflammatory Drugs

20.3.1.4.1 Piroxicam

Overexpression of COX, specifically the COX2 isoenzyme, occurs in a variety of tumor types, especially epithelial neoplasms. Examples of tumors reported to overexpress COX in people (Chan et al. 1999; Half et al. 2002; Reddy and Rao 2002; Ristimaki et al. 1997; Specht et al. 2002) include colorectal cancer and squamous cell, bladder, thyroid, and mammary carcinomas, while examples in dogs (Dore et al. 2003; Khan et al. 2000; Kleiter et al. 2004; Mohammed et al. 2001; Pestili de Almeida et al. 2001; Tremblay et al. 1999) include transitional cell, prostatic, squamous cell, nasal, and mammary carcinomas. COX expression has not been as well documented in feline neoplasias (Beam et al. 2003). COX2 expression promotes tumorigenesis, is a pharmacological target, and serves as a prognostic indicator in some cancers (Baek et al. 2009; Boonsoda and Wanikiat 2008). For example, COX2 expression can be prognostic in patients with colorectal cancer (Spugnini et al. 2005).

Of the available NSAIDs, piroxicam (a nonselective COX inhibitor) is the most widely studied NSAID, and it is used for its antineoplastic properties in dogs. For example, piroxicam is commonly used as a sole palliative agent or part of multidrug protocols to treat transitional carcinoma (Henry et al. 2003; Knapp et al. 1994, 2000; Mohammed et al. 2002, 2003). Its use in transitional cell carcinoma in dogs is based on data showing that piroxicam combined with cisplatin significantly improved tumor response compared with cisplatin alone (Knapp et al. 2000). In dogs, piroxicam may also be used to treat squamous cell carcinomas, oral malignant melanoma, and mammary carcinomas (Boria et al. 2004; Knapp et al. 1992; Schmidt et al. 2001).

20.3.1.4.2 Toceranib (Palladia®)
Toceranib is a tyrosine kinase inhibitor that is FDA approved for treating grade 2 and 3 mast cell tumors in dogs. Similar to tyrosine kinase inhibitors used in human medicine, toceranib targets dysfunctional tyrosine kinases that promote unregulated cell growth. These dysfunctional tyrosine kinases are associated with certain types of cancer in people, dogs, and cats. A number of tyrosine kinase inhibitors are FDA approved for use in people and are clinically active against a variety of tumor types. Toceranib is a multi-targeted tyrosine kinase inhibitor that has both antiangiogenic and antitumor activity, similar to sunitinib used in human medicine. In people, sunitinib is used in the treatment of a diverse group of cancers, including neuroendocrine, colon, as well as breast, and is considered the standard of care in treatment of metastatic renal cell carcinoma (Chow and Eckhardt 2007). In dogs, toceranib is used in the treatment of a variety of tumor types, most notability mast cell tumors but also sarcomas, carcinomas, and melanomas (London et al. 2003, 2009; Pryer et al. 2003). In cats, toceranib has been used to treat carcinomas, but data regarding its safety and efficacy in cats are largely limited to anecdotal experience (Merrick et al. 2017). *Because of potential differences in tyrosine kinase receptor binding (pharmacodynamic differences) and potential pharmacokinetic differences, human tyrosine kinase inhibitors should not be substituted for toceranib to treat dogs or cats.* Such a substitution might adversely affect both safety and efficacy.

20.3.1.4.3 Melanoma Vaccine
For dogs, melanomas occurring in the oral cavity and digits tend to have a high metastatic rate (60% and 40%, respectively), resulting in limited effective treatment options (Oncept 2012; Spangler and Kass 2006). In a variety of species, including dogs, immunotherapy is a means to help control local disease, targeting the overexpression of tyrosinase associated with melanomas (Bouchard et al. 1994; Phillips et al. 2012; Ramos-Vara and Miller 2011). For example, a canine melanoma vaccine (Oncept®) is available for the treatment of dogs with stage II or III oral melanoma (Oncept 2012).

This DNA (human-derived) vaccine against tyrosinase, the melanosomal glycoprotein essential for melanin synthesis, is used to generate an anti-tyrosinase response (Grosenbaugh et al. 2011; Oncept 2012). The vaccine is most efficacious for patients in which the primary tumor has been surgically excised or irradiated and there is no evidence of metastasis (Ottnod et al. 2013). Limited data are available on the vaccine's efficacy in patients with the presence of macroscopic lesions. The vaccine is provided by the manufacturer only to specialty veterinary hospitals. It is administered via a proprietary delivery system.

20.3.1.4.4 Corticosteroids
Corticosteroids are a component of most chemotherapy protocols for treating lymphoma in dogs and cats. Corticosteroids have cytotoxic activity against neoplastic lymphocytes. However, use of corticosteroids as a sole treatment for lymphoma is generally not recommended by veterinary oncologists for several reasons. First, unless the disease is fully characterized (via biopsy and histologic typing), treatment with corticosteroids is likely to interfere with important aspects of the diagnostic process that guide treatment strategies and provide prognostic information. Second, corticosteroid treatment alone has a lower remission rate and achieves shorter remission durations relative to combination chemotherapy protocols. Last, and perhaps most important, treatment with corticosteroids alone is thought to contribute to chemotherapeutic resistance – not only corticosteroid resistance but also resistance to many other classes of chemotherapeutic drugs. However, if the

owner elects not to pursue a full chemotherapy treatment protocol (e.g. due to cost limitations, concerns about their pet's quality of life during chemotherapy, or inability to bring their pet in for frequent veterinary appointments), prednisone can be used as a sole treatment for lymphoma, as long as the owner is fully aware of the drawbacks. Prednisone *may* manage the disease for a month or two, usually providing the animal with a good quality of life. Adverse effects of corticosteroids are discussed in Chapter 14.

20.4 Adverse Effects of Anticancer Drugs in Veterinary Species

Adverse effects shared between people and veterinary patients will be listed, but those that are unique to a particular veterinary species or for which a particular species is more susceptible will be emphasized. In addition to describing adverse effects of chemotherapeutic agents that pharmacists might dispense (i.e. orally administered drugs), this section will include adverse effects of injectable chemotherapeutic drugs since many chemotherapy protocols include both injectable agents (administered by the veterinarian) and oral drugs. Since pharmacists may interact with owners of patients undergoing chemotherapy, it is important for pharmacists to appreciate species differences in not only the type and frequency of adverse drug effects in veterinary patients but also how they might manifest in a veterinary patient in contrast to people who can verbalize symptoms. Last, this section also includes information on life-or-death pharmacogenetic influences and drug–drug interactions that pharmacists should recognize and help prevent.

20.4.1 Common Adverse Drug Reactions

20.4.1.1 Myelosuppression
With few exceptions, the chemotherapeutic drugs used in veterinary medicine can cause myelosuppression (i.e. neutropenia, thrombocytopenia, and/or anemia).

Mandatory monitoring
For all drugs that can cause myelosuppression, a complete blood count should be performed at the drug nadir.

Complications resulting from decreased neutrophils, platelets, and red blood cells include susceptibility to infections, bleeding, and low oxygen carrying capacity, respectively. Because veterinary patients can't communicate early symptoms associated with infection, it is important for pharmacists to educate pet owners on ways to monitor for infection. Likewise, because most dogs and cats are furry, minor bruising may not be noticed by the owner. However, pharmacists can encourage owners to examine their pet's skin and mucous membranes for signs of bleeding. People with anemia often describe being easily fatigued. Since veterinary patients cannot verbalize that, pharmacists can instruct owners to check the color of their pet's mucous membranes (pale mucous membranes may indicate anemia). By taking a picture of the mucous membrane color before chemotherapy begins, the owner has a reference point with which to compare once chemotherapy has started. Treatment options available for veterinary patients experiencing neutropenia, thrombocytopenia, and anemia are similar to those for human patients (i.e. recombinant human granulocyte colony stimulating factor, transfusions), but since most veterinary patients are not covered by insurance, owners must pay out of pocket. Therefore, chemotherapy doses tend to be lower in veterinary patients than in people to avoid severe adverse drug reactions that might require hospitalization.

20.4.1.2 Alopecia
Compared to people, alopecia in most dogs and cats tends to be minor. Hair that has been clipped or shaved for diagnostic procedures (e.g. ultrasounds or placement of intravenous catheters) is slow to regrow.

Dogs and cats may lose their whiskers. Some dog breeds with a continuously growing haircoat (e.g. Poodles, Schnauzers, curly-coated terrier breeds, and others) will experience more pronounced alopecia than others. Once chemotherapy has been completed, the fur will grow back, although it may be a slightly different color and texture. The reason that chemotherapy-induced alopecia in dogs and cats is milder is that their hair follicles are in different phases of the growth cycle. In humans, 80–90% of hair follicles are in the anagen (actively growing) phase at a given time and are therefore susceptible to cytotoxic effects of chemotherapy drugs. In dogs and cats, the telogen (resting phase) is the dominant phase. Since there are no actively dividing cells in the hair follicle during the telogen phase, these cells are resistant to the cytotoxic effects of chemotherapy.

20.4.1.3 Gastrointestinal

Vomiting and diarrhea are common with chemotherapy and can result from stimulation of the chemoreceptor trigger zone, cytotoxic effects on the GI epithelium, alteration of taste, modulation of motility, and other causes. Some chemotherapeutic classes are more likely to cause vomiting (e.g. platinum compounds), while others are more likely to cause diarrhea or colitis (e.g. doxorubicin). As in people, antiemetics, appetite stimulants, and antidiarrheal agents are used to alleviate GI adverse effects. Pharmacists should be aware of the antiemetics (i.e. maropitant or Cerenia®) and appetite stimulants (i.e. capromorelin or Entyce®) that are FDA approved for dogs and/or cats (with no human equivalent). The over-the-counter (OTC) antidiarrheal agent loperamide should be avoided in some dogs because of a deficient blood–brain barrier (a pharmacogenetic defect in P-glycoprotein; see Chapter 5).

20.4.1.4 Reproductive

Because most antineoplastic agents target rapidly dividing cells, reproductive organs can be targeted. Transient or permanent infertility is a potential outcome of chemotherapy in veterinary patients. Teratogenicity and loss of pregnancy are potential outcomes in pregnant animals receiving chemotherapy. In the USA, a large number of veterinary patients that are treated with chemotherapeutic drugs are neutered, but the pharmacist should request that information from the pet owner to provide the appropriate counseling and medication warnings.

20.4.2 Specific Adverse Reactions by Drug Class

20.4.2.1 Concerns for Pet Owners or Caretakers

Many anticancer drugs are mutagenic and teratogenic, potentially posing risks for individuals handling the drug itself or even active drug excreted in urine or feces. When pharmacists dispense chemotherapeutic drugs for owners to administer, pharmacists should provide education and counseling on safe handling of the drug for the pet owner. In addition, pharmacists must advise pet owners on safe handling of the pet's urine, feces, and other body fluids while the animal is being treated with cytotoxic drugs.

20.4.2.2 Vinca Alkaloids

The vinca alkaloids vincristine, vinblastine, and vinorelbine are all used in veterinary medicine. They must be administered by careful intravenous administration because they are vesicants (can cause extensive tissue damage) if extravasation occurs. Intravenous administration in veterinary patients is almost always more challenging than it is in people because veterinary patients are often smaller, have smaller veins, and are often less cooperative than people. Vinca alkaloids can cause peripheral and central neuropathies in both veterinary and human patients. However, these are usually diagnosed at a later stage in veterinary patients than in people (since veterinary patients are unable to verbalize neurologic sensations), so they will take longer to resolve after treatment is discontinued. Some neurological abnormalities may not be reversible.

Vinca alkaloids are substrates for P-glycoprotein. Dogs and cats with mutations in the ABCB1 (MDR1) gene are exquisitely sensitive to adverse effects caused by vinca alkaloids (i.e. myelosuppression, GI effects, and central neuropathy). Genetic testing is available for both dogs and cats to determine their ABCB1 genotype because animals with functional ABCB1 mutations require dose reduction to avoid severe toxicity. The ABCB1-1Δ mutation occurs in 50% or more of dogs in some breeds (herding), and the ABCB1 1930_1931del TC mutation occurs in about 4% of cats. Chapter 5 provides more details about the ABCB1 genotypes in dogs and cats.

20.4.2.3 Doxorubicin

While other anthracyclines may be used in human cancer patients, doxorubicin is by far the most common one used in veterinary patients (Figure 20.4). Doxorubicin shares some characteristics with vinca alkaloids, such as its vesicant properties and the fact that it is also a P-glycoprotein substrate. Thus, extreme care must be used for intrave-

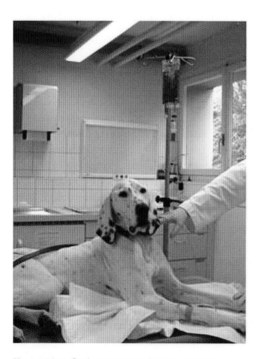

Figure 20.4 Canine cancer patient receiving a doxorubicin infusion. *Source:* Photo courtesy of Dr. Janean Fidel, Washington State University.

nous administration in veterinary patients, and dogs and cats should be genotyped for ABCB1 mutations to determine if dose reductions based on ABCB1 (MDR1) genotype are necessary.

Cumulative myocardial toxicity is a potential problem in veterinary patients, as it is in people, but the cumulative lifetime dose is lower. The maximum lifetime dose of doxorubicin for dogs is $250\,mg/m^2$, while that in people is $450–550\,mg/m^2$. Doxorubicin is often associated with diarrhea and colitis in dogs.

20.4.2.4 Platinum Compounds (Carboplatin and Cisplatin)

The most common adverse effects of cisplatin in dogs (aside from myelosuppression) are vomiting and nephrotoxicity. Pretreatment with antiemetics and saline diuresis is commonly used to prevent or at least mitigate these potential adverse effects.

> **Dramatic difference**
>
> A highly unusual adverse effect of cisplatin has been reported in cats. **Cisplatin causes acute, fulminant pulmonary edema in cats – it is absolutely contraindicated in cats.**

Carboplatin causes less vomiting and is less likely to cause nephrotoxicity in dogs than cisplatin. Importantly, it does not cause pulmonary toxicity in cats.

20.4.2.5 5-Fluorouracil (5-FU)

Pharmacists should be made aware of adverse effects of 5-fluorouracil not because the drug is used frequently in veterinary patients, but because it can cause fatal neurotoxicity to dogs and cats when used by pet owners. 5-FU 5% topical cream is indicated for the treatment of actinic keratosis and some superficial skin tumors in people. Accidental ingestion can occur if dogs gain access to and chew on the container or when dogs or cats lick the owner at the site of drug application. Numerous fatalities have resulted due to refractory seizures (acutely) or myelosuppression (if the animal survives the acute neurotoxicity). In one report, only 14 of

70 dogs survived after accidental exposure to 5-FU (Dorman et al. 1990). Animals that have been exposed to 5-FU should be referred for emergency medical care immediately.

20.4.2.6 Alkylating Agents

20.4.2.6.1 Chlorambucil

GI upset (i.e. anorexia and/or diarrhea) is the most common side effect of chlorambucil. This can occur even at metronomic doses (Table 20.2) (Schrempp et al. 2013). Other less common adverse effects reported include neurotoxicity in dogs (Giuliano 2013) and cats (Benitah et al. 2003) and acquired Fanconi's syndrome in cats (Reinert and Feldman 2016). Cytotoxic myelosuppression can occur when chlorambucil is dosed at the maximum tolerated dose (Table 20.2).

20.4.2.6.2 Cyclophosphamide

At metronomic doses (see Table 20.1), cyclophosphamide may cause low-grade GI upset. The MTD can cause more severe GI upset and is more likely to cause myelosuppression. The inflammatory metabolite of cyclophosphamide, acrolein, is associated with the development of sterile hemorrhagic cystitis in dogs and cats, limiting its use in some patients (Cox 1979). Sterile hemorrhagic cystitis in dogs has been caused by the MTD (Marin et al. 1996) and metronomic protocols (Elmslie et al. 2008; Lana et al. 2007).

Mandatory monitoring

Dogs or cats receiving cyclophosphamide should undergo regular urinalyses to identify sterile hemorrhagic cystitis. Pharmacists should instruct owners to monitor their pet closely for signs of painful urination or hematuria.

Additionally, owners should be encouraged to allow their pet to empty its bladder frequently (this may mean letting the dog out or taking the dog on short walks every few hours). Additional strategies to reduce the risk of developing cyclophosphamide-induced sterile hemorrhagic cystitis in veterinary patients include initiating measures

to dilute the urine, such as concurrent administration of furosemide (Best and Fry 2013; Setyo et al. 2017), or corticosteroids as part of metronomic protocols (Morais et al. 1999; Vieira et al. 2003), or treatment with mesna (i.e. cytoprotectant that inactivates acrolein) (Laberke et al. 2014).

20.4.2.6.3 Lomustine (CCNU)

Lomustine-induced adverse effects (myelosuppression, GI toxicosis, and hepatotoxicity) occur with greater frequency in dogs treated at MTD protocols than in those treated with metronomic doses, but they can occur in patients receiving lomustine at either the MTD or metronomic doses. Additionally, adverse effects tend to be more severe (i.e. higher grade) with MTD lomustine. Toxicities requiring drug discontinuation associated with metronomic lomustine treatment in dogs include GI signs, thrombocytopenia, increased liver enzymes (i.e. alanine aminotransferase [ALT]), neutropenia, and azotemia (Tripp et al. 2011). In one study, dogs treated with lomustine that were concurrently treated with the supplement S-adenosyl-methionine (SAMe) and silybin (i.e. Denamarin‧) had less severe elevations in liver enzymes compared to dogs treated with lomustine alone. This suggests that glutathione and other potential antioxidant effects of Denamarin may provide hepatoprotection from lomustine-induced hepatotoxicity (Skorupski et al. 2011). More information about SAMe and silybin is provided in a later section of this chapter ("Nutritional Supplements for Neoplastic Disease in Veterinary Patients").

20.4.2.6.4 NSAIDs (Piroxicam)

The most common side effects associated with piroxicam and other NSAIDs are consequences of the roles that prostaglandins play in protecting the gastric mucosa, in regulating renal blood flow, and in platelet aggregation (Jones and Budsberg 2000). Adverse effects include GI irritation/ulceration and acute kidney injury (Henry et al. 2003). Co-administration of corticosteroids with NSAIDs is contraindicated due to the significant risk of GI ulceration or perforation (Laine et al. 2010). Dogs seem to be at greater risk than people for gastric ulceration, while cats seem to be at greatest risk for NSAID-induced nephrotoxicity.

20.4.2.6.5 Toceranib
As a nonselective split-kinase receptor inhibitor, toceranib inhibits a number of receptors in the tyrosine kinase family, including cell surface and angiogenic receptors to include vascular endothelial growth factor receptor (VEGFR), platelet-derived growth factor receptor (PDGFR), type I tyrosine kinase receptor (KIT), and fms-like tyrosine kinase 3 (FLT3) (Bernabe et al. 2013; London et al. 2003, 2009; Pryer et al. 2003). Because of this inhibition, GI toxicity (anorexia, vomiting, diarrhea, or GI ulceration) may be serious enough to require dose reduction or drug withdrawal. Treatment of GI toxicity requires symptomatic care (i.e. antiemetics and appetite stimulants) and supportive care. Concurrent administration of NSAIDs with toceranib should be avoided due to the significant risk of GI ulceration, including the risk of perforation. In the event that piroxicam metronomic treatment is desired, it should not be administered on the same day as toceranib (which is dosed on an every-other-day regimen) (London et al. 2015). Other side effects observed in dogs treated with toceranib include neutropenia, muscle pain, proteinuria, and hypertension (Tjostheim et al. 2016). The latter is responsive to angiotensin-converting enzyme (ACE) inhibitors and amlodipine. Side effects reported in cats include bone marrow suppression (most frequently reported), GI toxicity, azotemia, and increased ALT (less common) (Merrick et al. 2017).

20.4.2.6.6 Melanoma Vaccine
The most common adverse effects associated with vaccine administration in dogs are redness, swelling, and pain at the site of administration. Other less commonly reported side effects in dogs include lethargy, fever, and hypersensitivity reactions (Oncept 2012).

Depigmentation of the hair and skin near the site of administration can occur.

20.5 Nutritional Supplements for Neoplastic Diseases in Veterinary Patients

SAMe and silymarin (Denamarin), and numerous other "antioxidant" or nutritional supplements, are marketed OTC for veterinary cancer patients. There is some evidence that antioxidants may interfere with radiation therapy and/or certain types of chemotherapy. In some cases, antioxidant supplementation in cancer patients may be protective against chemotherapy (or drug) adverse effects or have no impact, positive or negative, on the cancer patient. For example, nutritional supplements that are marketed to pet owners as "cancer preventives" or as providing "cancer support" include Nutrocept[*] and Apocaps[*]. There is no evidence that either of these improves outcome or quality of life in dogs or cats with cancer.

Denamarin is an example of an antioxidant supplementation of clinical benefit to prevent hepatotoxicity (inferred by elevations in serum ALT) associated with lomustine treatment at either metronomic or cytotoxic doses. There is some evidence that lomustine-treated dogs concurrently treated with a proprietary product, Denamarin, were less likely to develop liver enzyme elevation (68% had increased ALT) than dogs receiving only lomustine (84% had increased ALT). Denamarin is thought to promote antioxidant activity, in part by enhancing glutathione stores. Pharmacists must ensure pet owners understand how to properly administer the nutritional supplement. Denamarin is formulated as an enteric-coated or chewable tablet and must be given one hour before meals or two hours after a meal (i.e. on an empty stomach) to ensure optimal oral bioavailability.

Pharmacists should encourage owners to discuss the pros and cons of antioxidant supplementation in their pets with the veterinary oncologist to ensure that it will not interfere with treatment efficacy. Additionally, pharmacists should encourage pet owners to inform the pet's oncologist if their dog or cat is receiving any nutritional supplement.

Abbreviations

ABCB1	ATP-binding cassette subfamily B member 1
ACE	Angiotensin converting enzyme
FLT3	Fms-like tyrosine kinase-3
GI	Gastrointestinal
KIT	Type I tyrosine kinase receptor
LDMC	Low-dose metronomic chemotherapy
MCT	Mast cell tumor
NSAIDs	Nonsteroidal anti-inflammatory drugs
PDGFR	Platelet-derived growth factor receptor
TKI	Tyrosine-kinase inhibitor
SHC	Sterile hemorrhagic cystitis
VEGFR	Vascular endothelial growth factor receptor

References

Baek, S.J., McEntee, M.F., and Legendre, A.M. (2009). Review paper: cancer chemopreventive compounds and canine cancer. *Vet. Pathol.* 46: 576–588.

Barrs, V.R. and Beatty, J.A. (2012). Feline alimentary lymphoma: 2. Further diagnostics, therapy and prognosis. *J. Feline Med. Surg.* 14: 191–201.

Beam, S.L., Rassnick, K.M., Moore, A.S. et al. (2003). An immunohistochemical study of cyclooxygenase-2 expression in various feline neoplasms. *Vet. Pathol.* 40: 496–500.

Benitah, N., de Lorimier, L.P., Gaspar, M. et al. (2003). Chlorambucil-induced myoclonus in a cat with lymphoma. *J. Am. Anim. Hosp. Assoc.* 39: 283–287.

Bernabe, L.F., Portela, R., Nguyen, S. et al. (2013). Evaluation of the adverse event profile and pharmacodynamics of toceranib phosphate administered to dogs with solid tumors at doses below the maximum tolerated dose. *BMC Vet. Res.* 9: 190.

Best, M.P. and Fry, D.R. (2013). Incidence of sterile hemorrhagic cystitis in dogs receiving cyclophosphamide orally for three days without concurrent furosemide as part of a chemotherapeutic treatment for lymphoma: 57 cases (2007–2012). *J. Am. Vet. Med. Assoc.* 243: 1025–1029.

Beumer, J.H., Salvatore, E.C., and Salamone, J. (2012). Body-surface area-based chemotherapy dosing: appropriate in the 21st century? *J. Clin. Oncol.* 20 (31): 3896–3897.

Boonsoda, S. and Wanikiat, P. (2008). Possible role of cyclooxygenase-2 inhibitors as anticancer agents. *Vet. Rec.* 162: 159–161.

Boria, P.A., Murry, D.J., Bennett, P.F. et al. (2004). Evaluation of cisplatin combined with piroxicam for the treatment of oral malignant melanoma and oral squamous cell carcinoma in dogs. *J. Am. Vet. Med. Assoc.* 224: 388–394.

Bouchard, B., Vijayasaradhi, S., and Houghton, A.N. (1994). Production and characterization of antibodies against human tyrosinase. *J. Invest. Dermatol.* 102: 291–295.

Bracha, S., Walshaw, R., Danton, T. et al. (2014). Evaluation of toxicities from combined metronomic and maximal-tolerated dose chemotherapy in dogs with osteosarcoma. *J. Small Anim. Pract.* 55: 369–374.

Burton, J.H., Mitchell, L., Thamm, D.H. et al. (2011). Low-dose cyclophosphamide selectively decreases regulatory T cells and inhibits angiogenesis in dogs with soft tissue sarcoma. *J. Vet. Intern. Med.* 25: 920–926.

Cancedda, S., Marconato, L., Meier, V. et al. (2016). Hypofractionated radiotherapy for macroscopic canine soft tissue sarcoma. A retrospective study of 50 cases treated with a 5 × 6 GY protocol with or without metronomic chemotherapy. *Vet. Radiol. Ultrasound* 57: 75–83.

Cannon, C.M. (2015). Cats, cancer and comparative oncology. *Vet. Sci.* 2: 111–126.

Chan, C.M., Zwahlen, C.H., de Lorimier, L.P. et al. (2016). Primary nodal hemangiosarcoma in four dogs. *J. Am. Vet. Med. Assoc.* 249: 1053–1060.

Chan, G., Boyle, J.O., Yang, E.K. et al. (1999). Cyclooxygenase-2 expression is up-regulated in squamous cell carcinoma of the head and neck. *Cancer Res.* 59: 991–994.

Chow, L.Q. and Eckhardt, S.G. (2007). Sunitinib: from rational design to clinical efficacy. *J. Clin. Oncol.* 25: 884–896.

Cox, P.J. (1979). Cyclophosphamide cystitis – identification of acrolein as the causative agent. *Biochem. Pharmacol.* 28: 2045–2049.

Dore, M., Lanthier, I., and Sirois, J. (2003). Cyclooxygenase-2 expression in canine mammary tumors. *Vet. Pathol.* 40: 207–212.

Dorman, D.C., Coddington, K.A., and Richardson, R.C. (1990). 5-fluorouracil toxicosis in the dogs. *J. Vet. Intern. Med.* 4 (5): 254–257.

Elmslie, R.E., Glawe, P., and Dow, S.W. (2008). Metronomic therapy with cyclophosphamide and piroxicam effectively delays tumor recurrence in dogs with incompletely resected soft tissue sarcomas. *J. Vet. Intern. Med.* 22: 1373–1379.

Fulton, L.M. and Steinberg, H.S. (1990). Preliminary study of lomustine in the treatment of intracranial masses in dogs following localization by imaging techniques. *Semin. Vet. Med. Surg.* 5: 241–245.

Giuliano, A. (2013). Suspected chlorambucil-related neurotoxicity with seizures in a dog. *J. Small Anim. Pract.* 54: 437.

Gordon, I., Paoloni, M., Mazcko, C. et al. (2009). The comparative oncology trials consortium: using spontaneously occurring cancers in dogs to inform the cancer drug development pathwa. *PLoS Med.* 6: e1000161.

Graham, J. and Myers, R. (1999). Pilot study on the use of lomustine (CCNU) for the treatment of cutaneous lymphomia in dogs [abstract]. *J. Vet. Intern. Med.* 13: 257.

Grosenbaugh, D.A., Leard, A.T., Bergman, P.J. et al. (2011). Safety and efficacy of a xenogeneic DNA vaccine encoding for human tyrosinase as adjunctive treatment for oral malignant melanoma in dogs following surgical excision of the primary tumor. *Am. J. Vet. Res.* 72: 1631–1638.

Half, E., Tang, X.M., Gwyn, K. et al. (2002). Cyclooxygenase-2 expression in human breast cancers and adjacent ductal carcinoma in situ. *Cancer Res.* 62: 1676–1681.

Harper, A. and Blackwood, L. (2017). Toxicity of metronomic cyclophosphamide chemotherapy in a UK population of cancer-bearing dogs: a retrospective study. *J. Small Anim. Pract.* 58: 227–230.

Henry, C.J., McCaw, D.L., Turnquist, S.E. et al. (2003). Clinical evaluation of mitoxantrone and piroxicam in a canine model of human invasive urinary bladder carcinoma. *Clin. Cancer Res.* 9: 906–911.

Jones, C.J. and Budsberg, S.C. (2000). Physiologic characteristics and clinical importance of the cyclooxygenase isoforms in dogs and cats. *J. Am. Vet. Med. Assoc.* 217: 721–729.

Kent, M.S. (2013). Cats and chemotherapy: treat as 'small dogs' at your peril. *J. Feline Med. Surg.* 15: 419–424.

Khan, K.N., Knapp, D.W., Denicola, D.B. et al. (2000). Expression of cyclooxygenase-2 in transitional cell carcinoma of the urinary bladder in dogs. *Am. J. Vet. Res.* 61: 478–481.

Kiselow, M.A., Rassnick, K.M., McDonough, S.P. et al. (2008). Outcome of cats with low-grade lymphocytic lymphoma: 41 cases (1995–2005). *J. Am. Vet. Med. Assoc.* 232: 405–410.

Kleiter, M., Malarkey, D.E., Ruslander, D.E. et al. (2004). Expression of cyclooxygenase-2 in canine epithelial nasal tumors. *Vet. Radiol. Ultrasound* 45: 255–260.

Knapp, D.W., Glickman, N.W., Denicola, D.B. et al. (2000). Naturally-occurring canine transitional cell carcinoma of the urinary bladder a relevant model of human invasive bladder cancer. *Urol. Oncol.* 5: 47–59.

Knapp, D.W., Richardson, R.C., Bottoms, G.D. et al. (1992). Phase I trial of piroxicam in 62 dogs bearing naturally occurring tumors. *Cancer Chemother. Pharmacol.* 29: 214–218.

Knapp, D.W., Richardson, R.C., Chan, T.C. et al. (1994). Piroxicam therapy in 34 dogs with transitional cell carcinoma of the urinary bladder. *J. Vet. Intern. Med.* 8: 273–278.

Laberke, S., Zenker, I., and Hirschberger, J. (2014). Mesna and furosemide for prevention of cyclophosphamide-induced sterile haemorrhagic cystitis in dogs – a retrospective study. *Vet. Rec.* 174: 250.

Laine, L., Curtis, S.P., Cryer, B. et al. (2010). Risk factors for NSAID-associated upper GI clinical events in a long-term prospective study of 24,701 arthritis patients. *Aliment Pharmacol. Ther.* 32 (10): 1240–1248.

Lana, S., U'Ren, L., Plaza, S. et al. (2007). Continuous low-dose oral chemotherapy for adjuvant therapy of splenic hemangiosarcoma in dogs. *J. Vet. Intern. Med.* 21: 764–769.

Lautscham, E.M., Kessler, M., Ernst, T. et al. (2017). Comparison of a CHOP-LAsp-based protocol with and without maintenance for canine multicentric lymphoma. *Vet. Rec.* 180: 303.

Leach, T.N., Childress, M.O., Greene, S.N. et al. (2012). Prospective trial of metronomic chlorambucil chemotherapy in dogs with naturally occurring cancer. *Vet. Comp. Oncol.* 10: 102–112.

Lingard, A.E., Briscoe, K., Beatty, J.A. et al. (2009). Low-grade alimentary lymphoma: clinicopathological findings and response to treatment in 17 cases. *J. Feline Med. Surg.* 11: 692–700.

London, C.A., Gardner, H.L., Mathie, T. et al. (2015). Impact of toceranib/piroxicam/cyclophosphamide maintenance therapy on outcome of dogs with appendicular osteosarcoma following amputation and carboplatin chemotherapy: a multi-institutional study. *PLoS One* 10: e0124889.

London, C.A., Hannah, A.L., Zadovoskaya, R. et al. (2003). Phase I dose-escalating study of SU11654, a small molecule receptor tyrosine kinase inhibitor, in dogs with spontaneous malignancies. *Clin. Cancer Res.* 9: 2755–2768.

London, C.A., Malpas, P.B., Wood-Follis, S.L. et al. (2009). Multi-center, placebo-controlled, double-blind, randomized study of oral toceranib phosphate (SU11654), a receptor tyrosine kinase inhibitor, for the treatment of dogs with recurrent (either local or distant) mast cell tumor following surgical excision. *Clin. Cancer Res.* 15: 3856–3865.

Marin, M.P., Samson, R.J., and Jackson, E.R. (1996). Hemorrhagic cystitis in a dog. *Can. Vet. J.* 37: 240.

Mason, N.J., Gnanandarajah, J.S., Engiles, J.B. et al. (2016). Immunotherapy with a HER2-targeting listeria induces HER2-specific immunity and demonstrates potential therapeutic effects in a phase I trial in canine osteosarcoma. *Clin. Cancer Res.* 22: 4380–4390.

Merrick, C.H., Pierro, J., Schleis, S.E. et al. (2017). Retrospective evaluation of toceranib phosphate (palladia(R)) toxicity in cats. *Vet. Comp. Oncol.* 15: 710–717.

Mohammed, S.I., Bennett, P.F., Craig, B.A. et al. (2002). Effects of the cyclooxygenase inhibitor, piroxicam, on tumor response, apoptosis, and angiogenesis in a canine model of human invasive urinary bladder cancer. *Cancer Res.* 62: 356–358.

Mohammed, S.I., Coffman, K., Glickman, N.W. et al. (2001). Prostaglandin E2 concentrations in naturally occurring canine cancer. *Prostaglandins Leukot. Essent. Fatty Acids* 64: 1–4.

Mohammed, S.I., Craig, B.A., Mutsaers, A.J. et al. (2003). Effects of the cyclooxygenase inhibitor, piroxicam, in combination with chemotherapy on tumor response, apoptosis, and angiogenesis in a canine model of human invasive urinary bladder cancer. *Mol. Cancer Ther.* 2: 183–188.

Morais, M.M., Belarmino-Filho, J.N., Brito, G.A. et al. (1999). Pharmacological and histopathological study of cyclophosphamide-induced hemorrhagic cystitis – comparison of the effects of dexamethasone and Mesna. *Braz. J. Med. Biol. Res.* 32: 1211–1215.

Oncept (2012). *Canine Melanoma Vaccine* [Package insert]. Duluth, GA: Merial Limited.

Ottnod, J.M., Smedley, R.C., Walshaw, R. et al. (2013). A retrospective analysis of the efficacy of Oncept vaccine for the adjunct treatment of canine oral malignant melanoma. *Vet. Comp. Oncol.* 11: 219–229.

Paoloni, M.C. and Khanna, C. (2007). Comparative oncology today. *Vet. Clin. N. Am. Small Anim. Pract.* 37: 1023–1032; v.

Penel, N., Adenis, A., and Bocci, G. (2012). Cyclophosphamide-based metronomic chemotherapy: after 10 years of experience, where do we stand and where are we going? *Crit. Rev. Oncol. Hematol.* 82: 40–50.

Pestili de Almeida, E.M., Piche, C., Sirois, J. et al. (2001). Expression of cyclo-oxygenase-2 in naturally occurring squamous cell carcinomas in dogs. *J. Histochem. Cytochem.* 49: 867–875.

Phillips, J.C., Lembcke, L.M., Noltenius, C.E. et al. (2012). Evaluation of tyrosinase expression in canine and equine melanocytic tumors. *Am. J. Vet. Res.* 73: 272–278.

Pryer, N.K., Lee, L.B., Zadovaskaya, R. et al. (2003). Proof of target for SU11654: inhibition of KIT phosphorylation in canine mast cell tumors. *Clin. Cancer Res.* 9: 5729–5734.

Ramos-Vara, J.A. and Miller, M.A. (2011). Immunohistochemical identification of canine melanocytic neoplasms with antibodies to melanocytic antigen PNL2 and tyrosinase: comparison with Melan A. *Vet. Pathol.* 48: 443–450.

Rassnick, K.M., Moore, A.S., Williams, L.E. et al. (1999). Treatment of canine mast cell tumors with CCNU (lomustine). *J. Vet. Intern. Med.* 13: 601–605.

Reddy, B.S. and Rao, C.V. (2002). Novel approaches for colon cancer prevention by cyclooxygenase-2 inhibitors. *J. Environ. Pathol. Toxicol. Oncol.* 21: 155–164.

Reinert, N.C. and Feldman, D.G. (2016). Acquired Fanconi syndrome in four cats treated with chlorambucil. *J. Feline Med. Surg.* 18: 1034–1040.

Ristimaki, A., Honkanen, N., Jankala, H. et al. (1997). Expression of cyclooxygenase-2 in human gastric carcinoma. *Cancer Res.* 57: 1276–1280.

Schmidt, B.R., Glickman, N.W., DeNicola, D.B. et al. (2001). Evaluation of piroxicam for the treatment of oral squamous cell carcinoma in dogs. *J. Am. Vet. Med. Assoc.* 218: 1783–1786.

Schmidt, M. (2016). Dose-dense chemotherapy in metastatic breast cancer: shortening the time interval for a better therapeutic index. *Breast Care (Basel)* 11: 22–26.

Schrempp, D.R., Childress, M.O., Stewart, J.C. et al. (2013). Metronomic administration of chlorambucil for treatment of dogs with urinary bladder transitional cell carcinoma. *J. Am. Vet. Med. Assoc.* 242: 1534–1538.

Setyo, L., Ma, M., Bunn, T. et al. (2017). Furosemide for prevention of cyclophosphamide-associated sterile haemorrhagic cystitis in dogs receiving metronomic low-dose oral cyclophosphamide. *Vet. Comp. Oncol.* 15 (4): 1468–1478.

Skorupski, K.A., Hammond, G.M., Irish, A.M. et al. (2011). Prospective randomized clinical trial assessing the efficacy of Denamarin for prevention of CCNU-induced hepatopathy in tumor-bearing dogs. *J. Vet. Intern. Med.* 25: 838–845.

Spangler, W.L. and Kass, P.H. (2006). The histologic and epidemiologic bases for prognostic considerations in canine melanocytic neoplasia. *Vet. Pathol.* 43: 136–149.

Specht, M.C., Tucker, O.N., Hocever, M. et al. (2002). Cyclooxygenase-2 expression in thyroid nodules. *J. Clin. Endocrinol. Metab.* 87: 358–363.

Spugnini, E.P., Porrello, A., Citro, G. et al. (2005). COX-2 overexpression in canine tumors: potential therapeutic targets in oncology. *Histol. Histopathol.* 20: 1309–1312.

Stein, T.J., Pellin, M., Steinberg, H. et al. (2010). Treatment of feline gastrointestinal small-cell lymphoma with chlorambucil and glucocorticoids. *J. Am. Anim. Hosp. Assoc.* 46: 413–417.

Tjostheim, S.S., Stepien, R.L., Markovic, L.E. et al. (2016). Effects of Toceranib phosphate on systolic blood pressure and proteinuria in dogs. *J. Vet. Intern. Med.* 30: 951–957.

Tremblay, C., Dore, M., Bochsler, P.N. et al. (1999). Induction of prostaglandin G/H synthase-2 in a canine model of spontaneous prostatic adenocarcinoma. *J. Natl. Cancer Inst.* 91: 1398–1403.

Tripp, C.D., Fidel, J., Anderson, C.L. et al. (2011). Tolerability of metronomic administration of lomustine in dogs with cancer. *J. Vet. Intern. Med.* 25: 278–284.

Vieira, M.M., Brito, G.A., Belarmino-Filho, J.N. et al. (2003). Use of dexamethasone with mesna for the prevention of ifosfamide-induced hemorrhagic cystitis. *Int. J. Urol.* 10: 595–602.

Wendelburg, K.M., Price, L.L., Burgess, K.E. et al. (2015). Survival time of dogs with splenic hemangiosarcoma treated by splenectomy with or without adjuvant chemotherapy: 208 cases (2001–2012). *J. Am. Vet. Med. Assoc.* 247: 393–403.

Withrow, S. and Vail, D. (2007). *Withrow & MacEwen's Small Animal Clinical Oncology*, 4e. St. Louis, MO: Saunders Elsevier.

Withrow, S.J., Vail, D.M., and Page, R.L. (2013). *Withrow and MacEwen's Small Animal Clinical Oncology*. St. Louis, MO: Saunders.

21

Introduction to Equine Pharmacotherapy

Jennifer L. Davis

Department of Biomedical Sciences and Pathobiology, Virginia-Maryland (VA-MD) College of Veterinary Medicine, Virginia Tech, Blacksburg, VA, USA

Key Points

- Significant differences exist in pharmacokinetics of drugs between horses and humans as well as between horses and other companion animals.
- Oral absorption of many drugs is lower in horses compared to other species.
- Drug distribution, metabolism, and elimination of many drugs differ in horses compared to humans and other companion animals.
- Horses are particularly sensitive to adverse gastrointestinal effects of drugs, especially antibiotics.
- Other adverse drug effects unique to horses include laminitis and right dorsal colitis.

21.1 Drug Absorption, Distribution, Metabolism, and Elimination in the Horse

Numerous differences in drug pharmacokinetics exist between horses and other species. These differences, particularly in oral drug absorption capability, can result in therapeutic failure as well as an increased risk for adverse events. The factors contributing to these differences are discussed in this section, with particular reference to differences between horses and humans.

21.1.1 Absorption

For a drug to be absorbed from the gastrointestinal (GI) tract, it must first go into solution. Solubility must occur over a range of pH values, based on the pH of the stomach and small intestine, which can vary among species. Reported pH values in the fasting human are 1.4–2.1 in the stomach, 4.9–6.4 in the duodenum, 4.4–6.6 in the jejunum, and 6.5–7.4 in the ileum (Yu et al. 2002). In horses, the gastric pH is highly variable, particularly in the fasted state, with pH values ranging from 1.0 to 7.5 (Baker et al. 1993). Additionally, episodes of spontaneous alkalinization are noted in horses, with sustained pH values of 6.0–7.5. This is thought to be caused by reflux of alkaline duodenal contents into the stomach (Merritt 1999). Other explanations include salivary intake or variable gastric acid secretion (Baker and Gerring 1993). The median pH of the intestinal tract in horses, as recorded at necropsy, was 5.4 and 3.3 in the anterior and posterior stomach, respectively;

Pharmacotherapeutics for Veterinary Dispensing, First Edition. Edited by Katrina L. Mealey.

6.7–7.9 in the small intestine; 7.0 in the cecum; and 7.4 in the colon (Kararli 1995).

An additional factor affecting solubility is drug concentration and the volume of fluid available for dissolution. The human GI tract is exposed to approximately 5–10 L of fluids per day (Davenport 1982), taking into account ingested fluids and gastroduodenal and pancreatic secretions. The horse, in contrast, normally ingests maintenance fluids of approximately 24 L combined with gastroduodenal secretions of 38–40 L (Merritt et al. 1996), for a total exposure of 62–64 L of fluids per day. This represents a huge increase in the total fluids available for drug dissolution in the horse compared to humans; however, one must also take into account the increase in total drug dose administered on a per kilogram basis. This greater total amount of drug affects the dose/solubility ratio as well as the volume of fluid required for drug dissolution. This difference becomes highly important when dealing with compounded drugs for horses, as the goal is often to create a more concentrated drug formulation than is commercially available for ease of administration.

The volume of fluid administered with an oral drug formulation is not standardized for veterinary species. In humans, medications can be taken with one cup (240 mL) of water to aid in dissolution. In horses, many pharmacokinetic studies mimic this by administering the drug through a nasogastric tube followed by 1–2 L of water. However, in equine clinical practice, most drugs are administered in an oral dosing syringe by dissolving tablets in 40–60 mL of flavored water (i.e. corn syrup or molasses). In studies assessing oral drug bioavailability in horses, this common practice likely overestimates drug solubility and, subsequently, impairs oral bioavailability of marginally soluble drugs. This issue is often exacerbated when using compounded drug formulations, as many practitioners and owners prefer a paste formulation, (with an even lower water-to-drug content ratio) because pastes are easier to administer to horses.

Feeding can affect both gastric pH and the solubility of drugs. Ingestion of a meal can increase the gastric pH of humans to a variable degree, with ranges from 3.0 to 7.0 (Dressman et al. 1998). As stated here, fasted horses have variable gastric pH with episodes of spontaneous alkalinization. Feeding blunts alkalinization, resulting in a mean gastric pH that is usually only 1–2 points higher in fed versus fasted adult horses (Sanchez et al. 1998). The increase in pH is much more dramatic in foals, where the pH varies from <1.0 in the fasted state to >6.0 following milk ingestion (Sanchez et al. 1998). In horses, feeding creates a layered pH effect, with pH values as high as 6–7 in the squamous (upper) portion of the stomach and as low as 1–2 in the glandular (lower, secretory) portion (Baker and Gerring 1993; Merritt 2003). In the small intestine in humans, feeding generally causes a slight decrease in the pH (Persson et al. 2005). In contrast to horses and people, feeding induces a larger increase in gastric acid secretion in dogs, and the pH decreases rather than increases after a meal (Kararli 1995).

Feeding also alters the gastric emptying rate, increasing contact time with the gastric contents and delaying delivery of the drug to the intestine for absorption. Increased retention time in the stomach may be beneficial for some drugs that have an improved solubility in acidic environments (e.g. itraconazole), but may be detrimental to drugs that are degraded at low pH values (e.g. omeprazole and penicillins). The effect of feeding on gastric emptying in horses differs from that in other monogastric species. There was no significant difference in the emptying of solid, nondigestible, radiopaque markers in ponies following feeding, whereas the emptying of similar markers is greatly delayed by the presence of food in humans (Baker and Gerring 1994). Lorenzo-Figueras et al. (2005) report no difference in the effect of fat supplementation on gastric motility in horses, which is also markedly different from other species.

In human medicine, it is often recommended that drugs be taken with food. This may not be applicable to the horse because the composition of diets varies so much between species. Most equine diets, such as hay or grasses, have a low fat content. This type of high-roughage diet may decrease drug solubility and absorption by creating a physical barrier between the gastric fluid and the drug (Toothaker and Welling 1980). Drugs may also adsorb to feed particles, preventing solubilization. This was demonstrated for trimethoprim–sulfachlorpyridazine combinations in the horse (Van Duijkeren et al. 1996). Decreased oral absorption of drugs in fed horses has been demonstrated for rifampin, erythromycin, and doxycycline (Baggot 1992; Lakritz et al. 2000; Davis et al. 2006).

Anatomical differences may also contribute to differences in drug pharmacokinetics between horses and other species (Table 21.1). Horses are a monogastric species, similar to dogs and humans, but unlike these other species, they are herbivores. Horses are hindgut fermenters, relying on microorganisms in the large intestine for the synthesis of many proteins, vitamins, and volatile fatty acids. Gastric anatomy also differs in that horses have a high surface area of squamous versus glandular epithelium in the stomach, which affords protection from their high-fiber diet. Fiber in the diet may decrease drug dissolution in the stomach, resulting in undissolved drug being delivered to the small intestine, where the higher pH may further interfere with drug dissolution (Martinez et al. 2002). Consequently, more drug absorption may occur in the large intestine of horses compared to humans and other animals. This may explain the biphasic absorption of some drugs that is seen in the horse (Baggot 1992), rather than true enterohepatic recirculation. Horses lack a gall bladder and therefore secrete bile continuously into the intestinal lumen. Interspecies differences in bile flow and bile salt composition can affect oral absorption of drugs solubilized in bile.

Table 21.1 Comparative fluid capacity of the gastrointestinal tract in adult horses, cattle, pigs, and dogs.

	Species	Absolute capacity (L)	Relative capacity (%)
Stomach	Horse	18.0	8.5
	Cattle	252.5	70.8
	Pig	8.0	29.2
	Dog	4.3	62.3
Small intestine	Horse	63.8	30.2
	Cattle	66.0	18.5
	Pig	9.2	33.5
	Dog	1.6	23.2
Cecum	Horse	33.5	19.8
	Cattle	9.9	2.8
	Pig	1.5	5.6
	Dog	0.1	1.4
Colon	Horse	96.3	45.5
	Cattle	28.0	7.9
	Pig	8.7	31.7
	Dog	0.9	13.1

Note: Values were determined at autopsy.
Source: Adapted from Kararli (1995).

21.1.2 Distribution

The volume of distribution (Vd) is the pharmacokinetic parameter that quantifies drug distribution throughout the body, and it relates the mass of drug (dose) to the volume in which it is diluted (Toutain and Bousquet-Mélou 2004a). Thus, two of the main factors affecting the Vd are the dose used and the "volume" of the animal to be dosed. The volume, including intravascular, intracellular, and extracellular fluids, increases as the weight of the animal increases. Ergo, the volume of fluid in horses is expected to be larger than the volume in dogs, cats, and humans. For example, plasma volume is estimated to be between 35 and 42 mL/kg in humans, and 66 mL/kg in horses (Hurley 1975; Naylor et al. 1993). This can be further affected by disease states and age. Many conditions in horses, such as colic and diarrhea, are characterized by volume contraction and dehydration, which affect the extracellular fluid volume. Neonatal foals have a higher percentage of body water than adult horses (80% vs. 60% total body water), and the extra 20% is primarily confined to the extracellular fluid. Drugs with high Vds are usually very lipid soluble and typically are not significantly affected by changes in body water status, so they do not require dosage adjustment. However, there are many conditions that affect the disposition of low-Vd drugs (e.g. nonsteroidal anti-inflammatory drugs [NSAIDs] and aminoglycosides) in a patient, so these drugs do require dosage adjustments because of their narrow therapeutic index.

Aside from volume, another major factor affecting drug distribution is protein and tissue binding, as only unbound drug is able to equilibrate between blood and tissues (Fura et al. 2008; Berry et al. 2011). After equilibration, drug may subsequently become bound to tissues as well. Interspecies differences in plasma and tissue protein binding have been reported and are actually relatively common (Berry et al. 2011). For example, protein binding of doxycycline is 81.6% in the horse, 75–86% in dogs, and 99% in cats (Davis et al.

2006). Protein binding may also change with age and disease. Young animals typically have a lower plasma protein content compared with older animals. Additionally, the same diseases causing severe dehydration and volume contraction in horses (e.g. colic and diarrhea) may also cause a profound loss of protein.

21.1.3 Metabolism

Compared to humans, dogs, and some laboratory species, drug metabolic pathways in the horse are less well defined. It has been speculated that herbivores have a higher hepatic metabolic capacity, which would increase the first-pass metabolism of lipophilic compounds, resulting in an overall decrease in oral bioavailability (Baggot 1992). *In vitro* hepatic microsomal assays have demonstrated species variability between horses and other laboratory or food-producing animals, including rats, rabbits, cattle, pigs, and chickens (Nebbia et al. 2003). Hepatic metabolizing enzyme activity in the horse is lower at birth and in the first year of life, and it slowly increases over a period of at least 15 years (Nebbia et al. 2004). Overall, horses had much higher cytochrome P450 (CYP) 1A and 2E1 isoenzyme activity, but lower CYP2B and CYP3A isoenzyme activity, when compared to other species.

As is the case with other species, CYP450 enzymes are also expressed in equine intestine and may contribute to metabolism of some drugs prior to oral absorption (Tyden et al. 2004). P-glycoprotein and other efflux pumps have been characterized in the apical cell membranes of enterocytes, and, in addition, P-glycoprotein staining was observed in the intestinal intraepithelial and lamina propria lymphocytes.

21.1.4 Elimination

The rate at which a drug is eliminated from the body after intravenous administration is represented by the pharmacokinetic parameter clearance. Plasma clearance is defined as the plasma volume cleared of drug per unit of time, and it is influenced by the rate of elimination and the plasma concentration. The rate of elimination is further influenced by the extraction ratio, which is a property of the drug used, and the cardiac output of the species to which the drug is administered. Cardiac output itself varies greatly between species, and it can be calculated by the equation $(180 \times$ body weight$)^{-0.19}$. This equation emphasizes the influence of body weight on cardiac output, which defines the maximum clearance (Cl_{max}) a drug may undergo. Thus, animals with larger body weights have a lower relative cardiac output and lower maximum clearance. For example, Cl_{max} in cats, based on cardiac output, is 146 mL/kg/min; in humans, it is 80 mL/kg/min; and in horses, 55 mL/kg/min (Toutain and Bousquet-Mélou 2004b). Maximum clearance may be lower for drugs that have a high hepatic extraction ratio, or higher if the drug undergoes a high first-pass metabolism by the lungs, as has been shown for pentoxifylline in horses (Crisman et al. 1993), or if there is direct drug metabolism in the blood (i.e. procaine metabolism by plasma esterases).

Other factors affecting clearance include plasma protein binding and route of administration. Only protein-unbound drug is available for elimination, and, as discussed in Section 21.1.2 ("Distribution"), protein binding may differ between species.

Clearance values can be useful in extrapolating therapeutic doses between species, and may explain some differences in drug doses between species. For example, the recommended dose of morphine for humans is about 0.17 mg/kg, for dogs it is 1 mg/kg, while for horses it is 0.1 mg/kg. The difference in morphine doses is due to different plasma clearances, which are 14.7, 85, and 8.64 mL/kg/min in humans, dogs, and horses, respectively (Stanski et al. 1978; Combie et al. 1983; Barnhart et al. 2000). This relationship is exemplified in the equation $Dose_{species2} = (Dose_{species1} \times Cl_{species2}) / Cl_{species1}$. and can be corrected for protein binding if it differs between species. *Note:* This equation is for illustrative

purposes only; doses must be corrected for species differences in protein binding, drug transporter expression and function, and pharmacodynamic differences.

21.2 Drugs Commonly Prescribed for Horses

The use of compounded products in equine medicine is a common practice due to the lack of US Food and Drug Administration (FDA)-approved drugs for horses and the dearth of convenient, palatable formulations. Despite their common use, there are few standardized formulas available to enable pharmacists to produce a quality compounded drug product for horses. Given the poor oral availability of drugs, particularly antibiotics, in horses, care should be taken to ensure potency and stability of any products used to avoid subtherapeutic plasma drug concentrations. This section gives examples of drugs commonly dispensed for use in horses by category.

21.2.1 Antibiotics

21.2.1.1 Aminoglycosides
Drugs in this class demonstrate age-dependent pharmacokinetics, and relative doses for neonatal foals are much higher than for adults. As in other species, aminoglycosides are associated with nephrotoxicity in horses.

Owner counseling: Owners should monitor water intake and hydration while on aminoglycoside antibiotics, particularly if the animal is concurrently receiving other nephrotoxic drugs (e.g. NSAIDs).

Amikacin: 8–10 mg/kg intramuscularly (IM) every 24 hours in adult horses; 20–25 mg/kg IM every 24 hours in foals <2 weeks of age; 15–17 mg/kg IM every 24 hours in foals 4–6 weeks of age; 500–1000 mg intra-articular.

Gentamicin: 6.6 mg/kg IM every 24 hours in adult horses; 12–14 mg/kg IM every 24 hours in foals <2 weeks of age.

Dramatic difference

Aminoglycoside doses are highly age-dependent. A higher volume of distribution in foals results in a lower maximum concentration, which may lead to decreased efficacy. Alternatively, doses used in foals may be toxic to adult horses.

21.2.1.2 Beta-Lactams

Dramatic difference

Unlike other species, oral absorption of drugs such as amoxicillin, amoxicillin clavulanate, and cephalexin is too low to reach therapeutic concentrations in adult horses. That, combined with a higher risk of the development of diarrhea with oral administration, limits their use in horses.

Cephalosporins: There are two FDA-approved ceftiofur products for horses, both of which are labeled for the treatment of respiratory infections caused by *Streptococcus zooepidemicus.* Ceftiofur sodium (Naxcel®, Zoetis) is the immediate-release formulation and, ceftiofur crystalline-free acid (Excede®, Zoetis) is the sustained-release formulation.

Ceftiofur sodium: 2.2 mg/kg IM every 24 hours
Ceftiofur crystalline-free acid: 6.6 mg/kg IM repeated once at 96 hours.

Adverse effects are rare with ceftiofur sodium, although pain during injection and diarrhea at higher than normal doses may be seen.

Owner counseling: Injection site reactions are the most frequent adverse effect of the sustained-release formulation in horses, and they can be severe. Extreme swelling, reluctance to move, and high fever can accompany injection site reactions. Owners should be counseled to monitor the site and contact their veterinarian if adverse effects are detected.

Penicillins: Procaine penicillin products are FDA approved for horses and labeled for the treatment of Gram-positive and anaerobic infections. The label dose (6600 IU/kg) is too low. Due to increasing resistance, antimicrobial susceptibility data suggest higher doses are needed to maintain therapeutic tissue and blood concentrations; therefore, extra-label use is recommended. Several of the FDA-approved products are combinations of procaine and benzathine penicillin. Benzathine penicillin is designed to be a long-acting product, providing detectable drug concentrations for two to three days. However, despite the drug being detectable, it is often present at subtherapeutic concentrations, and use of these combination products should be discouraged.

Owner counseling: In general, penicillin products are safe for use in horses, although allergic reactions can occur. The most common adverse effect with procaine penicillin products is associated with procaine rather than penicillin. Procaine reactions in horses can range from mild twitching and behavioral changes to violent seizures and even death. The reaction occurs if the drug is inadvertently injected into the blood rather than IM. Only owners well trained in administering IM injections to horses should be allowed to administer procaine penicillin.

Procaine penicillin: 22 000 IU/kg IM every 12 hours.

21.2.1.3 Amphenicols

Chloramphenicol can cause a dose-dependent, reversible bone marrow suppression in horses treated for prolonged periods of time (>2 weeks). Owners should be counseled to check a complete blood count after two weeks of therapy. Chloramphenicol has a very bitter taste. Some horses will resist administration or go off feed during treatment. Rinsing the mouth or following administration with a syringe of corn syrup may counter these problems. Because chloramphenicol clearance relies heavily on hepatic metabolism, which is delayed in foals <1 week of age and extremely delayed in premature foals (Adamson et al. 1991), it should be used with caution in those age groups. Due to its effects as a potent hepatic enzyme inhibitor, prolonged use can also result in unwanted drug–drug interactions.

Owner counseling: Humans may experience an idiosyncratic, irreversible bone marrow aplasia after exposure to even small amounts of chloramphenicol. Owners should be counseled to wear gloves during administration and to avoid inhalation, ingestion, or other physical contact with the drug. Tablets or capsules should be dissolved, rather than pulverized, when compounding paste or suspension formulations, to avoid aerosolizing the drug.

Florfenicol is structurally similar to chloramphenicol and is approved for use in food animals (see Chapter 22). *Florfenicol has an unacceptably high risk for causing diarrhea in horses and* **should not be used.**

Chloramphenicol: 35–50 mg/kg PO every six to eight hours.

21.2.1.4   Tetracyclines

Doxycycline is the most common tetracycline used in horses. Some horses will develop diarrhea as a result of treatment with doxycycline. If compounded into a solution or suspension, owners should be counseled to watch for any change in coloration that may indicate oxidation and drug degradation (Figure 21.1). Compounded solutions and suspensions have a very short (14-day maximum) shelf life.

Dramatic difference
Intravenous administration of doxycycline, at any dose, is associated with cardiac arrhythmias and possible sudden death in horses and **should not be used** (Riond et al. 1992).

Doxycycline: 10 mg/kg PO every 12 hours.

21.2.1.5   Fluoroquinolones

Enrofloxacin is the most common fluoroquinolone used in horses. A recipe for a compounded oral gel formulation of enrofloxacin made from the FDA-approved bovine injectable product (Baytril® 100, Bayer Animal Health) has been published (Table 21.2) and is used in clinical practice (Epstein et al. 2004). The bovine formulation itself cannot be directly administered orally, as it is highly irritating to the oral mucosa and its high pH may cause ion trapping in the stomach, impeding oral absorption of the drug.

Intramuscular injection is also irritating. The compounded gel formulation is intended to enhance palatability and decrease mucous membrane irritation; however, oral ulceration may still occur, so owners should be counseled to rinse the horse's mouth after administration. The gel may also be corrosive to plastic (Figure 21.2) and should be stored in a dark bottle at room temperature. Exposure to temperatures of 43 °C for one day caused a 90% drop in drug concentration from the original formulation.

Enrofloxacin is a relatively safe antibiotic in adult horses; however, fluoroquinolones can cause cartilage damage in young, growing animals. These lesions are more severe and less reversible in younger horses; however, milder changes can occur in horses up to four years of age. In addition to age, weight bearing and activity level also increase the severity of lesions. Young animals, particularly neonates, should be stall rested during and for several days after treatment with fluoroquinolones to minimize the risk. Ciprofloxacin, although less expensive than enrofloxacin and readily available in community pharmacies, **should not be used** in horses because it causes severe diarrhea.

Mandatory monitoring
Horses younger than two years of age that receive fluoroquinolone antibiotics should be stall rested and monitored for the development of joint effusion and lameness. If noted, the drug should be immediately discontinued to prevent permanent articular cartilage damage.

Enrofloxacin: 7.5–10 mg/kg PO every 24 hours.

21.2.1.6   Macrolides

Doses for commonly used oral macrolide antibiotics (azithromycin, erythromycin, and clarithromycin) in foals are listed in Table 21.3. The main indication for macrolides in horses is for treating *Rhodococcus equi* pneumonia, which occurs primarily in foals two to three months of age. Minimum

(a)

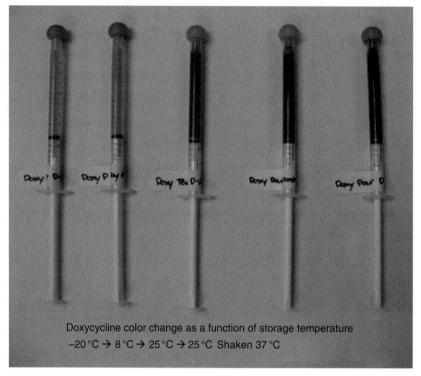

(b)

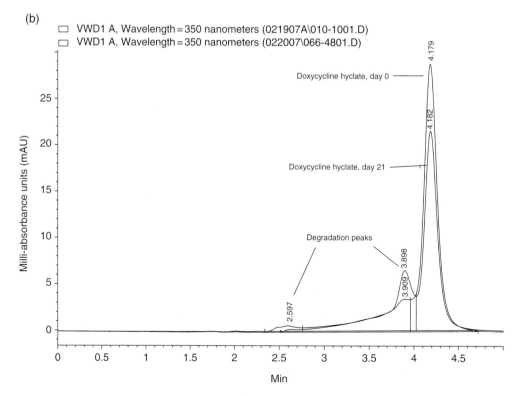

Figure 21.1 (a) Color change as a function of storage temperature in doxycycline suspension compounded from doxycycline tablets using Ora-Plus®. (b) The color change corresponds to the appearance of degradation peaks noted on the chromatograph (HPLC-UV) after 21 days of storage.

Table 21.2 Published formulation for a compounded palatable oral enrofloxacin gel for horses.

Compounded enrofloxacin oral gel formulation
To prepare 100 ml of the gel: • Pour 15 ml of injectable enrofloxacin (Baytril 100®) into a mortar. • Add 0.35 g stevia. • Add 0.6 ml apple flavor. • Mix to dissolve. • Sprinkle 2 g carboxymethylcellulose onto the solution to wet. • Mix well until smooth. • Gradually add the rest of the enrofloxacin injection while mixing (qs to 100 ml). The resulting concentration will be approximately 100 mg/ml.

Source: Epstein et al. (2004).

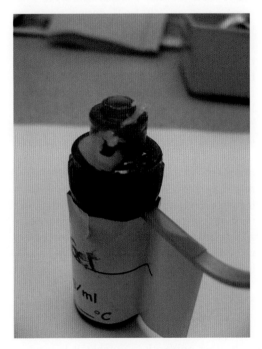

Figure 21.2 Corrosion of the plastic lid on a compounded gel formulation of enrofloxacin.

treatment duration is four weeks. Age is a critical factor when using macrolides in horses, as older foals, weanlings, and adult horses are likely to develop diarrhea if treated with macrolides. Diarrhea has even occurred in the mares of foals being treated with erythromycin, due to presumed environmental contamination (Båverud et al. 1998). Macrolide-induced diarrhea may be a result of changes in gut flora, or secondary to alter-ations in GI motility. Because erythromycin is a motilin receptor agonist in the intestinal tract, erythromycin lactobionate is sometimes used at low doses to stimulate intestinal motility (Roussel et al. 2000), particularly in horses with postoperative ileus.

Clinical experience suggests that diarrhea as a result of macrolide administration is more common with compounded formulations. The macrolides as a group are relatively insoluble in water, and attempts to compound a solution or suspension may result in precipitation of the drug (Figure 21.3). This may result in overdosing and increased risk for diarrhea as the drug is sampled from the lower portions of the container.

21.2.1.7 Potentiated Sulfonamides

There are several trimethoprim–sulfadiazine combination products that are FDA approved for use in horses, and they are available as powder or suspension formulations (Table 21.4). These products contain a 1:5 ratio of trimethoprim to sulfadiazine. Despite older label dose recommendations that indicate a once-daily dosing schedule, twice-daily dosing is currently required to achieve concentrations within the therapeutic range for most susceptible bacteria.

Trimethoprim–sulfadiazine combination products: 25 mg/kg PO every 12 hours (dose represents the quantity of trimethoprim plus sulfadiazine).

Human trimethoprim–sulfamethoxazole tablets are also frequently prescribed for use in

Table 21.3 Doses for oral macrolide antibiotics commonly used in foals for the treatment of *Rhodococcus equi* pneumonia.

Drug	Dose	Human drug formulation
Erythromycin estolate	25 mg/kg PO every 6–8 hours	Generic
Erythromycin phosphate	37.5 mg/kg PO every 12 hours	Generic
Azithromycin	10 mg/kg PO every 24 hours for 5–7 days, then every 48 h for 21–28 days	Zithromax®
Clarithromycin	7.5 mg/kg PO every 12 hours	Biaxin®

Note: Because these drugs are not FDA approved for horses, their use is considered extra-label.

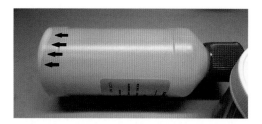

Figure 21.3 Clumping of compounded azithromycin at the bottom of the bottle (arrows), even after two minutes of vigorous shaking.

horses at a dose of 25–30 mg/kg PO every 12 hours. Although minor differences in susceptibility may exist, sulfamethoxazole is considered equivalent in activity to sulfadiazine for most important equine bacterial pathogens.

Pyrimethamine–sulfadiazine: This combination product is FDA approved as a treatment for equine protozoal myelitis. The ratio of ingredients is 1:20.

21.2.1.8 Miscellaneous Antibiotics

Metronidazole is not FDA approved for use in horses but is sometimes used in an extra-label manner. The optimum dosing regimen for metronidazole in horses is unknown. Veterinarians will vary treatments based on the horse's age and the type of infection being treated. Swain et al. (2015) demonstrated a longer elimination half-life and lower clearance in neonatal foals compared to older foals and adult horses, suggesting that neonatal foals should receive lower doses less frequently. The main adverse effect of metronidazole in horses is decreased feed

intake due to the bitter residual taste of the drug. Horses that go "off feed" during treatment should have their mouths rinsed with water or receive a syringe of corn syrup or molasses after metronidazole administration to remove the bitter taste. Other adverse effects are rare, but they may include ataxia and neurologic signs at high or prolonged doses. This can be extremely dangerous to owners if the horse falls while the owner is riding the horse or if the horse falls into the owner in a confined area. Diarrhea can also occur but is rare. All currently available pharmacokinetic studies of metronidazole in horses involve a metronidazole base. Because there are no studies using the more palatable metronidazole benzoate salt, compounded formulations using the benzoate salt should not be considered bioequivalent.

Metronidazole: 15–20 mg/kg PO every 8–12 hours.

Rifampin is rarely administered as a monotherapy in horses, but it is used in conjunction with other antibiotics. Notably, it is used in combination with macrolide antibiotics for the treatment of *R. equi* pneumonia. Rifampin is sometimes used in combination with potentiated sulfonamides or chloramphenicol. Co-administration of rifampin with macrolide antibiotics decreases oral bioavailability of the macrolide by up to 90% (Peters et al. 2011). These drugs are still used concurrently, however, due to synergistic antibacterial effects. Some clinicians advocate staggering dosing by one to two hours to help prevent this pharmacokinetic interaction.

Table 21.4 Potentiated sulfonamide combination formulations that are FDA approved for use in horses.

Drug (trade name; manufacturer)	Formulation	Individual drug concentrations	Label dose (combined drug weight)
Sulfadiazine; trimethoprim (Tribrissen® 48%; Merck, Di-Trim®; Zoetis)	Injection	400 mg/mL sulfadiazine and 80 mg/mL trimethoprim	2 mL/100 lb. (19.2 mg/kg) IV every 24 h for 5–7 days; dose can be split and administered in two doses
Sulfadiazine; trimethoprim (Tribrissen® 400 Oral; Merck, Di-Trim® 400; Zoetis)	Paste	333 mg sulfadiazine and 67 mg trimethoprim per gram of paste	3.75 g paste/110 lb. (30 mg/kg) PO every 24 hours for 5–7 days
Sulfadiazine; trimethoprim (Uniprim®; Neogen Corp., Tucoprim®; Zoetis)	Powder	333 mg sulfadiazine and 67 mg trimethoprim per gram of powder	3.75 g/110 lb. (30 mg/kg) in feed every 24 hours for 5–7 days
Sulfadiazine; trimethoprim (EQUISUL-SDT®; Aurora Pharmaceutical, LLC)	Suspension	333 mg/mL sulfadiazine and 67 mg/mL trimethoprim	24 mg/kg PO every 12 h for 10 days
Sulfadiazine; pyrimethamine (ReBalance®; Pegasus Laboratories)	Suspension	250 mg/mL sulfadiazine and 12.5 mg/mL pyrimethamine	4 mL/100 lb. (21 mg/kg) PO every 24 h for 90–270 days

---

Dramatic difference

The combination of doxycycline and rifampin used in foals resulted in hemolytic anemia and elevated liver enzymes (Venner et al. 2013). These effects have not been seen with doxycycline alone or with rifampin in combination with other drug classes.

Rifampin: 5 mg/kg PO every 12 hours.

Itraconazole is not FDA approved for use in horses, so human formulations are used in an extra-label manner. Oral bioavailability of itraconazole in horses is variable and highly dependent on formulation. The FDA-approved solution has an oral bioavailability of 60% compared with only 12% for the FDA-approved capsules. The discrepancy between the two formulations is due to the relative aqueous insolubility of the drug and the need for an acid environment for dissolution. The low pH of the solution circumvents these problems, and it therefore achieves greater oral bioavailability. Compounded itraconazole formulations, even solutions, are not orally bioavailable in horses, despite having the same concentration of active ingredient as the FDA-approved formulation (Figure 21.4). Therefore, compounded itraconazole should not be dispensed. *Ketoconazole* also has limited oral bioavailability in horses and does not achieve therapeutic concentrations. Other azole antifungal drugs, such as fluconazole and voriconazole, are well absorbed after oral administration to horses and are more suitable for use in compounded preparations. The pharmacist can play a key role in educating veterinarians about appropriate compounding of azole antifungals.

Itraconazole: 5 mg/kg PO every 24 hours.

Griseofulvin powder is FDA approved for use in horses for the treatment of dermatophytes. Teratogenic effects similar to those seen in other animals have been reported when the drug is administered to horses during pregnancy.

Griseofulvin: 2.5 g/500 kg PO every 24 hours (*Note:* the dose is not per kg but "per 500 kg").

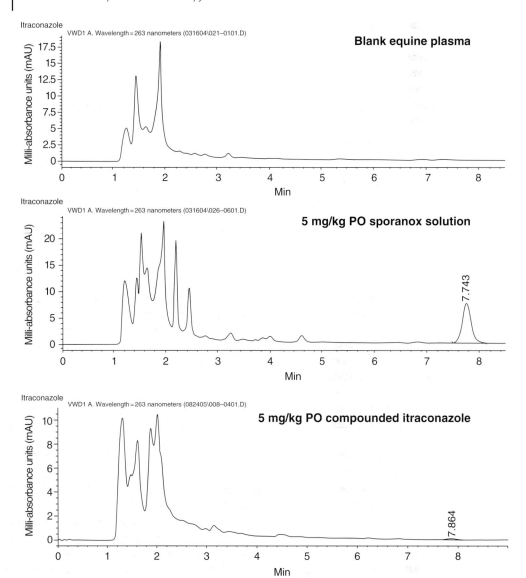

Figure 21.4 HPLC-UV chromatographs of extracted plasma from a horse administered no drug (blank equine plasma), a horse administered an FDA-approved (for people) solution of itraconazole, and a horse administered multiple doses of a compounded itraconazole formulation. The itraconazole peak appears on the right side of the chromatograph at approximately the eight-minute mark. The itraconazole plasma concentration was below the limit of detection (0.012 micrograms/mL) in the horse treated with compounded itraconazole.

21.2.2 Anti-inflammatory Drugs

21.2.2.1 Corticosteroids

As in other species, corticosteroids are used to treat a variety of inflammatory and allergic diseases. Most commonly, systemic corticosteroids are prescribed for the treatment of equine asthma, inflammatory/infiltrative bowel diseases, and allergic or immune-mediated dermatitis. Dexamethasone and prednisolone are the corticosteroids most commonly prescribed. Adverse effects of corticosteroids in the horse include potential GI ulceration, immunosuppression, iatrogenic hyperadrenocorticism and, unique to horses, *laminitis* (see Section 21.4, "Adverse Effects"). Increases in hepatic enzymes may occur in the horse; however, this seems to happen with less frequency than in dogs. Although horses are relatively insensitive to corticosteroids as a method of induction of parturition, high doses or prolonged dosing should be used only when absolutely necessary in pregnant mares.

Dexamethasone: 0.1 mg/kg PO or IM every 24 hours, tapered to the lowest dose at the longest interval possible. There are many FDA-approved formulations of dexamethasone labeled for use in horses, including injectable aqueous solutions and suspensions and oral powders and boluses. The oral formulations are difficult to obtain at times due to manufacturing shortages. In those situations, compounded formulations may be prescribed. A compounded powder formulation was shown to have good oral bioavailability (66%); however, absorption was greatly affected by feeding, with oral bioavailability decreasing to 28% in fed horses (Grady et al. 2010).

Prednisolone: 1 mg/kg PO every 24 hours, tapered to the lowest dose at the longest interval possible. Prednisolone may be less effective at clinically relevant doses than dexamethasone for inflammatory diseases in the horse but subjectively carries less risk for adverse effects. Because a single dose of prednisolone using commercially available 10 mg tablets would require 50 tablets for a 500 kg horse, prednisolone is often compounded to provide a higher strength of the drug in capsule form, for more convenient dosing.

Prednisone: Similar to cats, this drug is not effective after oral administration to horses. The active metabolite, prednisolone, is not detectable after oral administration of prednisone to horses (Peroni et al. 2002).

21.2.2.2 Nonsteroidal Anti-inflammatory Drugs

NSAIDs are prescribed frequently for horses to manage both acute (e.g. colic and fever) and chronic (e.g. osteoarthritis) diseases. There are many FDA-approved NSAIDs for use in horses, including injectable, oral, and topical formulations. The drugs licensed in the USA, available dosage forms, and recommended doses are summarized in Table 21.5. Because there are so many options, there is limited justification for compounding NSAIDs for horses. The few situations when compounding NSAIDS might be indicated include improving the taste for ease of administration or creating a more dilute dosage form for use in miniature horses or foals. Adverse effects – including renal disease; oral, gastroduodenal, and colonic ulcers (see Section 21.4, "Adverse Effects"); and injection site reactions – are relatively common. Bleeding disorders are less common in horses than in other species and typically do not occur at clinically relevant doses.

Acetaminophen: 20–30 mg/kg PO every 8–12 hours. Acetaminophen is often administered in conjunction with NSAIDs, or in animals that do not tolerate NSAIDs.

> **Dramatic difference**
>
> In contrast to dogs and cats, acetaminophen appears to be a very safe option for use in the horse.

Aspirin: 10–20 mg/kg PO every 24–48 hours. Aspirin is rarely used in horses to treat inflammation. However, it is used for its antiplatelet properties in horses with laminitis. Antiplatelet doses are well below analgesic or anti-inflammatory doses. Although there are products that are marketed for horses, none of these products are FDA approved.

Diclofenac: An FDA-approved topical product is available for horses for application directly over areas of inflammation, such as an injured joint. Due to manufacturing obstacles, product availability has sometimes been limited. Although the human product (Voltaren®) has been used as an alternative, there is some evidence (unpublished) to suggest that it is not bioequivalent to the equine product, which is formulated in a liposomal vehicle to enhance absorption.

Firocoxib: Firocoxib is most commonly used for long-term management of osteoarthritis.

Table 21.5 Label information for nonsteroidal anti-inflammatory drugs (NSAIDs) that are FDA approved for use in horses.

Drug (trade name; manufacturer)	Dose forms	Label dose
Diclofenac (Surpass®; Boehringer Ingelheim)	Topical liposomal cream (1%)	Apply a 5 in. ribbon twice daily over the affected joint for up to 10 days.
Firocoxib (Equioxx®; Merial)	Intravenous injection (20 mg/mL)	0.09 mg/kg IV every 24 hours for up to 5 days
	Oral paste (57 mg/tube) Oral tablet (57 mg/tablet)	0.1 mg/kg PO every 24 hours for up to 14 days*
Flunixin meglumine (Banamine®; Merck, generics also available)	Intravenous or intramuscular** injection (50 mg/mL) Oral paste (1500 mg/tube) Oral granules (250 mg/packet)	1.1 mg/kg IV every 12 hours for up to 3 days 1.1 mg/kg PO every 24 hours for up to 5 day.
Ketoprofen (Ketofen®; Zoetis)	Intravenous injection (100 mg/mL)	2.2 mg/kg IV every 24 h for up to 5 days
Phenylbutazone (Butazolidin®; Merck, generic)	Intravenous injection (200 mg/mL) Oral paste (6, 12 or 20 g/tube) Oral tablets (1 g/tablet) Oral powder (1 g/scoop)	2.2–4.4 mg/kg IV daily in three divided doses for up to 5 days*** 2.2–4.4 mg/kg PO daily in three divided doses; high dosage level for the first 48 h, and reduce to the lowest dosage capable of producing the desired clinical response.***

* A loading dose of 0.3 mg/kg once is recommended to achieve rapid therapeutic concentrations.
** Although intramuscular administration is on-label use, this route is contraindicated due to the risk of clostridial myositis.
*** Twice-daily dosing using the same total dose is more commonly used in equine practice.

It is the only FDA-approved COX2-selective inhibitor for horses. It is highly specific for COX2, with a COX1/COX2 IC$_{50}$ ratio of 263–643 in the horse (Kvaternick et al. 2007). The half-life of firocoxib is long (>29 hours), and therefore a loading dose of 0.3 mg/kg PO is recommended for the initial dose to reach therapeutic concentrations within 24 hours. In neonatal foals, clearance is higher, resulting in a shorter half-life, so a loading dose is not needed. However, higher doses and shorter dosing intervals are often recommended. The optimal dose for use in foals has not been established, but the drug does appear to be a safer option in neonates than many other NSAIDs (Hovanessian et al. 2014; Wilson et al. 2017). Despite the improved safety profile of the COX2 inhibitors in horses, firocoxib has been associated with renal disease and GI ulceration, particularly when administered at higher than label doses for an extended time period.

Flunixin meglumine: Clinical indications for flunixin meglumine include acute colic (as an analgesic), as an antipyretic, and at lower doses (0.25 to 0.5 mg/kg every 6–12 hours) it is used in horses that are suspected to have sepsis or endotoxemia. Flunixin has been purported to have "anti-endotoxin" properties. Despite label directions that this drug can be administered IM, it is highly irritating and is one of the drugs most frequently associated with clostridial myositis after injection (Figure 21.5). Although the FDA-approved injectable formulations can be administered orally (bioavailability of 72%; Pellegrini-Masini et al. 2004), the formulations can be bitter

(a)

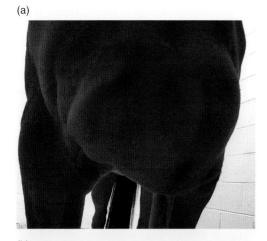

(b)

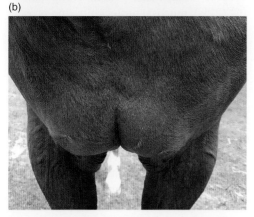

Figure 21.5 (a) Large swelling in the left pectoral muscle of a horse that received intramuscular flunixin meglumine and subsequently developed clostridial myositis. (b) A photograph of the pectoral muscles of a normal horse is included for comparison.

and irritating, and may be associated with decreased feed intake and oral ulceration.

Ketoprofen: Ketoprofen is most often used for fever that is unresponsive to other NSAIDs. It has been shown to be less ulcerogenic than flunixin meglumine and phenylbutazone at label doses (Mozaffari et al. 2010). It is also more water soluble than the other NSAIDs and less irritating for intramuscular injection.

Phenylbutazone: Phenylbutazone is typically used for horses with musculoskeletal pain and/or lameness. It is considered the most ulcerogenic of the NSAIDs at commonly used doses. Contact erosions can form on the oral mucosa and upper GI tract. Perivascular injection is highly irritating and associated with severe skin and tissue necrosis. The therapeutic goal should be to use the lowest possible dose that is effective. Horses should never receive more than 8.8 mg/kg/day (approximately 4 g per day in an average-sized adult horse), and this dose should not be maintained for more than three to five days without appropriate veterinary supervision. The pharmacokinetics of phenylbutazone are nonlinear, and plasma half-life will increase at higher doses, creating the potential for drug accumulation and increased risk for adverse effects (Tobin et al. 1986).

21.2.2.3 Intra-articular Therapies

As osteoarthritis is a common problem in equine athletes, many therapeutic agents are targeted toward local (intra-articular) administration, with the intent of achieving greater efficacy with fewer risks of systemic adverse effects. This potential benefit must be balanced with the risk of iatrogenic joint infection following intraarticular administration. Drugs that are injected intraarticularly must be sterile. Therefore, compounded products should not be substituted for FDA-approved injectable products for intraarticular use in horses. Pharmacists can play a key role in advising veterinarians and owners about the risks of using compounded products for intraarticular administration. Horses that have received an intraarticular injection should be stall rested for several days after the injection.

Corticosteroids: Triamcinolone acetonide (6–18 mg per joint), methylprednisolone acetate (20–40 mg/joint), and betamethasone acetate–sodium phosphate combination formulations (3–18 mg/joint) are all approved for intraarticular use in the horse. Despite their "local" use, systemic adverse effects can occur. Suppression of endogenous cortisol concentrations and even laminitis has been reported after intraarticular corticosteroid administration. Repeated intraarticular injections of corticosteroids can actually damage cartilage and hasten pathologic fusion of the joint. Iatrogenic joint sepsis is another serious adverse effect of intraarticular corticosteroids. To prevent this, some clinicians will concurrently inject an antibiotic. Although aminoglycosides are used most frequently for this purpose, precipitation may occur when these products are combined in the same syringe, limiting their efficacy.

Disease-modifying agents of osteoarthritis: This class of drugs is considered chondroprotective and includes products containing glycosaminoglycans and hyaluronic acid. Several injectable products are labeled for use in the horse, and multiple oral supplements are available.

21.2.2.4 Antihistamines

Antihistamines are typically used in horses to treat dermatitis or respiratory disease. Although they are used frequently, antihistamines are only minimally to moderately effective. Use should be limited to mild disease or as a preventative in horses with identified seasonal allergic disorders. Adverse effects are unlikely when administered orally, although sedation may be noted. High doses, particularly for injected antihistamines, can cause excitement, tremors, seizures, colic, and loss of appetite.

Cetirizine: 0.2–0.4 mg/kg PO every 12 hours

Chlorpheniramine: 0.25–0.5 mg/kg PO every 6–12 hours

Hydroxyzine: 0.5–1 mg/kg PO every 8 hours

Pyrilamine maleate: 0.66 mg/kg IM or subcutaneously every 6–12 hours (FDA approved for horses)

Tripelennamine hydrochloride: 1.1 mg/kg IM every 6–12 hours. Warm the solution prior to injection, and inject only into large muscle masses, such as the cervical or hind limb musculature (FDA approved for horses).

21.2.3 Anti-ulcer Drugs

Gastric ulcers are a common malady in horses, occurring in up to 90% of sport horse populations. Equine gastric ulcer syndrome (EGUS) is a general term to describe erosive and ulcerative diseases of the stomach, consistent with the use of the term peptic ulcer disease (PUD) in humans (Sykes et al. 2015). Equine squamous gastric disease (ESGD) and equine glandular gastric disease (EGGD) are terms that more specifically describe disease in the upper and lower anatomic regions of the stomach, respectively. The pathophysiology, predisposing factors, treatment recommendations, and prognosis for complete resolution for ESGD and EGGD differ, with EGGD being a more severe form of the disease. Multiple classes of drugs are used to treat EGUS, including H_2-histamine receptor antagonists, proton pump inhibitors (PPIs), mucosal protectants, and prostaglandin E analogs. These drugs are associated with very few adverse effects in horses.

21.2.3.1 H$_2$-Receptor Antagonists

These drugs are occasionally still used for treating either ESGD or EGGD, but they have fallen out of favor with the availability of PPIs. Rarely, a horse that does not respond to a PPI will respond to an H_2-receptor antagonist. Drugs in this class may be used for the initial few days of treatment combined with a PPI, because maximal acid suppression by omeprazole may be delayed for up to three to five days. The oral bioavailability and duration of action vary among drugs.

Ranitidine: 6.6 mg/kg PO every 8 hours. This is the most frequently prescribed H_2 receptor antagonist because of its consistent bioavailability and acid suppression. Prokinetic effects have also been ascribed to ranitidine, which may be beneficial in horses with ileus.

Cimetidine: 40–60 mg/kg PO every 8 hours. Cimetidine is rarely used for EGUS due to unreliable acid suppression and potential drug–drug interactions. It is, however, used occasionally for its immunomodulating effects. Cimetidine can block H_2-receptors on suppressor T-lymphocytes, inhibiting their function and potentially increasing responses to mitogen stimulation. It is therefore sometimes used for the treatment of melanomas in horses, although controlled clinical studies are lacking.

Famotidine: 0.5 to 2 mg/kg PO every 8 hours. This drug is used infrequently orally in horses, as it is a less effective acid suppressant in horses than ranitidine.

21.2.3.2 Proton Pump Inhibitors

PPIs are the treatment of choice for ESGD; however, EGGD is less likely to respond to treatment. For treatment of EGGD, PPIs should be combined with sucralfate.

Omeprazole: 1–2 mg/kg PO every 24 hours for ulcer prevention; 4 mg/kg PO every 24 hours for 3 weeks for treatment of ESGD or for 8–12 weeks for treatment of EGGD. There are two FDA-approved formulations of omeprazole for horses, one for ulcer prevention and one for ulcer treatment. Omeprazole is acid-labile and oral absorption is minimal, unless it is administered in a buffered vehicle. The FDA-approved products are appropriately buffered, allowing omeprazole to survive the acidic environment of the stomach. The drug then undergoes dissolution and absorption in the more alkaline small intestine. Compounded formulations are generally not appropriately buffered and are often ineffective or (at best) have a fraction of the efficacy of the FDA-approved products. For this reason, compounded omeprazole should not be substituted for FDA-approved products (Figure 21.6). Because feeding also decreases oral absorption, omeprazole should be administered 30 minutes prior to a meal. In horses, an all-hay diet dramatically decreases oral absorption and therefore efficacy of omeprazole (Sykes et al. 2017).

The most common adverse effect of omeprazole in horses is lack of efficacy. The side effects frequently seen in humans (e.g. fever, stomach pain) are not associated with omeprazole use in horses. Long-term use of PPIs and their association with malabsorption and increased risk of infection as seen in humans have not been documented in horses.

21.2.3.3 Mucosal Protectants

Sucralfate: 12–20 mg/kg PO every 6–12 hours. Sucralfate as monotherapy is

(a)
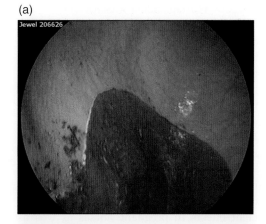

(b)
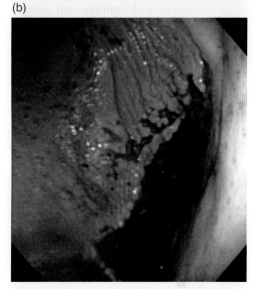

Figure 21.6 (a) Endoscopic view of normal equine gastric squamous mucosa, compared to (b) the severely ulcerated gastric squamous mucosa of a horse that received unbuffered compounded omeprazole for 30 days.

not successful in treating gastric ulceration in adult horses. Therefore, it is commonly used in combination with either ranitidine or omeprazole. As in humans, sucralfate can be involved in drug interactions limiting oral bioavailability of concurrently administered drugs. Separating oral drug doses from sucralfate administration by at least 2 hours is recommended to prevent drug interactions.

21.2.3.4 Prostaglandin E Analogs

Misoprostol: 5 micrograms/kg PO every 8–12 hours. Misoprostol has historically been used only for NSAID-associated ulceration. However, recent evidence suggests that it may be superior to omeprazole for treating EGGD (Varley et al. 2016). There is no evidence supporting its use in ESGD. Misoprostol can cause mild to moderate abdominal pain, colic, and diarrhea in horses. There are no data determining the safety of its use in pregnant mares. Owners should be counseled on misoprostol's possible abortifacient effects in pregnant horses as well as potential risks for pregnant women even when handling the drug.

21.2.4 Miscellaneous Drugs

Acepromazine: 0.044–0.088 mg/kg, IM or subcutaneously. Acepromazine is FDA approved as an injectable sedative/tranquilizer in horses. Its use as a sedative is favored by some clinicians because of its relatively long duration of effect (four to six hours). It can be used in combination with opioids and α-2 agonists (i.e. xylazine and detomidine); however, lower doses are advised (0.02 mg/kg) to avoid oversedation. Acepromazine is also used as a vasodilator in horses with laminitis. Adverse effects include profound sedation, decreased red and white blood cell counts, decreased hemoglobin and hematocrit (Parry et al. 1982; Hashem and Keller 1993), hypotension, and prolonged penile prolapse and priapism.

n-Acetylcysteine: The FDA-approved human product (20% solution) is administered to horses topically, within the guttural pouch, every 24 hours for the treatment of chondroids. For different indications, see Section 21.3, "Drugs Commonly Compounded for Horses."

> **Dramatic difference**
>
> Horses are one of the few species that have guttural pouches, which are sacs of air that expand from the eustachian tubes, one on each side of the head. Passing through each guttural pouch are critical structures, including the internal and external carotid arteries, several cranial nerves (CN IX, X, XI, and XII), and the vagosympathetic trunk. These structures are subject to trauma, inflammation, and damage with diseases that affect the guttural pouch. Additionally, any drugs instilled into or applied to the guttural pouch can cause chemical damage or irritation of these nerves, resulting in difficulty swallowing or breathing, and changes in facial expression and head posture.

Albuterol: 0.05 mg/kg PO as needed. Oral albuterol may be used as a bronchodilator for horses with asthma; however, its efficacy is questionable and likely decreases over time due to tolerance. Co-administration of corticosteroids may prolong efficacy. Inhalation is a much more effective route of administration. There is an FDA-approved albuterol metered-dose inhaler for horses (Chapter 25). The dose is 3–6 puffs (120 micrograms/puff), up to 4 times daily for a 1000-pound horse.

Although beta-adrenergic agonists are considered relatively safe drugs, adverse effects including sweating, muscle tremors, tachycardia, hypotension, and restlessness may occur, particularly at high doses. Beta-adrenergic agonists may antagonize the effects of prostaglandin $F_{2\alpha}$ and oxytocin and are occasionally used to prevent early parturition in mares. They should not be used in normal pregnant mares near term, however, as they may delay labor.

Altrenogest: 44–88 micrograms/kg PO every 24 hours. Altrenogest is FDA approved for use in horses and is used to suppress estrus or maintain pregnancy in mares. Adverse effects in horses are minimal, but humans handling the drug can experience adverse effects. Altrenogest is photosensitive and must be kept protected from light.

> **Mandatory monitoring**
>
> Owners (and pharmacists) must be counseled to wear nonpermeable gloves when handling altrenogest. Pregnant women or

> those who suspect they may be pregnant should not handle this drug. Altrenogest is readily absorbed through the skin and can result in disruption of the estrus cycle, cramping, and prolonged gestation in humans. In the case of accidental contact, the skin should be washed off immediately with soap and water.

Clenbuterol: An FDA-approved oral (syrup) formulation of clenbuterol is available for horses. The recommended dose is 0.8–3.2 micrograms/kg PO every 12 hours. Clenbuterol is prohibited for use in food animals and is not approved for use in people in the USA. It is considered a performance-enhancing drug; therefore, diversion is a potential problem that the pharmacist should be aware of. Adverse effects are similar to those described for albuterol.

Dipyrone: 25–30 mg/kg PO every 8 hours. There are currently no dipyrone products available in the USA, although there are multiple formulations labeled for horses either alone or combined with N-butylscopolamine in Canada, Europe, and other countries. It is mainly used for treating acute colic and as an anti-pyretic. It is not legal to use in food animals in the USA, as it has been linked to blood dyscrasias and teratogenesis in humans.

Pergolide: 2–4 micrograms/kg PO every 24 hours. Pergolide is a dopaminergic agonist used to treat equine Cushing's disease (hyperadrenocorticism). The FDA-approved human products have all been removed from the market due to an association with development of cardiac valvular diseases (Tran et al. 2015). Shortly after pergolide was pulled from the market in the USA, the FDA issued a limited exemption allowing pergolide products to be compounded from bulk substance. However, an FDA-approved pergolide product for horses has been available since 2011. *The FDA has since rescinded this exemption, and any compounded products must be made from the proprietary formulation.* Pergolide is not stable when exposed to heat or light (Davis et al. 2009). Compounded pergolide formulations should be stored in a dark container, protected from light, and refrigerated, and they should be discarded not later than 30 days after they are compounded. Formulations that have undergone a color change have likely undergone degradation and should be discarded immediately.

Dramatic difference

Dopamine agonists are not used to treat Cushing's disease in dogs or humans because the pathophysiology of the disease differs. While the disease in each of these species involves excessive adrenocorticotropin (ΛCTH) secretion by the pituitary gland, the region of the pituitary gland secreting ACTH differs. Horses with Cushing's disease experience pituitary pars intermedia dysfunction, while in dogs and humans it is usually the pars distalis that is involved. Dopamine inhibits ACTH secretion from the pars intermedia but does not affect ACTH secretion from the pars distalis.

21.3 Drugs Commonly Compounded for Horses

Acepromazine: Indications for acepromazine were discussed earlier in the chapter (injectable acepromazine). While there is no need to compound injectable acepromazine, there is sometimes a need to compound acepromazine for oral administration to horses. Oral bioavailability is approximately 50%, and doses higher than parenteral doses are often used (0.5–0.8 mg/kg). Oral administration appears to be safer than parenteral administration and avoids most of the common side effects. FDA-approved acepromazine tablets are available for dogs and should be used rather than bulk drug for compounding oral acepromazine formulations for horses.

Cisplatin: 1 mg/cm^3 of tumor intralesionally every two to four weeks for four treatments or until resolution of the tumor without regrowth. Cisplatin is mainly used to treat dermal tumors, such as sarcoids, melanomas, and sometimes squamous cell carcinomas. Carboplatin is sometimes substituted for cisplatin, depending on the availability of either compound. FDA-approved products for humans are only available as IV infusion formulations. For treatment of skin tumors in horses, a slow-release formulation that can be directly injected into the tumor is preferred to provide high concentrations at the tumor site while minimizing high systemic concentrations (to decrease the risk of adverse effects). To provide a depo effect, cisplatin is either mixed with sterile sesame oil or delivered in a biodegradable, implantable bead. The beads are being investigated for FDA approval, and clinical trials have been performed under an investigational new animal drug application (Matrix III Cisplatin Beads; Royer Biomedical). Reports indicate that intralesional use of cisplatin does not cause systemic side effects. Local side effects are reported to resolve quickly. Treatment is often in conjunction with surgical debridement and/or cryotherapy.

Dantrolene: 4 mg/kg PO or via nasogastric tube 90 minutes prior to exercise and within four hours of feeding. Dantrolene is used to prevent acute rhabdomyolysis and post-anesthetic myositis in susceptible horses. There is evidence to support its efficacy in decreasing muscle damage, but it can also decrease cardiac output and predispose horses to hyperkalemia and arrhythmias if used concurrently with anesthetic agents.

Isoxsuprine: 1.2 mg/kg PO every 8–12 hours, increasing the dosing interval to every 48 hours over time. Parenteral administration is associated with central nervous system (CNS) excitement and sweating. Although there is a tablet form of the drug that is FDA approved for use in people, it is not conducive for treating horses because each dose would require 60 tablets. Owner compliance and accuracy could become limiting factors, so when this drug is used, many veterinarians prefer to have it compounded into a more user-friendly formulation for horse owners.

Methocarbamol: 4.4–5.5 mg/kg PO as needed. Methocarbamol is used as a muscle relaxant. An FDA-approved intravenous product for horses has previously been available,

---

Practiced but not proven
Isoxsuprine is used to treat navicular disease, a common cause of lameness in horses. Because oral bioavailability is low, plasma concentrations necessary to cause vasodilation are unlikely to be achieved when the drug is administered orally (Erkert and Macallister 2002).

but is currently not marketed, and use of the human product IV is cost prohibitive. Higher doses are used for more severely affected cases, but can be associated with adverse effects such as sedation and ataxia. Because a convenient dosing form for horses is not available, it has been compounded in a suspension formulation.

Misoprostol: In addition to its use for gastric ulcer disease, misoprostol is also used as a compounded suspension that is topically applied to the cervix to aid in cervical dilation when inducing parturition. Owners must be counseled on possible abortifacient effects in pregnant women handling the drug.

n-Acetylcysteine: Several indications for n-acetylcysteine require compounding because commercial products are not available at the desired concentration. For example, a 5% solution for intrauterine administration is used for treating endometritis in mares; 8 g of n-acetylcysteine is combined with sodium bicarbonate (20 g), diluted in 200 mL of water, and administered intrarectally in foals as needed for the treatment of meconium impactions. Local irritation may occur but is typically minimal, and topical application is generally considered safe.

Pentoxifylline: 8.5–10 mg/kg PO every 12 hours. In horses, pentoxifylline is used as an adjunct therapy to treat laminitis and navicular disease, vasculitis, placentitis, and dermatitis. Absorption is rapid after oral administration, but elimination is variable. Serum concentrations decrease with repeated dosing, potentially necessitating an increase in the dosage (Liska et al. 2006). Oral dosing is well tolerated.

Practiced but not proven

An intravenous formulation of pentoxifylline can be compounded by dissolving drug in sterile water to a concentration of 50 mg/mL. Although this has been used for treatment of sepsis and endotoxemia in foals and horses, there is no evidence to support its safety or efficacy.

Pyrimethamine: Compounded pyrimethamine plus toltrazuril (poultry antiprotozoal) combinations have been used for treating equine protozoal myelitis, although toltrazuril is not approved for use in any form in horses. Care must be taken to ensure proper ratios are maintained. In 2014, a number of horses developed severe neurological toxicity (seizures and death) after being treated with a compounded pyrimethamine–toltrazuril formulation. Instead of the intended 416 mg/mL of toltrazuril and 17 mg/mL pyrimethamine, analysis revealed that the drug concentrations were reversed, and the formulation contained 416 mg/mL pyrimethamine and 17 mg/mL toltrazuril. *With several FDA-approved drugs for treating equine protozoal myelitis, it is difficult to justify dispensing a compounded drug for this disease.*

Reserpine: 2–8 micrograms/kg PO every 24 hours. Reserpine is used as a long-term oral sedative in horses on stall rest or with certain behavioral vices. The most common adverse effects are lack of efficacy, oversedation, colic, and diarrhea. Adverse effects are more common when the drug is administered IM; therefore, this route is used less frequently. Since there is not an FDA-approved reserpine formulation, compounded products are used.

Mandatory monitoring

Caution should be used when reserpine is administered to horses prior to anesthesia. Anecdotal reports of severe hypotension, prolonged recovery, and even death in horses anesthetized while on reserpine have occurred. These effects may last up to six weeks after withdrawal of the drug. Owners should be instructed to inform any veterinarian that their horse has been treated with reserpine prior to any anesthetic event.

21.4 Adverse Effects of Selected Drugs Specific to Horses

21.4.1 Antibiotics and Diarrhea

Antimicrobial-associated diarrhea (AAD) is the most frequently reported adverse effect of antibacterial drugs in horses. In a retrospective study of equine patients, from three referral veterinary hospitals in the USA, diarrhea developed in only 0.6% (32/5251) of horses treated with antibiotics for non-GI conditions. However, horses that did develop AAD had an 18.8% (6/32) mortality rate (Barr et al. 2013). The pathophysiology of AAD likely involves a change in GI and colonic microbial flora. Horses may be more susceptible to AAD than other animals due to low oral absorption, with subsequent increased delivery of active drug to the intestine and colon. Diarrhea is not limited to oral antibiotic administration, however, and injectable drugs have been implicated in AAD (Costa et al. 2015). This is likely due to biliary excretion of active drug into the small intestine. Bacteria most often associated with AAD are *Salmonella* and *Clostridium* spp.; however, an etiologic agent is not always identified. Alteration of GI motility may be another pathophysiologic mechanism for AAD in horses, as is the case with erythromycin.

Although any antibiotic can cause diarrhea, there are some antibiotics that should never be administered to horses by any route because of their strong association with severe, life-threatening diarrhea. The lincosamides (clindamycin and lincomycin) cause a severe, often-fatal diarrhea so predictably that they have even been used to

Table 21.6 Antibiotics most frequently associated with causing diarrhea in horses.

Antimicrobial-associated diarrhea	
Severe or frequent	**Mild or infrequent**
Clindamycin	Trimethoprim–sulfonamide (TMS) combinations
Lincomycin	Penicillin
Ciprofloxacin	Doxycycline
Moxifloxacin	Enrofloxacin
Neomycin	Gentamicin (often combined with penicillin or TMS)
Oxytetracycline (oral)	
Erythromycin (in adult horses)	
Florfenicol	
Tylosin	

create an experimental model for colitis in the horse. The human fluoroquinolone ciprofloxacin, if administered intravenously or orally, causes severe AAD, even though the veterinary fluoroquinolones enrofloxacin and marbofloxacin are tolerated by horses. Macrolide antibiotics, while safe to administer in young foals (two to three months of age), often cause diarrhea in older foals, weanlings, and adults. Other antibiotics associated with colitis are listed in Table 21.6.

> **Mandatory monitoring**
>
> All horses for which an antibiotic is dispensed should be monitored for signs of colic and diarrhea. If noted, the antibiotic should be discontinued and a veterinarian contacted immediately.

21.4.2 Corticosteroids and Laminitis

Laminitis, also known as "founder," is a disease in which the laminae of the foot become damaged and destroyed. The laminae are soft tissue structures that attach the coffin bone (distal phalanx) of the foot to the hoof wall. Loss of the laminae creates instability of the coffin bone and may result in separation of and rotation or sinking of the coffin bone within the hoof wall. In the most severe cases, the coffin bone may rotate through the bottom of the hoof, or the hoof wall may separate and slough (Figure 21.7). Laminitis is a crippling, excruciatingly painful condition of horses that can necessitate humane euthanasia in severe cases. Once a horse has experienced one episode of laminitis, that animal remains susceptible to future episodes. Lifelong monitoring and management are required.

Corticosteroid-associated laminitis in horses has long been clinically recognized but has not been experimentally reproduced (Bailey 2010). There are many other potential causes of laminitis, and it is likely that other predisposing factors may need to be present for corticosteroids to induce the disease. Predisposing factors include grain/carbohydrate overload, septicemic or endotoxic conditions (e.g. retained placenta in mares), trauma, lameness in one limb causing increased load bearing on a supporting limb, and obesity. In the author's experience, obese horses are most at risk for developing laminitis following corticosteroid administration. This may be due to the relationship between obesity and insulin resistance seen in horses with equine metabolic syndrome, a disease that parallels type 2 diabetes in humans. Persistent hyperinsulinemia has been shown to cause laminitis in horses (de Laat et al. 2010), and corticosteroids are renowned for their ability to cause insulin resistance in any mammalian species.

(a)

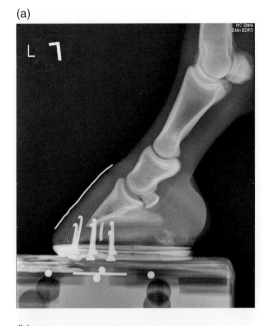

(b)

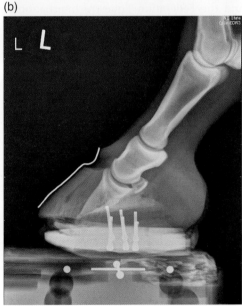

Figure 21.7 (a) Lateral radiograph of a normal equine hoof with a metal strip attached to the front of the hoof to demonstrate normal alignment of the hoof wall with the coffin bone. In contrast, (b) a lateral radiograph of an equine hoof with severe rotation and sinking (due to corticosteroid-associated laminitis). Note that the coffin bone is essentially protruding from the bottom of the foot. Despite aggressive treatment, the horse was euthanized.

Triamcinolone and dexamethasone (relatively potent and intermediate to long acting) are the two corticosteroids most commonly associated with inducing laminitis in horses. Systemic administration is thought to carry the highest risk, whereas local administration (e.g. inhalation or intraarticular) is considered safer. Recommendations for dosing should include a tapering schedule to reach the lowest dose and longest dosing interval that achieve an acceptable therapeutic effect.

Mandatory monitoring
All horses for which systemic corticosteroids are dispensed should be monitored for lameness, increased heat in the hoof, or increased pulses palpable in the arteries of the foot.

21.4.3 NSAIDS and Right Dorsal Colitis

Like other species, horses are susceptible to gastroduodenal ulceration and renal toxicity following exposure to NSAIDs. Unique to horses is the development of a syndrome called right dorsal colitis. Right dorsal colitis is associated with mucosal ulceration, edema, neutrophilic inflammation, and mural thickening of the right dorsal colon, a segment of the large colon located in the upper right quadrant of the horse's abdomen (Davis 2017). It is not known why this particular segment of the intestine is affected to a greater extent than other anatomic areas. The etiology is thought to be similar to gastric ulceration and related to a decrease in PGE_2 production.

Right dorsal colitis has been diagnosed most often in horses given excessive doses of NSAIDs, in particular phenylbutazone. However, it may also occur in horses receiving recommended doses. It has been reported not only with phenylbutazone, but also with flunixin meglumine and firocoxib. It appears to be precipitated by dehydration and anorexia;

therefore, NSAIDs should be used with caution in horses that are not eating or drinking adequately. Co-administration of two NSAIDs may also increase the risk of right dorsal colitis, and this practice should be discouraged.

Horses with right dorsal colitis will show signs of depression, lethargy, colic, and diarrhea, and they almost invariably have a low plasma protein concentration. Ventral (dependent) edema may also develop and may be the first sign noted by owners. Diagnosis is confirmed by ultrasonography, which reveals a thickened (>1 cm) right dorsal colon. Treatment involves prompt discontinuation of all NSAIDs, dietary changes, and colloidal and fluid support. Misoprostol can be administered orally to help increase colonic mucosal blood flow, which may enhance healing. Prognosis of horses with right dorsal colitis is usually guarded, unless the diagnosis is made early and all NSAID treatment is stopped. Death may occur acutely from colonic rupture or chronically as a consequence of colonic stricture and associated chronic colic.

Mandatory monitoring

All horses for which an NSAID is dispensed should be monitored for the development of colic, diarrhea, and ventral edema. Owners should ensure the horse is eating well during NSAID treatment and drinking at least 25 L of water per day (adult horse). Blood chemistries (creatinine and albumin) should be evaluated at least once weekly when animals are treated for longer than label dosing recommendations.

21.5 Regulatory Drug Restrictions for Performance Horses

An important consideration when the pharmacist is dispensing drugs for horses is the regulatory aspect of drug use in performance horses. Horses that are used for show or racing must follow regulations set forth by the relevant governing bodies of the sport. These guidelines have been put in place not only to ensure a level playing field but also to make sure that horses are not pushed beyond their physiologic capabilities, thus preserving the health and well-being of the animal. Multiple agencies may be involved in regulating drug use in horses, depending on the level of competition, the event, the location of the event, and the breed of the horse. Therefore, it can be challenging to determine if a particular drug is prohibited for a particular horse at any given time.

There are three main governing bodies overseeing drug use regulation in performance horses in the USA: the Association of Racing Commissioners International (ARCI), the United States Equestrian Federation (USEF), and the Fédération Equestre Internationale (FEI). ARCI is the umbrella organization for professional horse and greyhound racing in North America and parts of the Caribbean. USEF oversees drug regulations for multiple breeds and disciplines and implements drug-testing rules for state and national groups. FEI is an international governing body and is involved in high-level international competitions held in the USA.

In addition to these agencies, individual breed or discipline associations or state governments may have different rules. Unfortunately, in some cases, these rules are conflicting. Other organizations with their own unique regulations include the American Quarter Horse Association (AQHA), the United States Polo Association (USPA), and the American Endurance Ride Conference (AERC).

In general, drugs used in preventative medicine are allowed in most competitions. For example, anthelmintic medications and insect repellants are not prohibited. However, exceptions exist (levamisole and tetramisole). Anti-ulcer medications are also allowed, given the frequency of EGUS in competition horses. Antibiotics and antiprotozoals are allowed in certain circumstances.

Table 21.7 Selected websites for organizations that regulate drug use in performance and/or racehorses.

Organization	Website
ARCI	http://www.arci.com
USEF	http://www.usef.org/contentPage2.aspx?id=ruleshome
FEI	http://www.feicleansport.org
AERC	https://www.aerc.org/static/DrugRuleAppendices.pdf
AQHA	https://www.aqha.com/media/9467/aqha-handbook-2016.pdf
USPA	https://www.uspolo.org/assets/docs/2016-EDMP-Rules.pdf
American Association of Equine Practitioners (AAEP)	http://www.aaep.org/medication_rules.htm

Procaine penicillin is not allowed in some cases, as the procaine component may act as a performance-enhancing substance. Topical drugs and oral or parenteral joint therapies are not prohibited; however, FEI prohibits intraarticular drugs.

There is also a somewhat graded system for drug use. Although some drugs are permitted, others are restricted/controlled, and still others are banned/forbidden. Restricted or controlled substances are those drugs that have true therapeutic purposes in equine medicine but are forbidden in competition. Examples include clenbuterol and NSAIDs. A withdrawal time prior to competition must be assigned to these drugs. Additionally, the veterinarian may need to provide documentation justifying the use of a particular drug. Banned substances are those considered to have no therapeutic benefit in the horse but may be used for "doping" (pure performance enhancement) purposes. Examples include amphetamines, cocaine, and opiates. This prohibition may also extend to known active drug metabolites in order to prevent the use of designer drugs that may be compounded from substances not commercially available. "Natural" plant-based compounds, or nutraceuticals, are not regulated by the FDA as drugs; however, they may appear on the FEI and USEF forbidden-substance lists.

A list of all the regulated drugs for competition horses is beyond the scope of this chapter. However, pharmacists dispensing drugs for use in horses should be aware of these regulations and have access to resources that define the use of these drugs. A list of websites detailing this information is available in Table 21.7. Several resources are also available to review this particular topic (Gowen and Lengel 1993; Short et al. 1998).

Finally, although it is illegal to sell horsemeat for human consumption in the USA, there is a market for horsemeat in many other countries. Therefore, all drugs dispensed for equine patients in the USA should bear the statement "Do not use in horses intended for human consumption."

21.6 Nutritional Supplements Used in Horses

Numerous so-called "nutraceutical" products are used in horses. Most commonly, these are joint supplements; however, anti-oxidants, calming agents, gastroprotectants, and probiotics are also used. This section is a brief summary of some of the nutritional supplements for horses that a pharmacist may be asked about.

Pentosan polysulfate sodium (125 mg/mL) is a joint supplement available in several countries for the treatment of osteoarthritis. It is one of the more commonly compounded products used for horses with osteoarthritis in the USA. It is often combined with N-acetyl glucosamine (200 mg/mL). It is marketed as a sterile postsurgical lavage designed to replace synovial fluid lost during arthroscopy, but it is often used systemically (IM) for the treatment of joint damage and joint disease. Controlled studies establishing efficacy are lacking.

Other "joint supplements" are administered orally and include chondroitin sulfate, glucosamine, methylsulfonyl-methane (MSM), or some combination thereof. These products are safe and are thought to have a mild to moderate effect on joint pain and lameness.

Anti-oxidants: Products containing vitamin E and selenium are commonly used for anti-oxidant effects, as well as to treat or prevent neurologic and muscle-related diseases in horses that are genetically predisposed. They may also be used in geographical areas of the country where the forage is deficient in vitamin E or selenium. Vitamin E toxicity has not been documented in horses. The type of vitamin E must be considered when determining the appropriate dose. Natural non-racemic vitamin E in a micellized (non-acetate) form has a higher activity and bioavailability compared to synthetic forms (Finno and Valberg 2012). In contrast to vitamin E, selenium can be toxic and even fatal at high doses. A single oral dose of 3.3 mg/kg (even less for injectable products) can cause signs of toxicity, including pulmonary edema, hypotension, unconsciousness, and death. In 2008, 21 polo ponies died following administration of a compounded vitamin and mineral supplement prior to a competition. Forensic analysis revealed that the cause of death was a massive overdose of selenium (Desta et al. 2011). Further investigation revealed that the compounding pharmacy had been attempting to replicate a product available overseas that *should have contained 0.1 g selenium, but the compound contained 10 g instead.*

"Calming" agents: Calming agents often contain magnesium, because nervousness is one of many clinical signs of magnesium deficiency in horses. However, magnesium deficiency is not common in horses, so magnesium supplementation is not likely to be effective as a calming agent for the majority of horses. While magnesium supplementation is unlikely to cause toxicity, it can be associated with visual disturbances, ataxia, and weakness. *Alpha-casozepine*, a derivative of bovine milk casein, has calmative anxiolytic-like properties in humans and other species, including horses. At least one study has shown that alpha-casozepine holds promise as an aid to improve efficiency of handling and training horses (McDonnell et al. 2013).

Gastroprotectants: Due to the high prevalence of EGUS and the high cost of treatment with anti-ulcer drugs, many owners will use nutritional supplements that are purported to aid in digestion and may help prevent ulcers from forming. Common ingredients in these types of formulations include *aloe vera*, antacids (e.g. calcium carbonate), and amino acids (e.g. glutamine and glycine). Of the supplements tested, pectin–lecithin combination products appear to be more efficacious than others.

Client counseling: Owners should be made aware that these supplements are not substitutes for FDA-approved drugs in horses with EGUS. If symptoms persist while the horse is on these supplements, the horse should be examined by a veterinarian.

Probiotics: Probiotics are often administered to horses when sudden dietary changes are introduced, during stressful conditions (e.g. transport or a new environment), or if the horse has a GI disease that is likely to result in diarrhea. Most products contain *Lactobacillus* sp. and *Saccharomyces boulardii*. There is little evidence supporting the use of probiotics in horses (Schoster *et al.* 2014). Of the studies published to date, minimal to no beneficial effects have been documented in adult horses. Studies in foals have even suggested a potentially harmful effect, including an increased risk of diarrhea (Schoster et al. 2015).

References

Adamson, P.J., Wilson, W.D., Baggot, J.D. et al. (1991). Influence of age on the disposition kinetics of chloramphenicol in equine neonates. *Am. J. Vet. Res.* 52 (3): 426–431.

Baggot, J.D. (1992). Bioavailability and bioequivalence of veterinary drug dosage forms, with particular reference to horses: an overview. *J. Vet. Pharmacol. Ther.* 15 (2): 160–173.

Bailey, S.R. (2010). Corticosteroid-associated laminitis. *Vet. Clin. N. Am. Equine Pract.* 26 (2): 277–275.

Baker, S.J. and Gerring, E.L. (1993). Technique for prolonged, minimally invasive monitoring of intragastric pH in ponies. *Am. J. Vet. Res.* 54 (10): 1725–1734.

Baker, S.J. and Gerring, E.L. (1994). Gastric emptying of solid, non-digestible, radiopaque markers in ponies. *Res. Vet. Sci.* 56 (3): 386–388.

Baker, S.J., Gerring, E.L., and Fox, M.T. (1993). Twenty-four hour gastric pH monitoring and blood gastrin concentrations in fasted ponies. *Res. Vet. Sci.* 55 (2): 261–264.

Barnhart, M.D., Hubbell, J.A., Muir, W.W. et al. (2000). Pharmacokinetics, pharmacodynamics, and analgesic effects of morphine after rectal, intramuscular, and intravenous administration in dogs. *Am. J. Vet. Res.* 61 (1): 24–28.

Barr, B.S., Waldridge, B.M., Morresey, P.R. et al. (2013). Antimicrobial-associated diarrhoea in three equine referral practices. *Equine Vet. J.* 45 (2): 154–158.

Båverud, V., Franklin, A., Gunnarsson, A. et al. (1998). Clostridium difficile associated with acute colitis in mares when their foals are treated with erythromycin and rifampicin for *Rhodococcus equi* pneumonia. *Equine Vet. J.* 30 (6): 482–488.

Berry, L.M., Li, C., and Zhao, Z. (2011). Species differences in distribution and prediction of human Vss from preclinical data. *Drug Metab. Dispos.* 39 (11): 2103–2116.

Combie, J.D., Nugent, T.E., and Tobin, T. (1983). Pharmacokinetics and protein binding of morphine in horses. *Am. J. Vet. Res.* 44 (5): 870–874.

Costa, M.C., Stämpfli, H.R., Arroyo, L.G. et al. (2015). Changes in the equine fecal microbiota associated with the use of systemic antimicrobial drugs. *BMC Vet. Res.* 11: 19.

Crisman, M.V., Wilcke, J.R., Correll, L.S. et al. (1993). Pharmacokinetic disposition of intravenous and oral pentoxifylline in horses. *J. Vet. Pharmacol. Ther.* 16 (1): 23–31.

Davenport, H.W. (1982). Intestinal absorption of water and electrolytes. In: *Physiology of the Gastrointestinal Tract*, 5e (ed. H.W. Davenport). Chicago: Year Book Medical Publishers.

Davis, J.L. (2017). Nonsteroidal anti-inflammatory drug associated right dorsal colitis in the horse. *Equine Vet. Educ.* 29 (2): 104–113.

Davis, J.L., Kirk, L.M., Davidson, G.S. et al. (2009). Effects of compounding and storage conditions on stability of pergolide mesylate. *J. Am. Vet. Med. Assoc.* 234 (3): 385–389.

Davis, J.L., Salmon, J.H., and Papich, M.G. (2006). Pharmacokinetics and tissue distribution of doxycycline after oral administration of single and multiple doses in horses. *Am. J. Vet. Res.* 67 (2): 310–316.

Desta, B., Maldonado, G., Reid, H. et al. (2011). Acute selenium toxicosis in polo ponies. *J. Vet. Diagn. Invest.* 23 (3): 623–628.

Dressman, J.B., Amidon, G.L., Reppas, C. et al. (1998). Dissolution testing as a prognostictool for oral drug absorption: immediate release dosage forms. *Pharm. Res.* 15 (1): 11–22.

Epstein, K., Cohen, N., Boothe, D. et al. (2004). Pharmacokinetics, stability, and retrospective analysis of use of an oral gel formulation of the bovine injectable enrofloxacin in horses. *Vet. Ther.* 5 (2): 155–167.

Erkert, R.S. and Macallister, C.G. (2002). Isoxsuprine hydrochloride in the horse: a review. *J. Vet. Pharmacol. Ther.* 25 (2): 81–87.

Finno, C.J. and Valberg, S.J. (2012). A comparative review of vitamin E and associated equine disorders. *J. Vet. Intern. Med.* 26 (6): 1251–1266.

Fura, A., Vyas, V., Humphreys, W. et al. (2008). Prediction of human oral pharmacokinetics using nonclinical data: examples involving four proprietary compounds. *Biopharm. Drug Dispos.* 29 (8): 455–468.

Gowen, R.R. and Lengel, J.G. (1993). Regulatory aspects of drug use in performance horses. *Vet. Clin. North Am. Equine Pract.* 9 (3): 449–460.

Grady, J.A., Davis, E.G., Kukanich, B. et al. (2010). Pharmacokinetics and pharmacodynamics of dexamethasone after oral administration in apparently healthy horses. *Am. J. Vet. Res.* 71 (7): 831–839.

Hashem, A. and Keller, H. (1993). Disposition, bioavailability and clinical efficacy of orally administered acepromazine in the horse. *J. Vet. Pharmacol. Ther.* 16 (3): 359–368.

Hovanessian, N., Davis, J.L., McKenzie, H.C. 3rd et al. (2014). Pharmacokinetics and safety of firocoxib after oral administration of repeated consecutive doses to neonatal foals. *J. Vet. Pharmacol. Ther.* 37 (3): 243–251.

Hurley, P.J. (1975). Red cell and plasma volumes in normal adults. *J. Nucl. Med.* 16 (1): 46–52.

Kararli, T.T. (1995). Comparison of the gastrointestinal anatomy, physiology, and biochemistry of humans and commonly used laboratory animals. *Biopharm. Drug Dispos.* 16 (5): 351–380.

Kvaternick, V., Pollmeier, M., Fischer, J. et al. (2007). Pharmacokinetics and metabolism of orally administered firocoxib, a novel second generation coxib, in horses. *J. Vet. Pharmacol. Ther.* 30 (3): 208–217.

de Laat, M.A., McGowan, C.M., Sillence, M.N. et al. (2010). Equine laminitis: induced by 48 h hyperinsulinaemia in Standardbred horses. *Equine Vet. J.* 42 (2): 129–135.

Lakritz, J., Wilson, W.D., Marsh, A.E. et al. (2000). Effects of prior feeding on pharmacokinetics and estimated bioavailability after oral administration of a single dose of microencapsulated erythromycin base in healthy foals. *Am. J. Vet. Res.* 61 (9): 1011–1015.

Liska, D.A., Akucewich, L.H., Marsella, R. et al. (2006). Pharmacokinetics of pentoxifylline and its 5-hydroxyhexyl metabolite after oral and intravenous administration of pentoxifylline to healthy adult horses. *Am. J. Vet. Res.* 67 (9): 1621–1627.

Lorenzo-Figueras, M., Preston, T., Ott, E.A. et al. (2005). Meal-induced gastric relaxation and emptying in horses after ingestion of high-fat versus high-carbohydrate diets. *Am. J. Vet. Res.* 66 (5): 897–906.

Martinez, M., Amidon, G., Clarke, L. et al. (2002). Applying the biopharmaceutics classification system to veterinary pharmaceutical products. Part II. Physiological considerations. *Adv. Drug Deliv. Rev.* 54 (6): 825–850.

McDonnell, S.M., Miller, J., and Vaala, W. (2013). Calming benefit of short-term alpha-casozepine supplementation during acclimation to domestic environment and basic ground training of adult semi-feral ponies. *J. Equine Vet. Sci.* 33 (2): 101–106.

Merritt, A.M. (1999). Normal equine gastroduodenal secretion and motility. *Equine Vet. J.* 31 (S29): 7–13.

Merritt AM. (2003). The equine stomach: a personal perspective. In Proceedings of the 49th Annual Convention of the American Association of Equine Practitioners, New Orleans, LA.

Merritt, A.M., Burrow, J.A., Horbal, M.J. et al. (1996). Effect of omeprazole on sodium and potassium output in pentagastrin-stimulated equine gastric contents. *Am. J. Vet. Res.* 57 (11): 1640–1644.

Mozaffari, A.A., Derakhshanfar, A., Alinejad, A. et al. (2010). A comparative study on the adverse effects of flunixin, ketoprofen and phenylbutazone in miniature donkeys: haematological, biochemical and pathological findings. *N.Z. Vet. J.* 58 (5): 224–228.

Naylor, J.R., Bayly, W.M., Schott, H.C. 2nd et al. (1993). Equine plasma and blood volumes decrease with dehydration but subsequently increase with exercise. *J. Appl. Physiol.* 75 (2): 1002–1008.

Nebbia, C., Dacasto, M., and Carletti, M. (2004). Postnatal development of hepatic oxidative, hydrolytic and conjugative drug-metabolizing enzymes in female horses. *Life Sci.* 74 (13): 1605–1619.

Nebbia, C., Dacasto, M., Rossetto Giaccherino, A. et al. (2003). Comparative expression of liver cytochrome P450-dependent monooxygenases in the horse and in other agricultural and laboratory species. *Vet. J.* 165 (1): 53–64.

Parry, B.W., Anderson, G.A., and Gay, C.C. (1982). Hypotension in the horse induced by acepromazine maleate. *Aust. Vet. J.* 59 (5): 148–152.

Pellegrini-Masini, A., Poppenga, R.H., and Sweeney, R.W. (2004). Disposition of flunixin meglumine injectable preparation administered orally to healthy horses. *J. Vet. Pharmacol. Ther.* 27 (3): 183–186.

Peroni, D.L., Stanley, S., Kollias-Baker, C. et al. (2002). Prednisone per os is likely to have limited efficacy in horses. *Equine Vet. J.* 34 (3): 283–287.

Persson, E.M., Gustafsson, A.S., Carlsson, A.S. et al. (2005). The effects of food on the dissolution of poorly soluble drugs in human and in model small intestinal fluids. *Pharm. Res.* 22 (12): 2141–2151.

Peters, J., Block, W., Oswald, S. et al. (2011). Oral absorption of clarithromycin is nearly abolished by chronic comedication of rifampicin in foals. *Drug Metab. Dispos.* 39 (9): 1643–1649.

Riond, J.L., Riviere, J.E., Duckett, W.M. et al. (1992). Cardiovascular effects and fatalities associated with intravenous administration of doxycycline to horses and ponies. *Equine Vet. J.* 24 (1): 41–45.

Roussel, A.J., Hooper, R.N., Cohen, N.D. et al. (2000). Prokinetic effects of erythromycin on the ileum, cecum, and pelvic flexure of horses during the postoperative period. *Am. J. Vet. Res.* 61 (4): 420–424.

Sanchez, L.C., Lester, G.D., and Merritt, A.M. (1998). Effect of ranitidine on intragastric pH in clinically normal neonatal foals. *J. Am. Vet. Med. Assoc.* 212 (9): 1407–1412.

Schoster, A., Staempfli, H.R., Abrahams, M. et al. (2015). Effect of a probiotic on prevention of diarrhea and *Clostridium difficile* and *Clostridium perfringens* shedding in foals. *J. Vet. Intern. Med.* 29 (3): 925–931.

Schoster, A., Weese, J.S., and Guardabassi, L. (2014). Probiotic use in horses – what is the evidence for their clinical efficacy? *J. Vet. Intern. Med.* 28 (6): 1640–1652.

Short, C.R., Sams, R.A., Soma, L.R. et al. (1998). The regulation of drugs and medicines in horse racing in the United States. The Association of Racing Commissioners International Uniform Classification of Foreign Substances guidelines. *J. Vet. Pharmacol. Ther.* 21 (2): 145–153.

Stanski, D.R., Greenblatt, D.J., and Lowenstein, E. (1978). Kinetics of intravenous and intramuscular morphine. *Clin. Pharmacol. Ther.* 24 (1): 52–59.

Swain, E.A., Magdesian, K.G., Kass, P.H. et al. (2015). Pharmacokinetics of metronidazole in foals: influence of age within the neonatal period. *J. Vet. Pharmacol. Ther.* 38 (3): 227–234.

Sykes, B.W., Hewetson, M., Hepburn, R.J. et al. (2015). European College of Equine Internal Medicine Consensus Statement – equine gastric ulcer syndrome in adult horses. *J. Vet. Intern. Med.* 29 (5): 1288–1299.

Sykes, B.W., Underwood, C., and Mills, P.C. (2017). The effects of dose and diet on the pharmacodynamics of esomeprazole in the horse. *Equine Vet. J.* 49 (5): 637–642.

Tobin, T., Chay, S., Kamerling, S. et al. (1986). Phenylbutazone in the horse: a review. *J. Vet. Pharmacol. Ther.* 9 (1): 1–25.

Toothaker, R.D. and Welling, P.G. (1980). The effect of food on drug bioavailability. *Annu. Rev. Pharmacol. Toxicol.* 20: 173–199.

Toutain, P.L. and Bousquet-Mélou, A. (2004a). Volumes of distribution. *J. Vet. Pharmacol. Ther.* 27 (6): 441–453.

Toutain, P.L. and Bousquet-Mélou, A. (2004b). Plasma clearance. *J. Vet. Pharmacol. Ther.* 27 (6): 415–425.

Tran, T., Brophy, J.M., Suissa, S. et al. (2015). Risks of cardiac valve regurgitation and heart failure associated with ergot- and non-ergot-derived dopamine agonist use in patients with Parkinson's disease: a systematic review of observational studies. *CNS Drugs* 29 (12): 985–998.

Tyden, E., Olsen, L., Tallkvist, J. et al. (2004). CYP3A in horse intestines. *Toxicol. Appl. Pharmacol.* 201 (2): 112–119.

Van Duijkeren, E., Kessels, B.G., Sloet van Oldruitenborgh-Oosterbaan, M.M. et al. (1996). In vitro and in vivo binding of trimethoprim and sulphachlorpyridazine to equine food and digesta and their stability in caecal contents. *J. Vet. Pharmacol. Ther.* 19 (4): 281–287.

Varley, G., Bowen, I.M., Nicholls, V. et al. (2016). Misoprostol is superior to combined omeprazole and sucralfate for healing glandular gastric lesions. *Equine Vet. J.* 48 (S50): 11–12.

Venner, M., Astheimer, K., Lämmer, M. et al. (2013). Efficacy of mass antimicrobial treatment of foals with subclinical pulmonary abscesses associated with *Rhodococcus equi. J. Vet. Intern. Med.* 27 (1): 171–176.

Wilson, K.E., Davis, J.L., Crisman, M.V. et al. (2017). Pharmacokinetics of firocoxib after intravenous administration of multiple consecutive doses in neonatal foals. *J. Vet. Pharmacol. Ther.* 40 (6): e23–e29.

Yu, L.X., Amidon, G.L., Polli, J.E. et al. (2002). Biopharmaceutics classification system: the scientific basis for biowaiver extensions. *Pharm. Res.* 19 (7): 921–925.

22

Introduction to Food Animal Pharmacotherapy

Virginia R. Fajt

Veterinary Physiology and Pharmacology, College of Veterinary Medicine & Biomedical Sciences, Texas A&M University, College Station, TX, USA

Key Points

- To ensure a safe food supply, drug use in food animals is subject to legal regulations and restrictions that pharmacists must be aware of before dispensing drugs for use in food animal species.
- Cattle, pigs (including pot-bellied or mini-pigs), chickens, turkeys, sheep, goats, and food fish such as catfish and salmon should always be considered food animals.
- Deer, pheasant, quail, rabbits, camelids, and other species that are sometimes hunted or raised for food *might* be considered food animals, and the prescribing veterinarian should be queried.

- Intent of the owner of the animal does *not* define whether an animal is a food animal.
- Withdrawal time is the amount of time an animal or its edible products (e.g. milk or eggs) must be withheld from the food supply after drug administration.
- Use of drugs in a manner not included on the approved label may be legal, but there are additional requirements for drugs used extra-label in food animals.
- Some drugs are restricted from extra-label use in food animals under any circumstances.

22.1 Introduction

Food animals are animals from which edible products are harvested, such as milk, eggs, or meat from muscle and organs. Although the federal government does not explicitly codify in a single regulation the definition of a food animal, it can be inferred from guidance documents and regulations from the US Department of Agriculture (USDA) and the US Food and Drug Administration's (FDA) Center for Veterinary Medicine (CVM) that the following species are considered food animals for the purposes of drug dispensing and administration: cattle, pigs, chickens, turkeys, sheep, goats, and food fish such as catfish and salmon. Other species may be considered food animals, depending on their disposition (Table 22.1). Although horses are consumed by humans in some countries, horses are not considered food animals in the USA.

When drugs are administered to food animals, food products from those animals must not be contaminated with unsafe levels of drugs. This chapter focuses on what the pharmacist needs to know when dispensing drugs to food animals in order to maintain a

Pharmacotherapeutics for Veterinary Dispensing, First Edition. Edited by Katrina L. Mealey.
© 2019 John Wiley & Sons, Inc. Published 2019 by John Wiley & Sons, Inc.

Table 22.1 Animal species that, in terms of drug use, are considered food animals.

Animal species that should ALWAYS be considered food animals

Pigs (including pot-bellied pigs that are kept as pets)
Cattle
Sheep
Goats
Poultry: Chickens, turkeys, and ducks (including backyard pets and small flock)
Fish: Catfish, salmon, and tilapia

Animal species that may be considered food animals[a]

Rabbits
Pheasants
Camelids (llamas, alpacas, and vicunas)
Deer, reindeer, red deer, and other antelope
Bison

---

[a] Consult prescribing veterinarian for confirmation.

Table 22.2 Definitions for selected terminology used to describe food animal species.

Term	Definition
Barrow	A castrated male pig
Broilers	Chickens being raised for meat
Gilt	A female pig that has not yet given birth
Heifer	A female of the cattle species that has not given birth. Female cattle can be referred to as heifers from birth until their first calving.
Lactating cow	Any female dairy animal that has calved is considered a lactating cow, whether she is currently lactating or between one lactation and another (a "dry" cow).
Layers	Chickens being raised to produce eggs or those hens that are currently producing eggs
Steer	A castrated male of the cattle species
Wether	A castrated male sheep or goat

safe food supply. To start with, pharmacists dispensing drugs intended for food animals may not be familiar with some of the terms used in the production animal industry. Table 22.2 lists terms that might be encountered by a pharmacist.

22.2 Food Safety and Withdrawal Times

To keep the food supply safe, drug sponsors are required to provide information on drug labels; farmers (including those with "hobby farms"), ranchers, and veterinarians must follow rules designed to prevent unsafe levels of drugs in edible animal products; and government personnel test animal products (or a marker tissue) for drug residues to determine if they exceed the legal limit.

Dramatic difference

Drugs dispensed for food animals must include an appropriate withdrawal time on the label.

The obligation of drug sponsors is to include on the label a science-based "withdrawal time" for any drug with a label indication for any species of food animal (US Food and Drug Administration [FDA] 2006). Withdrawal time is the time between the last dose of drug that a particular animal received and when that animal or its product (meat, milk, or eggs) entered the food supply (at time of harvest or slaughter). Sponsors perform a number of studies during the approval process for food animal drugs in order to estimate the doses at which there would be no effect on humans. This is accomplished by performing acute and chronic toxicity studies, reproductive toxicity studies, and genotoxicity studies in laboratory animals such as rodents and dogs. No-observed-effects doses or levels, or similar measures, are then divided by a safety factor (usually, 10–100), and this number becomes the acceptable daily intake of the drug for humans. Based on the acceptable daily intake, human body weight, and expected food consumption values (e.g. 1500 ml of milk per day), a safe drug concentration is calculated. The safe drug concentration, along with other information related to distribution of the drug into specific tissues and organs and related to drug metabolism, is used to establish the final "tolerance" of the drug. Tolerance is the legal limit of drug (or its marker residue) that can be found in the tested sample at slaughter; tolerances are published in the Code of Federal Regulations for all legally approved food animal drugs. Once the tolerance has been established, sponsors perform the tissue residue studies necessary to estimate the time it will take for the drug to be below the tolerance for an estimated 99% of the population of treated animals with a 95% confidence interval (Riviere et al. 1998). This is the withdrawal time. Withdrawal times may be in hours (for milk or eggs), days (for meat), or even weeks for some drugs. The withdrawal time is typically included on the drug label in the section entitled "Warnings."

There is a legal obligation for farmers, ranchers, and veterinarians to observe the withdrawal time. Both the pharmacist and the veterinarian should ensure that the animal owner or caretaker is aware of the withdrawal time of drugs administered. This should be done via counseling and labeling, so that the animal owner or caretaker observes the withdrawal time. Veterinarians have the legal right to use drugs in an extra-label manner under certain circumstances, as provided in the Federal Food Drug and Cosmetic Act via the Animal Medicinal Drug Use Clarification Act of 1994 (AMDUCA) and its regulations. These regulations describe permissible and nonpermissible extra-label uses of drugs in animals. If a drug is used extra-label in a food animal, veterinarians are responsible for the establishment of an extended withdrawal time based on scientific data on drug disposition. In the USA, a joint USDA–university entity known as FARAD (Food Animal Residue Avoidance Databank; http://farad.org) employs various algorithms using published and unpublished pharmacokinetic data to provide an estimate of withdrawal intervals for drugs used in an extra-label manner to aid veterinarians. FARAD also regularly publishes *FARAD Digests*, which summarize the data and provide recommendations for specific drugs or groups of drugs (e.g. Payne et al. 1999; Smith 2013). Most of these publications are available

on the FARAD website. Pharmacists should not be expected to estimate withdrawal times for veterinarians, since AMDUCA specifically identifies the veterinarian as the responsible party. Pharmacists should be prepared to contact the prescribing veterinarian if a prescription indicates extra-label drug use and the veterinarian has not provided an extended withdrawal time.

The government is obligated to inspect tissues from animals slaughtered for meat, and this is performed by the USDA Food Safety Inspection Service (FSIS). A statistically determined random sample of animals are tested for a battery of drugs ("scheduled samples") (FDA 2017). Additional samples may be collected and carcasses withheld until testing is completed if animals appear grossly diseased or if there is evidence of drug administration suggesting recent treatment ("inspector-generated samples"). Animals with drug concentrations above the legal limit in tested tissues are removed from the food supply, and the seller is notified. Milk is also tested for drug residues, and milk production is a tightly regulated process, as dairies are inspected regularly for their animal production practices and milking routines. Repeat offenses can result in warning letters from the FDA, and eventually the offenders can be prohibited from selling animals, milk, or eggs. Examples of warning letters that have been listed are publicly available on the following website: https://www.fda.gov/ICECI/EnforcementActions/Warning Letters/default.htm.

An important concept related to tolerances of a particular drug is what the USDA FSIS considers violative. There are some situations for which there is no established acceptable drug level. In those situations, the USDA FSIS interprets the presence of any detectable amount of drug to be violative. This is especially problematic when drugs are used in an extra-label manner, in which case there may not be an established tolerance (DeDonder et al. 2013). For example, the tolerance may have been established for a different class of animal, such as in beef cattle, but the drug was used in dairy cattle. Because there is not an established tolerance level for dairy cattle, the FSIS would therefore determine that detection of any level of drug would result in a violation. The take-home message is that extra-label drug use requires careful consideration of the drug label (indicated species, indicated animal class within species, withdrawal time, dose, route of administration, and even site of administration) so that violative levels are not detected at slaughter. Practically speaking, a pharmacist would not need to know tolerances or be capable of establishing withdrawal times (in fact, it is the veterinarian's responsibility under AMDUCA to provide an extended withdrawal time on the prescription). However, it is useful for pharmacists to understand this process.

If the patient is a food animal (regardless of whether or not the owner considers it a pet) and no withdrawal time was provided, the pharmacist should contact the veterinarian to request one. Veterinarians, particularly those who work primarily with companion animals rather than food animals, are not always aware of the legal considerations for drug use in food animals. Food animals that are often considered pets include pot-bellied pigs, backyard poultry, bees, sheep, and goats (see also Table 22.1). Owners may take these "pets" to a companion animal veterinarian rather than a food animal veterinarian. The pharmacist can play an important role in ensuring appropriate food animal regulations are followed when dispensing drugs for these animals.

22.3 Drug Absorption, Distribution, Metabolism, and Elimination in Food Animals

As described in other chapters, drug disposition may differ across species of animal, and this is no less true for food animal species. These differences may be a result of anatomic or physiologic differences, particularly between what are called monogastric species (humans, pigs, and companion animals

such as cats and dogs) and ruminants (cattle, goats, and sheep), and between monogastrics and birds (e.g. poultry). Keep in mind that disposition differences impact drug regimens but also impact expected withdrawal times for meat, milk, and eggs. Factors that contribute to differences in drug absorption, distribution, metabolism, and elimination (ADME) in food animal species, particularly ruminants, are discussed in this section and have been reviewed more extensively elsewhere (Short 1994).

ADME differences between poultry and other species will not be discussed in detail herein, but they may be quite different (Goetting et al. 2011). On the other hand, some drugs may be dosed similarly across species, such as meloxicam (Souza et al. 2017).

22.3.1 Absorption

With regard to oral drug absorption, the ruminant digestive system features unique challenges. Ruminants are animals that have additional forestomachs (not four stomachs!) that act as fermentation vats for feedstuffs such as grass and hay (Figure 22.1). Between the esophagus and the abomasum (comparable to the stomach in people, in which gastric acid and pepsin are secreted), there are three distinct organs, the most important of which is the rumen. The rumen contains a microbial ecology of protozoa and bacteria that ferments grass and hay to make fatty acids that the animal can absorb as nutrients. The rumen of sheep can contain 5–10 gal of fluid, and that of a dairy cow can contain 40–50 gal! Drugs that are administered orally to ruminants must make it out of the voluminous rumen, through the reticulum and omasum to the true stomach, the abomasum. Thus, the forestomachs of a ruminant may be an impediment to effective oral drug absorption. It is not surprising, therefore, that the mere presence of a rumen can dramatically impact drug absorption rates and bioavailability after oral dosing. Unfortunately, no blanket rules apply to help predict rates of oral absorption or bioavailability in these

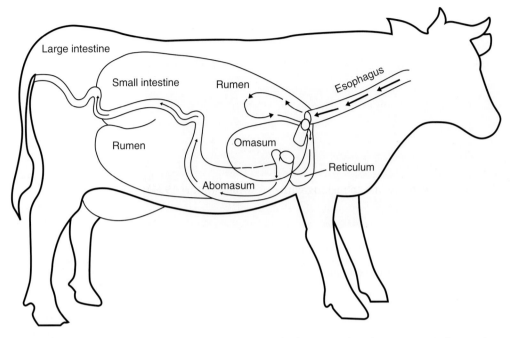

Figure 22.1 The ruminant gastrointestinal tract depicting the forestomaches: the rumen, reticulum, and omasum. Ingested food or orally administered medication is delivered from the esophagus to the rumen (essentially a fermentation vat that can contain 40–50 gal of fluid in an adult bovine). If a drug is not inactivated in the rumen, it would then proceed to the reticulum, to the omasum, and, finally, to the abomasum which is the true stomach. *Source:* Courtesy of Chris Long, Texas A&M University.

species; they must be determined empirically for each drug product in each ruminant species. However, it should be expected that oral dosing in these species is not likely to result in the same rate or extent of absorption as in nonruminants. Formulations approved in other species, including humans, require evidence of adequate oral absorption in ruminants before assumptions about efficacy can be made.

Pharmaceutical companies have exploited ruminant physiology and developed specific dosage forms that are designed to be delivered to the rumen, where they become trapped. These formulations are intended to essentially sink to the bottom of the rumen, and the specially designed encapsulation system provides a consistent, sustained drug release (i.e. antibiotic, corticosteroid, or other). This design is called a rumen bolus (Figure 22.2), and the bolus is often administered with a bolus gun or balling gun (Figure 22.3).

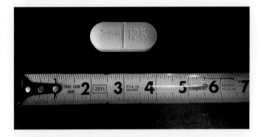

Figure 22.2 An example of a rumen bolus. This bolus contains dexamethasone and trichlormethiazide (a diuretic) and was indicated for the treatment of udder edema in dairy cows. Although this product is no longer marketed, it demonstrates the size of bolus that can be administered that allows the formulation to sink to the bottom of the rumen. *Source:* Courtesy of Dr. Meredyth Jones, Texas A&M University.

Alternatives to oral dosing include subcutaneous or intramuscular injections, which are often used in ruminants due to relative ease of administration. However, the site of injection has important implications that are

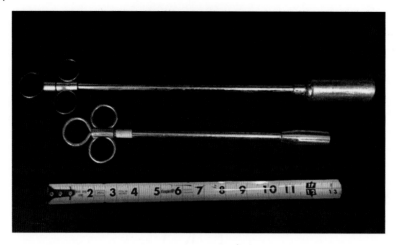

Figure 22.3 Balling gun or bolus gun – a device used to administer oral drugs to cattle. Single tablets, capsules, or boluses may be as large as the cup at the distal end of the balling gun. *Source:* Courtesy of Dr. Meredyth Jones, Texas A&M University.

not considered in human patients. For example, intramuscular injection can damage muscle tissue, resulting in what are called injection site lesions. Cattle carcasses with injection site lesions can cost the beef industry. General recommendations are to avoid intramuscular injections into the more expensive cuts of meat. Programs in the beef industry (e.g. the Beef Quality Assurance Program; https://www.bqa.org) have been created with the goal of decreasing the occurrence of injection site lesions. In terms of the rate and extent of absorption, intramuscular and subcutaneous routes should not be assumed to be equivalent (Korsrud et al. 1993; Papich et al. 1993). Drugs should always be administered in accordance with the labeled route, site, and drug volume per injection site to ensure therapeutic effect and expected withdrawal times. This is particularly well illustrated with ceftiofur, a third-generation cephalosporin (see Tables 21.5 and 21.6). There are four different formulations of ceftiofur that have been approved for use in cattle. The crystalline-free acid formulation, Excede˚, requires particular attention to label information or to published extra-label pharmacokinetic and dosing information, for two reasons: First, specific restrictions on cephalosporins exist for food

animals (see later discussion in "Dispensing Considerations"); and, second, the product must be injected in a specific location at the base of the ear for the desired prolonged absorption rate and prolonged duration of action after a single dose. This site and route also ensure that the withdrawal time on the label will actually result in adequate depletion prior to slaughter for this particular product. In contrast, a different ceftiofur formulation, Naxcel˚, is labeled for intramuscular or subcutaneous injection (not at the base of the ear). Thus, pharmacists should be exceedingly cautious about substituting one drug product for another if dispensing drugs for food animals.

Although often assumed to be related to absorption, the disposition of trimethoprim is quite different in adult ruminants than it is in dogs, cats, humans, or horses, leading to much shorter elimination half-lives and questionable therapeutic efficacy (Pashov et al. 1997). Potentiated sulfonamides, therefore, should not be expected to provide extended coverage of bacteria compared to sulfonamides alone in ruminants.

One additional route of administration that is unique to ruminants is the intramammary route, which is used for treating mastitis in dairy cattle. The absorption characteristics of this route and of the formulations developed specifically for this route are important to differentiate due to differences in withdrawal time, for both milk and meat. Even with the same drug, there may be an extended-release and an immediate-release formulation. For example, immediate-release formulations of cephapirin (a first-generation cephalosporin) are used in lactating dairy cows, for which milk withdrawal time must be short, since this milk must be discarded rather than consumed. The extended-release formulation of cephapirin is then used when milk is no longer being harvested from the animal and the cow is "dry." Cows are typically "dry" for 60 days immediately before they calve again, to allow for mammary tissue involution and regeneration. Similarly, lactating-cow and dry-cow formulations exist for hetacillin, cloxacillin, and penicillin, with the typical salt differences being sodium (more rapid release for lactating-cow therapy) versus benzathine (more extended release for dry-cow therapy).

22.3.2 Distribution

Although volumes of distribution may vary across species, there are no rules of thumb that can be used to predict these differences. Knowledge of volume of distribution by itself is not particularly useful when reviewing drug regimens or prescriptions, although this information may help explain differences in elimination half-life for some drugs (see the "Elimination" section). As with other species, young animals are expected to have a larger proportion of total body water than adults, which can lead to increased volumes of distributions in younger animals (Brown et al. 1996). This does not necessarily translate to a requisite change in dosing regimens, however.

Drug distribution into a human mother's milk is a major concern in human medicine because of the potential for an infant's exposure. In veterinary medicine, drug distribution into milk is a major concern in dairy cattle and goats because of the risk for human exposure to drugs through milk or milk products (cheese, butter, etc.). Predicting milk/plasma concentration ratios is complex, involving factors such as lipid solubility, pH, protein binding, the presence of inflammation, and the affinity of drugs for transporters. Surprisingly, even pharmacogenetics influences the amount of drug present in bovine milk. For example, lactating cows with the ABCG2 polymorphism Y581S have substantially higher concentrations of fluoroquinolones in milk compared to lactating wildtype cows (Otero et al. 2013). The ABCG2 transporter is thought to represent the main mechanism for active drug transport into milk, and ABCG2 Y581S is a gain-of-function polymorphism that is present in some cattle. When dispensing drugs to lactating dairy animals, including "pet" goats or cows, the pharmacist should be aware of the potential for drug distribution into milk.

22.3.3 Metabolism

The rate of drug metabolism in ruminants often differs from that in nonruminants. For example, the elimination half-life of salicylic acid is less than one hour in cattle, while it is six hours in pigs and humans, nine hours in dogs, and even longer in cats. Even among ruminants, there may be differences in drug disposition: Drug doses for goats may be higher or regimens may differ than those for cattle, because drugs that undergo oxidative metabolism may be metabolized faster in goats than cattle. For phase II metabolism, pigs and horses have been shown to have higher glucuronidation capacity than cattle (Toutain and Ferran 2010). However, obvious differences in a single pharmacokinetic parameter may not translate into a need for different doses between species (Taha et al. 1999). The impact of one particular variable may not be predictable across all animals in a given species. Additionally, as is the case with aspirin in ruminants, delivery by a slow-release oral formulation may counteract the rapid elimination half-life. Therefore, pharmacists should not attempt to calculate dosage regimens for one species by extrapolations based on the elimination rate of another species, even if both species are ruminants.

An important difference between ruminants and nonruminants, as mentioned in this chapter, is the rapid metabolism of trimethoprim, which is thought to explain most of the variation in elimination half-life of this drug across species.

Dramatic difference

While trimethoprim–sulfonamide formulations are commonly used in humans and companion animals (dogs and horses) for treating bacterial infections, they are not a rational choice for ruminants. Essentially, trimethoprim–sulfonamide combinations would be expensive sources of sulfonamides in ruminants since the trimethoprim is not available to potentiate the sulfonamide.

22.3.4 Excretion

Drugs that are not approved in ruminant species should *not* be assumed to be eliminated at the same rate or to the same extent as in other species. Differences in volume of distribution and clearance may result in changes in elimination and therefore in dose recommendations across species. On the other hand, among ruminants (cattle, sheep, and goats), drugs that are excreted unchanged via glomerular filtration are likely to be eliminated at similar rates and therefore have similar dosing regimens (Short 1994). The prescribing veterinarians should be consulted if there is a question about a dose or dosing interval, rather than assuming that the veterinarian made a mistake.

In contrast to human and companion animals, many drug products for food animals are used to treat large populations of animals in a short timeframe. From an economic and feasibility perspective, it is highly desirable to administer a single dose of antibiotic, for example, that remains active for several days instead of having to administer daily doses over the same time period. One

mechanism for accomplishing this is use of sustained-release injectable formulations. As a result of prolonged absorption in certain sustained-release formulations, "flip-flop" kinetics may result, in which prolonged absorption leads to longer measured elimination half-lives. The overall result of these formulations is that a single dose of drug can result in effective concentrations for several days. Examples of sustained-release formulations approved for cattle include ceftiofur crystalline-free acid (e.g. Excede) and oxytetracycline (e.g. LA-200). In contrast, the macrolide antibiotic tulathromycin actually has a prolonged elimination half-life in many species as a result of a large volume of distribution (Villarino et al. 2013), similar to the human macrolide azithromycin (Swainston Harrison and Keam 2007).

22.3.5 Other

Dramatic difference

Cattle, sheep, and goats require one-tenth of the dose of tranquilizer/analgesic alpha-2 adrenergic agonists such as xylazine, detomidine, and romifidine compared to horses, dogs, cats, and pigs.

This is not a pharmacokinetic difference, but likely a pharmacodynamic difference. Even though pharmacists are not likely to dispense these injectable alpha-2 adrenergic agonists from a community pharmacy, this serves as a striking example of the startling species differences that exist.

22.4 Drugs Commonly Prescribed for Food Animals

The vast majority of drugs approved for use in food animals are antibiotics or antiparasitics. Other commonly used drugs include nonsteroidal anti-inflammatory drugs (NSAIDs) and anesthetic drugs, including local anesthetics. Diseases commonly treated in food animals include infectious respiratory disease, mastitis, skin and soft tissue infections, gastrointestinal (GI) parasites, and ectoparasites such as ticks and mites. Common surgical procedures for which local and systemic anesthetics might be used include castration and dehorning (ruminants), teeth and tail clipping (pigs), and GI, orthopedic, and skin and soft tissue surgeries. Elective procedures (neutering, dehorning, and teeth and tail clippings) may be performed by lay personnel under the direction of a veterinarian, so pharmacists may be asked to dispense local anesthetics and NSAIDs for these purposes.

Because food animals are often raised in groups, flocks, or herds, disease challenges often involve the entire herd or flock. In many cases, administering drugs to the group via feed or water may be the only feasible way to ensure that all animals are dosed. In other cases, drugs may be administered to individual animals (by injection, for example). Even in these situations, though, drugs will generally be dispensed for a group of animals rather than an individual. Creative formulations and routes of administration have been developed to enhance ease of administration, safe (to human handler) application, and/or prolonged duration of action (for less

Table 22.3 Routes of administration used for food animals that are not typically used for human patients.

Route of administration
Intramammary
Intrauterine
In water
In feed
Immersion (fish)
Egg dip
In ovo (direct injection into poultry eggs)
Pour-on
CIDR (controlled internal drug release intravaginal device)

Note: Although some approved drug products include these routes of administration on their label, caution should be exercised when a prescription calls for one of these routes and it is *not* listed on the label. Pharmacokinetics may be significantly altered when a drug is administered by a route not indicated on the label, resulting in violative drug residues.

frequent administration). Table 22.3 lists routes of administration that are used for food animals, many of which will likely be unfamiliar to pharmacists.

22.4.1 Antibiotics

Common bacterial diseases in food animals and the most likely pathogens associated with those diseases include pneumonia (*Mannheimia hemolytica*); interdigital phlegmon, also known as pododermatitis or "footrot" (*Fusobacterium necrophorum*); mastitis (many bacteria); gastroenteritis; and infectious keratoconjunctivitis or "pinkeye" (*Moraxella bovis*). Figures 22.4 and 22.5 demonstrate how severe bacterial infections can be in food animals. Antibiotics that pharmacists are very familiar with are used in food animals, such as penicillin and ampicillin, but there are a number of antibiotics labeled for use in food animals that are not labeled for use in humans (Table 22.6). Although the individual drugs may be unique to food animals, they often belong to the same chemical class as human drugs. For example, tilmicosin, tulathromycin, gamithromycin, and tildopirosin are in the same class (macrolides) as the human drugs erythromycin, clarithromycin, and azithromycin. Similarly, enrofloxacin is a fluoroquinolone in the same chemical class as the human drug ciprofloxacin.

22.4.2 Antiparasitics

Pharmacists have probably trained the least for the condition that food animals experience the most – parasitism. That is because in the USA, parasitic diseases are uncommon in humans, so pharmacists dispense very few antiparasitic drugs. Gastrointestinal nematodes (roundworms) are commonly treated or prevented because of their large impact on animal health and well-being as well as their economic impact in production animals. The feed efficiency or feed conversion ratio is a measure of how much milk is produced (or weight is gained) by an animal per unit of feed provided. Both internal and external parasites can negatively impact feed efficiency, so

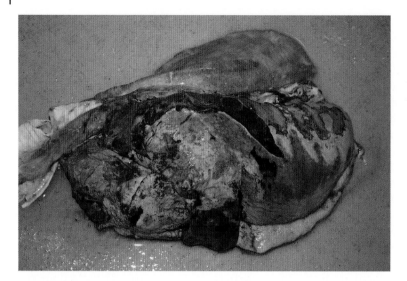

Figure 22.4 Necropsy specimen: Lungs from a steer with pneumonia. Pneumonia can be a consequence of "shipping fever" or bovine respiratory disease complex. The relatively healthy pink lung lobes at the top of the image are the right lobes; the left lobes at the bottom of the image are severely affected by diffuse pneumonia (tan, fibrinous tissue). Shipping fever is of great economic impact in the cattle industry. *Source:* Courtesy of Dr. Meredyth Jones, Texas A&M University.

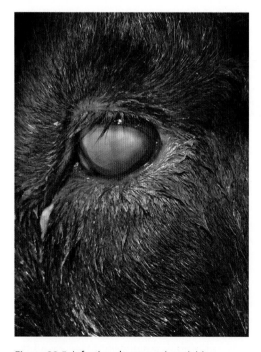

Figure 22.5 Infectious keratoconjunctivitis ("pinkeye") in a goat. *Source:* Courtesy of Dr. Meredyth Jones, Texas A&M University.

parasite control is of paramount importance in food animals.

The normal lifecycle of important nematode species such as *Haemonchus* and *Ostertagia* occurs on grass, so animals raised outside are particularly prone to parasitism since they consume grass. The discovery and development of ivermectin have largely reduced the burden of GI parasites because of its efficacy against many endoparasites and ectoparasites. However, resistance to ivermectin and other drugs in the same class, as well as other drug groups like benzimidazoles, is beginning to emerge. In some parts of the country, in sheep and goats, there are very few drug options left because of parasite resistance.

In some areas, lung nematodes are an important parasite. In cattle, these parasites sporulate in ponds and lakes, so animals with access to water can spread the organism. Lungworms are not as ubiquitous as GI parasites, but they are sporadically important in parts of the USA.

Other important parasites include ectoparasites, such as ticks, mites, and lice, most of which can be passed from animal to animal or from bedding to animal. Unique formulations (that go by the lay term "pour-ons") of ivermectin and eprinomectin have been developed to make management of parasites easier and safer for animal handlers. Some formulations are dosed by simply pouring a specified volume of the formulation onto the animal's back. The product is then absorbed cutaneously into the systemic circulation at concentrations sufficient to kill GI parasites as well as external parasites such as lice and mites.

Antiprotozoals should also be included with the antiparasitic drugs for food animals. Coccidia are obligate intracellular apicomplexan parasites that commonly infect animals that are housed together, including poultry and ruminants. Unique poultry drugs have been developed to address this common condition, but pharmacists would be unlikely to dispense them, since they are commonly delivered in feed or water. Coccidiosis in human patients is often treated with potentiated sulfonamides. There are a variety of drug classes used as coccidiostats in food animals (amprolium, diclazuril, monensin, and lasalocid) that have no human equivalent.

22.4.3 NSAIDs

In the USA, there is currently only one NSAID that has been approved for cattle, horses, and pigs, flunixin. Flunixin is labeled for use in these animals; there is no human equivalent. However, other NSAIDs, including meloxicam and occasionally phenylbutazone (labeled for human use decades ago, but withdrawn from the US market because of bone marrow toxicity), have been used extra-label to treat food animals. With increasing concerns for animal welfare of farm animals, the desire for pain control after routine procedures such as castration and dehorning or for disease conditions such as lameness has increased. In food animals, the desire for effective pain control must be balanced with the need for cost-effective and easy-to-administer drugs with short withdrawal times. It is currently an active area of research that could benefit from the expertise provided by pharmacists.

22.5 Dispensing Considerations

22.5.1 Labeling

As with other species, prescription drugs require instructions for the animal caregiver, and *in food animals, those instructions must either include the withdrawal time or state that no withdrawal time is needed.* Pharmacists receiving a prescription for a food animal patient may encounter unfamiliar terminology. Veterinarians may use terminology to indicate animal "classes" or to describe an animal's "signalment" – words that were not taught in the pharmacy curriculum. Examples and definitions for some of these are provided in Table 22.2. Additionally, the prescription may indicate a route of administration that is not used in human patients. Various routes of administration that are used in food animals are provided in Table 22.3.

Dramatic difference
Drugs dispensed for food animals have specific labeling requirements compared to human labeling requirements and companion animal labeling requirements.

Prescription drugs that are prescribed in an *extra-label* manner have additional federally mandated labeling requirements:

1) The name and address of the prescribing veterinarian. If the drug is dispensed by a pharmacy on the order of a veterinarian, the labeling shall include the name of the prescribing veterinarian and the name and address of the dispensing pharmacy, and may include the address of the prescribing veterinarian.
2) The established name of the drug or, if formulated from more than one active ingredient, the established name of each ingredient

3) Any directions for use specified by the veterinarian, including the class/species or identification of the animal or herd, flock, pen, lot, or other group of animals being treated, in which the drug is intended to be used; the dosage, frequency, and route of administration; and the duration of therapy
4) Any cautionary statements
5) The veterinarian's specified withdrawal, withholding, or discard time for meat, milk, eggs, or any other food that might be derived from the treated animal or animals (FDA 1996).

Over-the-counter (OTC) drugs that are being prescribed in an extra-label manner, such as human OTC drugs for a veterinary species, must bear this labeling as well; this is true whether or not the animal is a food animal. According to AMDUCA, if a drug is prescribed extra-label, regardless of its initial status as OTC, the drug must be labeled as above.

22.5.2 Veterinary Feed Directives

In many food animal species, one effective method of getting an animal to consume a drug is by adding it to feed, thereby successfully treating a group of animals without having to restrain and dose each animal individually. Although it is unlikely that pharmacists will encounter prescriptions for these types of drugs, it is important for pharmacists to have an understanding of the concept and process. Many individual drugs and drug combinations have been approved over the years for food animals, and until recently, many of the drugs were available OTC and could be ordered directly by a farmer or rancher (without the need for a prescription) to add to feed. Many of these drugs are medically important antibiotics, and this has resulted in literally tons of antibiotics fed to food animals in the USA on an annual basis. Recent concerns about antimicrobial resistance and the possibility of transfer of resistance elements from animals

to the food supply to humans have led to several initiatives within the FDA CVM to address the issue. For example, certain drugs or classes of drugs now have restrictions on use (see the "Prohibited Drugs" section and Table 22.4). Another example is the reclassification of certain antimicrobial drugs from OTC to a different category, the Veterinary Feed Directive (VFD). Starting in 2012, the FDA CVM asked drug sponsors to voluntarily remove growth promotion or feed efficiency indications from "medically important antimicrobials." According to FDA CVM Guidance for Industry #209, "The Judicious Use of Medically Important Antimicrobial Drugs in Food-Producing Animals," medically important antimicrobials are antimicrobial drugs that are deemed important for therapeutic use in humans (FDA 2012). Practically speaking, this includes all antimicrobial drugs that are "important," "highly important," or "critically important" in human medicine, as defined in FDA CVM Guidance for Industry #152 (FDA 2003, table A1) and summarized in Table 22.5. In addition to removing growth promotion claims from those drugs, the status of the drug was also modified from OTC status to VFD drug status. VFD drugs require a nonverbal order from the veterinarian to the feed mill or similar distributor to add the drug to feed and sell it to an animal owner for use in specifically identified animals. The VFD also requires the existence of a valid veterinarian–client–patient relationship, as defined in federal law in AMDUCA. VFD drugs also require specific labeling.

Pharmacists should be aware that a valid veterinarian–client–patient relationship is required not only for prescribing VFD drugs, but also for prescribing drugs in an extra-label manner. The federal definition of a veterinarian–client–patient relationship includes:

1) A veterinarian has assumed the responsibility for making medical judgments regarding the health of (an) animal(s) and the need for medical treatment, and the client (the owner of the animal or animals

Table 22.4 Drugs, families of drugs, and substances prohibited for extra-label use in food animals, as of November 1, 2017.

Drug	Specific prohibition (if applicable)	Rationale for prohibited use
Chloramphenicol		Risk of aplastic anemia
Clenbuterol		Reports of adverse effects in humans after consumption of contaminated products
Diethylstilbestrol		Potential carcinogen
Dimetridazole		Potential carcinogen
Ipronidazole		Potential carcinogen
Other nitroimidazoles (e.g. metronidazole)		Potential carcinogen
Furazolidone		Potential carcinogen
Nitrofurazone		Potential carcinogen
Fluoroquinolones		Risk of antimicrobial resistance
Glycopeptides (e.g. vancomycin)		Risk of antimicrobial resistance
Sulfonamides	Lactating dairy cattle	Residue risk
Phenylbutazone	Female dairy cattle >20 months of age	Risk of blood dyscrasias
Cephalosporins (excluding cephapirin)	In cattle, swine, chickens, or turkeys when used for disease prevention purposes; at unapproved doses, frequencies, durations, or routes of administration; or if the drug is not approved for that species and production class	Risk of antimicrobial resistance
Adamantanes and neuraminidase inhibitors (e.g. oseltamivir) approved for treating or preventing influenza A in humans	Only in chickens, turkeys, and ducks	Risk of antiviral resistance

Note: Prohibition of extra-label use may effectively be a complete ban on use if there is not a drug product and indication approved for the animal species (i.e. chloramphenicol, clenbuterol, diethylstilbestrol, furazolidone, nitrofurazone, metronidazole and other nitroimidazoles, glycopeptides, phenylbutazone, adamantanes, and neuraminidase inhibitors); or, if there is a drug product labeled for food animals, the drug cannot be used in an extra-label manner.
Source: Anonymous (2012) and Payne et al. (1999).

or other caretaker) has agreed to follow the instructions of the veterinarian.

2) There is sufficient knowledge of the animal(s) by the veterinarian to initiate at least a general or preliminary diagnosis of the medical condition of the animal(s).

3) The practicing veterinarian is readily available for follow-up in case of adverse reactions or failure of the regimen of therapy. Such a relationship can exist only when the veterinarian has recently seen and is personally acquainted with the keeping and care of the animal(s) by virtue of examination of the animal(s), and/or by medically appropriate and timely visits to the premises where the animal(s) are kept (FDA 1996).

Table 22.5 Example antimicrobial drugs that are "important," "highly important," or "critically important" in human medicine, as defined in FDA (2003).

Category	Example drugs or groups	Rationale
Critically important	Third-generation cephalosporins	Meningitis: necrotizing enteritis
	Fluoroquinolones	Infections due to multidrug-resistant Gram-negative rods
	Macrolides	Legionnaire's disease
	Trimethoprim–sulfonamides	Infection due to *Pneumocystis carinii*
Highly important	Natural penicillins	Neurosyphilis: serious infection due to Group A streptococci
	Aminopenicillins	Infections due to *Listeria monocytogenes*
	Carbapenems	Infections due to multidrug-resistant Gram-negative rods
Important	First-generation cephalosporins	
	Second-generation cephalosporins	

Note: "Critically important antimicrobial drugs": Are used to treat enteric pathogens that cause foodborne disease **AND** are the sole drug or one of few alternatives to treat serious human disease. "Highly important antimicrobial drugs": Are used to treat enteric pathogens that cause foodborne disease **OR** are the sole drug or one of few alternatives to treat serious human disease. "Important": Are used to treat enteric pathogens in nonfoodborne disease **OR** there is no cross-resistance or linked resistance with other drug classes **OR** resistance elements are difficult to transmit within or across genera of bacteria.
Source: FDA-CVM *Guidance for Industry #152* (FDA 2003, Table A1).

22.5.3 Prohibited Drugs

Although extra-label drug use in food animals may be legal under some conditions, it is important for pharmacists to understand that there are some drugs that are **absolutely prohibited** for use in food animals in an extra-label manner (see Table 22.4). Some of the prohibited drugs are not labeled for use in food animal labels, so their use is effectively banned in all food animals (e.g. chloramphenicol and clenbuterol). However, other drugs included in the regulation do have an approved food animal label indication. For the latter drugs, it is only the extra-label use that is illegal. For example, extra-label use of fluoroquinolones is illegal in food animals, but there are legal on-label uses of fluoroquinolones (i.e. enrofloxacin and danofloxacin) in cattle and swine. The same is true of sulfadimethoxine: it has labeled indications for lactating dairy cows, but any use that is not included on the label would be illegal in a lactating cow, whether the extra-label use is a different dose, a different route of administration, or to treat a condition that is not indicated on the label.

Other prohibitions included in AMDUCA are that drugs used in feed must never be used extra-label, laypersons may not use drugs in an extra-label manner except under the supervision of a veterinarian, and if use of a drug leads to a violative residue, that use is illegal.

22.5.4 Substitutions

Some drug products approved for food animals contain the same active ingredient as drug products approved for use in other species (i.e. human, equine, or companion animal drug products), so it may be tempting for the pharmacist to substitute one of these products for the food animal formulation. However, since the formulation may impact drug disposition, efficacy, tissue residues, and withdrawal times, substitutions should *never* be made by the pharmacist without explicit instructions from the veterinarian.

There are drugs used in food animals for which there are no human-labeled equivalents despite the fact that the same chemical is found in both food animal and human products (see Table 22.6). Substituting a human drug product for a food animal drug product should never be made without explicit directions from the veterinarian. It is important to note that most of the food animal products are formulated for a prolonged duration of action that would not be duplicated with human formulations.

22.5.5 Compounding

Compounding from bulk drugs is NOT acceptable for food animals (FDA 2015). Compounding from bulk drugs may alter the pharmacokinetics and withdrawal times in an unpredictable manner, and the primary concern of the veterinarian and pharmacist should be to protect the food supply. Even when using best practices and good manufacturing practices (GMP)-produced bulk drug, compounding from bulk drug for food animals should not be practiced.

Drugs compounded from approved products *may* be legal, but provisions for acceptable compounding are included in AMDUCA and in Chapter 3 of this book, and should be

Table 22.6 Selected drugs that are FDA approved for food animals with no human drug equivalent.

Drug	Class	Comments
Amprolium	Anticoccidial	
Ceftiofur	Antimicrobial (cephalosporin)	4 approved formulations, each of which has a different dose, different withdrawal time, or both
Dinoprost	Prostaglandin F2α analog	
Enrofloxacin	Antimicrobial (fluoroquinolone)	Cattle/swine formulation is different from small-animal formulation
Eprinomectin	Antiparasitic	
Fenbendazole	Antiparasitic	
Florfenicol	Antimicrobial (phenicol)	Same class as chloramphenicol without the risk of aplastic anemia
Flunixin	NSAID	Injectable and pour-on formulations available
Gamithromycin	Antimicrobial (macrolide)	
Isoflupredone	Glucocorticoid	Is less likely to cause abortions in pregnant cattle than dexamethasone
Moxidectin	Antiparasitic (ivermectin)	Available as sole drug in food animal formulations, and in single and combination products for small animals
Pirlimycin	Antimicrobial (macrolide/lincosamide)	Only available as intramammary formulation
Tildipirosin	Antimicrobial (macrolide)	
Tilmicosin	Antimicrobial (macrolide)	
Tulathromycin	Antimicrobial (macrolide)	

NSAID, Nonsteroidal anti-inflammatory drug.
Note: Additional drugs not labeled for humans are approved for use in *feed* for food animals, but because they are only approved for feed use, they are not included here. Pharmacists working with feed additives are encouraged to seek additional resources, such as the Feed Additive Compendium.

reviewed before compounded drugs are dispensed to food animals (FDA 1996).

22.6 Organic Production

The Organic Foods Production Act, enacted as part of the 1990 Farm Bill, establishes uniform standards for the production and handling of foods labeled as "organic." Although many drugs are not allowed in organic animal production, the National Organic Program does allow certain drugs to be used under particular circumstances, including the provision of extended withdrawal times. Pharmacists might need to be aware that the withdrawal time for drugs intended to be used for "organic" food production could be longer than the withdrawal time provided on the drug label. More information can be found at the National Organic Program website.

22.7 Summary

The dispensing and administration of drugs in food animals require particular attention to labeling requirements and withdrawal times to protect the food supply. It is important for pharmacists to know that laws and regulations that apply to drug use in food animals can change rapidly, and it is incumbent upon the pharmacist to keep abreast of the regulations.

References

Anonymous (2012). New animal drugs; cephalosporin drugs: extralabel animal drug use; order of prohibition. *Fed. Regist.* 77 (4): 735–745.

Brown, S.A., Chester, S.T., and Robb, E.J. (1996). Effects of age on the pharmacokinetics of single dose ceftiofur sodium administered intramuscularly or intravenously to cattle. *J. Vet. Pharmacol. Ther.* 19 (1): 32–38.

DeDonder, K.D., Gehring, R., Baynes, R.E. et al. (2013). Effects of new sampling protocols on procaine penicillin G withdrawal intervals for cattle. *J. Am. Vet. Med. Assoc.* 243 (10): 1408–1412.

Goetting, V., Lee, K.A., and Tell, L.A. (2011). Pharmacokinetics of veterinary drugs in laying hens and residues in eggs: a review of the literature. *J. Vet. Pharmacol. Ther.* 34 (6): 521–556.

Korsrud, G.O., Boison, J.O., Papich, M.G. et al. (1993). Depletion of intramuscularly and subcutaneously injected procaine penicillin G from tissues and plasma of yearling beef steers. *Can. J. Vet. Res.* 57 (4): 223–230.

Otero, J.A., Real, R., de la Fuente, A. et al. (2013). The bovine ATP binding cassette transporter ABCG2 Y581S SNP increases milk secretion of the fluoroquinolone danofloxacin. *Drug Metab. Dispos.* 41 (3): 546–549.

Papich, M.G., Korsrud, G.O., Boison, J.O. et al. (1993). A study of the disposition of procaine penicillin G in feedlot steers following intramuscular and subcutaneous injection. *J. Vet. Pharmacol. Ther.* 16 (3): 317–327.

Pashov, D.A., Lashev, L.D., Matev, I.B. et al. (1997). Interspecies comparisons of plasma half-life of trimethoprim in relation to body mass. *J. Vet. Pharmacol. Ther.* 20 (1): 48–53.

Payne, M.A., Baynes, R.E., Sundlof, S.E. et al. (1999). Drugs prohibited from extralabel use in food animals. *J. Am. Vet. Med. Assoc.* 215 (1): 28–32.

Riviere, J.E., Webb, A.I., and Craigmill, A.L. (1998). Primer on estimating withdrawal times after extralabel drug use. *J. Am. Vet. Med. Assoc.* 213 (7): 966–968.

Short, C.R. (1994). Consideration of sheep as a minor species: comparison of drug metabolism and disposition with other domestic ruminants. *Vet. Hum. Toxicol.* 36 (1): 24–40.

Smith, G. (2013). Extralabel use of anesthetic and analgesic compounds in cattle. *Vet. Clin. N. Am. Food Anim. Pract.* 29 (1): 29–45.

Souza, M.J., Bergman, J.B., White, M.S. et al. (2017). Pharmacokinetics and egg residues after oral administration of a single dose of meloxicam in domestic chickens (*Gallus domesticus*). *Am. J. Vet. Res.* 78 (8): 965–968.

Swainston Harrison, T. and Keam, S.J. (2007). Azithromycin extended release: a review of its use in the treatment of acute bacterial sinusitis and community-acquired pneumonia in the US. *Drugs* 67 (5): 773–792.

Taha, A.A., Elsheikh, H.A., Khalafalla, A.E. et al. (1999). Disposition kinetics of tylosin administered intravenously and intramuscularly in desert sheep and Nubian goats. *Vet. J.* 158 (3): 210–215.

Toutain, P.-L., Ferran, A., and Bousquet-Melou, A. (2010). Species differences in PK and pharmacodynamics. *Hdbk. Exper. Pharmacol.* 199 (199): 19–48.

US Food and Drug Administration (FDA) (1996). Extralabel drug use in animals: final rule, 21 CFR part 530. *Fed. Regist.* 61 (217): 57731–57746.

US Food and Drug Administration (FDA). (2003). Guidance for Industry #152: Evaluating the Safety of Antimicrobial New Animal Drugs with Regard to Their Microbiological Effects on Bacteria of Human Health Concern. US Food and Drug Administration, Center for Veterinary Medicine, Washington, DC.

US Food and Drug Administration (FDA). (2006). Guidance for Industry #3: General Principles for Evaluating the Safety of Compounds Used in Food-Producing Animals. US Food and Drug Administration, Center for Veterinary Medicine, Washington, DC.

US Food and Drug Administration (FDA). (2012). Guidance for Industry #209: The Judicious Use of Medically Important Antimicrobial Drugs in Food-Producing Animals. US Food and Drug Administration, Washington, DC. http://www.fda.gov/downloads/AnimalVeterinary/GuidanceComplianceEnforcement/GuidanceforIndustry/UCM216936.pdf

US Food and Drug Administration (FDA). (2015). Guidance for Industry #230: Compounding Animal Drugs from Bulk Drug Substances. US Food and Drug Administration, Center for Veterinary Medicine, Washington, DC. *(Guidance withdrawn and no longer available.)*

US Food and Drug Administration (FDA). (2017). National Residue Program for Meat, Poultry, and Egg Products 2017 Residue Sampling Plans. US Food and Drug Administration, Washington, DC.

Villarino, N., Brown, S.A., and Martin-Jimenez, T. (2013). The role of the macrolide tulathromycin in veterinary medicine. *Vet. J.* 198 (2): 352–357.

23

Pharmacotherapeutics for Nontraditional Pets

Valerie J. Wiebe[1] and Lauren Eichstadt Forsythe[2]

[1] Department of Medicine and Epidemiology, School of Veterinary Medicine, and Veterinary Medical Teaching Hospital, University of California, Davis, CA, USA
[2] Veterinary Medical Teaching Hospital, School of Veterinary Medicine, University of California, Davis, CA, USA

Key Points

- Pharmacokinetic and pharmacodynamic studies in nontraditional pets are lacking, and as a result, most drug dosages used in these species are based on anecdotal experience.
- Extreme differences in anatomic, physiologic, and metabolic characteristics of nontraditional species compared to humans make pharmacotherapeutics very challenging.
- Compared to humans, most drugs are not labeled for use in nontraditional species and must be used in an extra-label manner.

- Rabbits are sometimes raised for human consumption, which places them in the "food animals" category and its accompanying regulations on drug use (Chapter 21).
- Veterinary practitioners face daily challenges dosing small nontraditional species and often resort to compounded, non-FDA-approved pharmaceutical preparations.
- Cost is frequently a limitation in the pharmacotherapy of nontraditional species, and, unlike human patients, most drugs are not covered by insurance.

Treating all veterinary patients can be challenging due to the lack of US Food and Drug Administration (FDA)-approved drugs and well-controlled clinical trials relative to trials for human patients. However, treating nontraditional pets (also called exotic animals) is even more challenging than treating a cat or a dog. The FDA designates many nontraditional animals, including zoo animals, parrots, guinea pigs, ferrets, and ornamental fish, among others, as "minor species." Because a drug used to treat a minor species is generally not going to be profitable for a pharmaceutical company (called the drug sponsor in an FDA application), it is difficult to find drugs to treat diseases and prevent suffering in minor species. To address drug use in minor species, the Minor Use and Minor Species Animal Health Act of 2004 was signed into law. This is often referred to as the MUMS Act and was designed to make more drugs legally available to treat not only minor species but also uncommon diseases in major species. Most drugs intended for treating minor species do not undergo the traditional FDA drug approval process.

Pharmacotherapeutics for Veterinary Dispensing, First Edition. Edited by Katrina L. Mealey.
© 2019 John Wiley & Sons, Inc. Published 2019 by John Wiley & Sons, Inc.

The MUMS Act provides three alternative routes for bringing drugs to market compared to the traditional drug approval pathway. These alternate routes are Conditional Approval, Designation, and Indexing. Conditional Approval allows a drug sponsor to market a drug prior to collecting all necessary efficacy data. Instead, a reasonable expectation of efficacy is provided, and then additional data are collected while the drug is being marketed. The drug sponsor has up to five years to market the conditionally approved drug before full approval or removal from the market is required. Designation is modeled after the Orphan Drug Act for humans. Designated animal drugs are eligible for grants and incentives to support safety and efficacy testing. Designation status does not allow the drug to be marketed until the drug is either approved or conditionally approved. However, if the drug is eventually approved, the sponsor receives seven years of market exclusivity. Indexing is the route that is followed when a drug is intended for use in a species that is too rare or varied for adequate clinical trials. The drug and indication are then added to the Index of Legally Marketed Unapproved New Animal Drugs for Minor Species (https://www.fda.gov/AnimalVeterinary/DevelopmentApprovalProcess/MinorUseMinorSpecies/ucm125452.htm). Indexed drugs are limited to minor species that are not used for food. While these three provisions provide additional ways for drugs to be legally used and marketed for animals, conditionally approved drugs and indexed drugs must be used exclusively as indicated on the label (extra-label drug use is not allowed).

Because so little is known about many nontraditional species, some of the diseases that veterinarians treat in these animals are a result of overall ignorance of their normal physiology, dietary requirements, ultraviolet (UV) light requirements, body temperature regulation, exercise requirements, ability to handle stress, and so on. The debate as to whether or not some of these species should even be kept as pets is beyond the scope of this chapter. However, some of the information presented in this chapter relates directly to animal husbandry as a means of disease prevention – this is made available for those providing medications for nontraditional species.

Section 1: Rabbits, Birds, and Pet Rodents

23.1 Introduction

This section will address some of the unique aspects of pharmacotherapy of small exotic animals, including rabbits, hamsters, guinea pigs, mice and rats, and birds. It will briefly cover some of the anatomic, physiologic, and metabolic differences between species and how this impacts pharmacotherapeutics. The legal, ethical, and regulatory aspects of drug therapy, and the doses of many commonly used drugs, will be covered for each species.

Rabbits, hamsters, and guinea pigs are innately sensitive to many drugs commonly used in other species, particularly antibiotics and drugs that alter gastrointestinal motility. Stress incurred by restraint of these species for drug administration may outweigh the benefits of treatment. Instead of trying to force a tablet into a rabbit's mouth, they can be crushed in palatable food (e.g. bananas, jam, or peanut butter) that will be voluntarily ingested. Vehicles used to compound drugs for nontraditional species should be free of high-calorie oils and sugars. Both the volume of drug administered and the taste often limit the use of many commercially available human drug products, so compounded drugs are often a necessity for small exotic animals. Pharmacists interested in specializing in compounded drugs for nontraditional species should work closely with veterinarians that specialize in treating these animals. As is the case for all compounded drugs, pharmacists should inform owners about limitations of extra-label and compounded drugs relative to FDA-approved formulations used according to the label.

23.2 Rabbit Pharmacotherapeutics

23.2.1 Comparative Aspects of Rabbit Diseases

Rabbits traditionally were used commercially for research, meat, and fur, but are now more commonly household companions. In 2006, it was estimated that there were at least 6.1 million pet rabbits in the USA (Shepherd 2008)· Very few drugs are labeled for use in rabbits, so most drugs used in pet rabbits are used in an extra-label manner. Extra-label use of human and veterinary drugs is permitted under the Animal Medical Drug Use Clarification Act (AMDUCA) for therapeutic reasons. If a rabbit has the potential to be consumed as food by humans, it is considered a food animal, and special precautions must be taken to avoid drug residues in the animal's tissues. The Food Animal Residue Avoidance Databank (FARAD) can be contacted to help establish the meat withdrawal time for a particular drug (www.farad.org). It is a legal requirement that the meat withdrawal time be determined and included on the prescription label for drugs dispensed to any animal that even has the potential for human consumption.

While humans are considered omnivores, rabbits are herbivores, and their microflora consist primarily of Gram-positive and anaerobic bacteria. Because antibiotic agents used to treat omnivores are often not safe for herbivores, antibiotic choices are limited in rabbits, particularly if administered orally due to the potential for dysbiosis and enterocolitis. Anatomically, rabbits have simple stomachs and a very large (10-fold greater than stomach capacity) cecum that occupies much of the abdomen (Carpenter et al. 1995). Cellulose digestion primarily occurs in the cecum. Unlike humans, rabbits are coprophagic and re-ingest their own fecal pellets four to eight hours after eating. Ingested caecotrophs serve as a source of nutrients, including B vitamins, amino acids, and fatty acids (Carpenter et al. 1995)

Caecotrophs can also serve as a source of re-ingested active drug or metabolite for drugs excreted in feces. This can make for very interesting plasma drug concentration versus time curves (Figure 23.1).

The rabbit gastrointestinal tract has several other features that contribute to its susceptibility to disorders and ailments. In contrast to humans, but similar to horses, rabbits are physically unable to vomit (which is a protective reflex). Their narrow pyloric lumen predisposes rabbits to hair accumulation, causing hair balls (trichobezoars). Nutritional deficiencies and poor hygiene can result in hairballs, hair chewing, and enteric diseases. Rabbits are highly sensitive to stress. Their strong physiologic response to stress not only weakens their immune system but also can lead to impaired gastrointestinal motility, which may be detrimental, even fatal, to rabbits due to their sensitive gastrointestinal tracts. Restraint during drug administration, painful injections, unpalatable oral medications, and indwelling catheters may all be highly stressful to rabbits. The stress incurred may outweigh the benefits of treatment in some instances.

Rabbits have elodont teeth (continuously growing with no anatomic roots). Teeth grow up to 10–12 cm a year, so that overgrowth, particularly with malocclusion, is frequently seen in rabbits (Harkness 1989). Subsequently, dental abscesses are very common in rabbits and can be challenging to treat. In one study, acquired dental disease accounted for up to 40% of 167 pet rabbits presenting with clinical abnormalities (Makitaipale et al. 2015). Periapical infections, osteomyelitis of the jaw, unilateral exophthalmos, and facial abscesses are all seen with progressive dental disease (PDD) syndrome in rabbits (Capello 2016). Both anaerobic Gram-negative and aerobic Gram-positive pathogenic bacteria have been cultured from facial abscesses (Tyrrel et al. 2002; Gardhouse et al. 2015). Antibiotics alone are typically not effective for resolving facial abscesses due to their inability to sufficiently penetrate into the abscess, but they are an important adjunct to

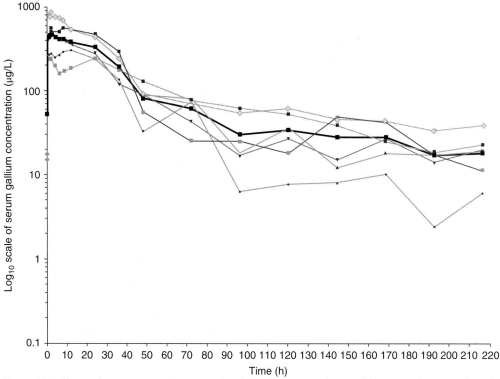

Figure 23.1 Plasma drug concentration versus time (nine days) curves for six rabbits treated once orally with gallium maltolate. Coprophagia causes numerous peaks and troughs in individual rabbit's plasma drug concentrations. *Source:* Image reproduced with permission from *Journal of Veterinary Pharmacology and Therapeutics* 2014;37(5):486–499.

surgical therapy. Aggressive surgical treatment is necessary to remove the abscess capsule, extract the diseased teeth, and address the focal osteomyelitis (Capello 2016) (Figure 23.2).

Similar to other animal species, rabbits can harbor bacterial, fungal, and parasitic diseases that can be transmitted to humans. Rabbits may have upper respiratory (sneezing, coughing, and nasal and ocular discharge) or lower respiratory (pneumonia) clinical signs due to *Bordetella bronchiseptia*, a Gram-negative rod-shaped bacterium that can also cause respiratory tract infections in humans. *Pasteurella multocida, Salmonella* sp., and *Francisella tularensis* may also cause significant clinical disease in both rabbits and humans. Ringworm (*Microsporum canis* or *Trichophyton* sp.) is an opportunistic fungal disease that causes skin lesions around the

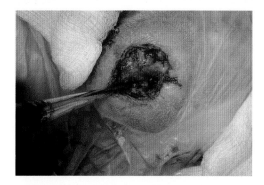

Figure 23.2 Facial abscesses are common in rabbits and are often a result of malocclusion. Abscesses do not respond well to systemic antibiotic treatment due to their thick-walled capsules. This rabbit's submandibular abscess was treated with surgical excision in combination with antibiotic therapy. Regular dental care was recommended to prevent reoccurrence.

head and ears of rabbits or raised erythematous plaques on human skin. Similar to other small mammals, rabbits frequently harbor fleas, ticks, and fur mites (*Cheyletiella* spp.).

23.2.2 Diagnostic Testing of Pet Rabbits

Rabbits are prey animals that often hide their illness, making it difficult for owners to detect health issues. Regular physical examinations by a veterinarian are advised, particularly in rabbits older than three years of age (Makitaipale et al. 2015). Physical examinations may identify common problems such as dental problems, abscesses, or intestinal abnormalities. Radiographs, computer tomography (CT) scans, blood work, and fecal and anaerobic and aerobic bacterial cultures may also be used for diagnostic purposes. Normal body temperature for rabbits is between 103.3 and 104 °F. Rabbits with temperatures <100.4 or >105 °F are cause for concern. Unlike humans, rabbits do not have elevated white blood cell (WBC) counts (leukocytosis) in response to infection. Sick rabbits are often anemic; therefore, low hemoglobin and packed cell volume (PCV) values are good indicators of illness. Rabbits have a much wider range of serum calcium concentrations (up to 16 mg/dL, whereas ~10 mg/dL is the upper limit of normal for dogs and cats), which may lead to an erroneous diagnosis of hypercalcemia

by veterinarians with little experience treating rabbits. Unlike most other mammals, rabbit urine is variable in color (yellow-red/brown) and clarity (clear to turbid), making overdiagnosis of urinary tract infections (UTIs) a common occurrence.

23.2.3 Pharmacologic Treatment of Common Rabbit Diseases

Antibiotics are probably the most common drug class prescribed for rabbits. As mentioned in this chapter, antibiotic choices are limited. Suppression of commensal enteric flora by some antibiotics allows proliferation of pathogenic bacteria, which can cause serious enteric disorders (Jenkins 1997). Antibiotics associated with dysbiosis, enteritis, and enterotoxemia in rabbits include amoxicillin, amoxicillin/clavulanic acid, ampicillin, cephalosporins, clindamycin, erythromycin, gentamicin, lincomycin, orally administered penicillin, tetracycline, and tylosin (Harkness and Wagner 1995; Jenkins 1997; Jekl et al. 2016). Antibiotics that are considered safe for rabbits include metronidazole, chloramphenicol, sulfonamides and potentiated sulfonamides, benzathine penicillin (this is an injectable formulation), and fluoroquinolones (Harkness and Wagner 1995; Jenkins 1997). Table 23.1 lists antibiotics and doses commonly used for treating bacterial infections in rabbits.

Table 23.1 Antibiotics commonly used to treat bacterial infections in rabbits.

Drug	Dose	Route	Frequency
Azithromycin	30 mg/kg	PO	Q 24 hours
Chloramphenicol	30–50 mg/kg	PO	Q 12 hours
Doxycycline	2.5 mg/kg	PO	Q 12 hours
Enrofloxacin	5–10 mg/kg	PO, IM, or SC	Q 12 hours
Marbofloxacin	2 mg/kg	PO	Q 24 hours × 5 days
Metronidazole	20–30 mg/kg	PO	Q 12 hours
Penicillin benzathine	42 000–60 000 IU/kg	IM	Q 48 hours

IM, Intramuscular; IU, International Units; SC, subcutaneous.

Mandatory monitoring
Rabbits treated with antibiotics should be monitored closely for any signs of gastrointestinal distress. Prolonged antibiotic courses of treatment should be avoided.

Abscesses are often polymicrobial involving anaerobic bacteria. Oral antibiotics including metronidazole, trimethoprim–sulfamethoxazole, or azithromycin, together with surgical lancing, cavitary lavage, and wound packing with synthetic gauze impregnated with antibiotics or polymethylmethacrylate (PMMA) antibiotic-impregnated beads, have shown some efficacy (Taylor et al. 2010). The most frequently prescribed fluoroquinolones in rabbits, enrofloxacin and marbofloxacin, do not have an adequate anaerobic spectrum.

Supportive care for rabbits often includes aggressive fluid therapy. Lactated Ringer's solution (LRS) or normal saline can be administered subcutaneously, although high volumes are typically required. Fluid rates in severely ill rabbits (10 ml/kg/hour) are higher than those administered to dogs and cats. Rabbits should receive appropriate analgesia to minimize stress, which will allow tissue healing. Mixed opioid agonist-antagonists such as buprenorphine and butorphanol are well tolerated and have fewer side effects than opioid agonists (e.g. oxymorphone and hydromorphone). Injectable buprenorphine can be dispensed to the owner to be administered to the rabbit orally (depositing the drug in the cheek pouch) for pain control. Drugs such as opioids can cause ileus or hypotension in rabbits. Table 23.2 lists analgesics and doses commonly used for treating rabbits.

Nonsteroidal anti-inflammatory drugs (NSAIDs) are used for chronic pain and inflammation in rabbits. Meloxicam has been administered long term for dental or arthritic pain. Rabbits should be monitored carefully for signs of gastrointestinal discomfort or ulceration with any NSAID. Although not helpful for preventing NSAID-induced gastrointestinal disease in dogs, there is evidence that sucralfate may help prevent NSAID-induced gastrointestinal irritation in rabbits (Schweitzer et al. 1985).

Rabbits are frequently the host for a variety of external parasites (fleas, ticks, mites, lice, and fly larvae). Fleas can be treated topically with imidacloprid. This is typically accomplished using a monthly flea preventive labeled for cats (Advantage II, Bayer Animal Health). Rabbits weighing less than 4 pounds can be dosed using the small-cat topical solution, while rabbits weighing over 4 pounds can be treated with the large-cat size. Similarly, a selamectin-containing product labeled for cats (Revolution, Zoetis) can be used, but because it is more rapidly cleared in rabbits it requires weekly (rather than monthly) application for effective flea control. Selamectin may also be used for treating lice and mites. Although a 1% ivermectin injectable cattle solution has been used in rabbits, it is not recommended because the product is highly concentrated, and it is difficult to safely and accurately measure

Table 23.2 Drugs commonly used as analgesics for rabbits.

Drug	Dose	Route	Frequency
Buprenorphine	0.01–0.05 mg/kg	SC, IM	Q 8–12 hours
Butorphanol	0.05–0.4 mg/kg	SC, IM	Q 8–12 hours
Carprofen	1.5 mg/kg	PO, SC	Q 12 hours
Meloxicam	1 mg/kg	PO, SC	Q 24 hours
Tramadol	11 mg/kg	PO	Q 8–12 hours

IM, Intramuscular; SC, subcutaneous.

Table 23.3 Drugs commonly used to treat/prevent parasitic diseases in rabbits.

Drug	Dose	Route	Frequency
Fenbendazole	10–20 mg/kg	PO	Repeat in 2 weeks
Ivermectin	0.2–0.4 mg/kg	SC	Repeat in 10–14 days
Praziquantel	5–10 mg/kg	PO, SC, IM	Repeat in 10 days
Lyme sulfa		Topical dip	Use weekly × 4–6 weeks
Imidacloprid/pyriproxyfen	Small cat for <4 lbs.	Topical	Q 4 weeks
(Advantage II™)	Large cat for >4 lbs.	Topical	Q 4 weeks
Selamectin	18 mg/kg	Topical	Q 7 days
(Revolution™)			

IM, Intramuscular; SC, subcutaneous.

out the volumes used to treat rabbits. Additionally, it is not a product that is typically stocked in retail pharmacies. Table 23.3 lists antiparasitic agents and doses commonly used to treat rabbits.

Rabbits have variable cytochrome P450 enzyme activity between different breeds and between individual animals, leading to variation in drug metabolism. They also have unique metabolic capacities that may affect some drugs. For example, rabbits have serum atropinesterase that greatly reduces the serum half-life of atropine relative to most mammalian species (Ecobichon and Comeau 1974). Vehicles such as propylene glycol that are used to dilute drugs can alter drug disposition and should be avoided when compounding drugs for rabbits (Walters et al. 1993).

23.2.4 Adverse Drug Effects in Rabbits

Rabbits have a very sensitive gastrointestinal tract that relies on a consistent microbiota and complex intestinal contractions. Drugs that disrupt digestive tract function in any way can be potentially fatal to rabbits by causing enterotoxemia. Orally administered antibiotics and drugs that disrupt appetite or gastrointestinal motility are examples. Owners must be educated to diligently monitor food intake and fecal output whenever administering drugs to their rabbit.

Corticosteroids are generally not prescribed for rabbits because they can cause severe immunosuppression and liver toxicity (Rosenthal 2004). Fipronil, the active ingredient in a number of topical flea and tick preventives for dogs and cats, should never be used on rabbits. If accidental exposure occurs, the rabbit should be bathed immediately with soap and water to remove as much of the drug as possible, and the rabbit should be examined by a veterinarian. Exposed rabbits that groom themselves may ingest the product, which could cause gastrointestinal signs (anorexia, hypersalivation, ileus, and adipsia) and depression. This may progress to tremors, seizures, or death (ASPCA AnTox Database).

23.2.5 Nutritional Supplements in Rabbits

Because rabbit gastrointestinal microflora are highly sensitive to changes in osmolarity, pH, and diet, nutritional supplements are not recommended. A rabbit's diet should include loose hay, high-quality dried grass provided ad libitum, and supplementation of dark, fibrous, leafy greens; fresh vegetables; and only a small amount of fresh fruit. Low intake of forage may contribute to the development of dental disease (Meredith et al. 2015). Diets or drug vehicles containing a large amount of simple carbohydrates can cause dysbiosis or even enterotoxemia (Carpenter et al. 1995). Baby rabbits (kits) may be given kitten or goat replacement formula twice daily until six weeks of age.

Trichobezoars (hair balls) can be prevented with a lubricating (petrolatum and mineral oil) laxative labeled for cats (Laxatone, Vetoquinol) administered orally every 12–24 hours for 5 days. Fresh pineapple juice (10 ml every 24 hours for 3–5 days every 2–3 months) has also been recommended (Carpenter et al. 1995).

23.3 Avian Pharmacotherapeutics

23.3.1 Comparative Aspects of Avian Diseases

Avian species are unique in many aspects of their anatomy and physiology, and they are more similar to their distant reptilian counterparts than to mammals. Their unique gastrointestinal, urogenital, and reproductive tracts predispose them to a variety of avian-specific diseases. For example, birds lack teeth, and their sharp beaks make it challenging to administer drugs orally. Oral medications may be administered directly by gavage, using a metal tube for larger birds or plastic catheter for smaller birds. Many birds have a crop, which is a thickened pouch that extends from the esophagus. Liquid medications should be administered directly into the crop and not into the upper esophagus, as this reduces the risk of regurgitation and aspiration. The maximum volumes that can be administered by gavage are dictated by the size of the bird and can be generalized to bird species: budgerigars (0.5 ml), cockatiels (2 ml), amazon parrots (5 ml), or macaws (10 ml). Birds can also be treated by adding drug to drinking water or feed. While this method has the advantage of being less stressful for the bird, it has its disadvantages. For one, sick birds tend to consume less food and water, which may result in subtherapeutic drug doses as well as dehydration if water intake is avoided

because of unpalatability. Nebulization is commonly used for administering drugs to treat respiratory tract or skin infections. Topically administered drugs are easily spread through preening and may damage plumage, which can cause loss of body heat – this is important because normal body temperature for birds (103–105 °F) is much higher than that of companion animals and humans.

Birds have a renal-portal system similar to that of reptiles. Blood from the caudal half of the body passes directly through the kidneys before joining the systemic circulation. Urine collected by the kidney is emptied into the cloaca through the ureters. The cloaca is the posterior orifice that serves as the common opening for the digestive, reproductive, and urinary tracts. Because of the renal-portal system, drugs injected into the leg muscles may actually get excreted before reaching the systemic circulation.

Unlike mammals, most pet birds are sexually dimorphic, so sex determination of a particular bird requires either endoscopic examination (requiring anesthesia) or DNA sexing. Most male birds do not have a phallus, so sperm is stored in the cloacal protuberance prior to copulation. Sperm is transferred when the cloacae touch and sperm enters the female reproductive tract. As eggs leave the ovary, they are fertilized before the shell is calcified in the oviduct. Reproductive disorders, including infertility, excessive egg production, dystocia, impacted oviduct, egg yolk peritonitis, and cloacal prolapse, are common in birds. Abnormal presentation of the egg can cause obstruction within the oviduct (dystocia) or "egg binding." Egg binding is defined as failure of the egg to pass through the oviduct within a normal time frame (48 hours) (Joyner 1994). Poor nutrition in the female (hen) can impair smooth muscle contraction or contribute to improper egg formation. Calcium, vitamin E, and selenium deficiency are key contributors to abnormal egg formation. Clinical signs include acute depression, sudden death, straining, drooped wings, coelomic distension, dyspnea, cloacal prolapse, paralysis, and unwillingness to perch.

Socially, birds exist in the wild as part of a flock. Captivity and isolation may lead to a variety of behavioral issues, such as feather plucking, aggression, and destructive behavior. These may reflect boredom as well as isolation in a species that is normally very social and flock-oriented. Chronic egg laying is the second most common behavioral problem in avian patients, and this may lead to a multitude of health issues (Gaskins and Bergman 2010).

Similar to human toddlers, birds seem to have a need to explore their environment with their mouths. This can lead to ingestion of potentially toxic substances, such as lead, zinc, pesticides, and drugs, which may cause toxicities in birds manifesting as lethargy, central nervous system signs, vomiting, and gastrointestinal disorders. Lead toxicosis is very common in birds that have chewed on blinds, costume jewelry, mirror backings, bird toys, and curtain weights. Lead accumulates in soft tissues and bone and is slowly released over time. Zinc toxicosis is less severe, but it occurs when birds chew on galvanized toys, chains, bells, keys, pennies, or galvanized wire. Birds also like to chew on plants, some of which (i.e. philodendrons) can irritate the tongue and pharynx.

Similar to other exotic species, birds are commonly treated for bacterial, fungal, and parasitic diseases. Respiratory, gastrointestinal, urinary tract, and reproductive tract infections are common in birds. The most common reported bacterial pathogens include Gram-negative enteric bacteria and Gram-positive cocci. Similar to humans, birds bitten by cats can become infected with *Pasteurella* sp. Pododermatitis (bumblefoot) is often associated with *Staphylococci*, which is usually a result of poor husbandry. Psittacosis is a zoonotic disease caused by *Chlamydia*, and it causes respiratory disease in birds and humans. Avian mycobacteriosis (*Mycobacterium avium* and *Mycobacterium genavense*) is not uncommon in psittacine species and manifests as anorexia, poor feather quality, lethargy, and diarrhea (Pollock 2006).

Fungal infections involving *Aspergillosis* spp. and *Candida* spp. are not uncommon in birds, particularly in birds that are stressed from travel, importation, overcrowding, and malnutrition (hypovitaminosis A). Prolonged antibiotic or corticosteroid treatments may also predispose birds to these opportunistic fungi, similar to other animal species (Dahlhausen 2006). Aspergillus infections tend to involve the nasal passages or deeper areas of the respiratory tract. *Candida albicans* more commonly affects the gastrointestinal tract, and infections are common in hand-reared neonatal birds.

Parasitic infections are common in birds, particularly if they are immunosuppressed. *Giardia psittaci* has been associated with feather-destructive behavior and diarrhea in cockatiels (Tully et al. 2009). Roundworms and tapeworms may be found in parrots that are housed outdoors. Mites (beak, face, legs, feathers, and airsacs) often cause crusting around the beak, cere (protuberance at the base of the bill), and legs in smaller birds (canaries, finches, and budgerigars).

23.3.2 Diagnostic Testing of Avian Pets

A thorough history of the bird's diet and husbandry, and the environmental stress under which the bird has been kept, is often valuable in determining a diagnosis, since disease is frequently related to these factors. A physical exam, complete blood count (CBC), and serum biochemistry are useful in diagnosis of metabolic diseases, renal compromise, infection, and inflammation. Increased serum concentrations of creatine phosphokinase (>600 IU/L) are indicative of muscle damage, which can occur with seizures, vitamin E or selenium deficiency, chlamydiosis, lead toxicity, or intramuscular (IM) injections. Elevated serum uric acid concentrations in birds are associated with renal disease, gout, dehydration, tissue damage, starvation, or hypervitaminosis. Unlike mammals, creatinine is not useful in determining renal function. Diagnostic imaging (e.g. radiographs and ultrasound) can be helpful in locating the position of an egg in "egg-bound" birds. Radiographs may reveal airsacculitis, granulomas, or severe pulmonary disease. CT scans or magnetic resonance imaging (MRI) may be used for diffuse disease. Use of molecular techniques such as polymerase chain reaction (PCR) can be useful for identifying specific infectious agents such as *Aspergillus*. Fecal examinations can be used for detecting gastrointestinal parasites. Mites may be seen on scrapings of crusts around the corners of the mouth, cere, or beak. Heavy metal toxicosis is diagnosed by determining plasma concentrations of the respective metals (e.g. lead or zinc).

23.3.3 Pharmacologic Treatment of Common Avian Diseases

Egg binding can be life-threatening in affected birds (Figure 23.3). Supportive care, fluids, analgesics, parenteral calcium, prostaglandins, or hormone therapy may be required (Scagnelli and Tully 2017). Chronic egg laying can be treated with dietary and environmental modifications in addition to pharmacologic manipulations. The synthetic human gonadotropin-releasing hormone agonist leuprolide acetate is commonly used to treat chronic egg laying in birds (Millam and Finney 1994; Klaphake et al. 2016). The "depo" formulations appear to work best (Deslorelin acetate, Suprelorin, and Virbac). Implants labeled for use in ferrets can be administered to Psittaciformes to suppress egg laying for up to three months (Mans and Pilny 2014; Summa et al. 2017).

Behavioral problems such as feather plucking have been treated with neuroleptics and antidepressants. Fluoxetine, amitriptyline, clomipramine, and haloperidol have all been used with some success. Drugs must be administered for three to four months before maximal efficacy is achieved, which can be discouraging to owners. The pharmacist can play a key role in client education in order to manage owner expectations and ensure owner compliance. Adding drugs to the drinking water by calculating the average daily water intake (50–150 ml water/kg body weight/day) may be of benefit in treating birds with oral medications. It is important to prepare medicated drinking water fresh

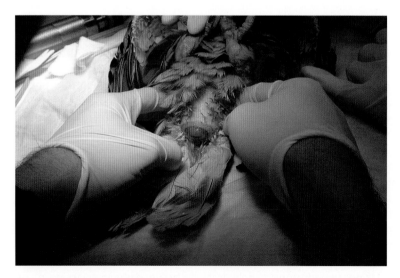

Figure 23.3 Egg-bound bird undergoing manual egg extraction. Egg binding is a common reproductive disorder in avian species that can be caused by obesity and diets poor in calcium and vitamins. Calcium, fluid therapy, oxytocin, and prostaglandins may assist in expulsion of the egg. If these fail, the veterinarian may extract the egg manually or surgically.

daily because drugs may degrade rapidly in aqueous solutions kept at room temperature.

Antibacterial therapy should be based on culture and sensitivity testing. Veterinary fluoroquinolones, such as enrofloxacin and marbofloxacin, can be compounded into flavored suspensions that can be administered to adult birds. Fluoroquinolones have bactericidal activity against many of the Gram-negative bacterial infections in birds (*Escherichia coli, Pseudomonas*, and *Serratia*) but should not be used in young birds. Ciprofloxin has highly variable absorption in veterinary species and should not be substituted for veterinary fluoroquinolones. The veterinary-approved amoxicillin/clavulanic acid product (Clavamox, Zoetis) is commonly administered for respiratory or skin infections caused by *Staphylococcus* or *Streptococcus* species. It may be diluted with half the volume of water stated on the label for a more concentrated suspension for smaller birds; however, the more concentrated solution has a shorter shelf life than if the product was diluted according to label directions. Prolonged courses of doxycycline are given for *Chlamydia psittaci*, although calcium and magnesium present in bird grit may impede oral absorption of doxycycline. Mycobacterial infections may be treated with azithromycin and ethambutol.

Common antifungal medications are listed in Table 23.4. Amphotericin B is the only fungicidal agent effective against *Aspergillus* sp. and may be administered by nebulization, nasal flush, intratracheal infusion, or intravenous (IV) injection. It must be diluted with sterile water since saline will decrease its potency. Oral terbinafine may be administered as an alternative. Nystatin or fluconazole are commonly used for *Candida* infections. Voriconazole is reserved for resistant organisms.

Giardiasis is typically treated with oral metronidazole (higher doses than for bacterial infections). Ivermectin, pyrantel pamoate, and fenbendazole are generally effective for treating roundworms, while praziquantel is used to treat tapeworm infections. Veterinary-labeled products are available in a variety of formulations (tablets, injectable, topical, oral, and spot-on products) and are preferred to human-labeled products. Mites may be treated with ivermectin or moxidectin.

Treatment of heavy metal toxicosis involves supportive care and chelation therapy. Calcium edetate disodium (Ca EDTA) is generally administered by injection while the bird is hospitalized. This is usually followed by oral treatment with dimercaptosuccinic acid (DMSA) or, less commonly, d-penicillamine for home treatment. Commercial availability of these products is sometimes questionable, so compounded products may be requested.

Table 23.4 Drugs commonly used to treat fungal infections in pet birds.

Drug	Dose	Route	Frequency
Amphotericin B	1 mg/kg	Intracheal	Twice daily
	0.25–1 mg/ml sterile	Nebulized water	10–20 minutes twice daily
Amphotericin B	100 mg/kg	PO	Q 12 hours × 30 days
Fluconazole	5–15 mg/kg	PO	Q 12 hours
Itraconazole	5–10 mg/kg	PO	Q 12–24 hours (Caution in African grays)
Ketoconazole	10–30 mg/kg	PO	Q 12 hours
Nystatin suspension	300 000–600 000 U/kg	PO	Q 12 hours
Terbinafine	10–15 mg/kg	PO	Q 12 hours
Voriconazole	12–18 mg/kg	PO	Q 12 hours

Midazolam, diazepam, and potassium bromide (compounded) are used for treating seizures in pet birds.

23.3.4 Adverse Drug Effects in Avian Patients

Antimicrobials can cause many adverse effects in exotic birds, particularly in finches, canaries, and soft bills. For example, potentiated sulfonamides may result in emesis or crop stasis, resulting in regurgitation one to three hours after oral dosing. Potentiated sulfonamides and aminoglycosides should be avoided in birds that are uricemic in order to prevent nephrotoxicity in dehydrated animals. Gentamicin seems to be more nephrotoxic than amikacin, and signs of nephrotoxicity (polyuria and polydipsia) are often encountered even when birds are treated with low doses. Cockatoos are particularly sensitive. African Gray parrots are very sensitive to gastrointestinal and hepatic adverse effects of itraconazole. Its use should be restricted to low doses only in conjunction with careful monitoring for regurgitation, anorexia, and hepatotoxicity. Fenbendazole may be toxic (e.g. causing intestinal necrosis and bone marrow suppression) to nestlings, growing birds, or those in molt. Ivermectin is toxic to finches, and it is toxic to budgerigars when administered parenterally but may be administered topically.

23.3.5 Nutritional Supplements in Avian Patients

Poor nutrition of the hen is a common contributor to both dystocia and egg binding. Calcium, vitamin E, and selenium deficiencies tend to be the most important causes (Joyner 1994). Obesity is also common in companion birds. High-fat table foods, seeds and nuts, too much food, and insufficient exercise contribute to obesity, hypercholesterolemia, and diabetes. A species-appropriate pellet diet should replace the table-food and seed/nut diet, and birds should be

encouraged to exercise by providing ropes and perches to encourage climbing. Bulk diets (with psyllium and peanut butter), which are sometimes recommended to enhance removal of lead from the gastrointestinal tract, should be used short term only. Predominantly seed diets may result in vitamin A deficiency and subsequent squamous metaplasia of the oral and respiratory epithelium, which predisposes to secondary fungal infections (Dahlhausen 2006). Vitamin A supplements can be sprinkled on food. Diets consisting of seeds only are deficient in iodine and can result in respiratory disease, causing stridor or wheezing. Lugol's iodine (1 drop/250 ml drinking water) can be used as a dietary supplement. Metabolic bone disease from nutritional secondary hyperthyroidism may be treated with supportive care, exposure to UV light, calcium gluconate (100 mg/kg, IM), and vitamin D supplementation. Iron storage disease from excessive iron intake is noted in toucans and mynahs with diets rich in vitamin C (citrus fruits) that increase iron absorption. Supplementation with chelators such as tannins, fiber, and phytates has been suggested. Although milk thistle (silymarin) and denamarin (S-adenosylmethionine and silybin–phosphatidylcholine complex) have been used in birds with elevated liver enzymes, there is no evidence as to their efficacy (Saller et al. 2001).

23.4 Rodent Pharmacotherapeutics

23.4.1 Comparative Aspects of Guinea Pig and Rodent Diseases

Guinea pigs, hamsters, mice, and rats are sometimes kept as household pets. Hamsters, mice, and rats belong to the mammalian order Rodentia. This is named after the Latin word *rodere*, which means "to gnaw." Guinea pigs and chinchillas are hystricomorph rodents from South America. Guinea pigs may also be considered food animals in some countries, such as those in South America, so when treating guinea pigs raised for food, all food animal restrictions must be followed (Chapter 22).

Because many of these species share similar anatomic and physiologic features, they will be addressed as a group. All are monogastric herbivores or omnivores and have continuously growing teeth, particularly the incisors, which can lead to dental problems if there is malocclusion. Rodents do not have sweat glands and are easily prone to heat exhaustion. To varying degrees, they are coprophagic, which serves as a good source of vitamin B. Total gastrointestinal drug transit time in guinea pigs may be up to 66 hours if coprophagy is taken into account (Ebino 1993) Unfortunately, little data exist as to how this affects the pharmacokinetics of drugs in these species.

Common disorders seen in pet rodents involve traumatic injuries from fighting with cage mates or predators (cats), nutritional deficiencies, and infectious diseases. Guinea pigs are unique among rodents (but similar to humans) in that they cannot metabolically convert glucose to ascorbic acid, so scurvy is a common disease. Guinea pigs with scurvy may have a rough hair coat, anorexia, diarrhea, lameness, and increased susceptibility to bacterial infections (Manning et al. 1984). Bacterial pneumonia involving *Bordetella bronchiseptica* and *Streptococcus pneumonia* is commonly seen in guinea pigs housed with dogs, cats, rabbits, or people harboring these organisms. While rodents can serve as a reservoir for diseases transmitted to other animals or humans, the reverse is also true. Pet rodents can be on the receiving end of diseases transmitted by humans or other animals.

Similar to rabbits, both guinea pigs and hamsters have a delicately balanced gastrointestinal microbiota that can be negatively impacted by antibiotics. Antibiotic-associated enterotoxemia may result from *Clostridium difficile* overgrowth, which can manifest as diarrhea, anorexia, dehydration, and hypothermia (Manning et al. 1984). Enteropathies are the most common ailment in hamsters for which a pharmacist might dispense drugs. Diarrhea can occur in hamsters of any age and is referred to as "wet-tail." Proliferative ileitis in young hamsters is associated with *Lawsonia intracellularis*, a Gram-negative obligate intracellular bacteria. Diarrhea in neonatal and adult mice is usually of viral origin.

Similar to humans, guinea pigs may develop urinary tract calculi. Older females (greater than three years old) are predisposed and may experience hematuria, dysuria, and a huddled or hunched posture (attributed to pain). Calcium oxalate stones often originate from a bacterial nidus in which calcium is deposited (O'Kewole et al. 1991). Urinary calculi are less common in mice. Chronic progressive nephrosis (CPN) is very common in pet and laboratory rats. Factors including sex, diet, age, and strain of rat will affect the likelihood that a rat will develop the disease as well as the age of onset and the rate of disease progression.

Many aged hamsters (>1.5 years) suffer from a genetically mediated cardiomyopathy. The disease can manifest as hyperpnea, tachycardia, and cyanosis. Atrial thrombosis may develop secondary to heart failure, and the incidence of arterial thrombosis is influenced by circulating androgens. Castrated male hamsters have an increased prevalence (Donnelly 1997).

Dermatologic infections in rodents may involve fungal organisms that cause ringworm (*Trichophyton mentagrophytes* and *M. canis*) or ectoparasites (mites, lice, and fleas). Animals with ringworm have pruritic lesions with alopecia and crusts of the face, forehead, and ears. Rodents with carcoptid mites often experience pruritus with excoriations on the thighs or back.

Guinea pigs may require treatment for cervical lymphadenitis (often called "lumps"), which is due to a *Streptoccoccus* infection of the mandible.

Similar to humans, dogs, and cats, rodents can develop neoplasia. Mammary neoplasms are common in both rats and mice, while hamsters are more likely to have neoplasia involving the scent gland.

23.4.2 Diagnostic Testing of Pet Rodents

Rodents are typically diagnosed after a thorough physical examination, an abbreviated CBC and/or blood chemistry, and a urinalysis. Large amounts of blood typically cannot be obtained from rodents, but a nail-clip or tail nick can provide enough blood for a smear and microhematocrit. Rectal temperatures may not be valid, since body temperature often increases during the examination. Unique to guinea pigs is that alanine aminotransferase (ALT) concentrations are low in hepatocytes, so it is not a good indicator of hepatocellular injury. Radiographs are useful for the diagnosis of scurvy, urinary calculi, and pulmonary changes consistent with pneumonia. Bacterial culture and susceptibility testing of bronchial secretions, mastitis, bite wounds, or infected cervical lymph nodes should be performed to guide antibiotic therapy. Ringworm can be diagnosed by fungal culture of plucked or scraped hair. Mite infestation can be diagnosed by cytologic examination of skin scrapings or identification of adult mites, nymphs, or eggs on hair shafts. Fecal smears or tape impression of the perianal skin can be used to diagnose pinworms. Blood urea nitrogen (BUN) can be estimated with the use of a blood dipstick for rats with CPN. Cardiomyopathy can be definitively diagnosed in hamsters by radiography and echocardiography.

23.4.3 Pharmacologic Treatment of Common Rodent Diseases

Disease prevention in pet rodents is important because pharmacological treatment of rodents is challenging. Good husbandry with balanced fresh food appropriate in caloric content, fresh water, a clean safe cage protected from extreme temperatures, and sunlight are basic needs. Rodents should be housed separate from other species to prevent interspecies pathogen transmission.

Administration of drugs to small rodents presents many unique challenges. Because commercially available drug formulations are generally not suitable for administration to very small animals, most drugs must be compounded. The oral route of administration is often the easiest route, as most rodents accept oral medications that have a sweet taste. For injectable medications, maximum volumes for drug administration are also very small and pose a limitation for some injectable drugs: IM (0.1 ml) and subcutaneous (SC) (2–5 ml).

The most common disease in guinea pigs that requires pharmacological treatment is scurvy. Vitamin C is administered by SC injection in the acute stage until the veterinarian determines that the patient can be adequately managed by oral vitamin C (vitamin C–fortified guinea pig chow). Antibiotic-associated enterotoxemia is best avoided in guinea pigs by avoiding inappropriate antibiotics and by *Lactobacillus* supplementation. Live culture yogurt (5 ml) per day can be administered to guinea pigs.

Guinea pigs diagnosed with urinary tract calculi are usually treated with antibiotics such as a potentiated sulfonamide, enrofloxacin, or chloramphenicol. Urinary acidifiers are typically not effective, since guinea pigs are not able to excrete acid loads (Harkness and Wagner 1995).

Depending on the severity of the disease, bacterial pneumonias in rodents may be treated with supportive care, including fluids, oxygen, force feeding, antibiotics, and vitamin C supplementation for guinea pigs. Antibiotics that are generally safe for guinea pigs include enrofloxacin, potentiated sulfonamides, or chloramphenicol. Bacterial respiratory infections are commonly treated with enrofloxacin or doxycycline (Donnelly 1997). Examples of drugs commonly used to treat guinea pigs are listed in Table 23.5.

Practiced but not proven

Although cardiomyopathy in hamsters is treated with the same classes of drugs often used to treat heart failure in other species (digoxin, pimobendan, diuretics, angiotensin-converting enzyme [ACE] inhibitors, and anticoagulants), there are no controlled studies to guide therapy.

Table 23.5 Drugs commonly used to treat guinea pigs.

Drug	Dose	Route	Frequency
Chloramphenicol	50 mg/kg	PO	Q 12 hours
Doxycycline	2.5 mg/kg	PO	Q 12 hours
Enrofloxacin	2.5 mg/kg	PO	Q 12 hours
Fenbendazole	20 mg/kg	PO	Q 24 hours × 5 days
Ivermectin	300 microgram/kg	SC	2 doses 8 days apart
Lyme sulfa 2.5% dip		Topical dip	Use weekly × 4–6 weeks
Miconazole cream		Topical	Use Q 24 hours × 2–4 weeks
Griseofulvin	25 mg/kg	PO	Q 24 hours × 3–5 weeks

SC, Subcutaneous.

Ringworm in guinea pigs can be treated topically with miconazole cream or lotion or systemically with griseofulvin (Hoefer 94). Ivermectin is frequently administered either subcutaneously or orally to treat mice with fur mites. A commercially available cattle formulation of ivermectin (1% solution) can be diluted with vegetable oil for oral administration. Housing mice on cedar or pine chips that have volatile hydrocarbons can provide ectoparasiticidal activity but may also induce cytochrome P450 enzymes, thereby enhancing the metabolism of some drugs (Donnelly 1997) – a unique drug–environment interaction.

23.4.4 Adverse Drug Effects in Rodents

Drugs known to cause enterotoxemia in guinea pigs and hamsters include penicillin, cephalosporins, ampicillin, clindamycin, erythromycin, tetracycline, bacitracin, vancomycin, and lincomycin. Rats and mice are less susceptible to antibiotic-induced gastrointestinal disturbances. However, streptomycin and dihydrostreptomycin have been reported to cause flaccid paralysis, coma, respiratory arrest, and death in rats and mice. As would be expected, rats with CPN should not be treated with nephrotoxic drugs.

23.4.5 Nutritional Supplements in Pet Rodents

Guinea pigs require supplemental sources of vitamin C. Pharmacists may recommend over-the-counter (OTC) vitamin C tablets. Vitamin C tablets are not highly stable in aqueous solution, so fresh vitamin C solution should be prepared daily (200–400 mg of vitamin C crushed in 1 L of deionized or distilled water). Aside from vitamin supplementation, so-called "nutraceuticals" are not recommended for pet rodents. A cross-section of commercial nutraceutical combinations showed no benefit and resulted in decreased lifespan in mice, suggesting they cause more harm than good (Spindler et al. 2014).

Section 2: Ferrets and Reptiles

23.5 Ferret Pharmacotherapeutics

Ferrets are popular pets throughout the USA. However, California and Hawaii have state laws that make it illegal to own ferrets within those states. There are also some cities with restrictions on owning ferrets despite the lack of statewide restrictions. Regardless of whether ferrets are considered legal pets, they can be found in all 50 states, so it is reasonable to assume that a pharmacist may come across a prescription for a ferret patient.

Ferrets have elongated bodies with short legs and have been described as otter- or weasel-like. Male ferrets are known as "hobs" and may be up to twice the size of females, known as "jills," with hobs growing to 2–4.5 pounds and jills reaching only 1–2.5 pounds. Unlike humans and dogs, ferrets are obligate carnivores. Their metabolic capacity for converting many xenobiotics found in plants is likely low, similar to cats, which are also obligate carnivores. This also affects their ability to metabolize drugs. For example, ferrets glucuronidate acetaminophen much more slowly than humans, dogs, or rats but at a similar rate to cats (Lewington 2000).

The ferret digestive tract is relatively short, resulting in passage of food within three to four hours (Lewington 2000). Therefore, oral drug transit time in ferrets is short relative to other species, which may impact the rate and extent of oral drug absorption. Because of their curious nature and nimble bodies, ferrets can gain access to purses, backpacks, cabinets, and other locations where OTC and prescription drugs are kept. The Animal Poison Control Center reported 43 cases of ibuprofen toxicosis in ferrets over a four-year period. Affected ferrets were reported to be more sensitive to ibuprofen-induced gastrointestinal and neurological toxicity than dogs at equivalent dosage rates (dogs, in turn, are more sensitive than people).

Ferrets seem to have an affinity for rubbery textures and will chew/eat any rubbery item they can obtain. This includes shoes, rubber bands, pencil erasers, and even rubber syringe stoppers, making them prone to gastrointestinal obstruction. This makes it difficult to find toys that ferrets can safely play with (Judah and Nuttall 2017).

Although ferrets are generally friendly and enjoy human attention, they can bite when agitated. When administering medication to ferrets, the animal should be restrained as gently as possible. If restraint is necessary, it should not involve holding the hind limbs, as this is particularly stressful for ferrets. Scruffing the ferret similar to a cat can provide effective restraint. A ferret that is scruffed with all four paws off the ground will relax completely (Lewington 2000). Many ferrets can be taught to readily accept small volumes of flavored drug solutions or suspensions. Meat and sweet flavors are often appropriate.

23.5.1 Comparative Aspects of Ferret Diseases

Ferrets can contract a variety of illnesses, some of which can be spread to people or other pets. For example, ferrets can contract rabies. There are very few drugs or biologicals approved for treating ferrets, but one of the few approved biologicals is a rabies vaccine. In states where ferrets are legal, rabies vaccination is required. Other organisms that can affect ferrets as well as other species include internal and external parasites (heartworms, fleas, and ear mites), influenza (human influenza types A and B), salmonella, and giardia. Noninfectious diseases that are common in ferrets include cardiac disease (dilated cardiomyopathy) and primary hyperadrenocorticism.

23.5.2 Diagnostic Testing of Pet Ferrets

- Thorough history and physical examination
- CBC, biochemistry panel, and urinalysis
- For dermatologic diseases: skin scrapings, and fungal and bacterial cultures
- Basal and stimulated or suppressed serum hormone concentrations (for hyperadrenocorticism)
- Radiographs
- Advanced imaging (less common due to owner financial constraints): ultrasound, CT, and MRI.

23.5.3 Pharmacologic Treatment of Common Ferret Diseases

Despite the popularity of ferrets as pets, there are very few drugs approved for treating them. Extra-label use of human or veterinary drugs is a necessity. Pharmacists can be a valuable part of the veterinary medical team by providing appropriate compounding. Dilution and flavoring of FDA-approved human or veterinary drugs comprise the most common need. Because liquid formulations are easiest for owners to administer, it is important that pharmacists have a good understanding of drug stability in liquid formulations.

Flea infestations can be a problem for ferrets. Because there are no FDA-approved products for treating ferrets, extra-label use of feline topical or "spot-on" products is often used, even though safety and efficacy have not been evaluated. Fipronil and imidacloprid have both been recommended (Table 23.6). Ferrets should not be allowed to lick the area where the product was applied before it is completely dry (Oglesbee 2006). Flea collars and products containing pyrethrins and pyrethroids should be avoided.

Respiratory disease in ferrets can vary from self-limiting viral infections to serious bacterial pneumonia. Not only are ferrets susceptible to human influenza types A and

B, but also the virus can be transmitted from humans to ferrets or from ferrets to humans. Ferrets with respiratory infections should be isolated from humans and other ferrets to prevent disease transmission.

Practiced but not proven

Symptomatic treatment (antihistamines) and antivirals may be prescribed for ferrets with influenza, but there are no data to support their efficacy.

Heartworm disease, caused by infection with *Dirofilaria immitis*, can occur in dogs, cats, and ferrets. While dogs can have relatively large worm burdens, cats and ferrets often have only a few adult worms. However, even one or two adult heartworms can cause severe cardiac disease in a ferret's small heart. The only FDA-approved drug for treating adult heartworms (melarsomine) is labeled for administration by a veterinarian only, so pharmacists won't be dispensing it to owners. A "slow kill" method for treating heartworms has also been described for animals without signs of congestive heart failure (CHF). This method involves the drug ivermectin. Regardless of which method is used to treat heartworms, death of adult heartworms within the vascular system can

Table 23.6 Antibacterial, antivirals, and antiparasitic drugs used to treat ferrets (Oglesbee 2006).

Drug	Dose	Route	Frequency
Amantadine	6 mg/kg	PO	Q 12 hours
Amoxicillin	10 mg/kg	PO	Q 12 hours
Cephalexin	15–25 mg/kg	PO	Q 8–12 hours
Clarithromycin	12.5 mg/kg	PO	Q 8 hours
Enrofloxacin	10–20 mg/kg	PO, SC or IM	Q 24 hours
Fipronil	1/5–1/2 of a cat tube	Topically	Q 60 days
Imidacloprid	1 cat dose	Topically	Q 30 days
Ivermectin	0.05 mg/kg	PO	Q 30 days
Metronidazole	20 mg/kg	PO	Q 12 hours

IM, Intramuscular; SC, subcutaneous.

cause a substantial inflammatory response. Anti-inflammatory doses of corticosteroids are usually administered for several months to address complications arising from worm emboli. There are limited data on the safety and efficacy of these treatment regimens in ferrets. The prognosis is usually poor, especially in ferrets with overt symptoms of CHF (Oglesbee 2006).

Ferrets can also develop CHF that is not associated with heartworm disease. This is most commonly a result of dilated cardiomyopathy. Drugs used to treat CHF in ferrets are based on those used in other species and include furosemide (ferrets will generally accept the pediatric elixir willingly), enalapril, digoxin, and nitroglycerin. Ferrets are sensitive to the hypotensive effects of ACE inhibitors, making it crucial to start with every-other-day dosing of enalapril (Oglesbee 2006).

Surgical castration of ferrets is a common practice in the USA to prevent reproduction, decrease aggression with other ferrets, and decrease their musky odor. Spaying females not only prevents reproduction but provides the added medical benefit of preventing estrogen-induced bone marrow suppression caused by persistent estrus in nonbreeding jills. However, neutered/spayed ferrets are at a higher risk of primary hyperadrenocorticism. In humans and dogs with hyperadrenocorticism, cortisol is the hormone that is usually secreted in excess, while in ferrets, sex steroids including estradiol, 17-hydroxyprogesterone, and androstenedione are secreted in excess. Pharmacological treatment for hyperadrenocorticism in ferrets, therefore, is not the same as it is for humans or dogs with hyperadrenocorticism. Surgical removal of the affected adrenal gland, if possible, offers the highest chance of cure. If surgery is not an option, long-acting GnRH agonists such as leuprolide acetate or deslorelin have been used. Deslorelin implants are available as an index drug that is labeled for use in ferrets and marketed under the name Suprelorin F° (Wagner et al. 2005; Schoemaker et al. 2008; Lennox and Wagner 2012; van Zeeland et al. 2014). These drugs are administered by

veterinarians, so it is unlikely that pharmacists will be dispensing them.

Ferrets are prone to gastroduodenal ulcers. Like humans, but unlike dogs, cats, and horses, *Helicobacter* frequently plays a role (*Helicobacter mustelae*). Other potential causes of gastroduodenal ulcers include foreign bodies, anorexia, gastric neoplasia, metabolic disease, drugs such as NSAIDs, and stress or major illness. Symptoms of gastric ulceration include anorexia, diarrhea, melena, vomiting, abdominal pain, weight loss, and weakness. Treatment involves addressing the underlying cause. If *Helicobacter* infection is identified or strongly suspected, then appropriate therapy includes combination protocols such as amoxicillin, metronidazole, and bismuth subsalicylate *or* clarithromycin, ranitidine, and bismuth subsalicylate (Oglesbee 2006).

Additional drugs that may be helpful in treating gastric ulcers in ferrets include gastric acid secretory inhibitors. Ferrets, like horses, are continuous gastric acid secretors. Anorexia greatly increases the risk for gastric ulceration. Proton pump inhibitors and histamine receptor antagonists have been used to suppress gastric acid secretion. Sucralfate may be used in patients with gastric ulcers to prevent further ulceration and promote healing. However, there are no data confirming efficacy of any of these drugs in ferrets. Aside from the potential for drug interactions associated with H2 receptor antagonists (cimetidine in particular), omeprazole, and sucralfate, there is little risk in empirical treatment (Oglesbee 2006). Table 23.7 lists drugs used for gastrointestinal disease in ferrets.

23.5.4 Adverse Drug Effects in Ferrets

Ferrets are susceptible to similar drug-related adverse effects seen in other species, but metabolic differences mean that some medications that are safe in humans (and other species) can be extremely toxic to ferrets. This is the case with flea products containing pyrethrin, as mentioned in this chapter. Even some OTC products can be toxic to ferrets

Table 23.7   Gastrointestinal agents used to treat ferrets.

Drug	Dose	Route	Frequency
Bismuth subsalicylate	17–20 mg/kg	PO	Q 12 hours
Cimetidine	5–10 mg/kg	PO, SC, or IM	Q 8 hours
Famotidine	0.25–0.5 mg/kg	PO	Q 12–24 hours
Omeprazole	0.7 mg/kg	PO	Q 24 hours
Ranitidine bismuth citrate	24 mg/kg	PO	Q 8 hours
Sucralfate	25 mg/kg	PO	Q 8 hours

IM, Intramuscular; SC, subcutaneous.
Source: Oglesbee (2006).

(and other veterinary species, as discussed in Chapter 6). For example, even extremely low doses of acetaminophen and ibuprofen can cause serious adverse effects in ferrets despite their safety in humans (even small children).

23.5.5   Nutritional Supplements in Ferrets

Nutritional supplements are not commonly used in ferrets, with the exception of replacing a specific nutritional deficiency. For example, ferrets with vitamin A deficiency were more susceptible to canine distemper virus infection than ferrets that received vitamin A supplementation (Rodeheffer et al. 2007). An appropriate diet will ensure that nutritional deficiencies do not occur.

23.6   Reptile Pharmacotherapeutics

While many US households have a dog or cat, few in comparison have reptiles as pets. However, the reptile population in the USA is estimated to be 7.3 million (Mader 1996). This patient population is difficult for veterinarians to treat because of the paucity of evidence to support the safety or efficacy of pharmacological therapy. This is slowly changing, as more veterinarians are starting to treat captive reptiles. As a result, pharmacists are more likely to be asked to fill prescriptions for reptile pets. Because this will entail extra-label use that will often require compounding, owners should be apprised of the relevant risk, particularly with compounded formulations.

The reptile class encompasses a wide variety of species that differ greatly in size and physical appearance. Additionally, these species have evolved to exist in a wide range of natural habitats. Thus, there is likely tremendous physiologic differences between reptilian species that contribute to differences in drug disposition. Unfortunately, almost nothing is known about drug disposition differences between reptile species. Drug dosages reported in the literature come from pharmacokinetic studies or from metabolic scaling, or they are empirical. While pharmacokinetic data are ideal when determining a dose, few studies have been performed. To further complicate matters, the temperature at which the study is performed can limit the applicability of the results. The process of metabolic scaling uses drug doses from well-studied species to predict a drug dose for a less well-studied species based on metabolic size. Animals are grouped into five metabolic categories (one of which is reptiles), with each category represented by a mathematical constant that is used to convert metabolic scale between groups. There are a number of limitations to metabolic scaling, one of which is that it doesn't address species differences between animals in the same group (i.e. it treats all reptiles the same). Another limitation is that metabolic scaling emphasizes weight differences with the assumption that smaller animals have a greater metabolic rate. While that is true for endothermic animals, it has not been shown to be the case with ectotherms. Another limitation is that metabolic scaling does not take age into account. It is presumed that immature reptiles may require lower drug doses due to incompletely developed hepatic and renal functions, but there are no studies to guide dosing of immature reptiles. Empirical dosing is loosely determined based on dosages used in mammalian species and subsequently adjusted based on clinical experience (Mader 1996).

As with other pets, owners of sick reptiles prefer to treat their pet at home rather than have their pet treated as a hospitalized patient.

Dramatic difference

The mortality rate is much higher for reptiles that are treated as outpatients compared to reptiles undergoing treatment as inpatients. Some potential reasons for improved outcomes in hospitalized versus home-treated reptiles include more tightly controlled husbandry in-hospital, treatments provided at the appropriate times (not based on the owner's schedule), and ongoing monitoring for early detection of complications. Thus, unless the owner is highly experienced in reptile care, it is in the reptile's best interest not to be discharged from the hospital until its therapeutic requirements are minimal.

One of the most important factors to consider when selecting a particular drug to treat a reptile patient is the route of administration. For example, the oral route may be feasible in some reptiles but not in others. For example, the oral route is often preferred in turtles, but this can be difficult to accomplish. To administer oral medications to a turtle, the head has to be held in a position that does not cause harm while simultaneously preventing the head from retreating into the shell and keeping the turtle's mouth open. This is often a job for more than one person. Another consideration is that aquatic turtles have difficulty swallowing food while on land. Therefore, after oral drug administration, the mouth must be thoroughly rinsed to prevent aspiration. Many turtles will also gag and vomit almost anything that is put into their mouth. Currently, there is little information published regarding pharmacokinetics of orally administered drugs in reptiles. Differences between reptile species, including differences in gastrointestinal transit times, likely contribute to species differences in oral drug absorption. For example, carnivorous reptiles generally have faster gastrointestinal transit times than herbivores. How this affects oral drug absorption in reptiles has not yet been determined.

If a parenteral route of administration is chosen, IM injection is generally preferred to SC injection. Drugs that are irritating to tissues should not be injected subcutaneously.

Dramatic difference

When administering drugs by injection to reptiles and birds, they should not be injected anywhere in the caudal half of the body (rear limbs) because the renal-portal vascular system may clear drug from the bloodstream before it can enter the systemic circulation.

23.6.1 Comparative Aspects of Reptile Diseases

Reptiles can harbor a variety of bacterial, fungal, protozoal, and parasitic organisms that can infect people (zoonotic organisms). Individuals who are most susceptible to these infections include children and elderly or immunocompromised individuals. The pharmacist can play an important role in educating reptile owners about the potential for zoonotic disease. Even apparently healthy reptiles can harbor zoonotic pathogens such as salmonella, so it is important to take pre-cautions to prevent human infection (Longley 2010). Proper hygiene (wash hands after contact with pet or its cage; disinfect cage frequently; keep reptile away from locations where food is stored, prepared, or eaten; etc.) is necessary in households with pet reptiles.

Unlike mammals and birds, reptiles are ectotherms. They are unable to increase their body temperature based on physiological changes (they do not experience "fevers"). However, some species can develop a "behavioral fever" in response to bacterial endotoxins. These endotoxins cause the release of a hormone that acts on the hypothalamus, resulting in the reptile seeking out warmer areas of the habitat, increasing the reptile's core body temperature. Increased core body temperature augments the reptile's immune system. Although age can affect immunocompetence in any species, the immune system appears to develop early in some reptiles (as early as 24 hours of age), but this varies by species. Similar to other species, an excessive stress response can suppress the reptile immune system. A number of modifiable factors can induce a stress response in reptiles, including poor nutritional status, insufficient heat and lighting, lack of hiding areas, poor water quality, excessive handling, recent capture and/or transport, injury, and others. Modifying these factors through appropriate care and husbandry can contribute significantly to the therapeutic plan for sick or injured reptiles (Mader 1996). This information can be part of the owner counseling and education process when a prescription is filled for a reptile patient.

23.6.2 Diagnostic Testing of Pet Reptiles

- Thorough history and physical examination, including accurate weight to facilitate appropriate drug dosing
  Note: Information about husbandry and diet are often key elements in diagnosing disease in reptiles.

- CBC, biochemistry panel, and urinalysis (less beneficial than in mammals)
- Fecal flotation (urine and fecal matter are commonly expelled during the exam) for diagnosis of internal parasites
- Radiographs can be helpful in assessing vitamin D deficiency and pathologic fractures.
- Cytologic or histopathologic evaluation of shed skin, skin scrapes, and impression smears, and biopsies of scale, skin, shell, or other tissues
- Sampling of respiratory tract via transtracheal wash or endoscopy
- Bacterial or fungal cultures.

23.6.3 Pharmacologic Treatment of Common Reptile Diseases

Dehydration can be a serious problem that complicates many other diseases of reptiles. Administering fluids intravenously to reptiles can be difficult, so crystalloid fluids are more commonly administered by oral, intracoelomic, SC, or intraosseous routes. If the reptile is maintained at appropriate temperatures, the oral route works well using a stomach tube or ball-tipped feeding needle. Fluid options include lactated Ringer's solution + 2.5% dextrose, or OTC electrolyte drinks such as Gatorade™ or Pedialyte™. If the oral route is not an option, parenteral routes can be used by appropriately trained veterinary staff. It is important not to overhydrate a reptile. Since reptiles lack a diaphragm, large fluid volumes can compromise lung capacity and tidal volume (Mader 1996).

Respiratory infections are usually chronic and advanced by the time veterinary care is sought for a reptile pet, so long-term, multimodal, aggressive antimicrobial therapy is undertaken. To ensure adequate plasma concentrations, the parenteral route of administration is often used. Antibacterial and antifungal drugs used in reptiles are listed in Table 23.8. For outpatient treatment of respiratory disease in turtles, any medication that can administered by nebulization to a person or small mammal can generally be administered to a turtle by that

Table 23.8 Antimicrobial agents commonly used to treat reptiles.

Drug	Dose	Route	Frequency
Ceftazidime	20–40 mg/kg	IM	Q 48–72 hours
Ceftiofur sodium	5 mg/kg	SC, IM	Q 24–48 hours
Enrofloxacin	5–10 mg/kg	IM	Q 24–48 hours
Itraconazole	5–10 mg/kg	PO	Q 24 hours
Piperacillin	50–100 mg/kg	IM	Q 24–48 hours
Voriconazole	10 mg/kg	PO	Q 24 hours

IM, Intramuscular, IU, International Units; PO, oral; Q, every; SC, subcutaneous.
Source: Mitchell and Tully (2016).

route, causing relatively little stress for the patient. However, this route can also have its limitations due to the ability of turtles to "hold their breath" for extended time periods (Mitchell and Tully 2016).

Metabolic bone disease describes a group of disorders that affect the development, integrity, and function of bones. In reptiles, metabolic bone disease is often the result of an improper diet or renal disease. A diet that is deficient in calcium and vitamin D and with excessive phosphorus is the most common cause. Treatment involves supplementation of calcium and vitamin D. Calcium should be administered orally in the form of calcium glubionate after vitamin D deficiency has been corrected. The patient's diet should be corrected to prevent recurrent nutritional deficiencies (Mitchell and Tully 2016).

Hypovitaminosis A is also the result of an improper diet and is most common in reptiles that are insectivores. Hypovitaminosis A increases susceptibility to secondary infectious diseases because it interferes with normal immune function. Treatment is accomplished by supplementing oral vitamin A and correcting the diet (Mitchell and Tully 2016).

23.6.4 Adverse Drug Effects in Reptiles

Pharmacists should not recommend OTC products to treat reptiles for a number of reasons. If a reptile is sick enough to be exhibiting signs that an owner takes note of, it is likely the pet's disease is serious and/or advanced and requires veterinary care. Doses for OTC products are not established in reptiles. In addition to the adverse drug effects seen in mammals, there is one particular drug sensitivity worth noting. The antiparasitic drug ivermectin is contraindicated in chelonians (turtles, terrapins, and tortoises) due to extreme susceptibility to its neurological adverse effects. This is most likely related to a blood–brain barrier deficiency.

23.6.5 Nutritional Supplements in Reptiles

Specific vitamin supplements are used to treat deficiencies that are caused when inappropriate diets are fed to pet reptiles. For example, lizards are often fed crickets or mealworms because they are easily obtained and trigger normal feeding. However, they are low in calcium, so calcium supplementation should be provided. Commercial products are available as powders that can be dusted onto the insects. There is no evidence that nutritional supplements with claims that suggest health benefits (e.g. milk thistle) have efficacy in reptiles, as is the case with other species (Jepson 2009).

References

Capello, V. (2005). *Rabbit and Rodent Dentistry Handbook*. Ames, IA: Wiley-Blackwell.

Carpenter, J.W., Mashima, T.Y., Gentz, E.J. et al. (1995). Caring for rabbits: an overview and formulary. Symposium on rabbit medicine. *Vet. Med.* 340–364.

Dahlhausen, R.D. (2006). Implications of mycosis in clinical disorders. In: *Clinical Avian Medicine*, vol. vol. 2 (ed. G.J. Harrison and T.L. Lightfoot), 691–704. Palm Beach, FL: Spix Publishing.

Donnelly, T.M. (1997). Disease problems of small rodents. In: *Ferrets, Rabbits and Rodents. Clinical Medicine and Surgery* (ed. E.V. Hillyer and K.E. Quesenberry), 307–336. Philadelphia: WB Saunders.

Ebino, K.Y. (1993). Studies on coprophagy in experimental animals. *Exp. Anim.* 42: 1–9.

Ecobichon, D.J. and Comeau, A.M. (1974). Genetic polymorphism of plasma carboxylesterases in the rabbit: Correlation with pharmacologic and toxologic effects. *Toxicol. Appl. Pharmacol.* 27: 28–40.

Gardhouse S, Sanchez-Migallon Guzman D, Paul-Murphy J, et al. (2015). Microbiology and antimicrobial susceptibilities of odontogenic abscesses in domestic rabbits. In Proceedings of Exotics Conference, San Antonio, TX, p. 357.

Gaskins, L. and Bergman, L. (2010). Surveys of avian practitioners and pet owners regarding common behavioral problems in psittocine birds. *J. Avian Med. Surg.* 25 (2): 111–118.

Harkness, J.E. (1989). *The Biology and Medicine of Rabbits and Rodents*, 3e (ed. J.E. Wagner), 9–19. Philadelphia: Lea and Febiger.

Harkness, J.E. and Wagner, J.E. (1995). *The Biology and Medicine of Rabbits and Rodents*, 4e. Baltimore: Williams and Wilkins.

Jekl, V., Hauptman, K., Minarikova, A. et al. (2016). Pharmacokinetic study of benzylpenicillin potassium after intramuscular administration in rabbits. *Vet. Rec.* 179 (1): 18. doi: 10.1136/vr.103531.

Jenkins, J.R. (1997). Soft tissue surgery and dental procedures. In: *Ferrets, Rabbits and Rodents: Clinical Medicine and Surgery* (ed. E.V. Hillyer and K.E. Quesenberry), 230–239. Philadelphia: Saunders.

Jepson, L. (2009). *Exotic Animal Medicine: A Quick Reference Guide*, 2e. St. Louis, MO: Elsevier.

Joyner, K.L. (1994). Theriogenology. In: *Avian Medicine: Principles and Application* (ed. B.W. Ritchie, G.J. Harrison and L.R. Harrison), 748–775. Lake Worth, FL: Wingers Publishing.

Judah, V. and Nuttall, K. (2017). *Exotic Animal Care & Management*. Boston: Cengage Learning.

Klaphake, E., Fecteau, K., DeWit, M. et al. (2016). Effects of leuprolide acetate on selected blood and fecal sex hormones in Hispaniolan Amazon parrots (*Amazona ventralis*). *J. Avian Med. Surg.* 23 (4): 253–262.

Lennox, A.M. and Wagner, R. (2012). Comparison of 4.7-mg deslorelin implants and surgery for the treatment of adrenocortical disease in ferrets. *J. Exotic Pet. Med.* 21 (4): 332–335.

Lewington, J.H. (2000). *Ferret Husbandry, Medicine & Surgery*. Woburn, MA: Butterworth-Heinemann.

Longley, L. (2010). *Saunders Soluions in Veterinary Practice: Small Animal Exotic Pet Medicine*. St. Louis, MO: Elsevier.

Mader, D.R. (1996). *Reptile Medicine and Surgery*. Philadelphia: WB Saunders.

Makitaipale, J., Harcourt-Brown, F.M., and Laitinen-Vapaavuori, O. (2015). Healthy survey of 167 pet rabbits (*Oryctolagus cuniculus*) in Finland. *Vet. Rec.* 177 (16): 418.

Manning, P.J., Wagner, J.E., and Harkness, J.E. (1984). Biology and diseases of guinea pigs. In: *Laboratory Animal Medicine* (ed. J.G. Fox, B.J. Cohen and F.M. Loew), 149–181. Orlando, FL: Academic Press.

Mans, C. and Pilny, A. (2014). Use of GnRH agonists for medical management of reproductive disorders in birds. *Vet. Clin. N. Am. Exotic Anim. Pract.* 17: 23–33.

Meredith, A.L., Prebble, J.L., and Shaw, D.J. (2015). Impact of diet on incisor growth and attrition and the development of dental disease in pet rabbits. *J. Small Anim. Pract.* 56: 377–382.

Millam, J. and Finney, H. (1994). Leuprolide acetate can reversibly prevent egg laying in cockatiels. *Zoo Biol.* 13: 149–155.

Mitchell, M.A. and Tully, T.N. (2016). *Current Therapy in Exotic Pet Practice*. St. Louis, MO: Elsevier.

Oglesbee, B.L. (2006). *The 5-Minute Veterinary Consult: Ferret and Rabbit*. Ames, IA: Blackwell.

O'Kewole, P.A., Odeyemis, P.S., Oldummade, M.A. et al. (1991). An outbreak of *Streptococcus pyogenes* infection associated with calcium oxalate urolithiasis in guinea pigs (*Cavia porcellus*). *Lab. Anim.* 25: 184–186.

Pollock, C.G. (2006). Implications of mycobacteria in clinical disorders. In: *Clinical Avian Medicine*, vol. vol. 2 (ed. G.J. Harrison and T.L. Lightfoot), 681–690. Palm Beach, FL: Spix Publishing.

Rodeheffer, C., Messling, V.V., Milot, S. et al. (2007). Disease manifestations of canine distemper virus infection in ferrets are modulated by vitamin A status. *J. Nutr.* 137: 1916–1922.

Rosenthal, K.L. (2004). Therapeutic contraindications in exotic pets. *Sem. Avian Exotic Pet. Med.* 13 (1): 4448.

Saller, R., Meier, R., and Brignoli, R. (2001). The use of silymarin in the treatment of liver disease. *Drugs* 61 (14): 2035–2063.

Scagnelli, A.M. and Tully, T.N. (2017). Reproductive disorders in parrots. *Vet. Clin. Exotic Anim.* 20: 485–507.

Schoemaker, N.J., van Deijk, R., Muijlaert, B. et al. (2008). Use of a gonadotropin releasing hormone agonist implant as an alternative for surgical castration in male ferrets (*Mustela putorius furo*). *Theriogenology* 70 (2): 161–167.

Schweitzer, E.J., Bass, B.L., Johnson, L.F. et al. (1985). Sucrafate prevents the experimental peptic esophagitis in rabbits. *Gastroenterology* 88 (3): 611–619.

Shepherd, A.J. (2008). Results of the 2006 AVMA survey of companion animal ownership in US pet-owning households. *J. Am. Vet. Med. Assoc.* 232: 695–696.

Spindler, S.R., Mote, P.L., and Flegal, J.M. (2014). Lifespan effects of simple and complex nutraceutical combinations fed isocalorically to mice. *Age* 36 (2): 705–718.

Summa, N.M., Wils-Plotz, E.L., Guzman, D.S.M. et al. (2017). Evaluation of the effects of a 4.7 mg deslorelin acetate implant on egg laying in cockatiels (*Nymphicus hollandicus*). *Am. J. Vet. Res.* 78 (6): 745–751.

Taylor, M.W., Beaufrere, H., Mans, C. et al. (2010). Long-term outcome of treatment of dental abscesses with a wound-packing technique in pet rabbits: 13 cases (1998–2007). *J. Am. Vet. Med. Assoc.* 237: 1444–1449.

Tully, T.N., Dorrestein, G.M., and Jones, A.K. (2009). *Handbook of Avian Medicine*. Edinburgh, UK: Saunders Elsevier.

Tyrrel, K.L., Citron, D.M., Jenkins, J.R. et al. (2002). Peridontal bacteria in rabbit mandibular and maxillary abscesses. *J. Clin. Microbiol.* 40: 1044–1047.

Wagner, R.A., Piche, C.A., Jochle, W. et al. (2005). Clinical and endocrine responses to treatment with deslorelin acetate implants in ferrets with adrenocortical disease. *Am. J. Vet. Res.* 66 (5): 910–914.

Walters, K.M., Mason, W.D., and Badr, M.Z. (1993). Effect of propylene glycol on the disposition of dramamine in the rabbit. *Drug Metab. Dispos.* 21: 305–308.

van Zeeland, Y.R.A., Pabon, M., Roest, J. et al. (2014). Use of a GnRH agonist implant as alternative for surgical neutering in pet ferrets. *Vet. Rec.* 175 (3): 66.

24

Special Considerations for Service, Working, and Performance Animals

Katrina L. Mealey

College of Veterinary Medicine, Washington State University, Pullman, WA, USA

Key Points

- Service animals are trained to perform a wide variety of functions that often depend on special senses such as vision, hearing, and smell, as well as physical capabilities.
- Before dispensing drugs that can adversely affect the special senses (olfaction, vision, and hearing) of service or working dogs, the veterinarian should be alerted so that the risks versus benefits can be assessed.
- Drug classes and dose levels permitted in performance animals vary widely depending

on the type of competition, the governing body, the location/venue of the actual event, and the species involved.
- As is the case with human athletes, drug testing may be employed to detect animals not in compliance. Disqualification of that animal may have financial consequences for the owner and therefore legal ramifications for the prescribing veterinarian and/or dispensing pharmacist.

24.1 Introduction

There is, justifiably, some confusion in many people's minds as to what constitutes a service animal. What makes the issue even more confusing is that the definition may vary by state. According to the American Disabilities Act (ADA), a service animal is a dog that has been trained to perform specific tasks to benefit a person with a physical, sensory, psychiatric, or intellectual or other mental disability. Examples might include pulling a wheelchair, alerting a deaf person to sounds, reminding a person to take their medication, or retrieving items out of that person's reach. Emotional support animals, "comfort" animals, and

therapy animals are not considered service animals under the ADA definition. Animals of a variety of different species are used as emotional support animals. The bulk of this chapter will provide information about service dogs and military working dogs, but the information with respect to the potential for drugs to interfere with a dog's ability to accomplish its tasks may be equally applicable to emotional support animals. Table 24.1 gives examples of service dogs and military or police working dogs and the types of tasks they perform.

Use of working dogs by the military; the police; US federal agencies such as the Federal Bureau of Investigation (FBI),

---

Pharmacotherapeutics for Veterinary Dispensing, First Edition. Edited by Katrina L. Mealey.
© 2019 John Wiley & Sons, Inc. Published 2019 by John Wiley & Sons, Inc.

Table 24.1 Some examples of service dogs and their specialty training/skills.

Type of service dog	Training/skills
Guide dog or Seeing Eye® dog	Allows a visually impaired person to travel independently by negotiating everyday hazards (traffic, curbs, obstacles, etc.)
Hearing or signal dog	Alerts a hearing-impaired person to certain sounds (alarms, timers, doorbells, etc.)
Sensory signal or social signal dog (SSig dog)	Alerts a person with autism that he or she is making repetitive movements that may be distracting in social situations
Seizure response dog	Many tasks, including guarding/protecting the person during a seizure episode and seeking help for the person during a seizure; some dogs can even predict impending seizures, allowing the person to prepare in advance for the seizure.
Psychiatric service dog	Many tasks, including detecting the onset of a psychiatric episode, reminding the individual to take medication, performing safety checks, interrupting self-mutilation cycles, and guarding/protecting the person if he or she becomes disoriented

Transportation Security Administration (TSA), and Bureau of Alcohol, Tobacco, Firearms and Explosives (ATF); and other law enforcement or regulatory agencies has increased dramatically over the past decade. Working dogs are used to guard, patrol, and perform combat missions. Additionally, their remarkable olfactory system allows dogs to detect and discriminate scents on a scale many orders of magnitude superior to that of humans. Working dogs are routinely used to scent-detect explosives, landmines, narcotics, and cadavers. These scent detection dogs have been used by the military to prevent severe injuries to military personnel and civilians caused by improvised explosive devices in combat zones.

Breeding, screening, and training of service dogs and working dogs are intensive processes that require highly qualified personnel. The monetary value of service and working dogs can be in the tens of thousands of dollars. The emotional value of these dogs to their owners/handlers can be incalculable. As part of the healthcare team for service and working dogs, pharmacists can help ensure these dogs have a long working lifespan by preventing drug-induced damage to critical special senses, such as vision, hearing, and olfaction.

24.2 The Role of Special Senses for Service Dogs and Working Dogs

To function successfully, service and working dogs must be physically fit with keen vision, sharp hearing, and high-acuity olfaction. Relative to humans, dogs are considered to have lower visual acuity, somewhat superior hearing, and vastly superior olfactory acuity. Detecting defects, particularly partial defects, in vision, hearing, and olfaction is much more difficult in animals than it is in people. A routine physical examination in a veterinary patient can detect catastrophic losses of special senses, but specialized testing is necessary to detect partial losses. This is an important problem, since even partial loss of vision, hearing, or olfactory acuity might impede the ability of a service or working dog to perform its job. The consequences could be devastating. Thus, it is important for pharmacists to bear in mind a drug's potential to interfere with function of the special senses.

The canine and human visual systems have evolved for very different purposes and therefore have different strengths and weaknesses. Dogs could be considered to be inferior with respect to depth perception, color perception, and visual acuity compared to people.

On the other hand, dogs have a greater field of view, superior night vision, and a greater ability to detect motion than people do (Miller and Murphy 1995). In ways that are not completely understood, it is obvious that service dogs and working dogs rely on vision to perform their duties. The fact that the military uses protective eyewear for many military working dogs emphasizes the importance of their visual system. German Shepherd dogs, one of the most common breeds used in the military, are susceptible to chronic superficial keratitis (pannus) that can result in blindness. Exposure to ultraviolet (UV) light is a risk factor for pannus. Protective canine goggles (sometimes referred to as "doggles") may help prevent pannus. Protective goggles can also prevent corneal injuries from foreign bodies (sandstorms, projectiles from explosions, etc.). It therefore seems reasonable to avoid drug-induced visual defects in working and service dogs.

Compared to humans, dogs can hear a greater range of sounds, particularly sounds at higher frequency. In terms of hearing sensitivity, dogs (and cats too, actually) can best detect sounds with frequencies between 5000 and 8000 cycles, while humans can best detect sounds with frequencies between 200 and 3000 cycles (Dworkin et al. 1940). Dogs, like humans, can sustain hearing loss from exposure to noise (explosive blasts, gunfire), and this can substantially limit the dog's function and shorten its time in the field. Because military working dogs are such highly valued assets, the US Department of Defense is soliciting grant applications for the development of hearing protection devices for military working dogs (https://www.sbir.gov/sbirsearch/detail/1254433). This underscores the importance of minimizing iatrogenic (i.e. drug-induced) ototoxicity in working dogs as well as service dogs.

Olfactory acuity is defined as the lowest concentration of a particular odorant that can be detected consistently (Lazarowski et al. 2015). Olfactory acuity in dogs is several orders of magnitude greater than that in people. The surface area of the nasal turbinates,

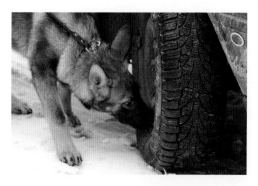

Figure 24.1 Military and law enforcement working dogs are trained to use their highly developed olfactory system to detect explosives, human remains, and illicit drugs.

which contain olfactory epithelium, is more than 100-fold greater in typical working dog breeds such as German Shepherds and Labrador Retrievers than it is in people. This is but one feature of the highly developed canine olfactory system that enables dogs to perform such feats as detecting cancer, tracking endangered species by the odor of their feces, and detecting narcotics or explosives (Figure 24.1).

It is important that working and service dogs can not only detect an odorant, a sound, or a command but also recognize it and react appropriately in response to it. Cognitive function in dogs is an ongoing area of research. Studies have shown that dogs can outperform apes and other primates in some cognitive-based skills. In particular, when dogs can use human cues, they demonstrate sophisticated cognitive skills (Hare et al. 2002). What this means for service dogs and working dogs is that medications that impair cognition might interfere with their ability to perform their job.

24.2.1 Drug-Induced Injury to the Special Senses

24.2.1.1 Vision

Permanent damage to the human visual system is an uncommon adverse drug reaction. Drug-induced optic neuritis has been reported in humans treated systemically with chloroquine, vigabatrin, digoxin, sildenafil, amiodarone, and other drugs (Dettoraki and Moschos 2016). The ability of human patients to communicate visual disturbances early in the disease process can prevent permanent retinal damage and visual dysfunction. Because early visual disturbances in dogs are unlikely to be detected, the best approach would be to limit use of drugs with ocular adverse effects in working dogs and service dogs.

Fluoroquinolones can cause severe, irreversible phototoxic retinal degeneration in cats that results in blindness (Ford et al. 2007). The US Food and Drug Administration (FDA) recently reported retinal degeneration in human patients who received intravitreal moxifloxacin injections. Thus, it is reasonable to exercise caution when considering the need for high doses of fluoroquinolones in working dogs, especially when they are subject to intensive UV light exposure. Phenothiazines have caused severe phototoxic retinopathy in humans (Li et al. 2008), but this has not been reported in veterinary patients. However, it is worth noting that a commonly used tranquilizer for dogs is a phenothiazine (acepromazine). Corticosteroids can cause several ocular adverse effects (e.g. they interfere with corneal wound healing, or lead to glaucoma) but are often life-saving drugs. Pharmacists can play an important role in discussions regarding the risks and benefits of drugs with the potential to cause ocular toxicity in working and service dogs.

24.2.1.2 Olfaction

Drug-induced olfactory dysfunction in humans is a relatively common occurrence but receives less attention than drug-induced visual or auditory impairment. This is probably because humans rely less on their sense of smell than they do on visual and auditory clues to navigate their environment. This is not to say that loss of olfaction is inconsequential in people. Chemotherapy consistently causes deterioration in olfactory threshold, discrimination, and identification in human cancer patients (Riga et al. 2015).

This is one of many factors that contribute to a decreased quality of life in cancer patients and is currently an active area of research.

Olfactory dysfunction can be drug-induced in dogs as well. In the early 1990s, the corticosteroids dexamethasone and hydrocortisone were shown to decrease olfactory acuity in dogs (Ezeh et al. 1992). More recent studies have focused on odorants of interest for military working dogs. The investigators discovered that metronidazole (a drug commonly used to treat gastrointestinal disease and giardia in dogs) adversely affected the detection threshold for two of three explosives (ammonium nitrate and trinitrotoluene) in trained explosive detection dogs (Jenkins et al. 2016). Half of the dogs had a degradation of performance in response to at least one explosive odorant. Metronidazole-induced olfactory dysfunction was reversible. On the other hand, the investigators identified no significant olfactory degradation after doxycycline administration.

Use of metronidazole (or other drugs that degrade olfactory function) should be carefully considered in explosive detection dogs and possibly other working dogs and service dogs as well. If the pharmacist believes another drug could be used to treat the dog's disease/condition, he or she should communicate that to the veterinarian and owner/handler.

24.2.1.3 Hearing

Military and working dogs experience not only combat-related injuries but can suffer from routine illnesses and injuries as well. Similarly, service dogs are not immune to the same health problems that pet dogs suffer from. For example, one of the most common non-combat-related conditions requiring veterinary care in military working dogs is otitis externa (Takara and Harrell 2014). Many "topical" (otic) drug products indicated for treating canine otitis externa contain drugs that can be ototoxic if the tympanic membrane is not intact. Unless the veterinarian has visualized an intact tympanum, potentially ototoxic drugs (Table 24.2) should be avoided.

Table 24.2 Potentially ototoxic drugs that should not be instilled into the ear unless the tympanum is intact.

Antibacterial drugs	Antiseptics	Cleansers/ceruminolytics
Aminoglycosides	Benzalkonium chloride	Detergents
Chloramphenicol	Chlorhexidien	Propylene glycol
Polymyxin	Iodophors/iodine	Salicylate
Vancomycin		Surfactants

Systemically administered drugs used to treat heart disease (furosemide), inflammation (salicylates), cancer (cisplatin), and infections (aminoglycoside antibiotics) can also cause ototoxicity (Pickrell et al. 1993). Use of alternate drugs should be considered before dispensing these drugs to service or working dogs. If it is determined that an ototoxic drug is considered necessary, it may be worthwhile to suggest brainstem auditory evoked response (BAER) testing periodically during treatment. Early auditory damage can be detected by BAER, and the drug can be discontinued before complete hearing loss occurs.

24.2.1.4 Cognitive Function

One last thing to consider in working dogs is the potential for drugs to interfere with cognitive function. Drugs that cause drowsiness may interfere with the ability of a service dog or working dog to perform at full capacity. The same drugs that affect a person's ability to safely operate a motor vehicle may impair cognition in a dog. Whether or not this affects the dog's performance is unknown. The author could not find any information in the literature specifically addressing drug-induced cognitive impairment in dogs, but it would be prudent for pharmacists to make owners/handlers of service or working dogs aware of this potential problem.

24.3 Performance Animals

Competitive events for animal athletes are as numerous and varied as they are for human athletes. Drug abuse by elite human athletes,

in order to gain a performance edge, is an occurrence reported in the news cycle on a weekly basis. Similarly, performance-enhancing drugs are sometimes used by owners and trainers of equine and canine athletes to gain a competitive advantage. Drug testing of performance animals (blood and/or urine) is regulated by the governing body that oversees a particular competition. In general, drugs that may affect the performance of an animal by calming it (sedatives/tranquilizers) or energizing it (stimulants) are prohibited. While it may seem counterintuitive, analgesics such as nonsteroidal anti-inflammatory drugs (NSAIDs) may be prohibited or have a dose-level restriction because of animal welfare issues. This is because, shortly before a horse race, a veterinarian examines all race entrants to ensure that the horses are healthy enough to compete safely. A horse with an underlying musculoskeletal injury that has been treated with an analgesic may not display lameness during the pre-race physical examination and thus be "cleared" by the veterinarian. That horse may then suffer a catastrophic injury if it is allowed to race.

Some horse owners will even medicate a horse prior to selling it in order to get a better price. Analgesics might be used to make a lame horse appear sound; behavior-modifying drugs might be used to make an excitable horse look gentle or to make an older horse appear spirited. For more information about prohibited substances in horses, including a list of websites that regulate drug use in performance horses, see Chapter 20.

Abbreviations

ATF   Bureau of Alcohol, Tobacco, Firearms and Explosives

FBI   Federal Bureau of Investigation
TSA   Transportation Security Administration

References

Dettoraki, M. and Moschos, M.M. (2016). The role of multifocal electroretinography in the assessment of drug-induced retinopathy: a review of the literature. *Ophthalmic Res.* 56 (4): 169–177.

Dworkin, S., Ktatzman, J., Hutchinson, G.A. et al. (1940). Hearing acuity of animals as measured by conditioning methods. *J. Exp. Psychol.* 26 (3): 281–298.

Ezeh, P.I., Myers, L.J., Hanrahan, L.A. et al. (1992). Effects of steroids on the olfactory function of the dog. *Physiol. Behav.* 51: 1183–1187.

Ford, M.M., Dubielzig, R.R., Giulano, E.A. et al. (2007). Ocular and systemic manifestations after oral administration of a high dose of enrofloxacin in cats. *Am. J. Vet. Res.* 68 (2): 190–202.

Hare, B., Brown, M., Williamson, C. et al. (2002). The domestication of social cognition in dogs. *Science* 298: 1634–1636.

Jenkins, E.K., Lee-Fowler, T.M., Angle, T.C. et al. (2016). Effects or oral administration of metronidazole and doxycycline on olfactory capabilities of explosives detection dogs. *Am. J. Vet. Res.* 77 (8): 906–912.

Lazarowski, L., Foster, M.L., Gruen, M.E. et al. (2015). Olfactory discrimination and generalization of ammonium nitrate and structurally related odorants in Labrador retrievers. *Anim. Cogn.* 18 (6): 1255–1265.

Li, J., Tripathi, R.C., and Tripathi, B.J. (2008). Drug-induced ocular disorders. *Drug Saf.* 31 (2): 127–141.

Miller, P.E. and Murphy, C.J. (1995). Vision in dogs. *J. Am. Vet. Med. Assoc.* 207 (12): 1623–1634.

Pickrell, J.A., Oehme, F.W., and Cash, W.C. (1993). Ototoxicity in dogs and cats. *Semin. Vet. Med. Surg.* 8 (1): 42–49.

Riga, M., Chelis, L., Papazi, T. et al. (2015). Hyposmia: an underestimated and frequent adverse effect of chemotherapy. *Support Care Cancer* 23 (10): 3053–3058.

Takara, M.S. and Harrell, K. (2014). Noncombat-related injuries of illnesses incurred by military working dogs in a combat zone. *J. Am. Vet. Med. Assoc.* 245 (10): 1124–1128.

25

Counseling for Owners of Veterinary Patients

Katrina L. Mealey

College of Veterinary Medicine, Washington State University, Pullman, WA, USA

Key Points

- Pharmacists are highly qualified to counsel human patients on all aspects of pharmacotherapeutics; however, most pharmacists are unprepared to counsel animal owners on veterinary pharmacotherapeutics.
- Because many veterinary patients do not voluntarily ingest their medication(s), dosage forms, routes of administration, and techniques used for drug administration to veterinary patients can differ substantially from those used for human patients.

- Veterinary patients do not "self-monitor" their pharmacotherapy, so pharmacists need to convey appropriate monitoring parameters to the animal's owner.
- Veterinary patients are unable to verbally communicate symptoms (e.g. pain, nausea, and blurred vision), so pharmacists will need to teach owners what clinical signs an animal might exhibit if experiencing a particular symptom.

25.1 Introduction

Pharmacists are depended upon by the public as well as all members of the human healthcare profession to educate and counsel patients in order to enhance pharmacotherapeutic outcomes. This is because, of all healthcare professions, pharmacists have received the most extensive training in human pharmacology, pharmaceutics, and pharmacotherapeutics. Their expertise in these scientific fields makes pharmacists the logical choice for counseling patients on their medications. In fact, some contend that pharmacists are obligated to warn patients of adverse effects and potential drug interactions (American Society of Health-System Pharmacists 1997).

Pharmacists are one of the most accessible members of the healthcare profession, allowing them to interact more frequently with patients. Collectively, a pharmacist's expertise, communication skills, and accessibility have led to numerous new healthcare roles for pharmacists. These expanded roles include medication management, immunizations, preventive screenings, and managing and improving population health such as tobacco cessation and diabetes management.

Pharmacotherapeutics for Veterinary Dispensing, First Edition. Edited by Katrina L. Mealey.
© 2019 John Wiley & Sons, Inc. Published 2019 by John Wiley & Sons, Inc.

Another expanded role that many pharmacists are undertaking is dispensing drugs to veterinary patients. However, pharmacy schools currently provide no core (required) courses that prepare pharmacists for this role. Regardless, the public still expects pharmacists to provide the same quality of patient counseling for a veterinary patient as they provide for human patients. The American Society of Health-System Pharmacists (ASHP) has published guidelines for effective patient education and counseling. The ASHP elements to include in an education and counseling session for human patients are listed in the remainder of this chapter, along with important differences with respect to counseling animal owners. This chapter will focus primarily on counseling owners of dogs and cats. In some ways, counseling the pet owner is similar to counseling for human infants. For example, the patient is small, is unable to verbally communicate, and may not be cooperative when the caregiver attempts to administer the drug.

25.2 ASHP List of Contents for an Education and Counseling Session – Veterinary Perspectives

25.2.1 The Medication's Trade Name, Generic Name, Common Synonym, or Other Descriptive Name(s) and, When Appropriate, Its Therapeutic Class and Efficacy

Pharmacists will have to learn new drug trade names, generic names, and even new therapeutic classes. For some drugs, the same generic name is used in the veterinary and human formulation, but the trade name differs. Table 25.1 lists some examples. The therapeutic class may also differ since some drugs belong to more than one therapeutic class, and the indication for the human formulation may differ from that for the veterinary formulation. For example, the

human formulation of butorphanol is primarily considered an analgesic, while the veterinary tablet is considered primarily an antitussive.

25.2.2 The Medication's Use and Expected Benefits and Action. This May Include Whether the Medication Is Intended to Cure a Disease, Eliminate or Reduce Symptoms, Arrest or Slow the Disease Process, or Prevent the Disease or a Symptom

Pharmacists need to have an understanding of diseases that are managed pharmacologically in veterinary patients in order to appropriately counsel pet owners. As discussed in the majority of chapters in this book, some veterinary diseases share characteristics with the corresponding disease in humans, but other diseases do not. Another critical factor that pharmacists must understand is the difference between a symptom and a clinical sign. A symptom is what a patient experiences or perceives, while a sign is something that another individual (e.g. the owner, veterinarian, or physician) observes. A human patient can describe symptoms such as pain, nausea, blurry vision, heart palpitations, and many more. Veterinary patients may experience symptoms but are unable to verbalize them. Animal owners and even veterinarians describe signs and often try to interpret them as symptoms, but this can be inaccurate. For example, a cat that refuses food can be said to be anorexic (a clinical sign), but to determine if the anorexia is due to nausea, oral pain, or anosmia (all symptoms), the veterinarian would have to pursue the cause by performing additional diagnostic testing that could reveal confirmatory signs such as azotemia (which is a known cause of nausea and inappetence), a tooth root abscess (which can cause pain when eating), or a brain tumor (which could cause anosmia). Simply assuming the cat was nauseated and treating it with an antinausea drug would be

Table 25.1 Examples of generic drugs with different trade names for the human versus the veterinary formulation.

Generic name	Trade name (human)	Trade name (veterinary)
Amoxicillin–clavulanic acid	Augmentin	Clavamox
Butorphanol	Stadol	Torbugesic
Cefadroxil	Duricef	Cefa-tabs
Clindamycin	Cleocin	Antirobe
Clomipramine	Anafranil	Clomicalm
Fluoxetine	Prozac	Reconcile
Ivermectin	Stromectol	Heartguard
L-deprenyl (selegiline)	Eldepryl	Anipryl
Methimazole	Tapazole	Felimazole
Omeprazole	Prilosec	GastroGard
Triamcinolone acetonide	Kenalog	Vetalog

Note: It is important to note that these formulations are not necessarily interchangeable since drug ratios (for combination products) may differ and other differences in formulation may contribute to differences in bioavailability.

inappropriate and completely ineffective in two of the three described scenarios.

25.2.3 The Medication's Expected Onset of Action, and What to Do if the Action Does Not Occur

Since pharmacists understand how a drug's pharmacokinetics affect steady-state and therapeutic blood concentrations, it should be straightforward for pharmacists to be able to predict the expected onset of drug action as long as species and breed differences (Chapters 4 and 5) in drug disposition are accounted for. However, some drugs have a delayed onset of clinical action. The delayed effect may be due to slow pharmacokinetic accumulation, distribution to the site of action, binding to receptors, or multistep adaptations of physiological processes secondary to the drug's effect. The latter is thought to be the case for the delay in action associated with tricyclic antidepressants and selective serotonin reuptake inhibitors in both human and veterinary patients (Chapter 16).

25.2.4 The Medication's Route, Dosage Form, Dosage, and Administration Schedule (Including Duration of Therapy)

Pharmacists with a particular interest in veterinary pharmacy can be of tremendous benefit to pet owners and veterinarians by compounding prescribed drugs into formulations with enhanced palatability or alternate routes of administration (as long as bioavailability and drug action or stability are not adversely affected). More detailed information on compounding can be found in Chapter 3.

25.2.4.1 Oral Drug Administration

In human medicine, most outpatient prescriptions involve oral drug formulations (tablets, capsules, solutions, and suspensions). While human patients can generally be convinced or motivated to ingest these medications, veterinary patients present unique challenges. Animals may be larger, stronger, more aggressive, and better equipped with defense mechanisms (sharp claws and teeth; horns; hooves that can deliver deadly force) than their owner, making it difficult and potentially dangerous to forcefully administer medications. Terminology that veterinarians use to refer to administering a tablet or capsule to a dog or cat may be confusing to pharmacists and is worth mentioning. The word "pill" is often used as a verb, as demonstrated in the sentences "It is often difficult to 'pill' cats or 'Pilling' cats usually requires more than one person." Because it is difficult to administer oral medications to veterinary patients, pharmaceutical companies have come up with creative ways of orally dosing veterinary patients that pharmacists may not be familiar with. For example, "pastes," "boluses," (described in Chapter 22), and "drenches" are exclusively intended for oral use, not topically or intravenously as when these terms are applied to human dosage forms. Table 25.2 lists some examples of dosage forms used in veterinary

medicine that might not be familiar to pharmacists. Figure 3.2 depicts a typical oral dosing syringe for horses that allows the owner to "dial in" a dose based on the horse's body weight, thus allowing the owner to conveniently administer the correct dose (Figure 25.1).

25.2.4.2 Parenteral Injections

Parenteral routes of administration may be more appropriate for veterinary species compared to humans because of anatomic differences. For example, a large potential space exists subcutaneously in dogs and cats, as the subcutaneous layer is loosely attached to the underlying muscle. The subcutaneous space can accommodate relatively large volumes at a single administration site (30–60 mL for a cat or small dog), and is sometimes used quite effectively for parenteral fluid administration to treat or prevent dehydration in dogs and cats. Figure 4.1 illustrates a subcutaneous injection in a dog. Subcutaneous injection

Table 25.2 Examples of dosage forms in veterinary species that pharmacists may be less familiar with, the species most likely to be prescribed that dosage form, and specific characteristics of that dosage form that pharmacists should be aware of.

Dosage form	Route of administration	Species/type of animal	Other
Bolus	Oral	Ruminants	
Chewables	Oral	Dogs, some cats	Often beef flavored, are designed to be palatable like a dog "treat." Owners should keep these in a secure location since dogs have been known to seek out the container and consume the contents.
Drench	Oral	Ruminant (herds)	Used with a calibrated drench "gun" to repeatedly deliver a fixed volume of oral liquid medication to individual animals in a herd
Paste	Oral	Horses	Supplied in special syringes that usually allow the owner to deliver a fixed volume
Pill pockets	Oral	Dogs, cats, ferrets	Flavored pouches that a tablet or capsule is hidden inside; these also help mask the "drug smell," which is important for cats and ferrets
Topical	Applied to dermis	Dogs, cats	Many antiparasitics are applied in this manner, some of which are intended to be absorbed systemically to treat both internal and external parasites.
Transdermal gel	Transdermal	Cats that are difficult to "pill"	Usually compounded and applied to pinnae; bioavailability often limited

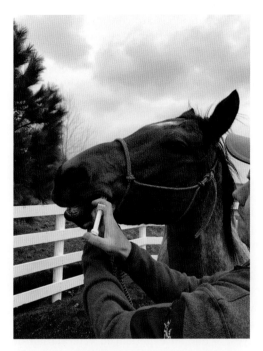

Figure 25.1 Administration of a paste to a horse. Ensure that the horse's mouth is empty. While the horse's head is restrained, the tip of the syringe is placed into the corner of the horse's mouth, preferably on the surface of the horse's tongue. The plunger is depressed to deliver the medication.

technique for a dog or cat is as follows: A fold of skin over the animal's neck or back is gently lifted, and the needle (25–22 G) is inserted perpendicularly to the skin fold. If performed correctly, the needle will pass easily through the skin. Release the fold of skin once the needle is inserted (this helps ensure that the needle tip did not penetrate through both folds of skin, which can happen with smaller needles). Before injecting, the plunger should be withdrawn to ensure that there is no blood and that there is negative pressure. Once the injection is complete, the area can be massaged gently, and the animal should be rewarded. The bioavailability of drugs administered subcutaneously compares favorably to drugs administered by the intravenous route. Pharmacists with veterinary expertise can help train dog and cat owners to administer subcutaneous medications so that parenteral drugs can be administered on an outpatient basis.

Intramuscular administration carries greater risks than subcutaneous injection, including accidental injection into blood vessels or nerves. Intramuscular injections are more likely to cause discomfort to the patient than subcutaneous injections, so the patient may move, increasing the risk of tissue damage (muscle, blood vessel, or nerve). Additionally, intramuscular injections are contraindicated in patients with coagulopathies. The muscles used for intramuscular injection in human patients are not the same as for veterinary patients, and the appropriate sites differ between species. Compared to the subcutaneous route, smaller volumes of fluid are administered by the intramuscular route of administration (up to 2 mL to cats or small dogs and up to 5 mL to very large dogs).

25.2.4.3 Feline Injection Site Sarcomas

Dramatic difference

Cats, compared to other species, are at greater risk of developing neoplasia, specifically sarcomas, at the site of injections than other species (Figure 25.2). These tumors were initially named vaccine-associated

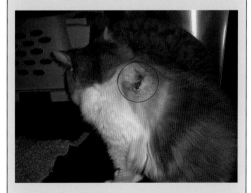

Figure 25.2 Feline injection site sarcoma (FISS) located near the scruff of the neck. FISS is a highly invasive tumor that infiltrates underlying muscle tissue and is poorly responsive to chemotherapy. Incisional biopsy had been performed to confirm the histologic type and grade of tumor. *Source:* Photo courtesy of Dr. Janean Fidel, Washington State University.

sarcomas until it was discovered that injection of drugs and microchips could also result in neoplastic transformation. They are currently referred to as feline injection site sarcomas (FISSs). FISSs were first described in over 300 cats in the early 1990s (Kass et al. 1993). The risk of sarcoma increased with the number of injections administered at the same site. At the time, feline immunizations were almost exclusively administered in the "scruff" of the neck or in the skin between a cat's shoulder blades. Sarcomas occurring at this site make treatment difficult because sarcomas are highly locally invasive, invading into underlying muscle and bone. At this site, it is impossible to achieve the recommended 5 cm surgical margins documented to improve survival. Subsequent (current) recommendations were to administer specific vaccines at specific anatomic sites (Table 25.3). This accomplished two important objectives. First, it provided further evidence that injections were responsible for inducing tumor formation. FISSs started occurring at these new injection sites where they had previously never been reported. Second, amputation of the involved limb allows for complete excision of the tumor, as long as the tumor involves only the distal limb, which is the most important prognostic indicator (Kobayashi et al. 2002).

Table 25.3 Vaccination site recommendations for cats to improve surgical treatment outcome for feline injection site sarcomas.

Vaccine(s)	Recommended[a] injection site
Feline parvovirus (FPV)	Below the right elbow
Feline herpesvirus-1 (FHV-1)	Below the right elbow
Feline coronavirus (FCV)	Below the right elbow
Feline leukemia virus (FELV)	Below the left stifle
Rabies	Below the right stifle

[a] *Source:* From Scherk et al. (2013).

Although FISSs are considered to be rare (~1/10 000 injections), pharmacists should instruct cat owners to monitor the sites where a cat has received a subcutaneous or intramuscular injection for the development of a lump that does not completely regress within three weeks of the injection. Cats that must receive frequent injections (i.e. insulin) should have the injection site rotated.

Intravenous drug administration to small animals is performed by or under the direct supervision of a veterinarian. Large-animal intravenous injections can sometimes be performed by lay personnel who have been appropriately trained.

25.2.4.4 Ocular Drug Administration

Pharmacists should instruct pet owners to wash their hands before administering eye drops or ophthalmic ointments to their pets' eyes. While an experienced veterinarian or veterinary technician (nurse) can administer eye drops to animals without assistance, most animal owners should seek assistance in restraining the animal. For cats and smaller dogs, wrapping the animal snugly (but not tightly) in a towel is helpful. All four limbs should be enclosed in the towel, with the head being the only body part that is exposed. Most animals will reflexively avoid objects placed near the eye by closing all three (yes, three!) eyelids (see Chapter 19 for additional information about the third eyelid), so holding the inverted bottle out of the pet's range of vision is helpful. One can rest the heel of the hand holding the eye drop bottle on the top of the pet's head and, without touching the tip of the bottle to the animal's eye, squeeze the correct amount of drops/ointment onto the eye. Eye drops disperse over the surface of the eye rapidly, but the owner may need to gently massage the animal's eyelids to disperse ointment. The animal should be rewarded. Cats can salivate profusely if the drug gains access to the oral cavity through the nasolacrimal system. This can cause treatment aversion. For this reason, it is sometimes preferable to use ocular ointments instead of drops for cats.

25.2.4.5 Rectal Drug Administration

Pharmacists may receive prescriptions for injectable anticonvulsants intended to be administered rectally in dogs with seizure disorders such as epilepsy. Rectal administration of diazepam (Mealey and Boothe 1995) and levetiracetam (Peters et al. 2014) has been shown to result in therapeutic drug concentrations after rectal administration of the injectable formulation to dogs. Because rapid seizure control is paramount to prevent morbidity and mortality associated with status epilepticus, the ability of owners to control seizures at home or *en route* to a veterinary hospital is highly desirable. In terms of owner education, pharmacists can improve the rate and extent of drug absorption by this route of administration by having owners digitally (wearing gloves) remove feces from the rectum, deposit the drug with the syringe (no needle) located in the distal one-third of the rectum, and hold down the tail to help prevent immediate expulsion of the drug. Drug absorbed from the proximal two-thirds of the rectum will be delivered to the portal circulation, while drug absorbed from the distal one-third of the rectum will be delivered to the caudal vena cava, bypassing first-pass hepatic metabolism. Interestingly, the bioavailability of diazepam is lower in dogs using the commercially available suppositories compared to the injectable formulation.

25.2.4.6 Transdermal Drug Administration

Many commercially available antiparasitic drugs for dogs and cats are formulated to be applied topically to prevent fleas and ticks, but many topical products are systemically absorbed in sufficient quantities to kill internal parasites as well. Systemic bioavailability after transdermal application varies widely between different drugs and between different species. For example, systemic bioavailability of topically applied selamectin in dogs is approximately 4% but is 74% in cats (Page 2008). Thus, pharmacists must make it clear to pet owners that transdermal products labeled for one species should not be used in a different species.

Application of commercially available topical products to cats and dogs is well explained in package inserts but will be summarized briefly here. Products are usually supplied as single-application tubes. The tip of the tube is applied to the skin on the back of the neck or between the shoulder blades (these locations help minimize the opportunity for the animal to ingest the drug while grooming). The tube is squeezed gently to expel the contents directly onto the skin. Drugs should not be applied to broken skin or if the hair coat is wet. Animals should not be allowed to lick the application site for one to two hours. The animal can be distracted by feeding, playing, being given a new toy, and so on. Pet owners should avoid contact with the animal while the application site is still wet (usually about one hour). In multiple-pet households, animals should be separated to prevent ingestion of drug by licking another animal's application site. Owners should wash hands thoroughly after applying the drug or if they accidentally come in contact with the application site while it is still wet.

Because of the relative ease of transdermal drug administration relative to oral drug administration to an animal that is frightened or intolerant of handling for any reason, veterinarians often turn to pharmacists to compound transdermal formulations of drugs that are commercially available only in oral or injectable formulations. This is particularly true for drugs that must be administered on a daily basis to cats for treatment of a chronic disease. An example of such a drug is methimazole, used for treating hyperthyroidism in cats. Transdermal formulations of methimazole in pluronic organogel have sufficient systemic bioavailability to effectively manage most hyperthyroid cats. Transdermal methimazole is applied to the inner pinna of the cat's ear while the owner is wearing impermeable gloves or a finger cot (Figure 25.3). Typically, a 0.1 mL dose is applied to alternate (left, then right) ears. Unfortunately, most other drugs are not

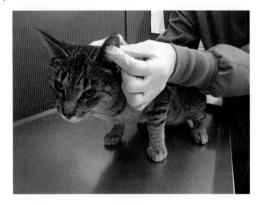

Figure 25.3 Transdermal gels are administered to cats by applying the gel to the inner pinna as demonstrated. Owners should be instructed to wear nonpermeable gloves or a finger cot. *Source:* Image courtesy of Dr. Sarah Wagner, North Dakota State University.

sufficiently bioavailable by the transdermal route to supply consistent systemic concentrations. Pharmacists can help educate veterinarians about the limitations with systemic bioavailability of transdermal drug delivery. Additional information about advantages and disadvantages of transdermal gels can be found in Chapter 3.

25.2.4.7 Aerosolized Drug Administration

Animals (dogs, cats, and horses in particular) with asthma and asthma-like diseases can be treated via inhalant delivery of aerosolized medications. This is accomplished using either nebulizers or human metered-dose inhalers, with modifications compared to how these drug delivery systems are used for human patients. Various types of commercially available nebulizers specifically for veterinary patients are available, including masks, tents, and aquarium-like containers that the pet is placed within. When weighing advantages and disadvantages of the options, the pharmacist should consider that the more removed the particle generator is from the respiratory tract, the less drug is delivered to the respiratory tract. Masks would certainly have the advantage if this were the only consideration. However, since we are dealing with animals, other factors might

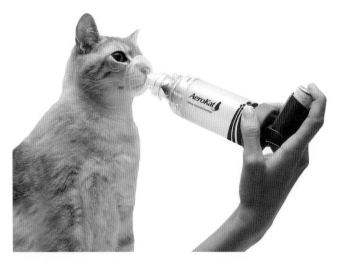

Figure 25.4 Demonstration of the use of a feline spacer device to be used in combination with a metered-dose inhaler to deliver inhalation therapy to feline asthma patients. *Source:* Image courtesy of Trudell Medical International.

prevail. Specifically, nebulizers are noisy, and many animals strongly resist having a noisy mask anywhere near their face. For these patients, a tent or tank might be the best option. The other inhalant delivery method is a metered-dose inhaler. While there are no veterinary-specific metered-dose inhalers, there are canine, feline (Figure 25.4), and equine (Figure 25.5) spacers that are intended to be used with human metered-dose inhaler products containing corticosteroids or bronchodilators.

25.2.4.8 Subconjunctival Sac Drug Administration

For most pharmacists, administration of drugs to the eye is limited to those drugs intended to treat ocular disease. While that is

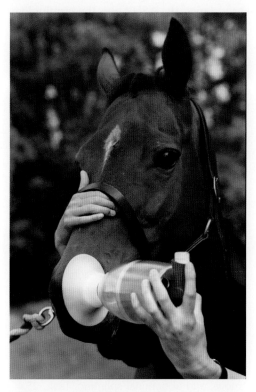

Figure 25.5 Demonstration of the use of a spacer device to deliver inhalation therapy to horses with reactive airway disease using a metered-dose inhaler. *Source:* Image courtesy of Erik Sethre Jorgensen Laboratories, Inc.

also the case in most instances for veterinary patients, there are two drugs that are administered into the subconjunctival sac of dogs that are intended to have systemic pharmacological action. Apomorphine is the drug of choice for "decontamination" (inducing emesis and administering activated charcoal) of dogs that have ingested potential toxins (see Chapter 6 for additional information). Apomorphine can be administered by injection or by instilling into the conjunctival sac. I prefer the latter method because once the dog has vomited, residual drug can be removed by gentle irrigation of the eye with sterile saline solution. That way, the dog is relieved of unnecessary vomiting and the residual sensation of nausea that will accompany parenteral apomorphine. The second drug that is conventionally delivered to the subconjunctival sac is desmopressin acetate (DDAVP), which is used for treating central diabetes insipidus.

25.2.5 Directions for Preparing and Using or Administering the Medication. This May Include Adaptation to Fit Patients' Lifestyles or Work Environments

Unless a "pet sitter" or animal caretaker is available, animals must be treated based on the owner's schedule, which may include full-time work, commuting, children, and other activities. Animals do not self-administer medication. Pharmacists can be of tremendous benefit to both veterinarians and pet owners by helping owners design rational but workable options for treating their pet.

25.2.6 Action to Be Taken in Case of a Missed Dose

Once a pharmacist understands the mechanism of action of veterinary drugs and the therapeutic strategy for a specific disease, that pharmacist can use the same approach that is used when counseling human patients.

25.2.7 Precautions to Be Observed during the Medication's Use or Administration and the Medication's Potential Risks in Relation to Benefits. For Injectable Medications and Administration Devices, Concern about Latex Allergy May Be Discussed

Similar to item 6 (Section 25.2.6), once a pharmacist understands the mechanism of action of veterinary drugs and the therapeutic strategy for a specific disease, a pharmacist can use the same strategy that is used when counseling human patients.

25.2.8 Potential Common and Severe Adverse Effects That May Occur, Actions to Prevent or Minimize Their Occurrence, and Actions to Take if They Occur, Including Notifying the Prescriber, Pharmacist, or Other Healthcare Provider

Pharmacists are highly proficient at providing counseling for adverse drug effects that might occur in human patients. However, unless they have received specific training in veterinary pharmacology, pharmacists may not have the competence to provide appropriate counseling for adverse drug effects in veterinary patients. The diverse metabolic capacities that occur not only between different species, but also between different breeds of the same species, lead to unique drug sensitivities or target organ toxicities that traditionally trained pharmacists are unaware of. For example, the presence of a drug transporter polymorphism that occurs in certain dog breeds can cause life-or-death differences in drug response. The antiparasitic drug ivermectin can be administered at a daily dose of 500 micrograms per kg for months to dogs without the polymorphism, but that same dose administered even once to a dog with the polymorphism can be fatal (see Chapter 5 for more detailed information). The intent of this book is to arm pharmacists with information about the key drugs used to treat the more common diseases in dogs and cats, the species that pharmacists are most likely to receive prescriptions for.

Additionally, some information is provided for other species, including food animals, horses, and nontraditional species such as birds, reptiles, and rodents.

25.2.9 Techniques for Self-Monitoring of Pharmacotherapy

Pharmacists play a key role in monitoring drug therapy for human patients and, with appropriate training, can play an equally important role for veterinary patients. Systematic monitoring of pharmacotherapy should include assessment for not only adverse drug events (see item 8) and drug–drug interactions (see item 10), but for therapeutic efficacy as well.

For veterinary patients, some key differences in monitoring are worth mentioning. For instance, the ASHP uses the terminology "self-monitoring." Obviously, this is not applicable to veterinary patients. Instead, pharmacists must counsel the animal owner to monitor the patient. Another major difference between human and veterinary patients (previously mentioned but worth repeating here) is the fact that veterinary patients are unable to verbally communicate symptoms.

Dramatic difference

Pharmacists cannot rely on veterinary patients to describe symptoms of adverse drug reactions, as is the case for human patients. Instead, pharmacists must help educate the owner to identify signs that their pet might exhibit if experiencing a particular symptom. For example, abdominal pain may be a *symptom* caused by an adverse reaction to nonsteroidal anti-inflammatory drugs (NSAIDs), causing the animal to exhibit *signs* of inappetence, vomiting, reluctance to move, and abdominal splinting. Table 25.4 lists some common symptoms of adverse drug events in human patients (Avery et al. 2011) and corresponding clinical signs that an animal might exhibit if experiencing that symptom. For human patients, pharmacists are accustomed to describing symptoms of adverse drug reactions (nausea, vertigo, pain, blurred vision, tingling, palpitations, etc.) rather than clinical signs. It is important that pharmacists adapt their patient-counseling skills to fit the needs of pet owners.

Table 25.4 Symptoms or types of adverse drug events experienced by humans, and corresponding clinical signs that an animal might exhibit if experiencing that symptom.

Symptom	Corresponding clinical sign to monitor in veterinary patients
Nausea	Inappetence (animal may approach food dish, but after sniffing or licking will walk away), drooling, frequent lip licking or smacking, inactivity, or listlessness
Itch (pruritis)	Frequent licking or chewing at parts of the body; rubbing up against stationary objects; rolling around on the floor/ground
Anaphylaxis	Wheals, urticaria (may have to part fur to visualize adequately), facial angioedema, vomiting, diarrhea, cough, wheezing, respiratory distress, and pale mucous membranes. Dogs are more likely to exhibit GI signs, while cats are more likely to exhibit respiratory signs.

Pharmacists are quite aware of the placebo effect in human patients, but they may not be aware of practitioner or owner placebo effects in monitoring drug response in veterinary patients. For cats in particular, the owner/caregiver placebo effect is quite high. In an analgesic clinical trial involving cats with pain associated with degenerative joint disease, owners judged 54–70% of placebo-treated cats to have had improvement in pain scores (Gruen et al. 2017). Providing monitoring parameters that are objective (e.g. is your dog able to walk up and down the stairs?) rather than subjective (e.g. does your dog seem to feel better?) are more likely to yield accurate assessments of drug response.

To effectively monitor pharmacotherapy in veterinary patients, pharmacists must possess a working knowledge of veterinary diseases, their progression, and appropriate monitoring parameters. Monitoring parameters for veterinary patients can differ dramatically from those used to monitor pharmacotherapy for human patients because of physiological differences. For example, body temperature might be used as a monitoring parameter to assess antimicrobial therapy. A human patient with a body temperature of 102.5 °F would be considered febrile, while that same temperature in a dog or cat would be considered normal. Heart rates, respiratory rates, and blood pressure also differ by species and by body size or breed within species. For example, larger dogs tend to have slower heart and respiratory rates than small dogs. The normal resting heart rate of a horse is 35–40 beats per minute, but fit horses can have resting heart rates of 25 beats per minute. That rate would be considered severe bradycardia in a human. Conversely, the resting heart rate in a (nonstressed) cat can vary from 140 to 180 beats per minute, which would reflect tachycardia in a human. Not only are the monitoring parameters different, but the methods for assessing these parameters vary by species. Heart rates, often determined by palpation of the neck (carotid artery) or wrist (radial artery) in human patients, are best determined by palpating the proximal inner thigh (femoral artery) for dogs and cats or the underside of the lower jawbone in horses (mandibular artery). Appendix C lists normal ranges for vital signs and other monitoring parameters in dogs, cats, and horses. Assessment of blood pressure in most veterinary patients requires specialized veterinary cuffs – using the wrong-sized cuff will yield erroneous results. Therefore, monitoring of blood pressure usually requires a visit to the veterinarian.

Therapeutic drug monitoring is another mechanism available for monitoring drug therapy in veterinary patients. Drug monitoring may be implemented for a veterinary patient for several possible reasons. Measuring blood concentrations may help determine if the owner is administering the drug appropriately (this has been used to determine if the owner is diverting controlled drugs, such as benzodiazepines or opioids). For other drugs prescribed to veterinary patients such as anti-epileptics or immunosuppressants, it is often important to determine if plasma concentrations are within the therapeutic range – doses can be adjusted accordingly to enhance efficacy or prevent toxicity. Several laboratories offer therapeutic drug monitoring for veterinary patients (Appendix G). Depending on the reason, a variety of samples from veterinary patients might be used for drug monitoring. For therapeutic assessment, blood is typically collected. For compliance or regulatory purposes, urine, saliva, blood, or hair may be sampled.

25.2.10 Potential Drug–Drug (Including Nonprescription), Drug–Food, and Drug–Disease Interactions or Contraindications

Community and hospital pharmacies are equipped with software designed to detect potential drug–drug interactions based on all drugs that have been dispensed to a particular patient. These systems are incredibly valuable for human patients. Unfortunately, these systems do not include veterinary drug products, so they are of less value for veterinary patients. Currently, there are no veterinary software systems to facilitate drug–drug interaction screening for veterinary patients. *This means that pharmacists must provide the screening necessary to prevent serious drug–drug interactions in veterinary patients.* There are several commonly used veterinary drugs (drugs that most pharmacists are not familiar with) that can cause serious drug–drug interactions. For example, spinosad, a once-a-month flea and tick preventive, is a P-glycoprotein inhibitor. When administered concurrently with P-glycoprotein substrates like ivermectin (used to treat mange), severe neurological toxicity has occurred. Ivermectin normally does not cross the blood–brain barrier, because it is exported by P-glycoprotein. However, inhibition of P-glycoprotein allows ivermectin to penetrate the blood–brain barrier, resulting in serious

neurological toxicity. Drug-interaction detection systems used in human medicine have no information about spinosad, and very little, if any, about ivermectin. What resources do pharmacists have for veterinary drugs to help predict drug interactions? The package insert/label for veterinary drugs often includes some information about potential drug interactions. Systems in place for human drug products may be helpful, since many drugs prescribed for veterinary patients are human drugs used in an extra-label manner. Additionally, since some veterinary drugs are from the same class as human drugs (e.g. fluoroquinolones, macrolides, and tyrosine kinase inhibitors), human–drug interaction information might be applicable to those veterinary drugs.

Drug interactions involving the cytochrome P450 (CYP) enzyme family can be fatal and have led to several human drugs being withdrawn from the US market, including terfenadine, astemizole, and cisapride (Lynch and Price 2007). Pharmacists will find that CYP-mediated drug interactions are particularly difficult to predict in veterinary patients as compared to human patients. The reasons for this are many. Each specific CYP enzyme is encoded by a different gene, which usually differs between species (see Chapter 4 for more detailed information). So, the ortholog of CYP3A4 in people is actually CYP3A12 or CYP3A26 in dogs. A drug that is metabolized by human CYP3A4 (i.e. midazolam) may not be metabolized by the orthologous enzymes in other species. Midazolam is primarily metabolized by CYP2B11 in dogs, for example. This means that CYP3A4 inhibitors/inducers could cause drug interactions with midazolam in humans, but not in dogs. However, CYP2B11 inhibitors/inducers could cause drug interactions with midazolam in dogs. Unfortunately, there is not a great deal of published information that indicates that drugs inhibit or induce CYP enzymes in dogs, cats, horses, or other veterinary species. Pharmacists are well aware that human drug labels indicate which, if any, CYP enzymes are involved in that drug's metabolism. That is not the case for veterinary drugs. Thus, there are many reasons why predicting CYP-mediated drug interactions in veterinary patients is challenging. Until more data become available, pharmacists should err on the side of caution when dispensing drugs that are CYP substrates, inducers, or inhibitors.

Lastly, with regard to drug interactions, pharmacists may be surprised to learn that there are veterinary specialists. These veterinary specialists, like human medical specialists, have received advanced clinical training in a particular area of medicine (e.g. cardiology, oncology, or neurology), limiting the scope of their practice. The reason why this is important is that pets may receive prescriptions from more than one veterinarian, potentially increasing the risk for drug–drug interactions since the general practitioner may not be aware of drugs that the specialist has prescribed and vice versa. By integrating pharmacists into the veterinary healthcare team, potential drug–drug interactions can be avoided because pharmacists, particularly those with adequate veterinary pharmacy training, are the most qualified profession to perform drug interaction screening assessments.

25.2.11 The Medication's Relationships to Radiologic and Laboratory Procedures (e.g. Timing of Doses and Potential Interference with Interpretations of Results)

As compared to human drug labels, this type of information is less likely to appear on labels of US Food and Drug Administration (FDA)-approved veterinary drugs. If there is a human drug in the same class, the information may be applicable to veterinary patients as well. Pharmacists and veterinarians should work closely and communicate frequently to ensure that potential drug interference is accounted for when interpreting results of diagnostic testing for a veterinary patient.

25.2.12 Prescription Refill Authorizations and the Process for Obtaining Refills

This process should be the same for human and veterinary patients.

25.2.13 Instructions for 24-Hour Access to a Pharmacist

Currently, it is difficult for pet owners to find a pharmacist with adequate training in veterinary pharmacology/pharmacotherapeutics. There are so few within the profession ensuring 24-hour access.

25.2.14 Proper Storage of the Medication

This information should be the same for human and veterinary patients. Veterinary drug labels include information about proper storage conditions (temperature and light). One additional factor to consider for all medications dispensed to homes with pets is to store drugs in cabinets or closets that are not accessible to pets (dogs especially). Hundreds of pet poisonings occur every year in the USA because pets ingest medications (usually by chewing through the container) that were left out on tabletops or countertops, or in purses or backpacks that were not securely closed. Unfortunately, childproof containers for dispensing medication are not "dog-proof."

25.2.15 Proper Disposal of Contaminated or Discontinued Medications and Used Administration Devices

These instructions would be similar for veterinary and human patients with one caveat. Animal owners should be counseled against discarding used containers of suspensions or pastes (pastes are often supplied in syringe-like devices for administration to horses) in trash cans or bins that dogs might have access to. It is easy for dogs to locate the scent of flavored suspensions and pastes, and many dogs are poisoned by the highly potent residual paste or suspension in containers discarded into trash bins around barns or stables.

25.2.16 Any Other Information Unique to an Individual Patient or Medication

Pharmacists should review Chapters 4 and 5 for information on species and breed differences in physiology that affect drug disposition. There are many unique and unpredictable species and breed susceptibilities to drugs that most pharmacists are unaware of because their pharmacology training was limited to one species (human).

The ASHP suggests that the following items may also be included as counseling points for human patients, depending on the pharmacist's role in the healthcare team for that particular patient.

1) **The disease state: whether it is acute or chronic and its prevention, transmission, progression, and recurrence.** For pharmacists that fill more than the occasional prescription for veterinary patients, additional training (i.e. a veterinary pharmacy fellowship, or veterinary pharmacology coursework) would be required to develop the expertise required to provide appropriate education and counseling to animal owners on their animal's disease state. There are simply too many differences between a particular disease in humans and its counterpart in veterinary medicine. Some of the more important differences of the most common diseases are provided in this book.

2) **Expected effects of the disease on the patient's normal daily living.** This is critically important for working animals (e.g. military, security, and police) and service animals (see Chapter 24 for more detailed information). For example, drugs that interfere with a working dog's special senses (hearing, vision, and olfaction) might endanger not only the dog, but also its handler and others who depend on that animal's ability to detect environmental information.

3) **Recognition and monitoring of disease complications.** To establish competency in providing counseling to animal owners on this topic, pharmacists will need to gain an understanding of the common diseases affecting the animal species that they will be working with. This information is currently not part of the core pharmacy curricula at any North American College of Pharmacy.

References

American Society of Health-System Pharmacists (1997). ASHP guidelines on pharmacist-conducted patient education and counseling. *Am. J. Health-Syst. Pharm.* 54: 431–434.

Avery, A.J., Anderson, C., Bond, C.M. et al. (2011). Evaluation of patient reporting of adverse drug reaction to the UK 'yellow card scheme': literature review, descriptive and qualitative analyses and questionnaire surveys. *Health Technol. Assess.* 15 (20): 1–234.

Gruen, M.E., Dorman, D.C., and Lascelles, B.D.X. (2017). Caregiver placebo effect in analgesic clinical trials for cats with naturally occurring degenerative joint disease associated pain. *Vet. Rec.* 180 (19): 473. doi:10.1126/vr.104168.

Kass, P.H., Barnes, W.G., Spangler, W.L. et al. (1993). Epidemiologic evidence for a causal relation between vaccination and fibrosarcoma tumorigenesis in cats. *J. Am. Vet. Med. Assoc.* 203: 396–405.

Kobayashi, T., Hauck, M.L., Dodge, R. et al. (2002). Preoperative radiotherapy for vaccine associated sarcoma in 92 cats. *Vet. Radiol. Ultrasound* 43 (5): 473–479.

Lynch, T. and Price, A. (2007). The effect of cytochrome P450 metabolism on drug response, interactions, and adverse effects. *Am. Fam. Physician* 76 (3): 391–396.

Mealey, K.L. and Boothe, D.M. (1995). Bioavailavility of benzodiazepines following rectal administration of diazepam in dogs. *J. Vet. Pharmacol. Ther.* 18 (1): 72–74.

Page, S.W. (2008). Antiparasitic drugs. In: *Small Animal Clinical Pharmacology*, 2e (ed.

J.E. Maddison, S.W. Page and D.B. Church), 198–260. St. Louis, MO: Elsevier.

Peters, R.K., Schubert, T., Clemmons, R. et al. (2014). Levetiracetam rectal administration in healthy dogs. *J. Vet. Intern. Med.* 28 (2): 504–509.

Scherk, M.A., Ford, R.B., Gaskell, R.M. et al. (2013). 2013 AAFP feline vaccination advisory panel report. *J. Feline Med. Surg.* 15: 785–808.

Appendix A

Veterinary Teaching Hospital Pharmacy Contact Information

Katrina L. Mealey

College of Veterinary Medicine, Washington State University, Pullman, WA, USA

Pharmacists employed by veterinary teaching hospitals can be a valuable resource for community pharmacists (see Table A.1).

Table A.1 Veterinary teaching hospitals, by state.

State	Institution	Phone number
Alabama	Auburn University College of Veterinary Medicine	334-844-6721
	Tuskegee University College of Veterinary Medicine	334-727-8436
California	University of California (Davis) School of Veterinary Medicine	530-752-0187
Colorado	Colorado State University College of Veterinary Medicine	970-297-1291
Florida	University of Florida College of Veterinary Medicine	352-294-4614
Georgia	University of Georgia College of Veterinary Medicine	706-542-5510
Illinois	University of Illinois College of Veterinary Medicine	217-333-2760
Indiana	Purdue University College of Veterinary Medicine	765-494-7622
Iowa	Iowa State University College of Veterinary Medicine	515-294-2427
Kansas	Kansas State University College of Veterinary Medicine	785-532-4127
Louisiana	Louisiana State University School of Veterinary Medicine	225-578-9504
Massachusetts	Tufts University School of Veterinary Medicine	508-887-4850
Michigan	Michigan State University College of Veterinary Medicine	517-353-1299
Minnesota	University of Minnesota College of Veterinary Medicine	612-625-6233
Mississippi	Mississippi State University College of Veterinary Medicine	662-325-1252
Missouri	University of Missouri College of Veterinary Medicine	573-882-7634
New York	Cornell University College of Veterinary Medicine	607-253-3231
North Carolina	North Carolina State University College of Veterinary Medicine	919-513-6570
Ohio	Ohio State University College of Veterinary Medicine	614-292-1010

(Continued)

Pharmacotherapeutics for Veterinary Dispensing, First Edition. Edited by Katrina L. Mealey.

Table A.1 (Continued)

State	Institution	Phone number
Oklahoma	Oklahoma State University College of Veterinary Medicine	405-744-7000
Oregon	Oregon State University College of Veterinary Medicine	541-737-6863
Pennsylvania	University of Pennsylvania School of Veterinary Medicine	215-898-7881
Tennessee	University of Tennessee College of Veterinary Medicine	865-974-5670
Texas	Texas A&M University College of Veterinary Medicine	979-845-9118
Virginia	Virginia-Maryland Regional, College of Veterinary Medicine	540-231-4626
Washington	Washington State University College of Veterinary Medicine	509-335-0711
Wisconsin	University of Wisconsin-Madison School of Veterinary Medicine	608-263-7600

Note: Several of these pharmacies offer Veterinary Pharmacy Fellowships.

Appendix B

Directional Anatomical Terminology of Bipeds Quadrupeds
Katrina L. Mealey

College of Veterinary Medicine, Washington State University, Pullman, WA, USA

Some anatomic terms are used interchangeably in humans and veterinary patients, but there are differences in others because humans are bipeds while most veterinary patients are quadrupeds. For example, a common knee injury in humans is an "ACL" tear (anterior cruciate ligament). Dogs can suffer the same knee injury, but it is called a "CCL" tear (cranial cruciate ligament) because the term "anterior" is not appropriate for veterinary species.

Human anatomic term: definition	Corresponding veterinary term: definition
Anterior • Situated toward the front part of the body	Ventral • Situated on the underside (abdominal) surface
Posterior • Situated toward the hind part of the body	Dorsal • Situated on the upper side (along the back) surface
Superior • Situated above another (reference) body part	Cranial • Situated toward the head
Inferior • Situated below another (reference) body part	Caudal • Situated toward the tail
Lateral • Situated toward the side	Same
Medial • Situated toward the midline	Same
Proximal • Situated nearer to the body or point of attachment of a limb to the body	Same
Distal • Situated away from the center of the body or away from the attachment of a limb to the body	Same
Rostral • Toward the nose	Rostral • Same – but the elongated muzzle of the dog means that this term is used more frequently in veterinary medicine than human medicine.

Pharmacotherapeutics for Veterinary Dispensing, First Edition. Edited by Katrina L. Mealey.

Appendix C

Vital signs and potential monitoring parameters for dogs, cats, horses, and ferrets

Katrina L. Mealey

College of Veterinary Medicine, Washington State University, Pullman, WA, USA

See Table C.1.

Temperature: Body temperatures are usually obtained rectally in veterinary patients. For large animals, it is important to keep hold of the thermometer (many veterinarians have a thermometer "leash"), because it is possible for the animal to exert enough negative pressure in the rectum to draw the thermometer completely into the rectum and exert enough pressure to break a glass thermometer.

Pulse/heart rate: Indicated as beats per minute. Assessing both heart rate (by palpation of the chest or stethoscope) and pulse is important to determine if arrhythmias or pulse deficits are present (these may indicate cardiovascular disease). In general, the larger the animal, the slower the resting heart rate. Because dogs vary tremendously in size, from under 5 pounds to over 200 pounds depending on the breed, the normal heart rate must be interpreted based on the dog's size and athleticism.

Respiratory rate: Respiratory rate can usually be determined by observing the expansion of the animal's thorax. A stethoscope can also be used to auscult for air movement. In addition to respiratory rate, respiratory effort should be noted. Open-mouth breathing can be an indication of respiratory difficulty, elevated body temperature, anxiety, or central nervous system diseases. Panting (rapid shallow breathing) is a normal thermoregulatory mechanism in dogs but is rare in other domestic species. Respiratory rates of a panting dog can be >200 breaths per minute! Corticosteroids can cause panting in dogs even when body temperature is normal. Signs of respiratory difficulty include wheezing or other respiratory noises, pronounced abdominal effort, or cyanotic mucous membranes.

Capillary refill time: Capillary refill time is determined by lifting the animal's upper lip, pressing on the mucous membranes (gums), and counting how long it takes for the pallor to resume its normal pink color.

Blood glucose: Portable glucose monitors allow pet owners to determine their pet's blood glucose values at home. These can be helpful for managing diabetic dogs and cats. Pharmacists are quite familiar with providing patient counseling for home blood glucose monitoring for human diabetics, and the same general rules apply to pets with one important caveat. The most important difference between human and veterinary patients is that the latter cannot verbalize the early symptoms of hypoglycemia. This increases the risk for severe hypoglycemic episodes. For this reason, target blood glucose nadirs in veterinary patients tend to be

Pharmacotherapeutics for Veterinary Dispensing, First Edition. Edited by Katrina L. Mealey.
© 2019 John Wiley & Sons, Inc. Published 2019 by John Wiley & Sons, Inc.

Table C.1 Vital signs and potential monitoring parameters for select veterinary species.

Monitoring/physiologic parameter[a]	Dog	Cat	Horse	Ferret
Rectal temperature (°F)	100–102.5	100–103	99–101	100–102.5
Pulse/heart rate (beats per minute)	65–145	110–140	26–42	280–300
Respiratory rate (breaths per minute)	12–30	20–30	9–15	32–38
Capillary refill time	<2 s	<2 s	<2 s	<2 s
Blood glucose (mg dl^{-1})	80–120	70–135	70–130	85–140
Approximate gestation period	63 d	63 d	330 d	42 d

ND = Not determined.
[a] Healthy adult animal in a relaxed state at ambient temperature.
[b] Packed cell volume is the same as hematocrit.

higher than those for human patients (often >90–100 mg/dL for dogs and >150 mg/dL for cats).

Approximate gestation period: The greatest risk of teratogenic effects of drugs in human patients (and likely for veterinary patients) is during the first trimester of pregnancy. The gestation periods of veterinary species are provided so that pharmacists have a baseline for comparison to human pregnancy.

Other Monitoring Parameters

Blood pressure: Cuffs used to measure blood pressure in human patients are not usually suitable for dogs or cats due to their size. Inappropriately sized cuffs will not yield accurate blood pressure readings. Systemic hypertension in dogs and cats may cause acute blindness due to retinal hemorrhage, as well as changes in mentation, seizures, photophobia, or epistaxis. Systemic hypertension is defined as sustained systolic blood pressure >160 mmHg and/or sustained diastolic blood pressure >95 mmHg.

Hydration status: Protrusion of the third eyelids (Chapter 19) may indicate dehydration but may be due to a variety of other conditions as well. Sunken eyes, dry or tacky mucous membranes, and abnormal skin "tenting" or skin turgor are signs of severe dehydration and are indications that the animal should be examined by a veterinarian immediately. For dogs and cats, the skin along the back of the neck (the "scruff") is typically used to assess hydration status.

Mucous membrane color: Normal mucous membrane color in animals is pink; however, some breeds have pigmented gums and tongue, so it is difficult to assess mucous membrane color in the mouth. Another site that can be evaluated is the conjunctiva. Anemia can cause pale or even white mucous membranes, methemoglobinemia can cause brownish mucous membranes, hyperbilirubinemia can cause jaundice (yellowish) mucous membranes (Figure C.1), hyperemic (bright red) mucous membranes might indicate shock or hyperthermia, and cyanotic (blueish or purplish) mucous membranes indicate hypoxemia.

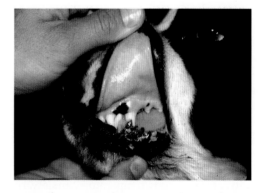

Figure C.1 Jaundiced mucous membranes of a Springer Spaniel with immune-mediated hemolytic anemia.

Appendix D

Auxiliary Labels Cross-referenced by Drug

Gigi Davidson

Clinical Pharmacy Services, College of Veterinary Medicine, North Carolina State University, Raleigh, NC, USA

Pharmacotherapeutics for Veterinary Dispensing, First Edition. Edited by Katrina L. Mealey.
© 2019 John Wiley & Sons, Inc. Published 2019 by John Wiley & Sons, Inc.

Auxiliary label column key

- L1 – MAY CAUSE DROWSINESS OR DIZZINESS
- L2 – DO NOT TAKE DAIRY PRODUCTS, ANTACIDS, OR IRON PREPARATIONS WITHIN ONE HOUR OF THIS MEDICATION
- L3 – Please provide access to plenty of fresh water while receiving this medication
- L4 – MAY CAUSE DISCOLORATION OF THE URINE OR FECES
- L5 – TAKE WITH FOOD
- L6 – To maximize effectiveness, administer 30–60 minutes prior to a meal
- L7 – FOR EARS
- L8 – FOR EXTERNAL USE ONLY
- L9 – FOR EYES
- L10 – PROTECT FROM LIGHT
- L11 – IMPORTANT: FINISH ALL THIS MEDICATION UNLESS OTHERWISE DIRECTED BY PRESCRIBER
- L12 – SHAKE WELL
- L13 – CAUTION: Federal law PROHIBITS the transfer of this drug to any person other than the patient for whom it was prescribed
- L14 – REFRIGERATE
- L15 – PACKAGE NOT CHILD RESISTANT
- L16 – KEEP OUT OF REACH OF CHILDREN
- L17 – Wash Hands After Use
- L18 – WEAR GLOVES
- L19 – CHEMOTHERAPY DRUG TOXIC — DISPOSE OF AS BIOHAZARD
- Specialty – Specialty Auxiliary Labels (Warning: Pregnant Women should avoid handling this medication)

Drug	L1	L2	L3	L4	L5	L6	L7	L8	L9	L10	L11	L12	L13	L14	L15	L16	L17	L18	L19	Specialty
Acetazolamide			🐾																	
Acepromazine Maleate	🐾																			
Aluminum hydroxide				🐾								🐾								
Amantadine					🐾															
Amitriptyline	🐾																			
Amlodipine																				
Ammonium Chloride																				
Amoxicillin											🐾									
Ascorbic Acid (Vitamin C)																				
Aspirin																				
Atenolol																				
Atovaquone					🐾															Shake Gently!; Pregnant
Azathioprine					🐾												🐾	🐾		Pregnant
Azithromycin		antacids									🐾									Susp—Empty Stomach
Benazepril																				
Bethanechol						🐾														
Budesonide																				
Buprenorphine													🐾							
Butorphanol	🐾												🐾							
Calcium (Tums)																🐾				
Calcitriol																				
Carprofen					🐾															
Carvedilol																				
Cefpodoxime					🐾						🐾									
Cephalexin											🐾									
Cetirizine	🐾																			
Chlorambucil (Leukeran)														🐾		🐾	🐾	🐾	🐾	Pregnant
Chloramphenicol											🐾					🐾	🐾	🐾		Chloramph; Pregnant
Chlorpheniramine	🐾																			
Ciprofloxacin		🐾									🐾									

Drug	May cause drowsiness or dizziness	Do not take dairy products, antacids, or iron preparations within one hour of this medication	Please provide access to plenty of fresh water while receiving this medication	May cause discoloration of the urine or feces	Take with food	To maximize effectiveness, administer 30–60 minutes prior to a meal	For ears	For eyes	Protect from light	Finish all this medication unless otherwise directed by prescriber	Shake well	Caution: Federal law prohibits the transfer of this drug	Refrigerate	Package not child resistant	Wash hands after use	Wear gloves	Chemotherapy drug toxic dispose of as biohazard	Specialty Auxiliary Labels
Cisapride						✓												
Clarithromycin																		
Clavamox					✓					✓								Clavamox
Clindamycin HCl					✓					✓								
Clomipramine HCl	✓				✓													
Clopidogrel																		
Colchicine				✓														Pregnant
Cosequin					✓													
Cyanocobalamin																		
Cyclophosphamide														✓	✓	✓	✓	
Cyclosporin (Atopica)					✓									✓	✓	✓		Pregnant
Cyclosporin (Optimmune)								✓						✓	✓			Pregnant
Cyproheptadine	✓		✓															
Darbepoetin alfa													✓					
Denamarin/Denosyl			✓			✓												Denamarin/Denosyl
Deracoxib					✓													
Desmopressin									✓				✓					
Dexamethasone																		Pregnant
Dexmedetomidine (Sileo)	✓																	Food ↑ Appt Urine
Diazepam			✓						✓			✓						
Diclofenac Topical Cream															✓	✓		
Diethylstilbestrol																✓		Pregnant
Digoxin														✓				
Diltiazem HCl														✓				Pregnant
Diphenhydramine HCl	✓																	
Docusate Na																		Horses – Molasses
Doxycycline		✓	✓		✓					✓								Horses – Molasses
Enalapril															✓	✓		
Enilconazole															✓	✓		Pregnant
Enrofloxacin (Baytril)		✓	✓							✓					✓	✓		Horses – Molasses

Auxiliary label legend (columns):
1. MAY CAUSE DROWSINESS OR DIZZINESS
2. DO NOT TAKE DAIRY PRODUCTS, ANTACIDS, OR IRON PREPARATIONS WITHIN ONE HOUR OF THIS MEDICATION
3. Please provide access to plenty of fresh water while receiving this medication
4. MAY CAUSE DISCOLORATION OF THE URINE OR FECES
5. TAKE WITH FOOD
6. To maximize effectiveness, administer 30–60 minutes prior to a meal
7. FOR EARS
8. FOR EXTERNAL USE ONLY
9. FOR EYES
10. PROTECT FROM LIGHT
11. IMPORTANT – FINISH ALL THIS MEDICATION UNLESS OTHERWISE DIRECTED BY PRESCRIBER
12. SHAKE WELL
13. CAUTION: Federal law prohibits the transfer of this drug to any person other than the patient for whom it was prescribed
14. REFRIGERATE
15. PACKAGE NOT CHILD RESISTANT
16. KEEP OUT OF REACH OF CHILDREN
17. Wash Hands After Use
18. WEAR GLOVES
19. CHEMOTHERAPY DRUG – TOXIC – DISPOSE OF AS BIOHAZARD
20. Specialty Auxiliary Labels

Drug	1	2	3	4	5	6	7	8	9	10	11	12	13	14	15	16	17	18	19	20 (Specialty)
Erythromycin											●									
Famciclovir																				
Famotidine																				
Fenbendazole suspension																				
Ferrous Sulfate/Fumarate												●								
Firocoxib					●															
Fish/Omega Fatty Acids			●		●											●				Refrigerate after opening
Fluconazole					●						●									
Fludrocortisone Acetate					●															
Flunixin			●		●															
Fluoxetine	●																			
Folic Acid																				
Furosemide			●																	
Gabapentin	●																			
Heparin																				
Hydrochlorothiazide (HCTZ)																				
Hydroxyurea			●													●	●	●	●	Pregnant
Hydroxyzine HCl	●																			
Isoxsuprine					●															
Itraconazole					●						●									
Ivermectin																				
Ketoconazole																				
Lactulose																				
Lanthanum Carbonate																				Lanthanum Carbonate
Leflunomide																●	●	●		Pregnant
Levetiracetam	●																			
Levothyroxine Sodium																				
Linezolid											●									
Lithium Carbonate	●																			
L-Lysine																				

Drug	May Cause Drowsiness or Dizziness	Do Not Take Dairy Products, Antacids, or Iron	Provide Access to Fresh Water	May Cause Discoloration of Urine or Feces	Take With Food	Administer 30–60 Minutes Prior to Meal	For Ears	For Eyes	Protect From Light	Finish All This Medication	Shake Well	Federal Law Prohibits Transfer	Refrigerate	Package Not Child Resistant	Wash Hands After Use	Wear Gloves	Chemotherapy Drug Toxic/Biohazard	Specially Auxiliary Labels
Paroxetine	🐾					🐾												
Ondansetron						🐾												
Omeprazole						🐾												
Oclacitinib (Apoquel)		ANTACIDS	🐾	🐾	🐾					🐾				🐾	🐾	🐾		Pregnant
Nitrofurantoin				🐾														Pregnant
Niacinamide					🐾													
Mycophenolate			🐾											🐾	🐾	🐾	🐾	Pregnant
Mitotane														🐾	🐾	🐾		Pregnant
Misoprostol																		Pregnant
Mirtazapine	🐾				🐾													
Minocycline	🐾	🐾	🐾		🐾	🐾				🐾				🐾	🐾	🐾		Horses – Molasses
Mexiletine					🐾					🐾								
Metronidazole						🐾												
Metoclopramide					🐾													
Methylprednisolone			🐾															Food ↑App↑Urine
Methotrexate														🐾	🐾	🐾	🐾	Pregnant
Methocarbamol	🐾																	
Methimazole			🐾		🐾					🐾				🐾	🐾	🐾		Pregnant
Methazolamide																		
Meropenem													🐾					
Melphalan														🐾	🐾	🐾		Glass; Pregnant
Meloxicam			🐾											🐾	🐾	🐾		Pregnant
Mefenoxam																		
Meclizine	🐾																	
Mastinib		🐾	🐾									🐾		🐾	🐾	🐾		Pregnant
Maropitant	🐾		🐾							🐾				🐾	🐾	🐾		Do not remove from foil
Marbofloxacin			🐾															
Lorazepam																		
Loperamide HCl																		
Lomustine (Cee-Nu)														🐾	🐾	🐾	🐾	Pregnant; Warning: Pregnant women should avoid handling this medication

Auxiliary label key (columns, left to right in the chart):

1. MAY CAUSE DROWSINESS OR DIZZINESS
2. DO NOT TAKE DAIRY PRODUCTS, ANTACIDS OR IRON PREPARATIONS WITHIN ONE HOUR OF THIS MEDICATION
3. Please provide access to plenty of fresh water while receiving this medication
4. MAY CAUSE DISCOLORATION OF THE URINE OR FECES
5. TAKE WITH FOOD / To maximize effectiveness, administer 30–60 minutes prior to a meal
6. FOR EARS
7. FOR EXTERNAL USE ONLY
8. FOR EYES
9. PROTECT FROM LIGHT
10. IMPORTANT — FINISH ALL THIS MEDICATION UNLESS OTHERWISE DIRECTED BY PRESCRIBER
11. SHAKE WELL
12. CAUTION: Federal law PROHIBITS the transfer of this drug to any person other than the patient for whom it was prescribed
13. REFRIGERATE
14. PACKAGE NOT CHILD RESISTANT
15. KEEP OUT OF REACH OF CHILDREN
16. Wash Hands After Use
17. WEAR GLOVES
18. CHEMOTHERAPY DRUG TOXIC — DISPOSE OF AS BIOHAZARD
19. Warning: Pregnant women should avoid handling this medication

Drug	Auxiliary labels indicated	Notes
Penicillamine	Take with food	
Pentoxifylline	Administer 30–60 min before a meal	
Pergolide Medylate		
Phenazopyridine	May cause discoloration of urine/feces; Take with food	
Phenobarbital	Federal law caution (transfer prohibited)	
Phenoxybenzamine	May cause drowsiness/dizziness; Take with food; Keep out of reach of children	
Phenylbutazone	Provide fresh water; Take with food	
Phenylpropanolamine (Proin)		
Phenytoin	May cause drowsiness/dizziness	
Pimobendan		
Piroxicam	Provide fresh water; Take with food; Keep out of reach of children; Wash hands after use	
Ponazuril	Finish all medication; Refrigerate	
Potassium Bromide		KBr/Invest; Pregnant
Potassium Citrate		Pot Citrate tablet
Potassium Gluconate		
Pradofloxacin	Do not take with dairy/antacids/iron; Take with food; Finish all medication; Shake well; Keep out of reach of children	
Prazosin		
Prednisolone		Food ↑App ↑Urine
Prednisone		Food ↑App ↑Urine
Propantheline Br		
Propranolol HCl		
Pyridostigmine Br	Take with food	
Pyrimethamine		
Ranitidine		
Rifampin	May cause discoloration of urine/feces; Administer 30–60 min before a meal	
Robenacoxib	Provide fresh water; Take with food; Finish all medication	
Rutin	Provide fresh water; Take with food	
Selegiline HCl	Take with food	
Sevelamer HCl		
Sildenafil		

Drug	MAY CAUSE DROWSINESS OR DIZZINESS	DO NOT TAKE DAIRY PRODUCTS ANTACIDS OR IRON PREPARATIONS WITHIN ONE HOUR OF THIS MEDICATION	Please provide access to plenty of fresh water while receiving this medication.	MAY CAUSE DISCOLORATION OF THE URINE OR FECES	TAKE WITH FOOD	To maximize effectiveness, administer 30-60 minutes prior to a meal	FOR EARS	FOR EXTERNAL USE ONLY	FOR EYES	PROTECT FROM LIGHT	IMPORTANT FINISH ALL THIS MEDICATION UNLESS OTHERWISE DIRECTED BY PRESCRIBER	SHAKE WELL	CAUTION: Federal law PROHIBITS the transfer of this drug to any person other than the patient for whom it was prescribed.	REFRIGERATE	PACKAGE NOT CHILD RESISTANT	KEEP OUT OF REACH OF CHILDREN	Wash Hands After Use	WEAR GLOVES	CHEMOTHERAPY DRUG TOXIC DISPOSE OF AS BIOHAZARD	Warning: Pregnant women should avoid handling this medication.
Silymarin																				
Sodium Bicarbonate																				
Sodium Bromide														🐾		🐾	🐾			KBr/Invest Pregnant
Sotalol HCl																				
Spironolactone			🐾																	
Sucralfate																				2 hr before/1 hr after
Sulfa/Trimeth			🐾								🐾									
Sulfadimethoxine			🐾								🐾									
Sulfasalazine				🐾	🐾															
Tacrolimus								🐾								🐾	🐾	🐾		Tacro sheet/Pregnant
Taurine															🐾	🐾				
Telmisartan																				Pregnant
Temaril-P	🐾																			Food ↑App↑Urine
Terbinafine					🐾						🐾									
Terbutaline Sulfate																				
Theophylline (Anhydrous)																				
Toceranib																🐾	🐾	🐾		Pregnant
Tramadol	🐾												🐾			🐾				
Trazodone	🐾																			
Triamcinolone																				Food ↑App↑Urine
Trilostane																🐾	🐾	🐾		Pregnant
Tylosin																				
Ursodiol					🐾															
Vitamin C																				
Vitamin K					🐾															
Warfarin																🐾				
Zonisamide	🐾																			

Appendix E

FDA Adverse Event Reporting Form

Gigi Davidson

Clinical Pharmacy Services, College of Veterinary Medicine, North Carolina State University, Raleigh, NC, USA

Pharmacotherapeutics for Veterinary Dispensing, First Edition. Edited by Katrina L. Mealey.
© 2019 John Wiley & Sons, Inc. Published 2019 by John Wiley & Sons, Inc.

DEPARTMENT OF HEALTH AND HUMAN SERVICES
Food and Drug Administration
Center for Veterinary Medicine

Form Approved: OMB No. 0910-0645
Expiration Date: 5/31/2019
(See mailer page for Burden Statement)

VETERINARY ADVERSE DRUG REACTION, LACK OF EFFECTIVENESS, OR PRODUCT DEFECT REPORT
(For VOLUNTARY Reporting)

NOTE: *This report is authorized by 21 U.S.C 352 (a) and (f). While you are not required to report, your cooperation is needed to assure comprehensive and timely assessment of product labeling.*

Individual Case Safety Report Number *(FDA Assigned Number)*	Submission Type
	☐ Initial ☐ Follow-up

Report Type
☐ Adverse Event   ☐ Product Problem   ☐ Both Adverse Event and Product Problem

Date of this Report *(mm/dd/yyyy)*	Date of Initial Report *(If this report is a follow-up) (mm/dd/yyyy)*
Month ☐ Day ☐ Year ☐	Month ☐ Day ☐ Year ☐

Sender Information

First Name	Last Name

Street Address

City	State or Province	Postal/ZIP Code

Country	Telephone Number	Telephone Number (Other)

Fax Number	Email Address

Sender Category
☐ Veterinarian   ☐ Animal Owner   ☐ Physician   ☐ Patient
☐ Other Health Care Professional   ☐ Other   ☐ Unknown

Sender Previously Reported to the Manufacturer?   ☐ Yes   ☐ No

If Yes, provide the Manufacturer's Case Number:

No Identity Disclosure   ☐ If you do NOT want your identity disclosed to the manufacturer, mark this box.

Preferred Method of Contact   ☐ Telephone   ☐ Email

Health Care Professional Information *(If different from Sender Information)*

First Name	Last Name

Street Address

City	State or Province	Postal/ZIP Code

Country	Telephone Number	Telephone Number (Other)

Fax Number	Email Address

Owner Information *(If different from Sender Information)*

First Name

Last Name

Street Address

City	State or Province	Postal/ZIP Code

Country	Telephone Number	Telephone Number (Other)

Fax Number	Email Address

Suspected Product Informatiom

Name of Suspected Product

Diagnosis and/or Reason for Use of the Product

Dosage Form (Chewable, liquid, tablet, topical, injection, etc.)

Date of First Exposure *(mm/dd/yyyy)*

Month   Day   Year

Date of Last Exposure *(mm/dd/yyyy)*

Month   Day   Year

Duration of Product Use

Product Use Information for Suspected Product

Dose Administered

Interval of Administration (Frequency)

Route of Administration

Product Administered By

☐ Veterinarian/Veterinary Staff   ☐ Owner   ☐ Other

Lot Number

Expiration Date *(mm/dd/yyyy)*

Month   Day   Year

Name of Manufacturer of Suspected Product

Adverse Event Information

Veterinarian's Level of Suspicion that Product Caused the Adverse Event

☐ High ☐ Medium ☐ Low ☐ Unknown

Treatment of Adverse Event *(Describe briefly)*

Did Adverse Event Abate After Stopping the Product?	Did Adverse Event Reappear After Reintroduction of the Product?
☐ Yes ☐ No ☐ Not Applicable	☐ Yes ☐ No ☐ Not Applicable

Outcome ☐ Recovered ☐ Died ☐ Other

Species and Related Information

☐ Budgerigar	☐ Cat	☐ Cattle	☐ Cockatiel	☐ Cockatoo
☐ Dog	☐ Ferret	☐ Fish	☐ Goat	☐ Guinea Pig
☐ Horse	☐ Human	☐ Parrot	☐ Pig	☐ Rabbit
☐ Sheep	☐ Other *(Specify)*:			

Breed	Gender ☐ Male ☐ Female
	☐ Male Neutered ☐ Female Neutered

Age: | Weight:

Overall Health Status When Suspected Product Given

☐ Excellent ☐ Good ☐ Fair ☐ Poor ☐ Critical

Number of Animals Treated:

Number of Animals Affected:

Adverse Event Occurrence

Date of Onset of Adverse Event *(mm/dd/yyyy)*

Month ☐ Day ☐ Year ☐

Length of Time Between First Exposure to Suspected Product(s) and Onset of Adverse Event	Length of Time Between Last Administration of Suspected Product(s) and Onset of Adverse Event

When the Adverse Event Occurred, Treatment with Suspected Product

☐ Had already been completed ☐ Was discontinued ☐ Was discontinued and replaced with another product

☐ Was discontinued and reintroduced later ☐ Was continued at an altered dose

☐ Other *(Specify)*:

Document Information

Attached Document Name *(Filename if Electronic)*

Attached Document Description

Attached Document Name *(Filename if Electronic)*

Attached Document Description

Attached Document Name *(Filename if Electronic)*

Attached Document Description

FORM FDA 1932a (7/16)   Page 3

Concurrent Clinical Problem(s)

Were There Concurrent Clinical Problems?

☐ Yes   ☐ No   ☐ Do not know   ☐ None

List Concurrent Clinical Problem(s).

Concurrent Product Information *(Excluding Treatment of Current Event)*

Please provide name(s), dose(s), interval(s), date(s) of treatment(s), and other relevant information to describe other products that the patient was taking at the time of the event. Either copy this section as needed (you may fill out this section in other copies of this form) or provide comments in the long narrative section that follows this one.

Were Concurrent Products Given?

☐ Yes   ☐ No   ☐ Do not know   ☐ None

List Names of Concurrent Products Administered.

Date of First Exposure *(mm/dd/yyyy)*

Month [ ]   Day [ ]   Year [ ]

Date of Last Exposure *(mm/dd/yyyy)*

Month [ ]   Day [ ]   Year [ ]

Duration of Product Use

Adverse Event/Product Problem *(Long Narrative)*

Describe the Adverse Event/Product Problem.

Appendix F

Veterinary Pharmacogenetics Testing Laboratories with Counseling Expertise

Katrina L. Mealey

College of Veterinary Medicine, Washington State University, Pullman, WA, USA

See Table F.1.

Table F.1 Pharmacogenetic testing laboratories that provide clinical pharmacology resources (i.e. drug-dosing adjustments or alternate drug options based on genotype) and genotyping.

Institution/organization	Laboratory	Contact information
Washington State University, College of Veterinary Medicine	Veterinary Clinical Pharmacology Laboratory	vcpl.vetmed.wsu.edu 509-335-3745
Mars Petcare	Wisdom Health^{TM}	Wisdompanel.com

Pharmacotherapeutics for Veterinary Dispensing, First Edition. Edited by Katrina L. Mealey.
© 2019 John Wiley & Sons, Inc. Published 2019 by John Wiley & Sons, Inc.

Appendix G

Therapeutic Drug Monitoring Laboratories

Katrina L. Mealey

College of Veterinary Medicine, Washington State University, Pullman, WA, USA

See Table G.1.

Table G.1 Therapeutic drug monitoring (TDM) laboratories for veterinary patients.

Name and location of laboratory	Phone	Website
Prairie Diagnostic Services, Inc. Saskatoon, Saskatchewan	306-966-7316	pdsinc.ca
Texas Veterinary Medical Diagnostic Laboratory College Station, TX	888-646-5623	tvmdl.tamu.edu
NMS Labs[a] Willow Grove, PA	866-522-2206	nmslabs.com
Clinical Pharmacology Laboratory, Auburn University Auburn, AL	334-844-7187	http://www.vetmed.auburn.edu/ veterinarians/clinical-labs
MiraVista Diagnostics (Veterinary Antifungal TDM) Indianapolis, IN	866-647-2847	https://miravistavets.com/vet-antifungal-tdm
LabCorp[a]		Labcorp.com

[a] Not specifically a veterinary laboratory, but will run samples from veterinary patients.

Pharmacotherapeutics for Veterinary Dispensing, First Edition. Edited by Katrina L. Mealey.
© 2019 John Wiley & Sons, Inc. Published 2019 by John Wiley & Sons, Inc.

Appendix H

Canine and Feline Body Surface Area Conversion Tables

Stephen W. Mealey

Washington State University, Pullman, WA, USA

The body surface area (BSA) conversionfactor for dogs and cats differs from that of humans. The body surface area conversiontables included here are the correct guide for canine and feline drug dosingbased on BSA. Do not use the human conversion factor or human scales/ tables forcalculating BSA for veterinary patients.

Canine body surface area conversion table.

Weight in pounds (lb)	Weight in kilograms (kg.)	Body surface area in meters squared (m^2)	Weight in pounds (lb)	Weight in kilograms (kg.)	Body surface area in meters squared (m^2)
2	0.91	0.095	42	19.09	0.72
4	1.82	0.151	44	20	0.75
6	2.73	0.198	46	20.91	0.77
8	3.64	0.239	48	21.82	0.79
10	4.55	0.278	50	22.73	0.81
12	5.45	0.31	52	23.64	0.83
14	6.36	0.35	54	24.55	0.86
16	7.27	0.38	56	25.45	0.88
18	8.18	0.41	58	26.36	0.90
20	9.09	0.44	60	27.27	0.92
22	10	0.47	62	28.18	0.93
24	10.91	0.50	64	29.09	0.95
26	11.82	0.53	66	30	0.97
28	12.73	0.55	68	30.91	0.99
30	13.64	0.58	70	31.82	1.01
32	14.55	0.60	72	32.73	1.03
34	15.45	0.63	74	33.64	1.05
36	16.36	0.65	76	34.55	1.07
38	17.27	0.68	78	35.45	1.09
40	18.18	0.70	80	36.36	1.11

(Continued)

Pharmacotherapeutics for Veterinary Dispensing, First Edition. Edited by Katrina L. Mealey.
© 2019 John Wiley & Sons, Inc. Published 2019 by John Wiley & Sons, Inc.

(Continued)

Weight in pounds (lb)	Weight in kilograms (kg.)	Body surface area in meters squared (m^2)	Weight in pounds (lb)	Weight in kilograms (kg.)	Body surface area in meters squared (m^2)
82	37.27	1.13	120	54.55	1.45
84	38.18	1.14	125	56.82	1.49
86	39.09	1.16	130	59.09	1.53
88	40	1.18	135	61.36	1.57
90	40.91	1.20	140	63.64	1.61
92	41.82	1.22	145	65.91	1.65
94	42.73	1.23	150	68.18	1.69
96	43.64	1.25	160	72.73	1.76
98	44.55	1.27	170	77.27	1.83
100	45.45	1.28	180	81.82	1.91
105	47.73	1.32	190	86.36	1.98
110	50	1.37	200	90.91	2.04
115	52.27	1.41			

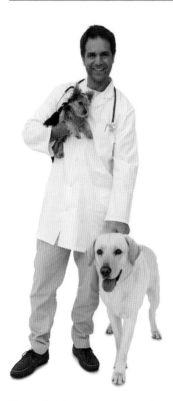

Figure H.1 For comparison, an 8 pound (3.64 kg) Yorkshire terrier would have a body surface area of 0.239 m^2 while an 80 pound (36.36 kg) Labrador Retriever would have a body surface area of 1.112 m^2. *Source:* CanStockPhoto, Halifax, NS, Canada.

Feline body surface area conversion table.

Weight in pounds (lbs)	Weight in kilograms (kgs)	Body surface area in meters squared (m^2)
1	0.45	0.059
2	0.91	0.094
3	1.36	0.123
4	1.82	0.149
5	2.27	0.173
6	2.73	0.196
7	3.18	0.217
8	3.64	0.237
9	4.09	0.256
10	4.55	0.275
11	5	0.293
12	5.45	0.311
13	5.91	0.328
14	6.36	0.344
15	6.82	0.361
16	7.27	0.376
17	7.73	0.392
18	8.18	0.407
19	8.64	0.422
20	9.09	0.437
21	9.55	0.451
22	10	0.465
23	10.45	0.480
24	10.91	0.493
25	11.36	0.507

Appendix I

Zoonotic Diseases of Dogs, Cats, and Horses

Katrina L. Mealey

College of Veterinary Medicine, Washington State University, Pullman, WA, USA

See Table I.1.

Table I.1 Examples of the more common zoonotic diseases[a] of dogs, cats, and horses in the USA (direct transmission, fecal-oral transmission, but not vector transmission)

Dogs	Cats	Horses
Bartonella henselae (bacteria)	*Bartonella henselae* (bacteria)	
Brucella canis (bacteria)		
Escherichia coli (bacteria)	*Escherichia coli* (bacteria)	*Escherichia coli* (bacteria)
Giardia spp. (protozoa)	*Giardia* spp. (protozoa)	
Leptospira spp. (bacteria)		*Leptospira* spp. (bacteria)
Microsporum canis (fungus)	*Microsporum* (fungus)	*Microsporum* (fungus)
Rabies (virus)	Rabies (viral)	Rabies (viral)
		Salmonella spp. (bacteria)
	Toxoplasma gondii (protozoa)	
Trichophyton (fungus)	*Trichophyton* (fungus)	*Trichophyton* (fungus)

[a] Bacterial, fungal, viral, protozoal.

Pharmacotherapeutics for Veterinary Dispensing, First Edition. Edited by Katrina L. Mealey.
© 2019 John Wiley & Sons, Inc. Published 2019 by John Wiley & Sons, Inc.

Index

Pharmacotherapeutics for Veterinary Dispensing, First Edition. Edited by Katrina L. Mealey.
© 2019 John Wiley & Sons, Inc. Published 2019 by John Wiley & Sons, Inc.